Medical Tomography

Medical Tomography

Editor: Steven Gray

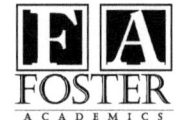

FOSTER
ACADEMICS

www.fosteracademics.com

www.fosteracademics.com

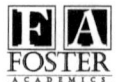

Cataloging-in-Publication Data

Medical tomography / edited by Steven Gray.
    p. cm.
Includes bibliographical references and index.
ISBN 978-1-63242-556-0
1. Tomography. 2. Radiography, Medical. I. Gray, Steven.
RC78.7.T6 M43 2018
616.075 72--dc23

© Foster Academics, 2018

Foster Academics,
118-35 Queens Blvd., Suite 400,
Forest Hills, NY 11375, USA

ISBN 978-1-63242-556-0 (Hardback)

Contents

Preface

I am honored to present to you this unique book which encompasses the most up-to-date data in the field. I was extremely pleased to get this opportunity of editing the work of experts from across the globe. I have also written papers in this field and researched the various aspects revolving around the progress of the discipline. I have tried to unify my knowledge along with that of stalwarts from every corner of the world, to produce a text which not only benefits the readers but also facilitates the growth of the field.

Medical tomography is the technique by which medical images of sections of the anatomy are obtained. X-ray devices are used alongside algorithms based on mathematical formulas for sectional reconstruction of the human body. Computerized axial tomography (CAT) and Positron emission tomography (PET) are two common forms of medical tomography. Most of the topics introduced in this book cover new techniques and the applications of this field. For all those who are interested in medical tomography, this book can prove to be an essential guide.

Finally, I would like to thank all the contributing authors for their valuable time and contributions. This book would not have been possible without their efforts. I would also like to thank my friends and family for their constant support.

Editor

Vessel Labeling in Combined Confocal Scanning Laser Ophthalmoscopy and Optical Coherence Tomography Images: Criteria for Blood Vessel Discrimination

Jeremias Motte[1], Florian Alten[2], Carina Ewering[1], Nani Osada[6], Ella M. Kadas[3], Alexander U. Brandt[3], Timm Oberwahrenbrock[3], Christoph R. Clemens[2], Nicole Eter[2], Friedemann Paul[3,4], Martin Marziniak[1,5]*

1 Department of Neurology, University of Muenster Medical Center, Muenster, Germany, 2 Department of Ophthalmology, University of Muenster Medical Center, Muenster, Germany, 3 NeuroCure Clinical Research Center and Experimental and Clinical Research Center, Charité University Medicine Berlin and Max Delbrück Center for Molecular Medicine, Berlin, Germany, 4 Department of Neurology, Charité University Medicine Berlin, Berlin, Germany, 5 Department of Neurology, Isar-Amper-Klinikum, Haar, Germany, 6 Institution of Medical Informatics, University of Muenster, Muenster, Germany

Abstract

Introduction: The diagnostic potential of optical coherence tomography (OCT) in neurological diseases is intensively discussed. Besides the sectional view of the retina, modern OCT scanners produce a simultaneous top-view confocal scanning laser ophthalmoscopy (cSLO) image including the option to evaluate retinal vessels. A correct discrimination between arteries and veins (labeling) is vital for detecting vascular differences between healthy subjects and patients. Up to now, criteria for labeling (cSLO) images generated by OCT scanners do not exist.

Objective: This study reviewed labeling criteria originally developed for color fundus photography (CFP) images.

Methods: The criteria were modified to reflect the cSLO technique, followed by development of a protocol for labeling blood vessels. These criteria were based on main aspects such as central light reflex, brightness, and vessel thickness, as well as on some additional criteria such as vascular crossing patterns and the context of the vessel tree.

Results and Conclusion: They demonstrated excellent inter-rater agreement and validity, which seems to indicate that labeling of images might no longer require more than one rater. This algorithm extends the diagnostic possibilities offered by OCT investigations.

Editor: Knut Stieger, Justus-Liebig-University Giessen, Germany

Funding: Novartis Germany has funded the OCT scanner (http://www.novartis.de) with an unrestricted grant. The funder had no role in study design, data collection and analysis, decision to publish, or preparation of the manuscript.

Competing Interests: The author disclosure information is as follows: Motte J, none; Alten F, Heidelberg Engineering, Novartis, Bayer, Allergan; Ewering C, none; Osada N, none; Kadas EM, none; Brand A, none; Oberwahrenbrock T, none; Clemens CR, Heidelberg Engineering, Novartis, Bayer, Allergan; Eter N, Heidelberg Engineering, Bayer, Novartis, Allergan, Pfizer, Bausch and Lomb; Paul F, Biogenldec, Teva, SanofiGenzyme, Merck, Novartis, Heidelberg Engineering; supported by German Research Foundation (DFG Exc 257), German Ministry for Education and Research (BMBF Competence Network Multiple Sclerosis); and Marziniak M, Biogenldec, Teva, SanofiGenzyme, Merck, Novartis.

* Email: Martin.Marziniak@kbo.de

Introduction

Optical coherence tomography (OCT) has come to be used increasingly to evaluate retinal degenerative changes involved in neurological diseases. Developed in the 1980s [1], today's modern spectral domain (SD) OCT scanners produce detailed cross-sectional and 3D-images of the eye. Thinning of the retinal nerve fiber layer (RNFL) measured by OCT has been widely described in patients with multiple sclerosis (MS) and MS-related optic neuritis [2–5]. Furthermore, some other neurodegenerative diseases, such as dementia, spinocerebellar ataxia or Parkinson's disease, were found to be associated with reduced thickness of the RNFL in SD-OCT scans [6–8], while others, such as amyotrophic lateral sclerosis, were not [9].

It is under discussion whether OCT has the potential to become a noninvasive, reproducible test for assessing axonal degeneration and whether it might be used as a valuable tool for measuring the therapeutic efficacy of potential neuroprotective agents [10]. This suggestion is based on the observation that retinal and cerebral atrophy are correlated [11–13].

In addition to RNFL thickness parameters, modern SD-OCT scanners provide additional information like confocal scanning laser ophthalmoscopy (cSLO) with infrared (IR) imaging. Additionally, the development of the eye tracker, which allows simultaneous investigation of the eye with two laser beams, ensures less eye-motion artifacts and highly comparable longitudinal examinations with reduced error rates.

Developments such as the ones outlined above enable us to collect a large number of data in a single examination, thus opening the door for multimodal examination of many neurological diseases.

Combining different technical approaches in a single investigation has numerous advantages:

- From the viewpoint of patients: combined confocal scanning laser ophthalmoscopy and optical coherence tomography is a non-radioactive examination that can be performed in less than 20 minutes. In this context, papillary dilation is no longer required to ensure high-quality results. The burden of OCT investigations on the patient is low, resulting in a high acceptance rate for longitudinal investigations.
- From the economic viewpoint: Compared to MRI scans, this approach can be handled with much less costly equipment and staff while also being faster.
- From the viewpoint of research, in particular: multimodality imaging opens the research spectrum and links different views on a particular disease.

Recently, consensus criteria for retinal OCT quality assessment (OSCAR-IB) have been published to increase the comparability and improve the quality management of OCT-images [14].

The main parameter analyzed in most studies is RNFL thickness, whereas lesser attention is paid to the retinal blood vessels. cSLO IR-imaging, however, is always combined with a OCT scan, which facilitates collection of additional information not only in patients with vasculopathy.

So far, there are no reliable and valid criteria for labeling blood vessels in cSLO IR-images recorded by OCT-scanners. Up to now, studies which describe labeling of retinal blood vessels refer to classical color fundus photography (CFP) images only.

A review of the ophthalmological literature yielded criteria originally developed for automatic analysis of CFP [15,16]. As a result of their shared embryology, cerebral and retinal blood vessels share similar anatomical and physiological properties. In the recent past, the eye, the "window to the brain", was used to investigate different neurological diseases. Changes in retinal vessels were detected in the context of many neurological diseases such as Alzheimer's disease or neuromyelitis optica [17,18]. Especially for Alzheimer's disease, retinal vascular image analysis was described as a potential screening tool. These examples demonstrate the huge potential of retinal blood vessels examination for detecting preclinical diseases and for evaluating clinical courses.

The aim of this study was:

1. to develop reliable and valid criteria for labeling retinal blood vessels in cSLO IR-images,
2. to investigate whether the criteria defined for automatic analysis of CFP can also be applied for cSLO IR-images,
3. to propose standard operating procedures for further studies in neurological diseases.

The study was comprised of three portions:
(1) an exploratory part, (2) an adaptation of the criteria based on the initial results, and (3) a validation study comparing the results with CFP.

Exploratory Study

Subjects

273 blood vessels in both (14) eyes of 7 healthy volunteers (6 males, mean age 50.9±13.9 years) were labeled by two independent raters (CE, JM).

All subjects had normal visual acuity (20/20), normal visual fields and no ocular, metabolic or neurological diseases. The whole study was conducted according to the principles expressed in the Declaration of Helsinki. The institutional review board of the ethics committee of the University of Berlin, Charite, approved the study with volunteers. Participants provide their written informed consent on a standardized informed consent form approved by ethics committee.

Methods

Retinal images were obtained using combined cSLO and SD-OCT imaging (Spectralis, Heidelberg Engineering, Software: Heidelberg EyeExplorer version 1.7.0.0) with the eye tracking function enabled.

Using automated eye tracking and image alignment based on cSLO images, the integrated software can be used to average a variable number of single images in real time (Automatic Real Time [ART] Module; Heidelberg Engineering), which significantly improves image quality. Furthermore, this technique ensures reliable follow-up measurements, as scans are recorded at exactly the same position as the baseline scan.

The IR-images were pseudonymized, exported by Heidelberg EyeExplorer, and uploaded to an ImagJ-Plugin for measuring vessel diameter (http://neurodial.de). Afterwards, blood vessels were labeled in cSLO images.

The inter-rater agreement between the two raters was measured using Cohen's kappa coefficient. According to Landis and Koch, strength of agreement was rated as poor (<0.00), slight (0.00–0.20), fair (0.21–0.40), moderate (0.41–0.60), substantial (0.61–0.80), or almost perfect (0.81–1.00) [19,20].

Test criteria

Criteria formerly reported in the literature, which had been developed for an automatic analysis of fundus images, were reviewed and eight criteria were selected for the exploratory analysis of the vessels and weighted equally to each other:

1. The central light reflex is wider in arteries and smaller in veins [15,16].
2. Arteries are brighter than veins [15], veins appear darker and deeper than arteries [16].
3. Arteries and veins alternate near the optic disc [15,16].
4. Arteries are 30% thinner than neighboring veins [15].
5. Arteries never cross arteries and veins never cross veins [16].
6. The angle between crossing vessels is almost 90°, and angles between outgoing vessels are between 30° and 45° [16].
7. Vessels should be seen in the context of the vessel tree [15].
8. Arteries take a straighter course than veins [16].

The raters labeled vessels with "A" for artery, "V" for vein and "U" for unknown.

Results

The inter-rater agreement of the exploratory study showed a kappa of 0.602. The two raters marked 20.5% or 38.8% of 273 vessels as unknown. The disagreement-rate was 27.5%.

Interpretation

The exploratory study showed a high rate of unknown vessels and substantial inter-rater agreement ($\kappa = 0.602$). There was a strikingly high difference between the raters for vessels labeled "unknown".

On the one hand, the main branches and bigger vessels were clearly labeled and the labeling left no space for interpretation. On the other hand, there are many vessels which leave some leeway

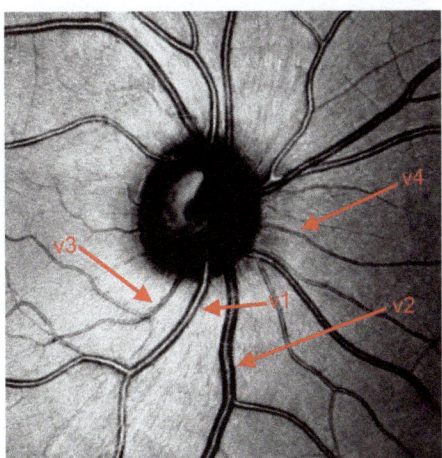

Figure 1. Vessels 1 (v1) and 2 (v2) are larger than vessel 3 (v3) and 4 (v4). V1 is an artery, v2 is a vein, v3 and v4 cannot be allocated clearly.

for interpretation. The smaller the vessels were, the harder clear labeling became (figure 1).

The results of this pre-test demonstrated the need to rate the criteria and to modify them. Originally, the criteria had been established for an automatic analysis of CFP images. Consequently, they needed to be adapted to the nature of cSLO IR-images. The images generated by OCT scanners are black and white pictures, and the relevant criteria did not seem to be transferable on a 1:1 basis.

Test Modification

In view of the above, our next step was to develop an algorithm for labeling blood vessels which could not be identified clearly. A non-hierarchical application of the criteria in the exploratory study was followed by a weighting of the criteria in a consensus meeting which included all authors from Münster. Decisions were based on the initial results, on anatomical and physiological facts, and on the different technical features of the OCT and cSLO IR-Images.

Main criteria

We defined two categories of criteria: main and additional criteria. Main criteria were based on anatomical or physiological correlates.

1. "The central light reflex is wider in arteries and smaller in veins."

Originally, this criterion was based on fundus images produced via the red channel mode, a special mode with colored filters in which veins show larger vessel edges and bigger color differences between the edge and the reflection zone in the middle of the vessel. In contrast, arteries appear lighter than veins (figure 2) [15].

The reason for the varying size of the light reflex is the difference of the vessel walls of arteries and veins. The central light reflex (CLR), which is caused by light reflection from vessel surfaces, is a phenomenon which was first observed in images produced by light of a 600 nm wavelength [21,22], but is also seen in 820 nm cSLO IR-images.

Moreover, arteries have solid walls built by the tunica media, the middle layer of an artery wall. They are rich in muscle fibers and reveal more reflection compared to the vessel wall of

veins. Veins show loosely packed vessel walls and the three layers of the wall, tunica intima, tunica media and tunica externa, merge with each other [23].

2. "Arteries are brighter than veins."

The brightness of arteries is also caused by the oxygen-enriched blood transported by them [15,21]. This effect also shows in IR images [21].

In contrast, the lumen of veins appears darker due to the circulation of deoxygenated blood (figure 3). In contrast to the first criterion, this criterion describes the brightness of the reflex rather than of its expansion (wider versus smaller).

3. "Arteries are up to 30% thinner than veins."

Because of the lower blood pressure, veins have bigger cross sections than their corresponding arteries. This is explained by the Hagen-Poiseuille equation ($\Delta P = 8\mu L Q / \pi r^4$). The volumetric flow rate (Q), the length of the pipe (L) and the dynamic viscosity (μ) do not change, which means that the cross section (r) will increase along with a decreasing blood pressure (figure 4).

In this context, it should be noted that the main criteria apply for vessels on the same level only and that comparing vessels in the periphery of a 30° image with vessels in the center close to the optic disc, or vessels leaving the upper half of the optic disc with vessels in the lower half is not acceptable in view of the fact that the vessels change their morphology in their course (becoming smaller or bigger) and because the illumination differs depending on the various parts of the image. In the cSLO image, three rings around the optic disc ensure consistent eccentricity for each vessel when grading it (figure 5). Furthermore, the three rings were created to be used by an upcoming automatic vessel analyzing software.

Additional criteria

Additional criteria are based on the experience of ophthalmologists and the raters' assessment. Their anatomical or physiological correlations are not as clear as for the main criteria.

1. "Arteries and veins alternate near the optic disc."

Near the optic disc, an artery runs next to a vein and vice versa. This means that an artery is surrounded by two veins and that a vein is surrounded by two arteries. It seems to be a very efficient differentiation criterion, because one labeled vessel is enough to specify the neighboring vessels.

The blood vessels in the periphery, however, do not strictly follow this rule—it only applies before blood vessels begin to branch out. In cSLO IR-images, the center of the optic disc is often outshined. Consequently, the blood vessels are indistinguishable. Furthermore, very small blood vessels do not show the typical CLR or variance of thickness and brightness (figure 6). Using this criterion alone could therefore lead to errors comparable to those produced by a frameshift mutation: all subsequent vessels would be labeled incorrectly.

2. "Arteries never cross arteries and veins never cross veins."

This criterion underlines that if two blood vessels cross each other, the darker one must be the vein and the lighter one the artery [16].

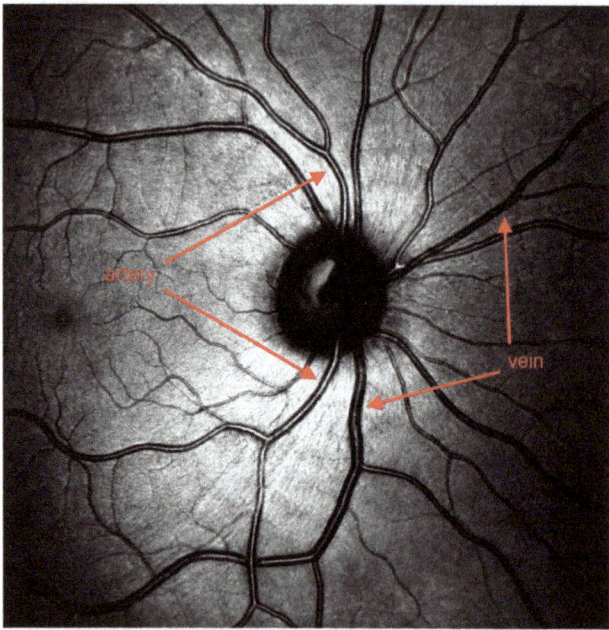

Figure 2. The artery shows a reflection-zone extending from the optic disc to the periphery of the retina. The reflection of the vein cannot be traced to the periphery. Compared to the venous cross section, the reflection is smaller. The venous vessel wall appears thicker.

3. "Vessels should be seen in the context of the vessel tree."

The idea of this criterion is to follow the course of vessels and find branchings. If a vessel can be labeled before the branching, it helps to determine the vessel parts after the branching; therefore unequivocal labeling of the part before the branching is absolutely necessary.

4. "Arteries take a straighter course than veins."

This observation is frequently cited and plausible in view of the physiological function of the arteries and veins. Veins drain the blood from wide tissue areas and a winding course will support this function.

For the rater, the aforestated rule leaves room for interpretation and therefore does not seem very reliable. Moreover, blood vessels near the optic disc, whether veins or arteries, generally tend to have a straight course. This is why the difference in straightness between arteries and veins might not be very pronounced in this region.

5. "The angles between crossing vessels are almost 90°, whereas the angles between outgoing vessels range between 30° and 45°."

Although this rule is found in the literature [16] and although examples for this case could be observed, our exploratory study often yielded deviation from this rule.

Based on the results of our exploratory study and the considerations indicated above, we reassessed the criteria in an attempt to answer the following questions:

1) Are the main criteria correct? How much of them are required for an unequivocal identification of a blood vessel?

2) How are the additional criteria to manage?

   a. Are additional criteria helpful if the main criteria are not adequate?

   b. Which additional criteria are correct and which are not?

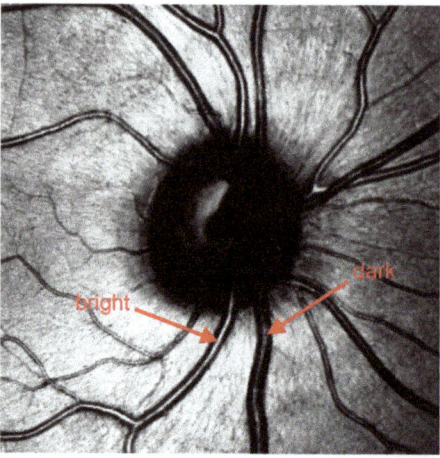

Figure 3. The darker vessel is a vein, the brighter an artery.

   c. How many of the additional criteria are required for correct labeling without using the main criteria?

3) Is the validity of the test impacted by modifying the test criteria?

To answer this questions, we developed a workflow for the main study:

- All vessels were reviewed using all main criteria. These were treated as equal.

- If unambiguous labeling based on the main criteria was impossible or if the main criteria were not detectable, the additional criteria were applied.

Main Study

Subjects

In the main study, 24 eyes from 12 healthy volunteers with 462 labeled vessels were investigated by two independent raters (JM, CE) (7 males, mean age 41.25 ± 13.23).

The inclusion criteria for the subjects were: normal visual acuity

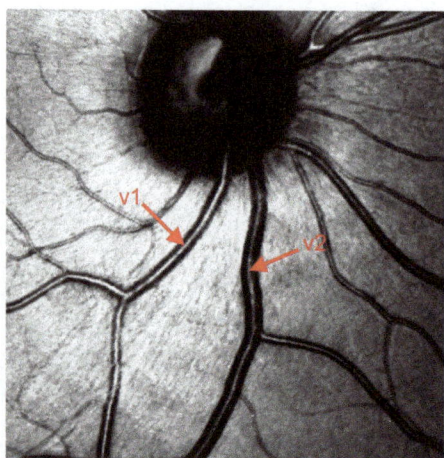

ǀure 4. An example of the difference in size can be observed tween vessel 1 and vessel 2. V1 is an artery, v2 is a vein.

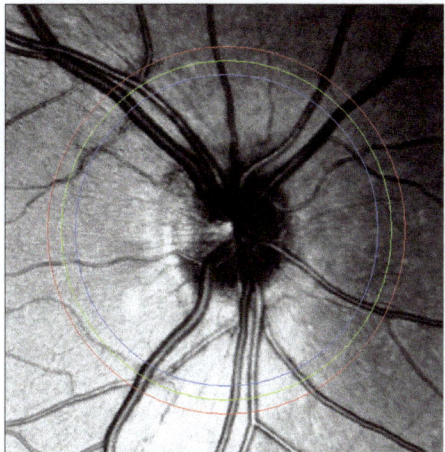

Figure 5. Three rings around the optic disc ensure vessel grading at consistent eccentricity for each vessel.

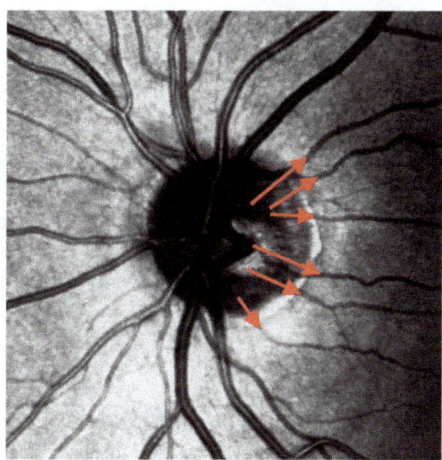

Figure 6. Alternate vessels with low variance of thickness and brightness.

(20/20), normal visual field and no ocular, metabolic or neurological diseases.

Methods

cSLO IR-Images were obtained and labeled as in the exploratory part of the study. All volunteers were examined by an ophthalmologist (FA). CFP imaging was performed using a 30° lens focused on the macula (Visucam, Carl Zeiss Meditech, Berlin, Germany). Photographs were viewed in the Zeiss Visupac 4.2. software (Carl Zeiss Meditech, Berlin, Germany). The vessels in these fundus images were labeled by the ophtalmologist and used as reference for the labeling of the cSLO IR images. Hand-labeling is an established method for finding a baseline [24].

The two cSLO-raters were blinded regarding the results of the CFP.

The criteria were used in the sequence indicated above until unequivocal labeling of the vessels became possible, starting with the main criteria and then using additional criteria, if needed. The number of criteria we applied ranged between one and eight. Each vessel was evaluated applying all main criteria supposing an equal status between the main criteria.

All steps of labeling were documented.

Moreover, using a two point system, we rated the image quality of all vessels as excellent (two points), medium (one point) or insufficient (zero points).

- picture sharpness: 1 point
- identifiability of the lumen of the vessel: 1 point

These ratings served to roughly reflect the cSLO picture quality.

Cohen's kappa was used to measure "inter-rater agreement" between the two raters to assess test reliability.

In the next step, we compared labeled cSLO IR-images and labeled CFP. If the two raters' results were identical, we compared them to the ophtalmologist's as reference. Analysis was performed by a fourfold table, chi-squared test and calculation of kappas to obtain a "test reference agreement". The test-reference agreement describes the agreement between our new test and the ophthalmologist's as reference. If the two raters (CE, JM) results were not identical, they were declared as a disagreement.

Cohen's kappa was used to measure a test reference agreement between the result of the test and the ophthalmologist's.

Additionally, Pearsons's chi-squared test and Fisher's exact test were used to recognize potential correlations.

Results

Inter-rater testing. In the first step, the reliability of our test was determined. The test reached a kappa of $\kappa = 0.840$ by labeling 462 vessels. In our control sample, the disagreement-rate between the test and the ophthalmologist's results was 8%. In 1.5% of the cases, vessels were labeled as unknown.

Inter-rater agreement in the main study was better than inter-rater agreement in the exploratory study (Kappa exploratory study: 0.602).

Our exploratory study revealed the difficulties involved in labeling smaller vessels in particular, since the three main criteria often were not applicable for these vessels.

To analyze the quality and the newly established hierarchy of the revised criteria, all vessels were subdivided into two groups to which the following criteria apply:

- 1st choice: The vessel is labeled based on two or three main criteria (MC). Complementary use of one to five additional criteria (AC) is possible, but not mandatory. ($\geq$ 2MC + X AC)
- 2nd choice: The vessel is labeled based on one or less (zero) main criteria. Complementary use of one to five additional criteria is possible, but not mandatory. ($\leq$ 1MC + X AC)

The above classification was selected based on the assumption that the main criteria were the most important ones (heuristic method).

The first and second groups were compared in a fourfold table (table 1).

Pearson's Chi-squared test and Fisher's exact test revealed a highly significant ($p<0.001$) difference between the groups and inter-rater agreement.

The Chi-squared test revealed a very high correlation between the use of first-choice criteria and inter-rater agreement. Also, we were able to demonstrate that application of second-choice criteria correlates with poorer inter-rater agreement.

To clarify this observation, kappa coefficients were calculated for the first- and second-choice groups separately:

Inter-rater agreement first choice: $\kappa = 0.976$

Inter-rater agreement second choice: $\kappa = 0.673$

Table 1. Inter-rater-agreement for 1st and 2nd choice.

inter-rater-agreement of the OCT-raters			no agreement	agreement	total
	1st choice	absolute	3	257	260
		relative	1.2%	98.8%	100%
	2st choice	absolute	34	168	202
		relative	16.8%	83.2%	100%
total			37	425	462
			8%	92%	100%

Further analysis of the first choice group revealed the importance of the additional criteria:

- In 50%, the blood vessel was labeled based on two main criteria plus additional criteria.
- In 15%, the blood vessel was labeled based on three main criteria plus additional criteria.

All in all, 65% of the vessels labeled based on the first-choice approach were labeled using additional criteria for support, therefore they play a crucial role for the analysis.

Validity of the test. The second step was to determine the validity of the test. The reference ophthalmologist labeled 85.8% (387 of 462) of the vessels as determinable. For the 387 vessels, Cohen's kappa between the ophthalmologist's result and the results of the cSLO raters was $\kappa = 0.803$.

The correlation respectively the values of kappa between the cSLO raters and the reference are the measure for the correctness of the test. The contingency table comparing the test and reference results is presented in table 2. Moreover, test sensitivity and specificity were calculated (table 3).

The cases were again divided into the first- and second-choice groups. Pearson's Chi-squared test and Fisher's exact test yielded a highly significant ($p<0.001$) difference between the first- and second-choice groups and the correct labeling result (table 4).

The first choice group included 257 (66%), and the second-choice group 130 of the identifiable blood vessels. Kappa values were calculated both for the first- and second-choice groups:

For the first-choice group, the test-reference agreement was $\kappa = 0.960$, and for the second-choice group $\kappa = 0.506$.

96% of the undeterminable vessels and 87% of the incorrectly labeled vessels were found in the second-choice group. This

distribution also revealed a very highly significant difference ($p<0.001$) between the groups.

Distribution of the criteria applied. To identify the criteria which correlated with incorrect results, we analyzed the frequency distribution of the results (table 5).

The result shows:

- In those cases where all three main criteria had been applied, all blood vessels were labeled correctly (0% incorrect or unidentifiable).
- If two main criteria were used, 6% of the vessels were labeled incorrectly or unidentifiable (8/135).
- Using one main criterion brought a colorful picture of results. In this case, 30% of the blood vessels were incorrectly labeled or unidentifiable (16/55).
- The use of zero main criteria resulted in:

   o a very high rate of unidentifiable vessels (42%; 62/147), and

   o a high rate of incorrectly labeled vessels (18%; 27/147).

Secondly, the **second-choice** cases were split into two groups (see column "cases" in table 5):

- the group **using one main criterion** to analyze the questions:

   o Are one or more of the additional criteria responsible for the wrong results?

   o Are one or more of the additional criteria responsible for the right results?

- the group **using zero main criteria** to answer three questions:

Table 2. Test-reference agreement of 387 identifiable vessels.

test-reference agreement		reference labeled		total
		artery	vein	
test labeled	artery	190	31	221
		86%	14%	100%
	vein	7	159	166
		4.2%	95.8%	100%
total		197	190	387
		50.9%	49.1%	100%

Table 3. Sensitivity, specificity and positive predictive value of the test.

test-sensitivity for arteries	0.964	(190/197)
test-sensitivity for veins	0.837	(159/190)
test-sensitivity for all vessels	0.902	(349/387)
test-specificity for arteries	0.837	
test-specificity for veins	0.964	
positive predictive value for arteries	0.860	(190/221)
positive predictive value for veins	0.958	(159/166)

○ Did one or more criterion have a falsifying effect?

○ Is the high rate of undeterminable vessels an indication of poor illustration quality?

○ Does labeling vessels without using any main criteria make sense?

The kappa values for the split second-choice group were calculated separately. If one main criterion and arbitrary additional criteria were used, the test-reference agreement was $\kappa = 0.712$. If zero main criteria and arbitrary additional criteria were used, the test-reference agreement was $\kappa = 0.361$.

Remember: The test-reference agreement of the second choice group as a whole amounted to: $\kappa = 0.506$. In table 6, the frequency of the additional criteria in the different cases was analyzed:

The overview shows that three of the five additional criteria were used very often (AC_1, AC_2, AC_3). The other two additional criteria were used significantly rarer [25]. Unlike in all other cases, AC_1 was the most often used criterion for the second-choice group. The frequencies of the three main criteria were calculated in the same way and did not reveal any significant differences in their distribution (table 7).

Analysis of the criteria used in the second-choice case. For the second-choice group, the rate of correct results showed no significant difference between using one or more additional criterion (p = 0.08), implying that more additional criteria did not improve the test result. Regarding the quality of the different additional criteria, we found a highly significant correlation between the number of correct results and the additional criterion used for the second-choice group (tables 8

and 9). Pearson's Chi-squared test and Fisher's exact test showed a highly significant (p<0.001) difference between the additional criterion applied and the test result for using one main criterion (table 8). This significant difference was also verifiable in case of using zero main criteria (table 9).

Tables 6, 8 and 9 show that the use of AC_1 correlated with a high rate of wrong results. AC_4 and AC_5 were sparely used and are statistically not evaluable, and the use of AC_2 and AC_3 correlated with correct results.

The kappas for application of one main criterion and zero main criteria were calculated excluding the use of the criteria AC_1, AC_4 and AC_5:

one main criterion: $\kappa = 0.940$

zero main criteria: $\kappa = 0.529$

Also, the test-reference agreement of the whole second-choice group without these criteria was calculated: $\kappa = 0.745$. The consequences of eliminating AC_1, AC_4 and AC_5 are summarized in table 10.

Because of the high frequency of AC_1 in the case of zero main criteria (table 9; AC_1 was used in 99/183 (54%) of cases), this additional criterion was considered separately. By using only AC_1, (while eliminating all other criteria), the test-reference agreement was $\kappa = 0.291$.

Discussion

Our study aimed to establish valid and reliable criteria for blood vessel labeling in cSLO IR-images, obtained by SD-OCT scanners used in parallel to OCT images. In doing so, we compared eight criteria extracted from the ophthalmological literature.

Table 4. Connection between the test results and the 1ˢᵗ and 2ⁿᵈ choice.

		Result			total
		incorrect	correct	unidenti-fiable	
1ˢᵗ choice	observed frequency	5	252	3	260
	expected frequency	21.4	196.4	42.2	260
	relative	1.9%	96.9%	1.2%	100%
2ⁿᵈ choice	observed frequency	33	97	72	202
	expected frequency	16.6	152.6	32.8	202
	relative	16.3%	48.1%	35.6%	100%
total	observed frequency	38	349	75	462
	expected frequency	38	349	75	462
	relative	8.2%	75.6%	16.2%	100%

Table 5. Correlation between main criteria and test results.

case	number of main criteria used	result			total
		incorrect	correct	unidentifiable	
2nd choice	0	27	58	62	147
	1	6	39	10	55
1st choice	2	5	127	3	135
	3	0	125	0	125
		38	349	75	462

We set up a hierarchy of these criteria with three main and five additional criteria.

Main criteria:

1. *The central light reflex is wider in arteries and smaller in veins.*
2. *Arteries are brighter than veins.*
3. *Arteries are thinner than veins.*

Additional criteria:

1. *Arteries and veins alternate near the optic disc.*
2. *Arteries never cross arteries and veins never cross veins.*
3. *Vessels should be seen in the context of the vessel tree.*
4. *Arteries take a straighter course than veins.*

5. *Angles between crossing blood vessels are almost 90°, whereas angles between outgoing vessels are between 30° and 45°.*

Moreover, blood vessels which were labeled applying two or more main criteria yielded better test results than vessels labeled based on less than two main criteria. These two cases were analyzed as first and second choice.

For the cases $\geq 2MC + X AC$ (first choice), an almost perfect inter-rater agreement ($\kappa = 0.976$), an almost perfect correctness rate ($\kappa = 0.960$) and a very low rate of unidentifiable vessels (1.15% (3/260)) was shown.

We demonstrated that the three main criteria were equally important and equally often used.

In case of using additional criteria we found, that for all correctly labeled vessels of the first-choice group, AC_2 and AC_3 led to correct results (table 6). However, only 66% of all potentially identifiable vessels were covered by the first choice. Consequently,

Table 6. Distribution of additional criteria, expected frequency means all AC are on an equal level, p-value for the difference between expected and observed frequency.

	criterion	relative frequency	observed frequency	expected frequency	p-value
all identifiable vessels (387)	AC_3	30.2%	117		0.0001
	AC_2	16.0%	62		0.0790
	AC_1	15.0%	58	50.8	0.2588
	AC_4	4.1%	16		0.0001
	AC_5	0.3%	1		0.0001
first choice (260)	AC_3	20%	52		0.0001
	AC_2	11.2%	29		0.0014
	AC_1	1.5%	4	17.2	0.0004
	AC_4	0.4%	1		0.0001
	AC_5	0%	0		0.0001
second choice (202)	AC_1	53%	107		0.0001
	AC_3	41%	83		0.0001
	AC_2	18.8%	38	50.0	0.0578
	AC_4	9.9%	20		0.0001
	AC_5	1%	2		0.0001
correctly labeled vessels (349)	AC_3	29.5%	103		0.0001
	AC_2	16.9%	59		0.0026
	AC_1	11.5%	40	41.6	0.7814
	AC_4	1.4%	5		0.0001
	AC_5	0.3%	1		0.0001

Table 7. Distribution of main criteria, expected frequency means all MC are on an equal level, p-value for the difference between expected and observed frequency.

	criterion	relative frequency	observed frequency	expected frequency	p-value
all identifiable vessels (387)	MC_1	60.5%	234		0.6264
	MC_2	59.4%	230	228	0.8712
	MC_3	56.8%	220		0.5164
first choice (260)	MC_1	86%	224		0.4522
	MC_2	86.9%	226	215	0.3582
	MC_3	75%	195		0.0948
second choice (202)	MC_1	6%	12		0.0700
	MC_2	4%	8	18	0.0032
	MC_3	17.3%	35		0.0001
correctly labeled vessels (349)	MC_1	66.5%	232		0.4436
	MC_2	64.8%	226	223	0.7844
	MC_3	60.2%	210		0.2986

using first choice only would leave one third of the vessels undetermined.

The second-choice group ($\leq 1MC + X\ AC$) presented a different picture of the test results and criteria frequencies. In an attempt to find a reason for the insufficient test results for the second-choice group, we subdivided this group into two subgroups, one using one main criterion and the other using zero main criteria.

It turned out that AC_2 and AC_3 were the only additional criteria which yielded good results in the second choice cases. Elimination of the other additional criteria caused the test-reference agreement of the second choice cases to increase significantly.

The test in its entirety

With the exception of the second-choice group, the additional criterion AC_3 was the most frequently used one (table 6) in all cases. Furthermore, analysis of frequencies suggests that AC_4 and

AC_5 might be irrelevant for first and second choice (whole test) (table 6).

In contrast to [16], we were able to demonstrate both statistically and empirically that criterion AC_5 is incorrect. To give an example, figure 7 shows blood vessels crossing at an angle of 45°, and blood vessels branching at a 90° angle. For the new test, AC_1, AC_4 and AC_5 were eliminated.

There are two different options for labeling:

1. The test should label all vessels based on the main criteria; if no main criterion can be detected or if non-ambiguous labeling is not possible, use of AC_2 and/or AC_3 is allowed.
2. The test should label only those vessels to which one or more main criteria apply. If no main criterion is detectable, the vessel should be classified as unidentifiable.

In connection with the first option, 18% ($n = 69$) of the potentially identifiable blood vessels remained undetected. The

Table 8. Correlation between application of additional criteria and test result based on one main criterion.

Using one main criterion in the second-choice group		result		total
		correct	incorrect or unidentifiable	
AC_1	observed frequency	3	5	8
	expected frequency	5.6	2.4	8
	relative	37.5%	62.5%	100%
AC_2	observed frequency	13	1	14
	expected frequency	9.8	4.2	14
	relative	92.9%	7.1%	100%
AC_3	observed frequency	31	9	40
	expected frequency	28.1	11.9	40
	relative	77.5%	22.5%	100%
AC_4	observed frequency	0	5	5
	expected frequency	3.5	1.5	5
	relative	0.0%	100%	100%

Table 9. Correlation between application of additional criteria and test results based on zero main criteria.

Using zero main criteria in the second-choice group		Result		total
		correct	incorrect or unidentifiable	
AC_1	observed frequency	33	66	99
	expected frequency	42.7	56.3	99
	relative	33.3%	66.7%	100%
AC_2	observed frequency	17	7	24
	expected frequency	10.4	13.6	24
	relative	70.8%	29.2%	100%
AC_3	observed frequency	24	19	43
	expected frequency	18.6	24.4	43
	relative	55.8%	44.2%	100%
AC_4	observed frequency	4	11	15
	expected frequency	6.5	8.5	15
	relative	26.7%	73.3%	100%
AC_5	observed frequency	1	1	2
	expected frequency	0.9	1.1	2
	relative	50%	50%	100%

kappa of the test-reference agreement was at $\kappa = 0.916$. For the second option, 25% (n = 98) of the potentially identifiable vessels were not detected by the test. The kappa of test-reference agreement was $\kappa = 0.957$.

The measured image quality of the missed blood vessels is shown in table 11.

Consequently, in the context of the first option, 91.1% of the missed vessels and 93.9% for the second option do not have a good quality. The quality of the detected vessels in the first possibility was good in 64%, in the second possibility in 70% of the cases.

A possible explanation for the fact that vessels are not identifiable is the different imaging technique of CFP and cSLO. The OCT scanner produces black-and-white cSLO IR images; the fundus image on the other hand is a colored photograph. A colored picture contains more information about the vessels, in particular on blood oxygenation.

Conclusion

Two new test forms with excellent results are possible:

In the first version, the test labels all vessels by the main criteria, and if no main criterion can be detected or if non-ambiguous labeling is not possible, using additionally criteria (AC_2 and/or AC_3) is allowed.

In the second version, only those vessels in the test to which one or more main criteria apply are subjected to labeling. If no main criterion can be detected, the vessel should be classified as unidentifiable.

The first version yields a higher rate of identifiable vessels, the second version a higher rate of security in labeling. In the first version, the kappa of $\kappa = 0.916$ remains almost perfect. So, to include as many vessels as possible, we prefer the first version of the test. This benefit outweighs the lower level of accuracy.

Ultimately, the user of the test has to define an objective before starting the test. This objective will depend on what the data will be used for. Before the labeling is run, the user will define whether the goal is a high rate of identifiable vessels or maximum test-accuracy. Figure 8 shows a hands-on workflow for vessel labeling and visualizes the different levels of test security.

The disadvantage of our method is that image resolution here does not attain the level reached via CFP. Moreover, cSLO-images are black-and-white shots only, so the level of information is technically limited. Moreover, the test did not determine all vessels which could be identified in the reference.

In spite of these curtailments, the method presented here, which involves using cSLO IR-images produced by an OCT scanner for the purpose of investigating blood vessels has many benefits:

Table 10. Test reference agreement of the second-choice group before and after elimination of AC_1, AC_4 and AC_5.

	before elimination of AC 1,4,5	after elimination of AC 1,4,5
whole second choice group	$\kappa = 0.506$	$\kappa = 0.745$
using one main criterion	$\kappa = 0.712$	$\kappa = 0.940$
using zero main criteria	$\kappa = 0.361$	$\kappa = 0.529$

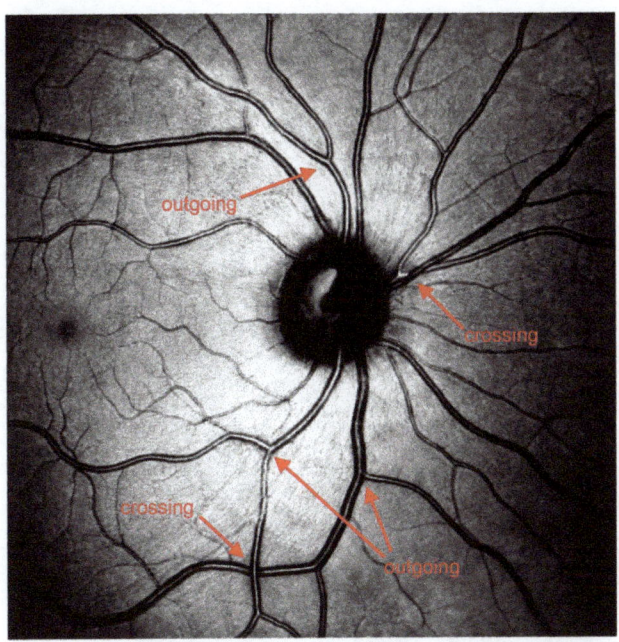

Figure 7. Both the crossing and the outgoing vessels show 90° and 30°-45° angles.

- high reliability ($\kappa = 0.840$)
- high validity ($\kappa = 0.957$)
- time-saving method – only one rater required.

The test was developed based on data from healthy subjects. This fact brings a few restrictions. In course of ethical reasons it was not possible to use fluorescein angiography in place of CFP as ophthalmologic reference. Moreover the small number of subjects in the study precludes a definite evidence. To get an impression of the test results in pathologic entities the workflow was tested additionally on four eyes of two patients. One was suffering from cerebral vasculitis, the other one was affected by giant-cell arteriitis. Diagnosis was made by cerebral MRI and vessel biopsy. Even in these pathological conditions it was possible to label the vessels using the developed workflow. The cSLO images of them are shown in figure 9. The characteristics of arteries and veins in the images of these sick two patients do not differ from healthy subjects. Thus, the workflow for vessel labeling could be applied exemplary in eyes with vascular diseases as well. To detect differences in the vessel morphology of sick and healthy subjects measurements, e.g. of the vessels' diameter, in cSLO images are necessary. This could be done in future studies. Recently, the workflow was also successfully used for vessel labeling in CADASIL patients [Alten et al., manuscript submitted].

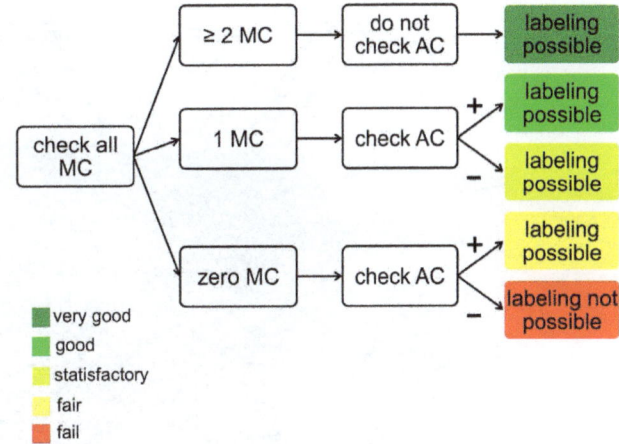

very good
good
statisfactory
fair
fail

Figure 8. Workflow for correct vessel labelling in cSLO images. The different levels of test security are visualized by five colours. MC = main criteria: The central light reflex is wider in arteries and smaller in veins. Arteries are brighter than veins. Arteries are thinner than veins. AC = additional criteria: Arteries never cross arteries and veins never cross veins. Vessels should be seen in the context of the vessel tree.

The examination of vessels in cSLO images offers a straightforward, practicable extension of the application of OCT technique into neurology without tying up further technical resources. Blood vessel examination and screening has a high clinical potential. Spectral domain optical coherence tomography using automated eye tracking and image alignment based on cSLO images is very fast, non-invasive and little personel intensive and combines several aspects of retinal examination in a single device.

Many clinical applications are conceivable; in particular vascular neurological diseases like cerebral vasculitis, CADASIL or cerebral micro-/macroangiopathies might be revealed in abnormal vessels in OCT and cSLO-images.

But since widespread diseases like dementia or stroke also have been shown to correlate with retinal vessel changes in CFP, SD-OCT technology has the potential to open an even wider field of medical applications as it combines knowledge on cerebral and retinal diseases in one application. The increasing use of SD-OCT imaging, originally used in ophthalmology, shows the increasing overlap between the different medical disciplines.

Author Contributions

Conceived and designed the experiments: JM FA CE NO EMK CRC FP MM. Performed the experiments: JM FA CE EMK AB TO CRC FP MM. Analyzed the data: JM FA CE NO EMK AB TO CRC NE MM. Contributed reagents/materials/analysis tools: JM FA CE NO EMK AB TO NE FP MM. Wrote the paper: JM FA CE NO EMK AB TO CRC NE FP MM.

Table 11. Quality of potentially identifiable missed vessels applying the 1st or 2nd test option.

Quality of missed vessels	1st option	2nd option
good	8.7% (6)	6.1% (6)
medium	24.6% (17)	25.5% (25)
bad	66.7% (46)	68.4% (67)

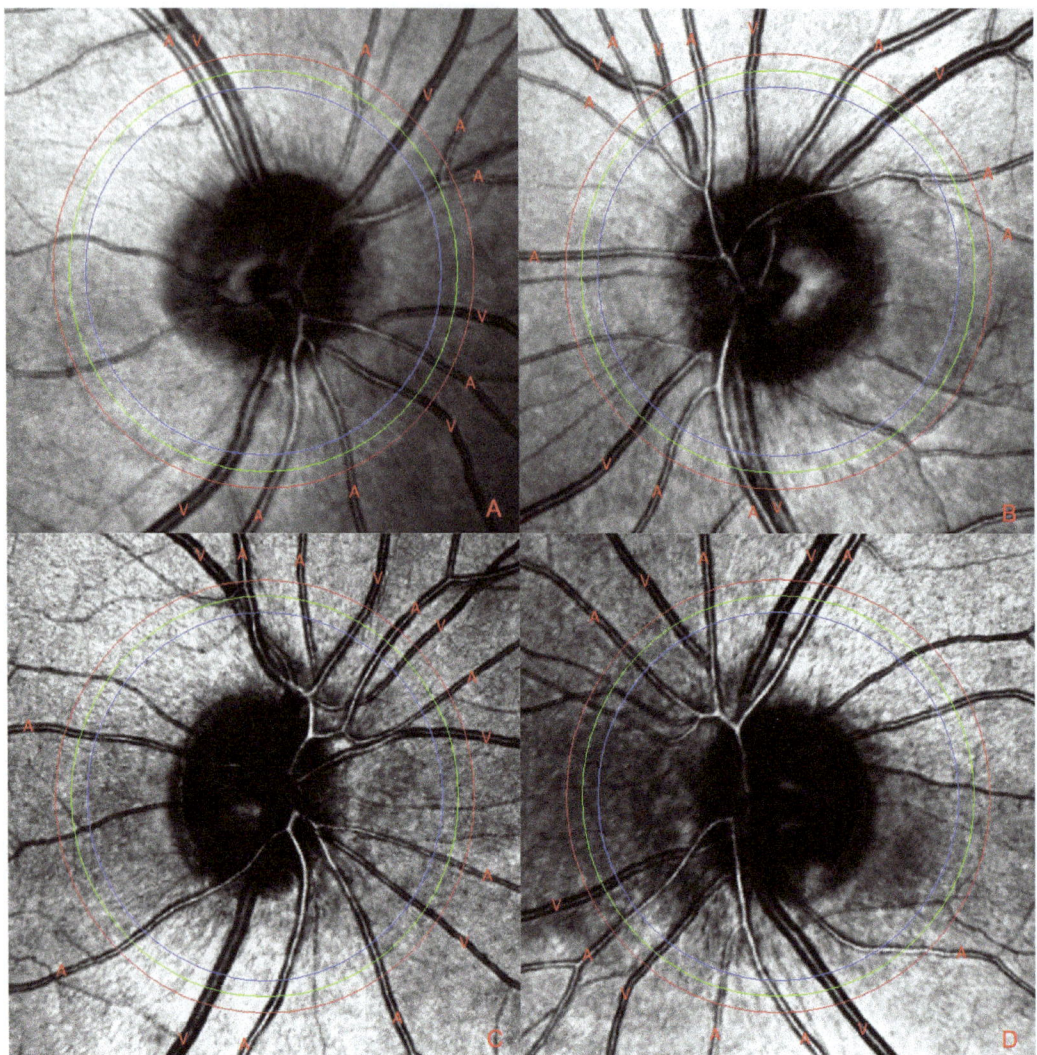

Figure 9. As an example for vascular diseases cSLO images of four eyes of two patients are shown. Picture A and B belong to a patient suffering from cerebral vasculitis. Picture C and D arise from a patient who is affected by giant-cell arteriitis. A change of vessel characteristics is not noticeable. Vessel labeling was performed using the new workflow.

References

1. Huang D, Swanson EA, Lin CP, Schuman JS, Stinson WG, et al. (1991) Optical coherence tomography. Science 254: 1178–1181.
2. Frohman EM, Fujimoto JG, Frohman TC, Calabresi PA, Cutter G, et al. (2008) Optical coherence tomography: a window into the mechanisms of multiple sclerosis. Nat Clin Pract Neurol 4: 664–675.
3. Petzold A, de Boer JF, Schippling S, Vermersch P, Kardon R, et al. (2010) Optical coherence tomography in multiple sclerosis: a systematic review and meta-analysis. Lancet Neurol 9: 921–932.
4. Oberwahrenbrock T, Schippling S, Ringelstein M, Kaufhold F, Zimmermann H, et al. (2012) Retinal damage in multiple sclerosis disease subtypes measured by high-resolution optical coherence tomography. Mult Scler Int 2012: 530305.
5. Oberwahrenbrock T, Ringelstein M, Jentschke S, Deuschle K, Klumbies K, et al. (2013) Retinal ganglion cell and inner plexiform layer thinning in clinically isolated syndrome. Mult Scler 19:1887–1895.
6. Subei AM, Eggenberger ER (2009) Optical coherence tomography: another useful tool in a neuro-ophthalmologist's armamentarium. Curr Opin Ophthalmol 20: 462–466.
7. Albrecht P, Muller AK, Sudmeyer M, Ferrea S, Ringelstein M, et al. (2012) Optical coherence tomography in parkinsonian syndromes. PLoS One 7: e34891.
8. Stricker S, Oberwahrenbrock T, Zimmermann H, Schroeter J, Endres M, et al. (2011) Temporal retinal nerve fiber loss in patients with spinocerebellar ataxia type 1. PLoS One 6: e23024.
9. Roth NM, Saidha S, Zimmermann H, Brandt AU, Oberwahrenbrock T, et al. (2013) Optical coherence tomography does not support optic nerve involvement in amyotrophic lateral sclerosis. Eur J Neurol 20: 1170–1176.
10. Greenberg BM, Frohman E (2010) Optical coherence tomography as a potential readout in clinical trials. Ther Adv Neurol Disord 3: 153–160.
11. Siger M, Dziegielewski K, Jasek L, Bieniek M, Nicpan A, et al. (2008) Optical coherence tomography in multiple sclerosis: thickness of the retinal nerve fiber layer as a potential measure of axonal loss and brain atrophy. J Neurol 255: 1555–1560.
12. Dorr J, Wernecke KD, Bock M, Gaede G, Wuerfel JT, et al. (2011) Association of retinal and macular damage with brain atrophy in multiple sclerosis. PLoS One 6: e18132.
13. Zimmermann H, Freing A, Kaufhold F, Gaede G, Bohn E, et al. (2013) Optic neuritis interferes with optical coherence tomography and magnetic resonance imaging correlations. Mult Scler 19: 443–450.
14. Tewarie P, Balk L, Costello F, Green A, Martin R, et al. (2012) The OSCAR-IB consensus criteria for retinal OCT quality assessment. PLoS One 7: e34823.
15. Kondermann C, Kondermann D, Yan M (2007) Blood vessel classification into arteries and veins in retinal images. Proceedings of SPIE Medical Imaging: 651247–6512479.
16. Chrástek R, Wolf M, Donath K, Niemann H, Michelson G (2002) Automated calculation of retinal arteriovenous ratio for detection and monitoring of cerebrovascular disease based on assessment of morphological changes of retinal

vascular system; Proceedings of IAPR Workshop on machine vision applications: 240–243.

17. Green AJ, Cree BA (2009) Distinctive retinal nerve fibre layer and vascular changes in neuromyelitis optica following optic neuritis. J Neurol Neurosurg Psychiatry 80: 1002–1005.

18. Frost S, Kanagasingam Y, Sohrabi H, Vignarajan J, Bourgeat P, et al. (2013) Retinal vascular biomarkers for early detection and monitoring of Alzheimer's disease. Transl Psychiatry 3: e233.

19. Fleiss JL, Levin B, Paik MC (2004) Statistical Methods for Rates and Proportions: Wiley.

20. Landis JR, Koch GG (1977) The Measurement of Observer Agreement for Categorical Data. Biometrics 33: 159–174.

21. Narasimha-Iyer H, Beach JM, Khoobehi B, Roysam B (2007) Automatic identification of retinal arteries and veins from dual-wavelength images using structural and functional features. IEEE Trans Biomed Eng 54: 1427–1435.

22. Gang L, Chutatape O, Krishnan SM (2002) Detection and measurement of retinal vessels in fundus images using amplitude modified second-order Gaussian filter. Biomedical Engineering, IEEE Transactions on 49: 168–172.

23. Welsch U (2006) Sobotta Lehrbuch Histologie: Elsevier, Urban & Fischer.

24. Hoover A, Kouznetsova V, Goldbaum M (2000) Locating blood vessels in retinal images by piecewise threshold probing of a matched filter response. Medical Imaging, IEEE Transactions on 19: 203–210.

25. Sachs L (2004) Angewandte Statistik: Anwendung statistischer Methoden; Springer-Verlag GmbH, Germany.

2

Non-Contrast-Enhanced Whole-Body Magnetic Resonance Imaging in the General Population: The Incidence of Abnormal Findings in Patients 50 Years Old and Younger Compared to Older Subjects

Andrzej Cieszanowski[1,2], Edyta Maj[1,2]*, Piotr Kulisiewicz[1,2], Ireneusz P. Grudzinski[3], Karolina Jakoniuk-Glodala[1], Irena Chlipala-Nitek[1], Bartosz Kaczynski[4], Olgierd Rowinski[1]

1 2nd Department of Clinical Radiology, Medical University of Warsaw, Warsaw, Poland, **2** Diagnostic Center, Medicover Hospital, Warsaw, Poland, **3** Department of Toxicology, Medical University of Warsaw, Faculty of Pharmacy, Warsaw, Poland, **4** Department of Medical Informatics and Telemedicine, Medical University of Warsaw, Warsaw, Poland

Abstract

Purpose: To assess and compare the incidence of abnormal findings detected during non-contrast-enhanced whole-body magnetic resonance imaging (WB-MRI) in the general population in two age groups: (1) 50 years old and younger; and (2) over 50 years old.

Materials and Methods: The analysis included 666 non-contrast-enhanced WB-MRIs performed on a 1.5-T scanner between December 2009 and June 2013 in a private hospital in 451 patients 50 years old and younger and 215 patients over 50 years old. The following images were obtained: T2-STIR (whole body-coronal plane), T2-STIR (whole spine-sagittal), T2-TSE with fat-saturation (neck and trunk-axial), T2-FLAIR (head-axial), 3D T1-GRE (thorax-coronal, axial), T2-TSE (abdomen-axial), chemical shift (abdomen-axial). Detected abnormalities were classified as: insignificant (type I), potentially significant, requiring medical attention (type II), significant, requiring treatment (type III).

Results: There were 3375 incidental findings depicted in 659 (98.9%) subjects: 2997 type I lesions (88.8%), 363 type II lesions (10.8%) and 15 type III lesions (0.4%), including malignant or possibly malignant lesions in seven subjects. The most differences in the prevalence of abnormalities on WB-MRI between patients 50 years old and younger and over 50 years old concerned: brain infarction (22.2%, 45.0% respectively), thyroid cysts/nodules (8.7%, 18.8%), pulmonary nodules (5.0%, 16.2%), significant degenerative disease of the spine (23.3%, 44.5%), extra-spinal degenerative disease (22.4%, 61.1%), hepatic steatosis (15.8%, 24.9%), liver cysts/hemangiomas (24%, 34.5%), renal cysts (16.9%, 40.6%), prostate enlargement (5.1% of males, 34.2% of males), uterine fibroids (16.3% of females, 37.9% of females).

Conclusions: Incidental findings were detected in almost all of the subjects. WB-MRI demonstrated that the prevalence of the vast majority of abnormalities increases with age.

Editor: Erica Villa, University of Modena & Reggio Emilia, Italy

Funding: The authors have no support or funding to report.

Competing Interests: The authors have declared that no competing interests exist.

* Email: jeczene@gmail.com

Introduction

Recent technological progress has enabled the implementation of whole-body magnetic resonance (WB-MR) screening in the general population. These technical developments include extended scanner table range, multiple input channels permitting parallel imaging, integrated high-resolution surface coils covering the whole body and high-quality sequences with short acquisition times [1–3]. Application of these hardware and software improvements facilitated a considerable reduction of the total imaging time without a significant decrease in image quality, which nowadays approaches the quality of dedicated examinations. Depending on the applied protocol, the imaging time of the whole body ranges from 20 to 90 minutes [1,4–6]. Magnetic resonance imaging (MRI) not only has the high sensitivity required for the detection of abnormalities in different body organs including the head, spine, abdomen, pelvis and bones, but also offers the ability to characterize disease correctly in a significant number of cases, decreasing the number of false-positive diagnoses when compared to other currently used modalities, such as computed tomography (CT) or positron emission tomography (PET) [7,8]. Due to its high sensitivity for the detection of tumor deposits, WB-MR imaging has been used effectively by many investigators in patients with different malignant diseases [8–14], however only a few centers have performed research on the utilization of this method for screening asymptomatic subjects [4–6, 15].

The main possible advantage of whole-body MRI in the general population is for the early detection of significant disease (e.g., malignant tumors, atherosclerosis) leading to rapid implementation of treatment and a likely improvement of the prognosis [2]. On the other hand, the shortcoming of such a screening is the depiction of a substantial number of incidental lesions, which cannot be accurately characterized based on WB-MR images [6,5,8,15,16]. These incidental findings often lead to the application of further investigation, not only generating additional costs, but also leading to severe psychological distress [17].

There is an additional and possibly beneficial aspect of whole-body imaging – MRI offers a unique opportunity to take an insight into the human body without considerable side effects. The majority of data regarding the prevalence of various abnormalities is based on anatomopathological postmortem studies. However in recent years, several papers, concerning incidental findings in patients undergoing different imaging examinations, including MRI of the brain and spine, have been published [18–24]. The current WB-MR techniques enable an estimation of the incidence of many abnormalities as well as – indirectly, by the analysis of their frequency in different age groups – an investigation of their natural history. Nevertheless, to date, no study analyzing the incidence of abnormalities found in WB-MR imaging in different age groups has been published.

Consequently, the aim of this study was twofold: firstly, to assess the incidence of significant abnormalities detected during non-contrast-enhanced WB-MR imaging; and secondly, to compare the incidence of abnormalities in two age groups: 50 years old and younger and over 50 years old.

Materials and Methods

This study was approved by the academic bioethics committee. As the study was retrospective, a written consent was not obtained from the subjects included in this analysis. Patient records were anonymized and de-identified prior to analysis.

Study population

The study group comprised 666 patients (465 male; 201 female) with a mean age of 46.4 years (age range 20–77 years), who underwent non-contrast-enhanced WB-MR screening at a private hospital between December 2009 and June 2013. The MRI examinations were contracted in accordance with special private health insurance, along with laboratory tests and other imaging studies, which were part of this screening program (chest X-ray, breast ultrasound or mammography, ultrasound of the abdomen and pelvis, cardiac CT for calcium score). All women underwent transvaginal ultrasound of the pelvis.

The inclusion criteria were as follows: age ≥ 18 years, willingness and ability to undergo MRI and participate in the screening. Exclusion criteria were contraindications to MRI (such as, peacemakers, metallic implants), severe claustrophobia, age < 18 years, significant artifacts during MRI, precluding reliable assessment of obtained images. Since the aim of this study was to assess the incidence of abnormalities in general population (asymptomatic subjects), patients with significant clinical symptoms or with known, active disease at the time of MR imaging were also excluded from the analysis. Overall, 24 subjects were excluded from the analysis due to presence of clinical symptoms or known, active disease at the time of MR examination (n = 15), contraindications to MRI (n = 3), severe claustrophobia precluding MR scanning (n = 4), low quality of obtained MR images (n = 2).

There were 451 patients 50 years old and younger (the mean age 40.9 years) including 315 men and 135 women, and 215 patients over 50 years old (the mean age 57.9 years), among them 149 men and 66 women.

In 31 patients, the following surgical procedures were performed: emplacement of breast-implant devices (n = 9), cholecystectomy (n = 6), hysterectomy (n = 5), resection of the prostate (n = 3), reconstruction of the anterior cruciate ligament (n = 3), strumectomy (n = 2), mastectomy (n = 1), resection of the cerebellopontine angle tumor (n = 1), resection of liposarcoma of the lower extremity (n = 1). Malignant tumors were diagnosed in 9 patients prior to WB-MRI: uterine cancer (n = 2), cervical cancer (n = 1), ovarian cancer (n = 2), prostate cancer (n = 1), breast cancer (n = 1), liposarcoma (n = 1), thyroid cancer (n = 1). All of them underwent surgery and the interval between the operation and MR imaging in all cases exceeded 3 years. At the time of examination, none of these patients had clinical or laboratory evidence of the recurrence of neoplastic disease.

MR imaging

Magnetic resonance imaging was performed on a 1.5-T system (Magnetom Avanto, Siemens Medical Solutions, Erlangen, Germany), using a phased-array multicoil system. The WB-MR imaging protocol consisted of the following sequences: T2-weighted short time inversion recovery (T2-STIR) of the whole body in the coronal plane, T2-STIR of the whole spine in the sagittal plane, T2-weighted turbo spin-echo (T2-TSE) sequence with fat-saturation of the neck and trunk in the axial plane, T2-weighted fluid attenuated inversion recovery (T2-FLAIR) of the head in the axial plane, 3D T1-weighted gradient recalled echo (3D T1-GRE) with fat saturation of the thorax in the coronal and axial planes, T2-TSE of the abdomen in the axial plane, 3D T1-GRE with fat saturation of the abdomen in the axial plane, chemical shift imaging of the abdomen in the axial plane. Selected parameters of the applied sequences are shown in table 1. The approximate examination time was 50 minutes.

Image analysis

The retrospective evaluation of all studies was performed by two radiologists with 15- and 10-years experience in interpreting MR images (and with 22 and 19 years of experience in general radiology, respectively), working at academic hospital. The assessment of WB-MR images was performed in MR reading room on a dedicated workstation. Readers were unaware of the patients' clinical data. All abnormal findings were documented and classified according to the organ of origin and the significance. The criteria for lesion classification were determined before starting the assessment of MRI scans. Detected abnormalities were categorized as: of low significance, moderately or potentially significant, and significant. The abnormalities were classified as insignificant or of low significance (type I) if they did not require further evaluation or treatment (e.g., old brain infarcts, renal cysts, hepatic or splenic cysts or hemangiomas, disc herniations without compression of nervous structures, adrenal adenomas). The abnormalities were classified as moderately or potentially significant lesions (type II) if they required further medical evaluation, could cause clinical symptoms or required treatment (e.g., multiple sclerosis, gallstones, pulmonary nodules, spondylolisthesis $\geq 2°$). A lesion was categorized as significant (type III) if it required immediate treatment or referral to verify its character.

In case of discrepancies between radiologists the final MRI diagnosis was based on consensus interpretation.

Table 1. Selected parameters of applied MR sequences.

Parameter	T2 STIR	T2 STIR	T2 TSE fat-sat	FLAIR	3D T1 GRE	3D T1 GRE	T2 TSE	In-Out GRE
Imaged area	whole body	whole spine	neck-trunk	head	thorax	abdomen	abdomen	abdomen
Plane	coronal	saggital	axial	axial	axial, coronal	axial	axial	axial
TR/TE (ms)	6400/108	3000/50	2200/125	9000/92	3.24/1.24	4.89/2.23	2110/125	130/2.2/4.9
Flip angle (°)	150	150	150	150	10	10	150	70
Turbo factor	25	11	50	16	–	–	50	–
NSA	1	1	1	1	1	1	1	1
FOV (mm)	500×500	500×500	380×380	230×175	400×300	380×285	360×360	380×285
Matrix	384×346	320×320	256×256	256×192	288×156	288×147	256×256	256×173
Slice thickness (mm)	6	3	6	5	3.5	3	6	6
Number of sections	4	2	3	1	1 (in each plane)	1	1	1
Total acquisition time (all sections)	10 min	2 min 48 s	6 min 40 s	2 min 24 s	15 s (for each plane)	17 s	2 min 30 s	26 s

Then, a separate evaluation was performed in two different age groups: 50 years old and younger and over 50 years old to compare the prevalence of abnormalities in these subjects.

All WB-MR reports were delivered to referring primary care physicians, who decided upon further management.

Follow-up and validation of significant imaging findings

The medical data of all subjects in whom significant abnormalities were demonstrated on WB-MR imaging was checked after, at least, a three-month interval following MRI. All information in terms of additional imaging, follow-up studies, implemented treatment and histopathological validation was recorded.

Overall, 695 of 3375 incidental findings (20.1%) reported by radiologists were confirmed, including 443 of 2997 type I lesions (14.8%), 237 of 364 type II lesions (65.1%) and all type III lesions (100%). In 5 patients with type III lesions, the reference standard for the diagnosis was histopathologic proof obtained intra-operatively. For 8 remaining type III lesions the confirmation was based on supplementary contrast-enhanced MRI, CT, ultrasound (abdominal and transvaginal) and follow-up studies.

Six hundred fifty-four of 680 confirmed type I and type II lesions were validated by other imaging studies, performed due to a private health insurance (chest X-ray, breast ultrasound or mammography, ultrasound of the abdomen and pelvis, cardiac CT for calcium score), whereas in 26 patients confirmation was based on the results of supplementary examinations (contrast-enhanced MRI, CT, ultrasound of the thyroid).

Statistical analysis

The statistical analysis was performed using Statistica software (version 10.0).

A χ^2 test was applied to compare the differences in the incidence of abnormalities (with the incidence of $\geq 1\%$ in the studied population) between two groups: subjects 50 years old and younger and subjects over 50 years old. A p-value of <0.05 was considered significant.

Results

The radiologists reported 124 different types of abnormalities. Overall, 3375 incidental findings were depicted in 659 (98.9%) of 666 subjects. Type I abnormalities (insignificant) constituted the highest number of incidental findings (n = 2997; 88.8%), followed by type II (moderately or potentially significant; n = 363; 10.8%) and type III lesions (significant; n = 15; 2.3%). Type I and type II lesions with an incidence of $\geq 1\%$ in the screened population as well as their prevalence in the two different age groups (50 years old and younger and over 50 years old) are listed in tables 2 and 3.

Fifteen lesions in 13 patients (2.0%) were categorized as significant (type III). Among them, there were nine types of malignant or possibly malignant lesions (in 7 patients) including 1 brain glioma (fig. 1), 1 bronchogenic carcinoma, 1 renal cell carcinoma, 1 complicated renal cysts (type 3 according to Bosniak classification), 1 ovarian tumor, 1 testicular Leydig cell tumor (fig. 2) and, in one patient, metastatic lesions in the lungs, liver and adrenal gland. Six benign lesions were also noted in this group: 3 meningiomas (fig. 3), 2 degenerative myelopathies and 1 lobar pneumonia. Five patients from this group were treated surgically (with glioma, bronchogenic carcinoma, renal cell carcinoma, Leydig cell tumor and meningioma), while in six of them (2 with meningiomas, 2 with degenerative myelopathy, 1 with metastatic disease and 1 with lobar pneumonia) conservative management was implemented. In the patient with metastatic lesions in lungs, liver and adrenal gland, no primary site of malignancy was

Table 2. The incidence of the most frequent type I lesions in two age groups.

Region	Imaging finding	≤50 years: number (frequency)	>50 years: number (frequency)	Statistically significant difference*	All: number (frequency)
Brain	Lesions with brain infarct pattern	85 (18.8%)	84 (39.1%)	Yes (p<0.00001)	169 (25.4%)
	Lesions suggestive of leucoaraiosis	1 (0.2%)	16 (7.4%)	Yes (p<0.00001)	17 (2.6%)
	Pineal gland cyst	10 (2.2%)	2 (0.9%)	No (p=0.19)	12 (1.8%)
	Arachnoid cyst	4 (0.9%)	6 (2.8%)	No (p=0.084)	10 (1.5%)
	Cerebral atrophy	0	8 (3.7%)	Yes (p=0.001)	8 (1.2%)
	Choroid plexus cyst	5 (1.1%)	2 (0.9%)	No (p=0.8)	7 (1.1%)
Head and neck	Sinus mucosal thickening	225 (49.9%)	103 (47.9%)	No (p=0.11)	328 (49.2%)
	Thyroid nodules/cysts	38 (8.4%)	43 (20%)	Yes (p=0.0002)	81 (12.1%)
	Nasal septum deviation	28 (6.2%)	11 (5.1%)	No (p=0.4)	39 (5.9%)
	Fluid in mastoid process	18 (4%)	10 (4.7%)	No (p=0.85)	28 (4.2%)
	Enlarged neck lymph nodes	16 (3.5%)	5 (2.3%)	No (p=0.29)	21 (3.2%)
Spine	Degenerative spinal disease (all)	391 (86.7%)	211 (98.1%)	No (p=0.27)	602 (90.4%)
	Degenerative spinal disease (small-moderate)	289 (64.1%)	111 (51.6%)	Yes (p<0.00001)	400 (60.1%)
	Degenerative spinal disease (significant)	102 (22.6%)	100 (46.5%)	Yes (p<0.00001)	202 (30.3%)
	Scoliosis	71 (15.7%)	46 (21.4%)	No (p=0.2)	117 (17.6%)
	Schmorl's nodes	65 (14.4%)	31 (14.5%)	No (p=0.62)	96 (14.4%)
	Spondylolisthesis	36 (8%)	25 (11.6%)	No (p=0.25)	61 (9.2%)
	Meningeal cysts	35 (7.8%)	25 (11.6%)	No (p=0.073)	60 (9%)
	Lesion with vertebral hemangioma pattern	25 (5.5%)	13 (6%)	No (p=1)	38 (5.7%)
	Lumbarization of S1	13 (2.9%)	16 (7.4%)	Yes (p=0.0165)	29 (4.4%)
	End plate fracture	5 (1.1%)	12 (5.6%)	Yes (p=0.0013)	17 (2.6%)
Thorax	Fibrosis/adhesions	17 (3.9%)	20 (8.7%)	Yes (p=0.0102)	37 (5.6%)
	Enlarged thoracic lymph nodes	24 (5.5%)	8 (3.5%)	No (p=0.25)	32 (4.8%)
	Breast cysts	16 (3.7%)	8 (3.5%)	No (p=0.89)	24 (3.6%)
Abdomen/GI	Liver lesions suggestive of cysts/hemangiomas	105 (23.3%)	79 (36.7%)	Yes (p=0.004)	184 (27.6%)
	Splenic lesions suggestive of cysts/hemangiomas	13 (2.9%)	6 (2.8%)	No (p=0.76)	19 (2.8%)
	Cystic lesions of the pancreas	3 (0.7%)	9 (4.2%)	Yes (p<0.00001)	12 (1.8%)
	Enlarged spleen	9 (2%)	1 (0.5%)	No (p=0.088)	10 (1.5%)
	Enlarged abdominal lymph nodes	4 (0.9%)	6 (2.8%)	No (p=0.0849)	10 (1.5%)
Retroperitoneum	Renal cysts	74 (16.4%)	93 (43.3%)	Yes (p=0.0032)	167 (25.1%)
	Perinephric inflammatory changes	3 (0.7%)	11 (5.1%)	Yes (p=0.0005)	14 (2.1%)
	Adrenal lesion suggestive of adenoma	4 (0.9%)	5 (2.3%)	No (p=0.16)	9 (1.4%)
Male pelvis	Enlarged prostate	16 (5.1%)	51 (34.2%)	Yes (p<0.00001)	67 (14.4%)
	Varicocele	19 (6%)	18 (12.1%)	No (p=0.0537)	37 (8%)
	Epididymal cyst	20 (6.3%)	7 (4.7%)	No (p=0.35)	27 (5.8%)
	Hydrocele testis	5 (1.6%)	3 (2%)	No (p=0.82)	8 (1.7%)
Female pelvis	Nabothian cysts	45 (33.3%)	19 (28.8%)	No (p=0.4)	64 (31.8%)
	Prominent pelvic veins	16 (11.9%)	4 (6.1%)	No (p=0.15)	20 (10%)
Musculoskeletal	Extra-spinal degenerative disease	98 (21.7%)	140 (65.1%)	Yes (p<0.00001)	238 (35.7%)
	Joint effusion	54 (12%)	29 (13.5%)	No (p=0.91)	83 (12.5%)
	Baker's cysts	40 (8.9%)	27 (12.6%)	No (p=0.29)	67 (10.1%)
	Non-cystic bone lesions (benign appearance)	32 (7.1%)	14 (6.5%)	No (p=0.56)	46 (6.9%)
	Bone marrow edema	23 (5.1%)	9 (4.2%)	No (p=0.42)	32 (4.8%)
	Solitary bone cyst	11 (2.4%)	3 (1.4%)	No (p=0.3)	14 (2.1%)

* χ^2 test was applied to compare the differences in the incidence of abnormalities.

identified and in another two patients (with ovarian tumor and complicated renal cysts) no medical data regarding management was available.

Analysis of the site of the depicted abnormalities revealed that 269 of them were located in the brain, 505 in the head and neck, 1072 in the spine, 102 in the lungs, mediastinum and breasts, 435 in the abdominal system and the gastrointestinal tract, 227 in the urinary tract, 91 in the male genital system, 157 in the female genital system, 494 in the musculoskeletal system and 23 in the cardiovascular system.

The most frequent (incidence >20%) were the following type I abnormalities: degenerative spinal disease (n = 602; 90.4%), sinus mucosal thickening (n = 328; 49.2%), hepatic cysts/hemengiomas (n = 184; 27.6%), brain infarcts (n = 169; 25.4%) and renal cysts (n = 167; 25.1%).

A separate analysis performed in order to compare the prevalence of incidental findings in two different age groups revealed that the great majority of them was less frequent in the subjects 50 years old and younger as compared to subjects over 50 years old (tables 2 and 3) and the difference reached statistical significance for the following type I abnormalities: lesions with brain infarct pattern (18.8% vs. 39.1%, respectively), lesions suggestive of leukoaraiosis (0.2% vs. 7.4%), cerebral atrophy (0.0% vs. 3.7%), thyroid cysts/nodules (8.4% vs. 20%), small/moderate degenerative spinal disease (64.1% vs. 51.6%), significant degenerative spinal disease (22.6% vs. 46.5%), lumbalization of of S1 (2.9% vs. 7.4%), vertebral end plate fracture (1.1% vs. 5.6%), thoracic fibrosis/adhesions (3.9% vs. 8.7%), extra-spinal degenerative disease (21.7% vs. 65.1%), liver cysts/hemangiomas (23.3% vs. 36.7%), cystic lesions of the pancreas (0.7% vs. 4.2%), renal cysts (16.4% vs. 43.3%), perinephric inflammatory changes (0.7% vs. 5.1%), enlarged prostate (5.1% vs. 34.2% of males), as well as, for some type II lesions: pulmonary nodules (5.0% vs. 16.2%), hepatic steatosis (15.8% vs. 24.9%), gallstones (3.2% vs. 7.0%) and uterine fibroids (16.3% vs. 37.9% of females) (fig. 4).

Only some abnormalities, including pineal gland cysts, splenic enlargement and ovarian cysts, were more frequent in subjects 50 years old and younger than in the older population. However, the differences in the incidence of these lesions were not statistically significant.

Discussion

The technical improvements in magnetic resonance imaging have enabled the application of this modality for the examination of the whole body. Obtaining both high contrast and high spatial resolution WB-MR images is now feasible within a reasonable acquisition time and the quality of the acquired images is approaching that of dedicated MR examinations [1,5]. Moreover, there is no exposure to ionizing radiation, contrary to other imaging techniques which could be implemented for whole-body examination, such as computed tomography, positron emission tomography or scintigraphy.

Consequently, WB-MR imaging was used for the assessment of various neoplasms and, when compared to other whole-body imaging techniques, was advantageous with regard to the identification of bone marrow involvement, staging of tumors with low metabolic activity, detection of brain and hepatic metastases, lack of ionizing radiation and imaging of the pediatric population [8,12,25]. Other studies aimed at the assessment of preexisting non-neoplastic diseases, such as diabetes and arteriosclerotic vascular disease (ASVD), with whole-body contrast-enhanced magnetic resonance angiography (MRA) [26–28], musculoskeletal disorders, body fat distribution, or even postmortem findings [29–31].

Despite the various benefits of WB-MR imaging, to date only a few centers have carried out research on the implementation of this technique for screening asymptomatic subjects [4–6,15]. Besides the economic aspects, one of the principal reasons of such caution is that whole-body screening of the general population with any modality still remains a controversial issue and the benefits of such imaging have never been proven [2,17]. Thus, some authors advocate limiting the screening to certain groups, in which early detection of a disease or its complications may have potential clinical consequences and enable early and effective treatment (e.g., diabetes mellitus, advanced atherosclerosis, neoplasms) [2,3,26–28]. Regarding the two most lethal conditions affecting the general population (atherosclerosis, malignant tumors), the early detection of malignancy appears to be more important in terms of the implementation of urgent treatment and increased survival time (e.g., renal cell carcinoma, bronchial carcinoma) [2]. For that reason, our WB-MR imaging protocol focused more on tumor detection than on the identification of cardiovascular disease, however, the optimal method of whole-body screening is still a matter for discussion.

The cost of whole-body MR examinations is another crucial issue. For an extended, multi-organ study, approaching 60 minutes as in the case of our examinations, the cost is commonly related to the time of scanner occupation and is usually close to twice or three times the price of a standard MRI (e.g., head, spine). Moreover, the cost of the whole procedure should include the expense of additional tests, such as ultrasound, mammography, computed tomography, positron emission tomography, endoscopy, follow-up MRI, biopsies and laboratory tests, implemented to verify potentially relevant WB-MR imaging findings.

Table 3. The incidence of the most frequent type II lesions in two age groups.

Region	Imaging finding	≤50 years: number (frequency)	>50 years: number (frequency)	Statistically significant difference*	All: number (frequency)
Thorax	Pulmonary nodule	22 (5%)	37 (16.2%)	Yes (p<0.00001)	59 (8.9%)
Abdomen	Hepatic steatosis	69 (15.8%)	57 (24.9%)	Yes (p=0.0044)	126 (18.9%)
	Gallstones	14 (3.2%)	16 (7%)	Yes (p=0.0247)	30 (4.5%)
Femele pelvis	Uterine fibroid	22 (16.3%)	25 (37.9%)	Yes (p=0.0047)	47 (23.4%*)
	Ovarian cyst (>2 cm)	16 (11.9%)	4 (6.1%)	No (p=0.15)	20 (10%*)
Vascular	Varicose veins	10 (2.3%)	7 (3.1%)	No (p=0.53)	17 (2.5%)

* χ^2 test was applied to compare the differences in the incidence of abnormalities.

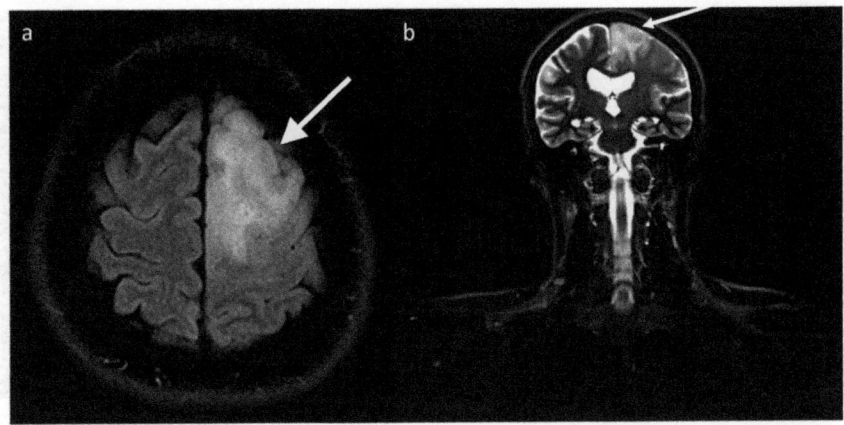

Figure 1. A 43-year-old male with cerebral glioma (arrows) confirmed histopathologically and excised. An axial T2-FLAIR image of the head shows a hyperintense area in the left frontal lobe (A). This lesion is also seen on a coronal whole-body T2-STIR image (B).

A further important consideration are the false-positive or undetermined MRI results. Despite the relatively high specificity of MRI for discrimination between benign and malignant lesions, there are a substantial number of cases, in which WB-MR imaging cannot confidently exclude malignancy. Incidental findings are a well-recognized problem in radiological screening programs [24], and the number of "incidentalomas" rises with an increase in the sensitivity of imaging modalities [22,23], leading to substantial psychosocial distress [17]. Moreover, Schmidt et al. have found strong disagreement between patients' and radiologists' recognition of the severity of reported abnormalities [17]. Thus, even some insignificant findings (e.g., liver or splenic hemangiomas/cysts, renal cysts) may lead to severe mental distress for a patient.

Based on previous reports, as well as on our subjective impression after evaluating over 600 studies, we assume that the assessment of abnormalities by WB-MR imaging varies for different body regions and different pathologies [4–6,15]. We presume that our scanning protocol of a non-contrast enhanced WB-MRI enabled the appropriate assessment of the majority of lesions in the brain, spine, paranasal sinuses, thyroid, lungs, abdominal parenchymal organs, adrenals, pelvis, testes and bones. Conversely, a detailed evaluation of the cardiovascular system, colon, joints, neck and prostate (except for its size and volume) could be compromised. Until recently, an important drawback of MRI was the compromised imaging of the lung. Currently, the improvement in MRI techniques, particularly the introduction of the 3D T1-GRE sequence, has helped to overcome this problem. According to published papers [32,33], as well as to our own experience, this technique enables the detection of clinical relevant pulmonary nodules with high sensitivity.

To date, there are results available from four other groups imaging asymptomatic subjects with WB-MR. In three of these

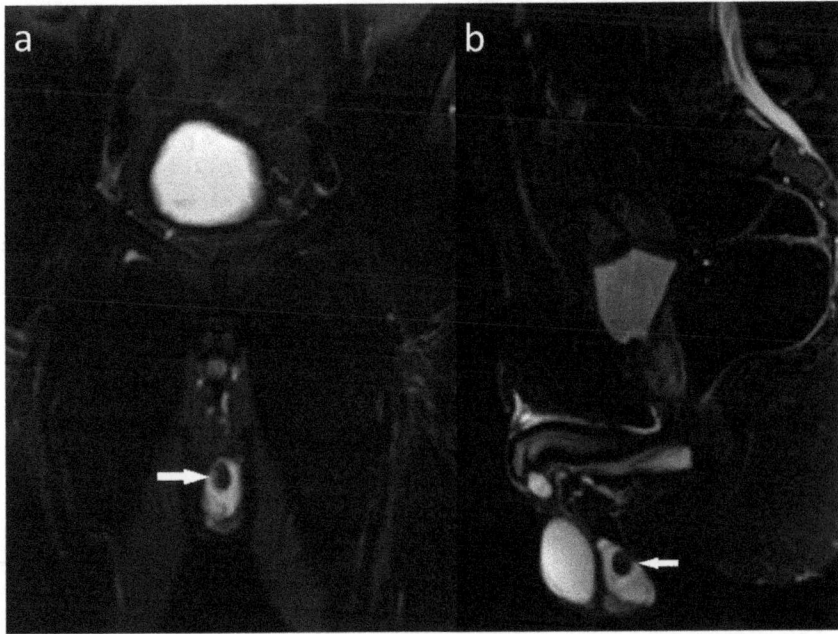

Figure 2. A 43-year-old male with confirmed Leydig cell tumor of the left testis seen as a hypointense lesion (arrows) on a coronal whole-body T2-STIR image (A) and a saggital whole-spine T2-STIR image (B).

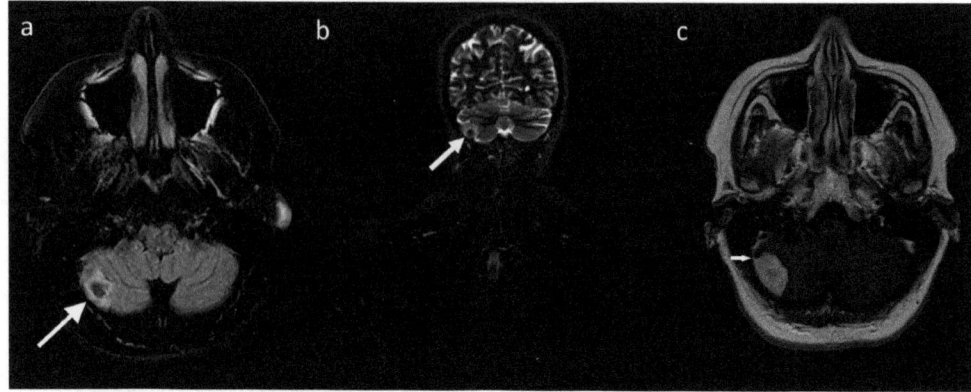

Figure 3. A 59-year-old female with surgically removed meningioma. A lesion of mixed signal intensity (arrows) is seen in the posterior fossa on a T2-FLAIR image of the head (A) and a coronal whole-body T2-STIR image (B). A supplementary, preoperative contrast-enhanced MR study (C) demonstrated enhancing lesion with a tail sign (arrow).

reports, the number of analyzed examinations was less than 300, thus our study group comprise the second largest number of subjects. Furthermore, we evaluated, for the first time, the prevalence of abnormalities in different age groups. The comparison of our results with the results of previous investigations is not straightforward, due to several factors including different MRI systems and protocols used for image acquisition, various methods of data analysis and a lack of standardization for the classifications of detected lesions [4–6,15]. Despite quite similar criteria for determining the significance of depicted abnormalities (e.g., "relevant findings", "might require further non-urgent evaluation or treatment", "requires prompt medical follow-up", "requires immediate referral") the final categorization was to some extent subjective. Furthermore, two studies assessed the prevalence of

cardiovascular disease, implementing, for that purpose, contrast-enhanced MRI [4,6], whereas two other groups focused on detection of other abnormalities and used no contrast agent [5,15].

The incidence of abnormalities detected in our group of subjects during WB-MR imaging (98.9%) was similar to that previously reported by Lo et al. and Hegenscheid et al. (>90%) [5,6]. The much lower detection rate noted by Morin et al. (29.1%), was probably due to the use of only two sequences (T1-weighted SE sequence in the axial plane and T2-weighted GRE survey sequence), inclusion of a young cohort of subjects with a median age of 36 years and the lack of detailed imaging of the spine and brain [15]. We presume that the implementation in our imaging protocol of several devoted techniques enabled the acquisition of detailed images of the head, spine, lungs and abdomen, facilitating

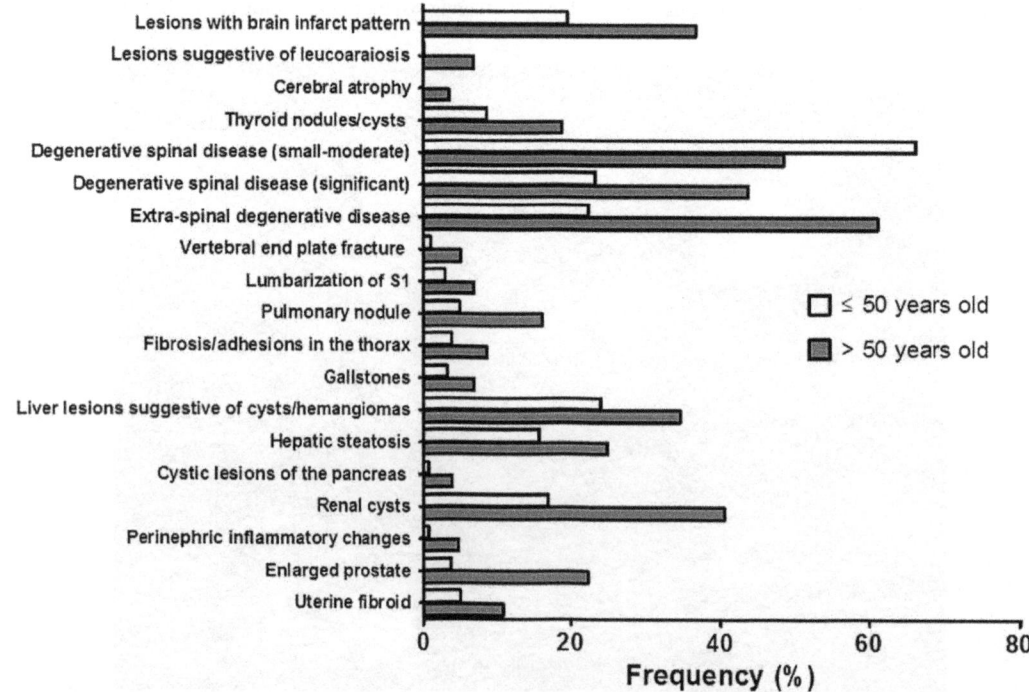

Figure 4. Graph illustrating the incidence of lesions, which reached statistically significant differences (p<0.05), in two different age groups.

a significant improvement in the detection rate of some common abnormalities (e.g., cerebral infarcts, degenerative spinal disease, pulmonary nodules, liver cysts/hemangiomas, renal cysts, uterine fibroids) as compared to Morin et al.

A comparison of our findings with that of Goehde et al. is even more difficult as they focused on imaging of the brain, cardiovascular system and colon, using for this purpose contrast-enhanced WB-MR angiography, cine true-FISP technique and MR colonography [4]. Our scanning protocol did not comprise contrast-enhanced techniques, however, it included several sequences dedicated to spinal, thoracic and abdominal imaging. Consequently, the incidence of such abnormalities as degenerative spinal disease, pulmonary nodules (fig. 4), hepatic cysts/hemangiomas, splenic cysts/hemangiomas, was clearly higher among our group of subjects.

The WB-MR protocol implemented in the present study was in some aspects similar to that used by Lo et al. [5], in terms of the number and type of sequences. Therefore, the detection rates of the major abnormalities including T2 hyperintense lesions in the liver (24.0% vs. 34.5% in our study group) and renal cysts (18% vs. 25% in our study group) are comparable. However, we cannot exclude that the application of two T2-weighted abdominal sequences (T2-TSE, T2-TSE fat-sat in axial planes) may have resulted in slightly higher detection rates in our material. The higher difference noted in the detection rates of pulmonary nodules (8.9% in our group, compared to 3% in the group studied by Lo et al. [5]) was probably related to the implementation of 3D T1-GRE sequence in our imaging protocol (fig. 5). This sequence was effective in detecting even small pulmonary nodules and similar results have been obtained previously by researchers focusing on lung imaging [32,33].

The protocol implemented in our study was shorter than that proposed by Hegenscheid et al. [6]. We omitted several techniques applied by Hegenscheid et al. for imaging of the brain (T2-TSE, T1-MPR, DWI, SWI, TOF angiography), thorax (T2-HASTE) and abdomen (3D MRCP, DWI). Thus, we could miss small aneurysms or other intracranial lesions, including small extra-axial meningiomas, as well as acute brain infarctions. On the other hand, we believe that the inclusion of the T2-FLAIR sequence, as in our study, facilitates detection of the majority of significant intra- and extra-axial lesions without the use of a contrast agent. As the incidence of intracranial aneurysms was only 0.2% on our WB-MR images, it is probable that due to the exclusion of the TOF MRA sequence from the protocol, we missed some of these lesions, as their reported incidence is 1.8–2.4% [6,19]. Alternatively, omitting DWI could result in overlooking acute brain infarction, even though its incidence in

the general population was very low (0.16%), according to Hegenscheid et al. [6]. Moreover, they are usually symptomatic.

As compared to the abdominal protocol used by Hegenscheid et al., our assessment of the biliary tree could be compromised, however, the application of two axial T2-TSE sequences (without and with fat saturation) enabled the detection of dilated bile ducts and the visualization of gallstones in a relatively high number of subjects (n = 30, 4.5%). Implementation of the DWI sequence could probably slightly improve the detection rate of focal hepatic and extra-hepatic lesions, although at the expense of prolonged imaging time. Alternatively, we applied chemical shift imaging of the abdomen, allowing the diagnosis of hepatic steatosis (incidence of 18.9% in our study group) and leading to the recommendation of the implementation of a proper diet and a reduction in the patient's cholesterol intake (fig. 6). This technique also facilitates the discrimination of adenomas (incidence of 1.4% in our study group) from other adrenal lesions and permits the detection of lipids in some hepatic tumors (hepatocellular carcinoma, hepatic adenoma, focal hepatic steatosis, hepatic angiomyolipoma, lipoma) as well as in extra-hepatic lesions (e.g., renal angiomyolipoma). In our material, it also assisted in confirming the diagnosis of benign pancreatic lipoma in two subjects.

We expect that the results of our study will add some valuable information towards the optimization of a WB-MR screening protocol. Such a protocol is always a compromise between the quality/number of images/sequences and the acquisition time. The results of our study support the inclusion of some dedicated MR techniques, such as T2-FLAIR (head), 3D T1-GRE (thorax) and chemical shift imaging (abdomen) into a WB-MR imaging protocol, along with whole-body and whole-spine sequences. We applied 2D FLAIR sequence with 5 mm slice thickness for imaging of the brain. The application of 3D FLAIR images would not only allow obtaining high-resolution images with isotropic voxel size of 1 mm, but also enable multi-planar imaging of the head devoid of cerebro-spinal fluid flow artifacts often visible on 2D images [34]. This would facilitate detection of higher number of lesions in cerebral hemispheric white matter and brainstem, however on the expense of prolonged both acquisition time and time needed for the evaluation of images.

Additional factors which may influence the protocol of WB-MR screening are the aims of the investigation (cardiovascular screening, tumor detection or both), the general type of the examined population, and the individual characteristics of the participants. Screening of diabetic patients or subjects with increased risk of ASVD may lead to the application of whole-body MR angiography. Taking into consideration individual factors, such as body mass index (BMI) and family history of

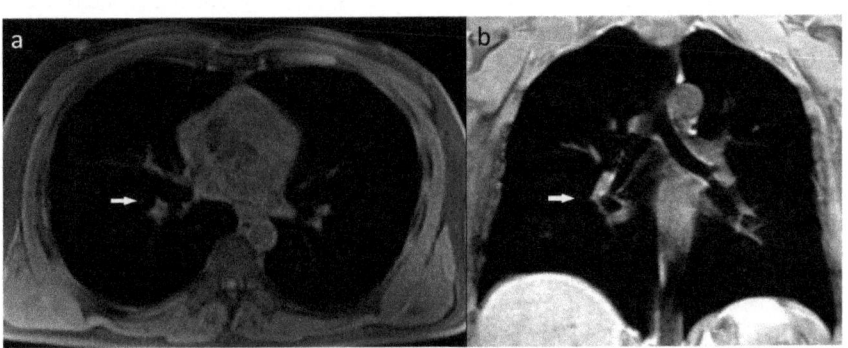

Figure 5. A 55-year-old female with a 5 mm nodule in the right lung (arrows). The lesion noted on both 3D T1-GRE axial (A) and coronal (B) images.

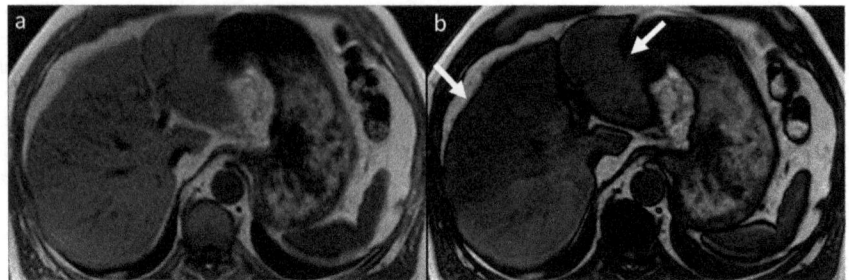

Figure 6. In-phase (A) and opposed phase (B) chemical shift MR images of a 51-year-old male demonstrate hepatic steatosis, consistent with areas of decreased signal intensity on an opposed-phase image. Steatosis is more pronounced it the left lobe and the anterior segments of the right liver lobe (arrows in B).

neoplastic disease, may lead to further personalization of the scanning protocol. In obese subjects application of Dixon technique facilitates segmentation of adipose tissue enabling its quantification and assessment of distribution [35]. Patients with known or suspected neoplasms as well as individuals with the family history of certain neoplasm require application of MR techniques sensitive for tumor detection, such as diffusion weighted imaging (DWI) [13,36]. In addition, the use of short-tau inversion recovery (STIR) sequence in patients with multiple myeloma or bone metastases enables identification of bone marrow involvement and increases the sensitivity for the detection of bone lesion [37,38].

The results of our study showed that non-contrast-enhanced WB-MR imaging facilitated the assessment of the incidence of numerous abnormalities in the general population and enabled the detection of significant findings in 2% of the patients, including 7 patients with malignant lesions (4 of whom were treated surgically). Even though the implemented imaging was beneficial for several subjects, the overall cost of WB-MR screening is high and might not be justified by the early detection of malignancy in a relatively small percentage of the scanned population.

The role of imaging modalities in the estimation of prevalence of various abnormalities considerably increased in recent years, mostly due to a significant increase in spatial resolution of CT and MRI. Based on imaging findings, the prevalence of a wide range of incidental findings such as silent brain infarcts, intervertebral disc degeneration, lung nodules, liver hemangiomas, adrenal adenomas, renal cell carcinomas and uterine fibroids, appeared to be more frequent than previously thought [18–24,39–41].

A good example is renal cell carcinoma (RCC), which accounts for 90% of primary renal neoplasms and represents 3% of all adult malignancies [39,40]. The incidence of this neoplasm has gradually risen during recent decades, mostly due to advances in imaging. Nowadays a classic clinical presentation triad of RCC (hematuria, flank pain, palpable abdominal mass) is seen in only 5–10% of cases. More than 60% of RCCs are now diagnosed incidentally by CT, MRI or ultrasound [40]. Since the majority of detected RCCs are currently smaller and of lower stage the number of partial or "nephron-sparing" nephrectomies has increased as compared to total nephrectomies. In addition, survival has improved, with an overall 5-year survival rate of 62%. The 5-year survival in higher for incidentally detected tumors (85%) than for symptomatic cases (53%) [40].

Solitary pulmonary nodule (SPN) is another abnormality, which occurs more frequently than previously thought. While it is found incidentally in only 0.09–0.2% of all chest radiographs, the reported incidence of SPN on CT scans is much higher, ranging from 8% to 51% [41–43]. The radiologic features of SPN, such as calcification or fat within a nodule, its size, margins, location and rate of growth help to determine the likelihood of malignancy in a majority of cases [41,44]. Nevertheless, the American College of Physicians recommended CT follow-up at 3, 6, 12, and 24 months for indeterminate SPN [44].

Monitoring SPNs and other suspicious lesions detected incidentally on imaging studies might lead to better outcomes by detecting early cancers, but on the other hand diagnosis of indeterminate mass often results in severe distress for a patient and additional imaging and follow-up.

A novel aspect of our study was the use of magnetic resonance imaging for the analysis of the occurrence of abnormalities in different age groups, which could assist in a better understanding of their natural history. We noted a higher incidence of the great majority of abnormal lesions, such as, vascular infarcts, significant degenerative spinal and extra-spinal disease, pulmonary nodules, liver cyst/hemangiomas, gallstones, renal cysts and uterine fibroids, in subjects over 50 years old. However, we observed several interesting exceptions, including pineal gland cysts, splenic enlargement and ovarian cysts (>2 cm), which were more frequent in subjects 50 years old and younger, although, in both cases, the differences were not statistically significant. Moreover, in this population, we noted a significant incidence (>10%) of some abnormalities presumed to be typical for older subjects (e.g., vascular infarcts, substantial degenerative spinal disease, renal cysts). As the natural history of many lesions is not fully known, the detailed statistical analysis of WB-MR data of large cohorts of asymptomatic subjects in narrow age groups, concerning not only the prevalence of different abnormalities, but also their number and size, may provide some valuable information without the implementation of invasive techniques or postmortem studies.

This study has certain limitations. Firstly, the subjects were not selected randomly, but had WB-MR examinations due to private health insurance, which, in general, reflected their better material status as compared to the average population. Therefore, we cannot exclude that their average health status may somewhat differ from that of randomly selected subjects. In addition, there is an important ethical consideration – if WB-MR screening proves to be feasible then it cannot be restricted to a group of individuals but it has to be accessible to all people independent of their socio-economic status [2].

Secondly, the presence and the character of the majority of incidental findings noted during WB-MR imaging (79.9%) was not confirmed by other tests and the final conclusion was based on the subjective opinion of the radiologist evaluating the study. For this reason, we could not assess the number of false-negative cases and the true sensitivity of the implemented MR technique for detecting abnormalities in various organs, nor determine its specificity for discrimination between different lesions. All abnormalities classified as significant (type III) underwent further comprehensive assessment, while the whole studied population underwent supplementary imaging being a part of their private health insurance (chest X-ray, breast ultrasound or mammography, ultrasound of the abdomen and pelvis, cardiac CT for calcium score), which supported the verification of a number of diagnoses (e.g., hepatic steatosis, gallstones, urinary tract calculi, uterine fibroid, prostatic enlargement). Even though, the majority of incidental findings was not validated. As this is a natural limitation of similar studies, investigators undertaking analogous research experienced the same problem [5,6,15].

Thirdly, the comparison of the prevalence of abnormalities in two different age groups should be regarded as a preliminary. For a more comprehensive evaluation, further studies are needed based on even larger number of subjects.

In a current study the use of relatively new technical applications such as extended scanner table range, parallel imaging combined with multiple input channel, high-resolution surface coils covering the whole body (total imaging matrix, TIM) and sequenced with short acquisition time enabled us to obtain high quality images of the whole body within acceptable time. We presume that in the future the role of high field systems (≥ 3T) for whole-body MR imaging may increase since they offer substantially higher signal-to-noise ratio (SNR) and contrast-to-noise ratio (CNR) than lower field systems. Increases in SNR and CNR can result in improving image resolution and shortening time of imaging [45]. However there are several potential drawbacks of imaging at high-field scanners, including limitation of energy deposition, increased magnetic susceptibility and chemical shift artifacts, marked increase in specific absorption rate (SAR) and problem with radio frequency (RF) and field inhomogeneity [45]. These technical limitations especially apply to imaging larger fields of view and for thoracic and abdominal scans may result in significant image distortion and signal loss related to soft-tissue and gas interfaces (e.g. bowel gas in the abdomen and pelvis, lung bases in the upper abdomen). Moreover, the cost of installation and upkeep of high-field scanners is substantially higher compared with 1.5T units [45].

There are other relatively new MRI techniques which could be used for a variety of MR imaging, such as functional magnetic resonance imaging (fMRI), diffusion tensor imaging (DTI), voxel based morphometry (VMB), positron emission tomography combined with magnetic resonance imaging (PET-MRI) or traveling wave MRI [46,47]. Functional MRI enables the indirect (based on hemodynamics) measurement of brain activation, DTI allows identification of white matter tracks (fiber tracking) in the brain and spine, which can be displayed as DTI maps, VBM facilitates monitoring changes in gray matter (related to aging, drug abuse, psychiatric disorders or other environmental and health factors) and PET-MRI, which yields information about biochemical processes, permits detection and staging of neoplastic diseases [46]. However, the above techniques are more suited for dedicated MR examinations and its role for screening in asymptomatic subjects currently appears to be limited. Traveling wave MRI is an interesting new technique, which relies on traveling radio-frequency waves sent and received by an antenna, allows more uniform coverage of samples that are larger than the wavelength of the MR signal [47]. Despite uniform coverage of larger volumes this technique requires very high magnetic fields and at this time cannot be implemented for whole-body screening [47].

In conclusion, the results of our study confirmed that non-contrast-enhanced WB-MR imaging is a reliable, safe and accurate method enabling the detection of disease throughout the entire body, including malignant tumors. They also support the incorporation of some dedicated MR techniques, in particular T2-FLAIR, 3D T1-GRE and chemical shift imaging into the screening protocol. The evaluation of the prevalence of abnormalities in different age groups showed that most of them increase with age. We believe that in the future such analyses may have an important cognitive aspect and facilitate the understanding of the natural history of different pathologies, especially their incidence and growth rates.

Author Contributions

Conceived and designed the experiments: AC EM PK IPG KJG ICN BK OR. Performed the experiments: AC EM IPG KJG ICN BK. Analyzed the data: AC EM PK IPG KJG ICN BK OR. Contributed reagents/materials/analysis tools: AC EM KJG ICN BK. Wrote the paper: AC EM IPG OR. Critical revision of the manuscript: AC EM PK IPG KJG ICN BK OR.

References

1. Kruger DG, Riederer SJ, Grimm RC, Rossman PJ (2002) Continuously moving table data acquisition method for long FOV contrast-enhanced MRA and whole-body MRI. Magn Reson Med 47: 224–231.
2. Ladd SC (2009) Whole-body MRI as a screening tool? Eur J Radiol. 70: 452–62.
3. Kramer H, Nikolaou K, Reiser MF (2009) Cardiovascular whole-body MRI. Eur J Radiol 70: 418–23.
4. Goehde SC, Hunold P, Vogt FM, Ajaj W, Goyen M, et al. (2005) Full-body cardiovascular and tumor MRI for early detection of disease: feasibility and initial experience in 298 subjects. AJR Am J Roentgenol 184: 598–611.
5. Lo GG, Ai V, Au-Yeung KM, Chan JK, Li KW, et al. (2008) Magnetic resonance whole body imaging at 3 Tesla: feasibility and findings in a cohort of asymptomatic medical doctors. Hong Kong Med J 14: 90–96.
6. Hegenscheid K, Seipel R, Schmidt CO, Völzke H, Kühn JP, et al. (2013) Potentially relevant incidental findings on research whole-body MRI in the general adult population: frequencies and management. Eur Radiol 23: 816–826.
7. Furtado CD, Aguirre DA, Sirlin CB, Dang D, Stamato SK, et al. (2005) Whole-body CT screening: spectrum of findings and recommendations in 1192 patients. Radiology 237: 385–394.
8. Ghanem NA, Pache G, Lohrmann C, Brink I, Bley T, et al. (2007) MRI and (18)FDG-PET in the assessment of bone marrow infiltration of the spine in cancer patients. Eur Spine J 16: 1907–1912.
9. Engelhard K, Hollenbach H, Wohlfart K, von Imhoff E, Fellner FA (2004) Comparison of whole-body MRI with automatic moving table technique and bone scintigraphy for screening for bone metastases in patients with breast cancer. Eur Radiol 14: 99–105.
10. Costelloe CM, Kundra V, Ma J, Chasen BA, Rohren EM, et al. (2012) Fast Dixon whole-body MRI for detecting distant cancer metastasis: a preliminary clinical study. J Magn Reson Imaging 35: 399–408.
11. Sohaib SA, Cook G, Allen SD, Hughes M, Eisen T, et al. (2009) Comparison of whole-body MRI and bone scintigraphy in the detection of bone metastases in renal cancer. Br J Radiol 82: 632–639.
12. Schmidt G, Schoenberg S, Schmid R, Stahl R, Tiling R, et al. (2007) Screening for bone metastases: whole-body MRI using a 32-channel system versus dual-modality PET-CT. Eur Radiol 17: 939–949.
13. Ohno Y, Koyama H, Onishi Y, Takenaka D, Nogami M, et al. (2008) Non-small cell lung cancer: whole-body MR examination for M-stage assessment - utility for whole-body diffusion-weighted imaging compared with integrated FDG PET/CT. Radiology 248: 643–654.
14. Qu X, Huang X, Yan W, Wu L, Dai K (2012) A meta-analysis of ^{18}FDG-PET-CT, ^{18}FDG-PET, MRI and bone scintigraphy for diagnosis of bone metastases in patients with lung cancer. Eur J Radiol 81: 1007–1015.
15. Morin SH, Cobbold JF, Lim AK, Eliahoo J, Thomas EL, et al. (2009) Incidental findings in healthy control research subjects using whole-body MRI. Eur J Radiol 72: 529–533.
16. Hegenscheid K, Kühn JP, Völzke H, Biffar R, Hosten N, et al. (2009) Whole-body magnetic resonance imaging of healthy volunteers: pilot study results from the population-based SHIP study. Rofo 181: 748–759.
17. Schmidt CO, Hegenscheid K, Erdmann P, Kohlmann T, Langanke M, et al. (2013) Psychosocial consequences and severity of disclosed incidental findings from whole-body MRI in a general population study. Eur Radiol 23: 1343–1351.

18. Morris Z, Whiteley WN, Longstreth WT Jr, Weber F, Lee YC, et al. (2009) Incidental findings on brain magnetic resonance imaging: systematic review and meta-analysis. BMJ 339: b3016. doi:10.1136/bmj.b3016.

19. Vernooij MW, Ikram MA, Tanghe HL, Vincent AJ, Hofman A, et al. (2007) Incidental findings on brain MRI in the general population. N Engl J Med 357: 1821–1828.

20. Takatalo J, Karppinen J, Niinimäki J, Taimela S, Näyhä S, et al. (2009) Prevalence of Degenerative Imaging Findings in Lumbar Magnetic Resonance Imaging Among Young Adults. Spine 34: 1716–1721.

21. Cheung KM, Karppinen J, Chan D, Ho DW, Song YQ, et al. (2009) Prevalence and pattern of lumbar magnetic resonance imaging changes in a population study of one thousand forty-three individuals. Spine 34: 934–40. doi: 10.1097/BRS.0b013e3181a01b3f.

22. Gore RM, Newmark GM, Thakrar KH, Mehta UK, Berlin JW (2010) Pelvic incidentalomas. Cancer Imaging 10 Spec no A: S15–26.

23. Tsui KH, Shvarts O, Smith RB, Figlin R, de Kernion JB, et al. (2000) Renal cell carcinoma: prognostic significance of incidentally detected tumors. J Urol 163: 426–430.

24. Woodward CI, Toms AP (2009) Incidental findings in "normal" volunteers. Clin Radiol 64: 951–953.

25. Ley S, Ley-Zaporozhan J, Schenk JP (2009) Whole-body MRI in the pediatric patient. Eur J Radiol 70: 442–451.

26. Weckbach S, Schoenberg SO (2009) Whole body MR imaging in diabetes. Eur J Radiol 70: 424–430.

27. Fenchel M, Scheule AM, Stauder NI, Kramer U, Tomaschko K, et al. (2006) Atherosclerotic disease: whole-body cardiovascular imaging with MR system with 32 receiver channels and total-body surface coil technology-initial clinical results. Radiology 238: 280–291.

28. Laible M, Schoenberg SO, Weckbach S, Lettau M, Winnik E, et al. (2012) Whole-body MRI and MRA for evaluation of the prevalence of atherosclerosis in a cohort of subjectively healthy individuals. Insights Imaging 3: 485–493.

29. Schmidt GP, Reiser MF, Baur-Melnyk A (2007) Whole-body imaging of the musculoskeletal system: the value of MR imaging. Skeletal Radiol 36: 1109–1119.

30. Brennan DD, Whelan PF, Robinson K, Ghita O, O'Brien JM, et al. (2005) Rapid automated measurement of body fat distribution from whole-body MRI. AJR Am J Roentgenol 185: 418–423.

31. Patriquin L, Kassarjian A, Barish M, Casserley L, O'Brien M, et al. (2001) Postmortem whole-body magnetic resonance imaging as an adjunct to autopsy: preliminary clinical experience. J Magn Reson Imaging 13: 277–287.

32. Frericks BB, Meyer BC, Martus P, Wendt M, Wolf KJ, et al. (2008) MRI of the thorax during whole-body MRI: evaluation of different MR sequences and comparison to thoracic multidetector computed tomography (MDCT). J Magn Reson Imaging 27: 538–545.

33. Biederer J, Hintze C, Fabel M (2008) MRI of pulmonary nodules: technique and diagnostic value. Cancer Imaging 19: 125–130.

34. Kitajima M, Hirai T, Shigematsu Y, Uetani H, Iwashita K, et al. (2012) Comparison of 3D FLAIR, 2D FLAIR, and 2D T2-weighted MR imaging of brain stem anatomy. AJNR Am J Neuroradiol 33: 922–7. J Magn Reson Imaging; Jan 22. doi: 10.1002/jmri.24509.

35. Ludwig UA, Klausmann F, Baumann S, Honal M, Hövener JB, et al. (2014) Whole-body MRI-based fat quantification: A comparison to air displacement plethysmography. J Magn Reson Imaging. 2014 Jan 22. doi: 10.1002/jmri.24509.

36. Low RN, Gurney J (2007) Diffusion-weighted MRI (DWI) in the oncology patient: value of breathhold DWI compared to unenhanced and gadolinium-enhanced MRI. J Magn Reson Imaging; 25: 848–858.

37. Shortt CP, Gleeson TG, Breen KA, McHugh, O'Connell MJ, et al. (2009) Whole-body MRI versus PET in assessment of multiple myeloma disease activity. AJR; 92: 980–986.

38. Hanrahan CJ, Christensen CR, Crim JR (2010) Current concepts in the evaluation of multiple myeloma with MR imaging and FDG PET/CT. RadioGraphics; 30: 127–142.

39. Dyer R, DiSantis DJ, McClennan BL (2008) Simplified imaging approach for avaluation of the solid renal mass in adults. Radiology 247: 331–343.

40. Ng CS, Wood HG, Silverman PM, Tannir NM, Tamboli P, et al. (2008) Renal cell carcinoma: diagnosis, staging, and surveillance. AJR 2008; 191: 1220–1232.

41. Khan AN, Al-Jahdali HH, Irion KL, Arabi M, Koteyar SS (2011) Solitary pulmonary nodule: A diagnostic algorithm in the light of current imaging technique. Avicenna J Med; 1: 39–51.

42. Swensen SJ, Jett JR, Hartman TE, Midthun DE, Sloan JA, et al. (2004) Lung cancer screening with CT: Mayo Clinic experience. Radiology; 226: 756–61.

43. Gohagan J, Marcus P, Fagerstrom R, Pinsky P, Kramer B, et al. (2004) Writing Committee, Lung Screening Study Research Group. Baseline findings of a randomized feasibility trial of lung cancer screening with spiral CT scan vs chest radiograph: the Lung Screening Study of the National Cancer Institute. Chest; 12: 114–21.

44. Tan BB, Flaherty KR, Kazerooni EA, Iannettoni MD (2003) American College of Chest Physicians. The solitary pulmonary nodule. Chest; 123 (1 Suppl): 89S–96S.

45. Chang KJ, Kamel IR, Macura KJ, Bluemke DA et al. (2008) 3.0-T MR Imaging of the abdomen: comparison with 1.5 T. RadioGraphics; 28: 1983–1998.

46. Bandettini PA (2009) What's new in neuroimaging methods? Ann N Y Acad Sci; 1156: 260–293.

47. Brunner DO, Zanche ND, Frohlich J, Paska J, Pruessmann KP (2009) Travelling-wave nuclear magnetic resonance Nature; 457: 994–999.

Reactions to Media Violence: It's in the Brain of the Beholder

Nelly Alia-Klein[1,2]*, Gene-Jack Wang[1,3], Rebecca N. Preston-Campbell[1], Scott J. Moeller[1,2], Muhammad A. Parvaz[1], Wei Zhu[4], Millard C. Jayne[3], Chris Wong[3], Dardo Tomasi[3], Rita Z. Goldstein[1,2], Joanna S. Fowler[5], Nora D. Volkow[3]

1 Department of Psychiatry, Friedman Brain Institute, Icahn School of Medicine at Mount Sinai, New York, New York, United States of America, 2 Department of Neuroscience, Friedman Brain Institute, Icahn School of Medicine at Mount Sinai, New York, New York, United States of America, 3 Laboratory of Neuroimaging, National Institute on Alcohol Abuse and Alcoholism, Bethesda, Maryland, United States of America, 4 Applied Mathematics and Statistics, SUNY, Stony Brook, New York, United States of America, 5 Medical Department, Brookhaven National Laboratory, Upton, New York, United States of America

Abstract

Media portraying violence is part of daily exposures. The extent to which violent media exposure impacts brain and behavior has been debated. Yet there is not enough experimental data to inform this debate. We hypothesize that reaction to violent media is critically dependent on personality/trait differences between viewers, where those with the propensity for physical assault will respond to the media differently than controls. The source of the variability, we further hypothesize, is reflected in autonomic response and brain functioning that differentiate those with aggression tendencies from others. To test this hypothesis we pre-selected a group of aggressive individuals and non-aggressive controls from the normal healthy population; we documented brain, blood-pressure, and behavioral responses during resting baseline and while the groups were watching media violence and emotional media that did not portray violence. Positron Emission Tomography was used with [18F]fluoro-deoxyglucose (FDG) to image brain metabolic activity, a marker of brain function, during rest and during film viewing while blood-pressure and mood ratings were intermittently collected. Results pointed to robust resting baseline differences between groups. Aggressive individuals had lower relative glucose metabolism in the medial orbitofrontal cortex correlating with poor self-control and greater glucose metabolism in other regions of the default-mode network (DMN) where precuneus correlated with negative emotionality. These brain results were similar while watching the violent media, during which aggressive viewers reported being more *Inspired* and *Determined* and less *Upset* and *Nervous*, and also showed a progressive decline in systolic blood-pressure compared to controls. Furthermore, the blood-pressure and brain activation in orbitofrontal cortex and precuneus were differentially coupled between the groups. These results demonstrate that individual differences in trait aggression strongly couple with brain, behavioral, and autonomic reactivity to media violence which should factor into debates about the impact of media violence on the public.

Editor: Jonathan A. Coles, Glasgow University, United Kingdom

Funding: Funding was provided by (1) Brookhaven National Laboratory under contract DE-AC02-98CH10886, http://www.bnl.gov/world/; (2) National Institute of Mental Health: R01MH090134 (NAK), http://www.nimh.nih.gov/index.shtml; and (3) National Institute of Mental Health NIDA and NIH K05DA020001 (JSF) and the National Institute of Alcohol Abuse and Alcoholism Intramural Program, http://www.drugabuse.gov/ and http://www.niaaa.nih.gov/. The funders had no role in study design, data collection and analysis, decision to publish, or preparation of the manuscript.

Competing Interests: The authors have declared that no competing interests exists.

* Email: nelly.alia-klein@mssm.edu

Introduction

While visual media is replete with images of violence, only a small minority in the population engages in real-life violent behavior. Critically, whether a person will act violently depends on individual trait variations which play a prominent role in how visual media is experienced and processed [1]. Therefore, understanding the neurobiological underpinnings of those with aggressive personality traits above the documented norms, is an important prerequisite to the ongoing debate about media impact on behavior [2]. Enduring trait aggression reflects self-report of retaliatory motivation, with high face validity, where individuals endorse questions regarding the degree of their readiness to hurt others. It is emerging in the literature that aggressive individuals differ from non-aggressive individuals in their baseline, trait-like, neurobiological architecture [3], suggesting involvement of the brain's default mode network (DMN) [4,5]. The DMN forms a distributed circuit of connected brain systems that shows high and coherent metabolic activity or blood flow during awake yet passive resting states which may represent internal and self-referential processing [4–7]. The DMN includes regions typically spanning the posterior cingulate cortex (PCC) and precuneus, lateral inferior parietal gyrus (IPG), medial temporal gyrus (MTG), and ventromedial prefrontal cortex, including the orbitofrontal cortex (OFC) [8]. We hypothesize that at resting baseline, individuals with high trait aggression will exhibit different brain metabolism patterns in the DMN including its ventromedial prefrontal regions, revealing fundamentally different internal preoccupations than those with normative trait aggression.

Stimuli with violent themes can prime, or perhaps facilitate existing trait tendencies [1,9]. The General Aggression Model (GAM) [10] outlines the processes by which exposure to violence can cause aggressive behavior through the interplay of enduring traits that drive internal states, coupled with congruent visual stimuli from the environment (e.g., violent media). Therefore, according to GAM, chronic exposure to violent images in the media reinforces existing aggressive traits, thereby preparing the individual towards future violence [11,12]. The OFC is specifically involved in elements of aggressive behaviors [13–15] through its role in prioritizing emotional cues according to intrinsic salience [16]. Likewise, gray matter deficits in the OFC have been observed in individuals with aggressive and violent behavior [17]. As such, we predict involvement of the OFC since it appears to be specifically involved in response to repeated media violence [18,19]. Individual differences in brain and behavior during visual media viewing can be further understood in the context of self-reported affective states and autonomic responses (or lack thereof) [20,21]. For example, self-reported distress and systolic blood pressure changes were observed in response to viewing violent media [1,21]. Cortical representations of emotion-dependent autonomic response (e.g., blood pressure) have been shown in the OFC, anterior cingulate, and insula in response to viewing violent media in healthy controls [22].

To test our hypotheses regarding baseline and media viewing differences as a function of trait aggression, we recruited a group of healthy aggressive individuals with a history of assault behavior and a group of non-aggressive healthy controls. Measurements of glucose metabolism with [18F]fluoro-deoxyglucose using positron emission tomography (PET) were obtained at three conditions: at resting baseline, during exposure to violent media, and during exposure to emotional, non-violent media. Blood pressure (BP) and behavioral ratings of state affect were collected intermittently during the movie presentations. We expected that aggressive individuals would have a distinct intrinsic brain activity pattern at resting baseline and during passive viewing of the violent media compared to emotional media.

Methods

Ethics Statement

This research protocol was approved by the ethical review board of Stony Brook University and conducted accordingly. All participants provided written informed consent prior to participation. Approval number BNL-381.

Participants

A total of 54 males who responded to advertisement for healthy controls and healthy individuals with history of physical fights, were evaluated for their physical assault tendencies and other inclusion/exclusion criteria. Individuals were initially screened by phone and then seen at Brookhaven National Laboratory by a physician for general exclusion criteria which included current or past psychiatric disorders (e.g., drug abuse or dependence), neurological disease, significant medical illness, current treatment with medication (including over the counter drugs) and head trauma with loss of consciousness >30 minutes. Normal physical examination and laboratory tests were required for entry and pre-scan urine tests ensured the absence of any psychoactive drugs. Individuals were classified as aggressive (Ag) or non-aggressive (Na) depending on their responses on the Physical Aggression subscale of the Buss-Perry Aggression Questionnaire (the physical aggres-

sion subscale correlates strongly with peer ratings of aggression demonstrating its concurrent validity) [23]. Of these 54 participants, only individuals who reported physical fights in the last year and scored at or higher than 75th percentile on the Physical Aggression scale (Ag, n = 12) or those who reported they did not engage in physical fights and scored at 50th percentile or below on the Physical Aggression scale (Na, n = 13) were chosen for the study (mean age 25.15) [23]. As planned, the participants differed on Physical Aggression (Ag, mean $\pm$ standard error 33.5±1.2; Na, 14.5±1.0, p<.0001). They also differed significantly on the other subscales of the Buss-Perry: Verbal Aggression (Ag, 18.8±1.0; Na, 11.6±1.2, p<.0001), Anger (Ag, 23.7±1.5; Na, 9.6±0.6, p< .0001), Hostility (Ag, 23.1±2.0; Na, 11.8±0.9, p<.0001) and the total score (Ag, 99.5±3.8; Na, 47.5±2.7, p<.0001). The two groups did not differ on age, handedness [24], socio-economic status [25], estimates of verbal and non-verbal intelligence [26,27], and depression symptoms [28]. Participants were asked about their media habits including the number of hours they watched TV per day on weekdays and on weekends (Table 1). The participants were monetarily compensated for their participation. It is important to note that the staff performing the media exposure, imaging, nursing, and questionnaire completion, were blind to the subject's assignment as aggressive or non-aggressive.

Personality and Behavioral Measures

In addition to the Buss-Perry Aggression Questionnaire, the Multidimensional Personality Questionnaire (MPQ) [29], a three-factor structural model of personality was used. As listed in Table 1, the MPQ models three higher order dimensions of personality: *Negative Emotionality* (NEM, or *Neuroticism*) reflecting tendency toward emotional distress, alienation from others and aggressive behavior; *Positive Emotionality* (PEM, or extraversion) reflecting enduring positive affect through interpersonal engagement, and *Constraint* measuring tendencies toward self-control. Several lines of evidence have shown that high levels of NEM as *Neuroticism* are robustly associated with violence and aggression [30]. Similarly, individuals with elevated scores of NEM tend to experience/report more frequent negative emotions such as anger and anxiety, perceive their environment as hostile/unfair, and often exhibit poor coping mechanisms in a stressful situation [31]. The three NEM sub-scales include *Stress Reaction* which is linked to low frustration tolerance; *Aggression* which reflects the tendency to respond with retaliatory response style; and *Alienation* which is the most predictive primary scale of aggressive behavior. We also assessed attention and inhibitory control using a performance based measure, the Attention Network Task (ANT), that captures reaction-time performance on Alerting (response readiness), Orienting (scanning and selection), and Conflict (inhibitory control) in attention [32].

Imaging Conditions and State Reactivity

There were three 40-minute imaging conditions: resting baseline, where participants were instructed to rest with eyes open, a video presentation of violent scenes, and a video presentation of emotional scenes not portraying violence. The two videos (violent and emotional) were edited from R-rated movies and documentary films. The violent media presentation contained 20 scenes of violent acts encompassing the depiction of intentional acts of violence from one individual to another (e.g. interpersonal, shootings, street fights). The emotional media presentation contained 19 emotionally intense and action filled but non-violent scenes (e.g. people interacting during a natural disaster, sudden failures during competitive sports). The length of each of the violent or emotional scenes was between 1–4 minutes;

Table 1. Demographics, personality, inhibitory control, and media exposure as a function of trait aggression.

Demographics[a]	Ag	Na	Statistics
Age	24.9±0.8	25.4±0.8	$t_{23}=-0.4$, P=0.69
Laterality Quotient	0.86±0.07	0.92±0.02	$t_{21}=-0.8$, P=0.42
SES	42.8±3.2	44.7±3.4	$t_{21}=-0.3$, P=0.69
WRAT-3	105.1±2.9	110.7±2.5	$t_{21}=-1.4$, P=0.16
MATRIX	10.7±0.7	12.5±0.6	$t_{21}=-1.8$, P=0.08
BDI	7.0±1.3	4.6±0.90	$t_{21}=-1.5$, P=0.15
Personality			
Negative Emotionality	**28.1±2.5**	**7.9±2.3**	$\mathbf{t_{21}=5.8}$, **P=0.0001**
Alienation	**7.1±1.4**	**1.7±0.57**	$\mathbf{t_{21}=3.7}$, **P=0.001**
Aggression	**13.7±1.0**	**3.6±1.1**	$\mathbf{t_{21}=6.3}$, **P=0.0001**
Stress Reaction	**7.1±0.95**	**2.5±0.90**	$\mathbf{t_{21}=3.5}$, **P=0.002**
Positive Emotionality	51.2±4.1	47.6±2.5	$t_{21}=.73$, P=0.463
Well Being	8.3±0.60	8.5±0.62	$t_{21}=-.15$, P=0.877
Social Potency	17.6±1.8	11.6±1.5	$t_{21}=2.5$, P=0.021
Social Closeness	13.0±1.9	14.0±1.9	$t_{21}=-.38$, P=0.706
Achievement	12.1±1.3	13.4±1.2	$t_{21}=-.68$, P=0.501
Inhibitory Control			
Constraint	44.4±3.9	51.1±2.8	$t_{21}=-1.40$, P=0.176
Control	**14.0±1.3**	**19.0±0.99**	$\mathbf{t_{21}=-2.98}$, **P=0.007**
Harm Avoidance	14.0±2.4	17.5±1.8	$t_{21}=-1.16$, P=0.256
ANT			
Alerting	35.8±19.0	26.5±6.8	$t_{21}=.55$, P=0.615
Orienting	26.3±8.2	44.6±8.9	$t_{21}=-1.45$, P=0.159
Conflict	**188.2±21.1**	**95.5±7.2**	$\mathbf{t_{21}=4.6}$, **P=0.002**
Media Exposure (hours of TV viewed per day)			
On weekdays	3.9±1.4	3.5±2.1	$t_{21}=.62$, P=0.798
On weekend	5.6±2.6	4.2±2.4	$t_{21}=1.05$, P=0.278
Most time in a given day	10.8±4.8	9.4±1.9	$t_{21}=1.21$, P=0.310

[a]Means ± Standard Error, SES: socioeconomic status, WRAT-3: estimate of verbal intelligence, MATRIX: estimate of non-verbal intelligence; BDI: Beck Depression Inventory; ANT attention network task.

these scenes were separated by a black screen that appeared for 30 seconds which signaled the next scene. The level of valence and intensity of each of the violent and emotional scenes was evaluated internally in the laboratory (data not shown) for valence and intensity and sequenced to optimize with the dynamics of FDG uptake (most intense scenes during the first 10 minutes of FDG uptake period). During the movie presentations, state levels of emotional reactivity were assessed using the Positive and Negative Affective Schedule (PANAS) with adjectives of mood states (ranked from 1, slightly to 5, extremely) [33]. The PANAS was completed by the subjects 5 minutes before the media presentations, 10 minutes into the presentations, and at the end of the media presentations. Table 2 shows PANAS adjectives where differences were found between the groups at p<0.05 during the violent as compared to emotional media presentations. Systolic and diastolic BP was monitored with a compression cuff that operated automatically (Propaq Encore) on the participant's non-dominant arm starting 5 minutes before the imaging and continued throughout the scanning sessions occurring at 5-minute intervals. For Figure 1 systolic BP data was first averaged within each group at each point in the time series during the violent and during the emotional media presentation. Then, the percentage changes in

BP (delta) were calculated from the emotional to the violent media within each group [(violent-emotional)/emotional].

PET Imaging

The 25 subjects were scanned 3 times with PET-FDG in counterbalanced order on separate days and under 3 conditions: resting baseline, violent scenes, non-violent emotional scenes. The scanning procedure is standardized and was described before [34]. The violent and neutral video presentations started 10 min prior to FDG injection and continued for a total of 40 min. PET imaging was conducted with a Siemens HR+ tomograph (resolution $4.5\times4.5\times4.5$ mm^3 full-width half-maximum, 63 slices) in 3D dynamic acquisition mode. Static emission scan started 35 min after FDG injection and continued for the next 20 min. Arterialized blood was used to measure FDG in plasma. During the uptake period of FDG, subjects were resting with eyes open (no stimulation) or watching a movie (violent or emotional) in a quiet dimly lit room with a nurse by their side to ensure that they did not fall asleep. Metabolic rates were computed using an extension of Sokoloff's model [35]. The emission data for all the scans were corrected for attenuation and reconstructed using filtered back projection.

Table 2. Statistical Parametric Mapping results showing the clusters where normalized brain metabolism was significantly different as a function of aggression.

Gyrus, Brodman Area (BA)	Talairach Coordinates (x, y, z)	Cluster size	Z-value[a]
BASELINE (no media)			
Ag≥Na			
Superior Temporal, BA 38	−36, 24, −36	210	4.79
Inferior Parietal, BA 40	−54, −46, 54	1960	5.75
Inferior Parietal, BA 40	42, −60, 44		5.16
Inferior Parietal	−32, −50, 50		5.43
Sensory Motor Area (SMA)	−8, −14, 64		4.13
Caudate	14, 26, −2	996	4.31
Posterior Cingulate, BA 30	−18, −58, 8		5.15
Precuneus	−14, −46, 44		5.03
Precuneus	4, −58, 50		4.73
Cuneus, BA 19	4, −76, 34	1500	5.46
Calcarine Gyrus	14, −76, 16		4.75
Superior Occipital Gyrus	−22, −72, 24		4.81
Cerebellum	−6, −88, −36		5.36
Ag<Na			
Orbitofrontal, BA 11	4, 50, −32	1849	5.27
Hippocampus	−18, 0, −38		4.98
Posterior Cerebellum	40, −66, −40	3795	4.31
Cerebellum V	14, −72, −36		4.13
VIOLENT MEDIA			
Ag>Na			
Superior Temporal, BA 38	52, 18, −28		4.68
Medial Temporal Pole	−36, 22, −36	613	5.11
Inferior Parietal, BA 40	−32, −36, 36	535	4.62
Fusiform Gyrus, BA 37	−34, −62, −8	2279	4.36
Superior Occipital Gyrus	−24, −76, 22		4.15
Lingual Gyrus	22, −54, 2		4.18
Caudate	14, 26, −2	436	4.38
Ag<Na			
Gyrus rectus, BA 11	2, 54, −30	924	5.20
Orbitofrontal, BA 11	22, 34, −26		3.91
Cerebellum	−8, −90, −36		6.12
EMOTIONAL MEDIA			
Ag>Na			
Lingual, BA 18	−20, −56, 4	2540	4.61

[a]Based on SPM8 cluster threshold of P<0.001, extent >100.

Image and Data Analyses

Prior to the analysis, each participant's PET image was mapped onto the Montreal Neurological Institute (MNI) template and smoothed via a Gaussian kernel with full width half maximum at 16 mm. Normalized metabolic images were analyzed using Statistical Parametric Mapping (SPM) [36]. The normalized images (relative images) were obtained by dividing the signal level of each voxel by the global mean, which was the average signal level of all voxels in the PET image. Analyses were performed in SPM8 with a flexible factor model design with one between-subject factor (Ag and Na groups) and one within-subject factor

(baseline, violent, emotional conditions). Main effects of group were tested separately (Figure 2) as well as group x condition interactions. The cluster threshold used was p<0.001, cluster extent >100; given the number of subjects, these parameters were chosen to ensure a minimum of t = 3.00 for each cluster reported. After the SPM results were obtained, cubic regions of interest (ROIs) with 125 voxels were centered at the peak coordinates of relevant activation clusters to compute average metabolic values within these ROIs. Pearson linear correlations were used to assess the association between average ROI measures and BP.

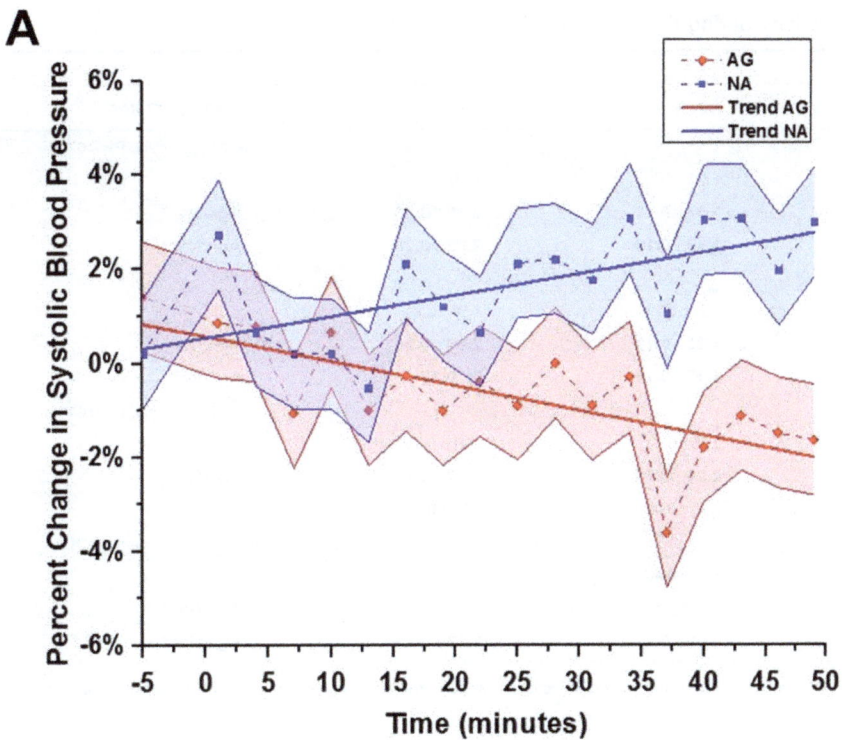

Figure 1. Systolic blood pressure response to violent media. Ag (red) individuals show reduction in systolic blood pressure while watching the violent media versus Na (blue) individuals who show progressive increase in systolic blood pressure. Systolic blood pressure measures were averaged for each group at each time point and a percent change and a trend line were calculated (Y-axis). Error bars (joined and filled) reflect the standard deviation of the data that are presented.

The behavior and personality indices (Table 1) were analyzed using independent-samples t-tests Bonferroni corrected for multiple comparisons [37]. The changes in BP (delta) were calculated from the emotional to the violent media within each group [(violent-emotional)/emotional] (Figure 1). We tested whether the progressive change in systolic BP was significantly different between the groups with a general linear model (GLM), where time points and group were independent variables while the BP

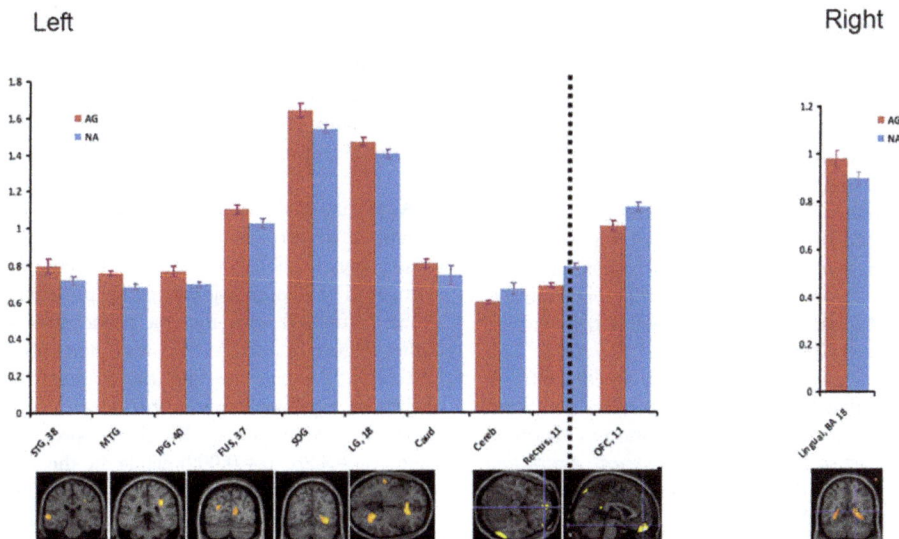

Figure 2. Glucose metabolism in response to media condition. Left panel: Relative glucose metabolism (Y-axis) in Ag (red) and Na (blue) in response to the violent media. On the left of the dotted line are results from Ag>Na contrast and on the right of the dotted line are results from the Ag<Na contrast. Right panel: Glucose metabolism results in response to the emotional media Ag>Na. There were no significant results for Ag<Na. Standard error is presented in the corresponding error bars.

Table 3. Emotional reactivity during the violent media presentation.

PANAS[a]	Ag	Na	F and post hoc
Upset			$F_{1,23} = 6.58$, P = 0.02
pre	1±0	1±0	
10 min.	**1.67±0.19**	**2.69±0.36**	**Ag<Na****
End	**1.33±0.19**	**2.08±0.26**	**Ag<Na****
Nervous			$F_{1,23} = 3.64$, P = 0.07
pre	1.58±0.29	1.54±0.24	
10 min.	**1.25±0.13**	**2.08±0.26**	**Ag<Na****
End	**1.33±0.14**	**2±0.25**	**Ag<Na***
Inspired			$F_{1,23} = 4.64$, P = 0.04
pre	2.58±0.34	2.31±0.31	
10 minutes	**2.25±0.39**	**1.31±0.17**	**Ag>Na***
End	2.33±0.45	1.61±0.24	
Determined			$F_{1,23} = 7.56$, P = 0.01
pre	3.42±0.40	2.62±0.33	
10 min.			**Ag>Na****
End	**3.08±0.47**	**1.77±0.28**	**Ag>Na****

[a]PANAS of response during violent media presentation using adjectives that demonstrated differences between the groups during the violent compared to emotional media; mean ± standard error.
*$p<0.05$,
**$p<0.01$.

Results

delta was the dependent variable. Two separate linear regression models were fitted within each group and used to test whether the delta in BP changed significantly over time and whether the slopes were significantly different between the groups. Analysis of PANAS responses to the violent and emotional media presentations was done by calculating differences in responses between violent and emotional presentations at 3 time points (pre, 10 min and end) using a GLM (Table 2).

Results

Traits, Inhibitory Control, and Resting Metabolism

As documented in Table 1, the groups were not different on demographics and media exposure and no differences were found on MPQ personality traits of PEM which includes the subscales *Well Being*, *Social Potency*, *Social Closeness* and *Achievement*. Not surprisingly, the groups were substantially different on *Negative Emotionality* and inhibitory control. Individuals from the Ag group, reported more NEM, with high scores on the NEM subscales, *Alienation*, *Aggression* and *Stress Reaction*. The Ag group also demonstrated poor inhibitory control, reporting less self-*Control* on the MPQ and also showed increased latency to respond specifically in the Conflict condition of the ANT. This performance measure of inhibitory control correlated with self-reported aggression such that more latency as a result of conflict in attention was seen in those with more trait aggression as measured by two different self-report scales (Buss-Perry *Physical Aggression* scale r = .76, P<0.0001, and MPQ *Aggression* (r = .66, P<0.001).

The normalized brain metabolic measures were characterized by robust group effects at resting baseline, involving hyperactivity in the DMN and caudate, and dampened OFC metabolism in Ag as compared to Na (Table 2). These resting metabolic measures in precuneus correlated positively across participants with NEM (R = .56, p<.01) and negatively with *Control* (R = −.46, 0<.05) whereas those in OFC showed the opposite pattern revealing a negative correlation with NEM (R = −.40, p<.05) and positive correlation with *Control* (R = .48, p<.05).

Glucose Metabolism and Mood Reactivity during Media Viewing

Listed in Table 2 are the main effects of group for each condition separately. These results show similar group differences at resting baseline than for the comparisons during violent media presentation, involving hyperactivity in the DMN and caudate, and dampened OFC metabolism in Ag than Na participants (Figure 2, left panel). While viewing the emotional media presentation, the only significant difference between groups was higher glucose metabolism in bilateral lingual gyrus in the Ag group (Figure 2, right panel). Group x condition interactions were not significant at our threshold or at a reduced threshold of p< 0.005.

As documented in Table 3, differences emerged between the groups in state reactivity 10 minutes into and at the end of the media presentations. During the violent media presentation as compared to the emotional media presentation, Ag participants when compared with the Na participants reported feeling less *Upset* (Figure 3) and *Nervous* and more *Inspired* and *Determined* (Table 3). In-line with the mood reactivity data, there were divergent responses between the groups in systolic BP across time. In the Na group, percent BP change progressively increased over time ($t_{16} = 3.26$, p = 0.002) while in the Ag group, systolic BP progressively decreased ($t_{16} = -4.23$, p = 0.0003) in response to the violent media as compared to emotional media (Figure 1). A comparison of the trend lines between the groups shows that the trend lines were significantly opposite ($F_{1, 32} = 27.60$, p<0.0001). Systolic and diastolic BP did not differ between the groups at resting baseline (p>0.05). Diastolic BP was not different between the groups in any of the conditions.

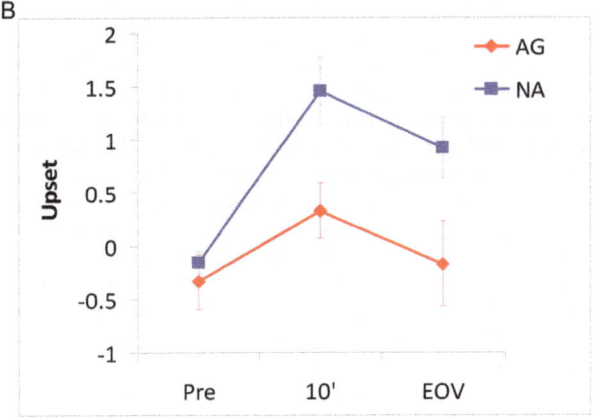

Figure 3. Time-course of emotional reactivity. Self-report of being *Upset* immediately before, during, and at the end (EOV) of the violent media viewing. Standard error is presented in the corresponding error bars.

To examine the coupling of BP with glucose metabolism between the groups, we conducted ROI analyses to assess the correlation between regional metabolism during the violent media exposure and changes in systolic BP at time 37 (when most accentuated differences in BP were found between groups, as shown in Figure 1). In the Na, increases in BP were positively associated with increased metabolism in the right OFC (x = 22, y = 34, z = -26; r = 0.74; p<0.005) whereas the correlation was negative in (r = -0.56, p<0.005) (Figure 4) in whom decreases in BP were also associated with metabolism in precuneus (R = -.81, p<.001). That is, in Na participants increases in BP were associated with higher metabolism in OFC whereas in Ag participants decreases in BP were associated with increased metabolism in the OFC and precuneus.

Discussion

This study documented brain, behavior, and blood-pressure response as a function of trait aggression. Results showed that Ag had heightened traits of NEM and poor inhibitory control compared to Na. These constitutional differences between the groups were apparent in their brain function at resting baseline and during the violent media viewing, where Ag had higher relative metabolism in the retrosplenial DMN, and lower relative metabolism in OFC, gyrus rectus, and posterior cerebellum. While watching the violent compared to emotional media, the Ag viewers reported being more *Inspired* and *Determined,* less *Upset* and *Nervous,* and showed a progressive decline in systolic blood-pressure compared with controls in whom systolic BP increased. Furthermore, the BP findings were differentially coupled with glucose metabolism between the groups. While viewing violent media, increased blood-pressure in Na was associated with increased metabolism in OFC; in Ag, the observed reduced blood-pressure was associated with increased metabolism in this same region and also in the precuneus.

The Value of Pre-Selection Based on Abnormal Aggression Traits

In pre-selecting participants based on trait aggression this study revealed important baseline differences in brain and behavior compared with controls. Elevated trait aggression is found specifically in individuals with associated disorders, such as antisocial personality disorder and intermittent explosive disorder, as it has straightforward face validity [38]. In addition to elevated trait aggression, Ag also reported more *Alienation* and *Stress Reaction* and demonstrated poor inhibitory control, as measured by the ANT conflict [39], which are part of externalizing behaviors in adults [40]. Studies show that inhibitory control (as documented here using the ANT) play an important role in violent media effects and aggression [41]. Similarly, high levels of NEM as *Neuroticism* have shown robust connections with violence and aggression [30]. These results on characterizing personality in trait

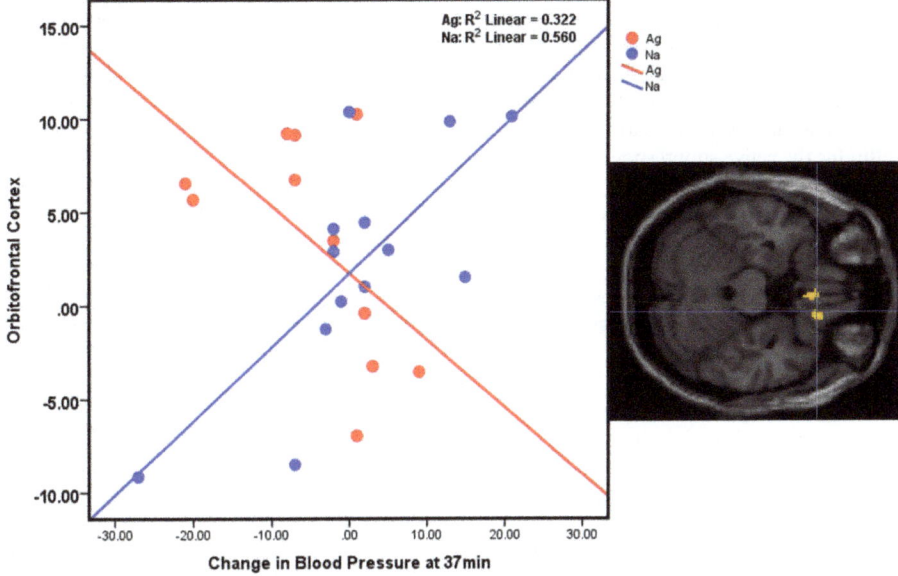

Figure 4. Coupling of blood pressure response with glucose metabolism in the OFC between the groups. On the y-axis is response in the OFC response to violent media compared with emotional media; on the x-axis is systolic BP change between violent media compared with emotional media at time 37 into the media viewing.

aggression, lend support to the GAM theory, documenting the specificity of trait aggression in its effects on other personality traits [42] and their potential cognitive substrates. Those who endorse few or no aggression items, hence, the Na group, scored at the norms in NEM and PEM, demonstrating that it is normative to endorse very few aggression questions, providing an adequate control for Ag. Importantly, PEM and its subscales were comparable between the groups, perhaps validating a characterization of trait aggression specifically involving NEM while having normative PEM [42]. Supportive of the GAM theory on the role of traits in media viewing, these trait results are important in setting the context of brain metabolism comparisons between the groups.

Characterization of Trait Aggression through Resting Brain Metabolism

The most robust finding in this study is relative hyperactivity of the DMN during resting baseline with relative hypoactivity of the OFC and cerebellum in Ag compared to Na. The documented over-activity in components of the DMN may reflect a neural marker of enduring traits fostering inwardly directed attention to self-referential information stemming from years of social and cognitive learning [43]. Each of the DMN nodes and their network is associated with awareness and conscious information processing [44], mental imagery, perspective taking, and autobiographical memory retrieval [45–47] needed to facilitate an enduring brain activity pattern of behavioral patterns (i.e., trait) [48,49]. Several studies mapped DMN regions with trait profiles; for example, *Neuroticism* (NEM in this study), was associated with lower volumetric measures and lower metabolism of the OFC [50,51] in line with our results of hypoactive OFC in Ag. Conducting direct correlations between resting metabolism and NEM as well as with trait *Control*, we found that the lower resting metabolism in the OFC the higher were NEM and lower *Control* scores. In contrast the higher resting metabolism in precuneus the higher was NEM and lower *Control* trait scores. Supporting this finding are recent findings of higher precuneus with reduced conscientiousness and openness [49] both associated with NEM and characteristic of those with high trait aggression.

Other over activated regions at baseline among Ag participants included the sensory motor area and caudate. One could speculate that this increased activity during rest would have a role in compromised responses during a cognitive task. A recent study proposed that striatal dopamine circuits, particularly the caudate, may provide a mechanism for the active suppression of the DMN under conditions that require increased processing of external stimuli (e.g., an attention demanding cognitive task) relative to internal, self-directed processing [52]. This might be related to a recent finding where heightened trait aggression is associated with reduced dopamine in striatum [53] and that striatal dopamine influences the DMN to affect shifting between internal states and cognitive demands [54].

Brain Metabolism during Violent Media Viewing

The fusiform gyrus was uniquely activated during violent media viewing in Ag, perhaps suggesting increased attention to facial representation of socially relevant cues [55]. Aside from the fusiform activation, while viewing the violent media presentation, the Ag participants compared with the Na showed similar patterns of activation as they had during resting baseline. As such, it appears that DMN regions are active during passive viewing of visual stimuli (e.g., movie) [56,57]. We postulate that the violent media condition reflects congruence between the trait and the visual stimuli, such that the stimuli are syntonic (oscillating

together) with internal processing, perhaps indicating personal experience with this material. Since resting baseline refers to mind wondering, it could be that participants in the Ag group have had aggressive thoughts that were instigating similar brain networks as during violent media viewing. A study in children during exposure to violent media documented engagement of the posterior cingulate and hippocampi, which was postulated to link memory and emotion to motor activation integrating existing aggression-related thoughts, thereby making them strongly accessible scripts over time [58]. The amygdala is a likely target for cortical arousal in violence viewing. Mathiak and Weber (2006) documented amygdala activation during active game-play in fMRI environment [59]. Their activation pattern showed signal decrease in the amygdala during players' virtual violent behavior. Our study did not document amygdala responses possibly as a result of the passive nature of the viewing violent media or alternatively, amygdala was not documented because of the temporal resolution differences between PET and fMRI.

Hypoactivity of the Orbitofrontal Cortex

In our study, the Ag participants showed a pattern of reduced OFC activity relative to the Na in the both resting baseline and violent media conditions. The OFC plays a role in externalizing/impulsive behavior, and regulating emotional and social behavior [13,60–64]. Specific damage to the OFC is associated with impulsive and aggressive behavior [64], and individuals with such damage show little control over their emotions as well as limited awareness of the moral implications of their actions, and poor decision making [65]. Impulsive aggressive personality disordered patients demonstrate impaired emotion regulation, and exhibit blunted prefrontal, including OFC, metabolism in response to a serotonergic challenge [66]. Deficits in the orbitofrontal lobes as represented by atrophy, lesion, or hypoactive metabolism have been observed across a number of psychiatric populations prone to aggression (e.g., antisocial personality disorder, psychopathy, borderline personality disorder, intermittent explosive disorder) [66–68] and suggest that OFC hypo-function may be a common mechanism underlying the pathophysiology of aggressive behavior in general (e.g., both impulsive and premeditated forms). Hypoactivity of the OFC in this study and its correlation with high NEM and low *Control* scores further support the reliable implication of OFC in the externalizing continuum.

This OFC hypoactivity is consistent with other studies where exposure to violent media is associated with decreased OFC activation. In a study that examined components of the fronto-parietal network in response to aggressive video cues, reduced levels of OFC activation were found [19]. It is possible that OFC hypoactivation reflects desensitization to violence and disrupts the process of moral evaluation of the violent visual stimuli [69].

Familiarity with violent material could breed desensitization [69–71]. It could be that Ag have exhibited reduced inhibition and blunted evaluative categorization of violent stimuli as supported in other studies [71] such that they demonstrate a response (physiological/behavioral/cortical) that is suggestive of an overall desensitization to media violence [72,73].

Under-reactive Emotional and Autonomic Response to Violent Media

There is further evidence in this study supporting the desensitization hypothesis. The Ag group reported being less *Nervous* and *Upset* and more *Inspired* and *Determined* during the media violence (compared with emotional media) while their systolic BP progressively decreased. In stark contrast, The Na mood and BP responses to the violent media may be associated with a threat evaluation producing sympathetic activation, resulting in BP increase in the Na group. In a study with healthy adolescents, participants viewing violent movie clips experienced increased BP compared to baseline; however, prior exposure to violence was associated with lowered BP [21]. Autonomic under-arousal to threat stimuli has been documented in individuals who exhibit low levels of fear [74]. Angered subjects permitted to commit aggression against the person who had annoyed them often display a drop in systolic blood pressure. They seem to have experienced a physiological relaxation, as if they had satisfied their aggressive urges [75,76].

Indeed, the documented pattern of BP under-reactivity in Ag was associated with hypoactivations in the OFC (Figure 3) and hyperactivation of the precuneus. Behaviorally-evoked changes in cardiovascular (e.g., blood pressure, heart rate) and cardiac-autonomic (e.g., heart rate variability) activity are correlated directly with neural activity within areas of the anterior cingulate cortex, OFC, medial prefrontal cortices, and the amygdala and often in interaction with activity in the insula, and relay regions of the thalamus and brainstem [22,77,78]. Based on neuroimaging and lesion evidence, a neurobiological model of cardiovascular reactivity shows that physiological and behavioral reactions are instantiated in the corticolimbic brains systems (e.g., medial/prefrontal corticies, insula, and amygdala) [79]. Afferent feedback, appraised by the OFC is integral in generation of somatic markers which trigger an emotional response, subsequently biasing overt behavior [80]. It is important to note here, that these results are relative to responses to emotional media viewing. It appears from our results that non-violent, yet emotionally salient action stimuli increase BP in the Ag individuals, whereas violent stimuli have the opposite effect of decreasing BP in these individuals. The specificity of hypo-response to violent content supports our assertion that the effects of violent media on individuals depend on theme-related traits, in this case aggression, and the brain of the beholder.

Caveats

There are several limitations in this study that constrain our interpretation power and generalizability. First, there may have been too few participants in the study to ascertain group by condition interactions and to conduct correlations between trait and brain measures. Second, the inclusion of males only in this study was done to control for potentially differential emotional reaction patterns of activation as a function of sex. However, this approach prevents us from making any claims about female response to violent media. Future studies must include females. Third, the experimental design did not include an acute test of aggression following the media condition. Future studies could include such a test to document aggressive responses following violent media as a function of brain response during the violent media. Fourth, there are brain activity results during violent video games finding anterior cingulate involvement [59,81]. These results may not be comparable to this study since playing video games requires task-dependent active attention compared to passive attention maintained during movie viewing as we show in our results; therefore more studies are needed to distinguish responses to media sources requiring active attention such as video games from those requiring only passive attention as movie scenes [82].

Acknowledgments

The authors gratefully acknowledge the contributions of all members of the Brookhaven PET team for advice and assistance in different aspects of this study.

Author Contributions

Conceived and designed the experiments: NAK NDV RZG JSF GJW. Performed the experiments: NAK MCJ CW DT. Analyzed the data: NAK MAP WZ CW. Contributed reagents/materials/analysis tools: WZ CW DT. Contributed to the writing of the manuscript: NAK SJM RPC RZG NDV MAP.

References

1. Bushman BJ, Geen RG (1990) Role of cognitive-emotional mediators and individual differences in the effects of media violence on aggression. J Pers Soc Psychol 58: 156–163.
2. Bushman BJ, Huesmann LR (2006) Short-term and long-term effects of violent media on aggression in children and adults. Arch Pediatr Adolesc Med 160: 348–352.
3. Siever LJ (2008) Neurobiology of aggression and violence. Am J Psychiatry 165: 429–442.
4. Shannon BJ, Raichle ME, Snyder AZ, Fair DA, Mills KL, et al. (2011) Premotor functional connectivity predicts impulsivity in juvenile offenders. Proc Natl Acad Sci U S A 108: 11241–11245.
5. Raichle ME, MacLeod AM, Snyder AZ, Powers WJ, Gusnard DA, et al. (2001) A default mode of brain function. Proc Natl Acad Sci U S A 98: 676–682.
6. Fox MD, Raichle ME (2007) Spontaneous fluctuations in brain activity observed with functional magnetic resonance imaging. Nat Rev Neurosci 8: 700–711.
7. Fox MD, Snyder AZ, Vincent JL, Raichle ME (2007) Intrinsic fluctuations within cortical systems account for intertrial variability in human behavior. Neuron 56: 171–184.
8. Tomasi D, Volkow ND (2010) Functional connectivity density mapping. Proc Natl Acad Sci U S A 107: 9885–9890.
9. Berkowitz L (1984) Some effects of thoughts on anti- and prosocial influences of media events: a cognitive-neoassociation analysis. Psychol Bull 95: 410–427.
10. Anderson CA, Bushman BJ (2002) Human aggression. Annu Rev Psychol 53: 27–51.
11. Bartholow BD, Bushman BJ, Sestir MA (2006) Chronic violent video game exposure and desensitization to violence: Behavioral and event-related brain potential data. Journal of Experimental Social Psychology 42: 532–539.
12. Anderson CA, Bushman BJ (2002) Psychology. The effects of media violence on society. Science 295: 2377–2379.
13. Bechara A, Damasio H, Damasio AR (2000) Emotion, decision making and the orbitofrontal cortex. Cereb Cortex 10: 295–307.
14. Christakou A, Brammer M, Giampietro V, Rubia K (2009) Right ventromedial and dorsolateral prefrontal cortices mediate adaptive decisions under ambiguity by integrating choice utility and outcome evaluation. J Neurosci 29: 11020–11028.
15. Spinella M (2002) Correlations among behavioral measures of orbitofrontal function. Int J Neurosci 112: 1359–1369.
16. Bechara AB, Damasio H, Damasio AR, Lee GP (1999) Different contributions of the human amygdala and ventromedial prefrontal cortex to decision-making. Journal of Neuroscience 19: 5473–5481.
17. Yang Y, Raine A (2009) Prefrontal structural and functional brain imaging findings in antisocial, violent, and psychopathic individuals: a meta-analysis. Psychiatry Res 174: 81–88.
18. Goyer PF, Andreason PJ, Semple WE, Clayton AH, King AC, et al. (1994) Positron-emission tomography and personality disorders. Neuropsychopharmacology 10: 21–28.
19. Strenziok M, Krueger F, Deshpande G, Lenroot RK, van der Meer E, et al. (2011) Fronto-parietal regulation of media violence exposure in adolescents: a multi-method study. Soc Cogn Affect Neurosci 6: 537–547.
20. Engelhardt CR, Bartholow BD, Saults JS (2011) Violent and nonviolent video games differentially affect physical aggression for individuals high vs. low in dispositional anger. Aggress Behav 37: 539–546.
21. Madan A, Mrug S, Wright RA (2014) The effects of media violence on anxiety in late adolescence. J Youth Adolesc 43: 116–126.
22. Gianaros PJ, Sheu LK, Remo AM, Christie IC, Crtichley HD, et al. (2009) Heightened resting neural activity predicts exaggerated stressor-evoked blood pressure reactivity. Hypertension 53: 819–825.
23. Buss AH, Perry M (1992) The aggression questionnaire. J Pers Soc Psychol 63: 452–459.
24. Oldfield RC (1971) The assessment and analysis of handedness: the Edinburgh inventory. Neuropsychologia 9: 97–113.
25. Hollingshead AB (1975) Four-factor index of social status. Unpublished paper.
26. Wilkinson G (1993) The Wide-Range Achievement Test 3: Administration Manual. Wilminton, DE: Wide-Range Inc.
27. Wechsler D (1999) Wechsler abbreviated scale of intelligence: San Antonio, TX: Psychological Corporation.

28. Beck AT, Steer RA, Brown GK. (1996) Beck Depression Inventory Manual. 2nd ed. San Antonio, TX: The Psychological Corporation.

29. Tellegen A, Waller NG (1997) Exploring personality through test construction: development of the multidimensional personality questionnaire. In: Briggs SR, Cheek JM, editors. Personality measures: development and evaluation. Greenwich: JAI Press.

30. Blonigen DM, Krueger RF. (2007) Personality & Violence: The unifying role of structural models of personality. In: Flannery DJ VA, Waldman ID (Eds.), editor. The Cambridge handbook of violent behavior. New York, NY: Cambridge University Press.

31. Hicks BM, Markon KE, Patrick CJ, Krueger RF, Newman JP (2004) Identifying psychopathy subtypes on the basis of personality structure. Psychol Assess 16: 276–288.

32. Fan J, McCandliss BD, Sommer T, Raz A, Posner MI (2002) Testing the efficiency and independence of attentional networks. Journal of Cognitive Neuroscience 14: 340–347.

33. Watson D, Clark LA, Tellegen A (1988) Development and validation of brief measures of positive and negative affect: the PANAS scales. J Pers Soc Psychol 54: 1063–1070.

34. Wang GJ, Volkow ND, Roque CT, Cestaro VL, Hitzemann RJ, et al. (1993) Functional importance of ventricular enlargement and cortical atrophy in healthy subjects and alcoholics as assessed with PET, MR imaging, and neuropsychologic testing. Radiology 186: 59–65.

35. Phelps ME, Hoffman EJ, Coleman RE, Welch MJ, Raichle ME, et al. (1976) Tomographic images of blood pool and perfusion in brain and heart. J Nucl Med 17: 603–612.

36. Friston KJ, Holmes AP, Worsley KJ, Poline JB, Frith CD, et al. (1995) Statistical parametric maps in functional imaging: a general approach. Human Brain Mapping 2: 189–210.

37. Stevens J (1992) Applied multivariate statistics for the social sciences. 2nd ed. Lawrence Erlbaum Associates: NewJersey.

38. Anderson CA, Buckley KE, Carnagey NL (2008) Creating your own hostile environment: a laboratory examination of trait aggressiveness and the violence escalation cycle. Pers Soc Psychol Bull 34: 462–473.

39. Thienel R, Voss B, Kellermann T, Reske M, Halfter S, et al. (2009) Nicotinic antagonist effects on functional attention networks. Int J Neuropsychopharmacol 12: 1295–1305.

40. Krueger RF, Markon KE, Patrick CJ, Benning SD, Kramer MD (2007) Linking antisocial behavior, substance use, and personality: an integrative quantitative model of the adult externalizing spectrum. J Abnorm Psychol 116: 645–666.

41. Swing EL, Anderson CA (2014) The role of attention problems and impulsiveness in media violence effects on aggression. Aggress Behav.

42. Hosie J, Gilbert F, Simpson K, Daffern M (2014) An examination of the relationship between personality and aggression using the general aggression and five factor models. Aggress Behav 40: 189–196.

43. Nagai Y, Critchley HD, Featherstone E, Trimble MR, Dolan RJ (2004) Activity in ventromedial prefrontal cortex covaries with sympathetic skin conductance level: a physiological account of a "default mode" of brain function. Neuroimage 22: 243–251.

44. Zhang S, Li CS (2012) Functional connectivity mapping of the human precuneus by resting state fMRI. Neuroimage 59: 3548–3562.

45. Raichle ME, Snyder AZ (2007) A default mode of brain function: a brief history of an evolving idea. Neuroimage 37: 1083–1090; discussion 1097–1089.

46. Dorfel D, Werner A, Schaefer M, von Kummer R, Karl A (2009) Distinct brain networks in recognition memory share a defined region in the precuneus. Eur J Neurosci 30: 1947–1959.

47. McDermott KB, Ojemann JG, Petersen SE, Ollinger JM, Snyder AZ, et al. (1999) Direct comparison of episodic encoding and retrieval of words: an event-related fMRI study. Memory 7: 661–678.

48. Wei L, Duan X, Zheng C, Wang S, Gao Q, et al. (2014) Specific frequency bands of amplitude low-frequency oscillation encodes personality. Hum Brain Mapp 35: 331–339.

49. Sampaio A, Soares JM, Coutinho J, Sousa N, Goncalves OF (2013) The Big Five default brain: functional evidence. Brain Struct Funct.

50. Wright CI, Williams D, Feczko E, Barrett LF, Dickerson BC, et al. (2006) Neuroanatomical correlates of extraversion and neuroticism. Cereb Cortex 16: 1809–1819.

51. DeYoung CG, Hirsh JB, Shane MS, Papademetris X, Rajeevan N, et al. (2010) Testing predictions from personality neuroscience. Brain structure and the big five. Psychol Sci 21: 820–828.

52. Kelly C, deZubicaray G, Di Martino A, Copland DA, Reiss PT, et al. (2009) L-dopa modulates functional connectivity in striatal cognitive and motor networks: a double-blind placebo-controlled study. J Neruosci 29: 7364–7378.

53. Schluter T, Winz O, Henkel K, Prinz S, Rademacher L, et al. (2013) The impact of dopamine on aggression: an [18F]-FDOPA PET Study in healthy males. J Neurosci 33: 16889–16896.

54. Dang LC, Donde A, Madison C, O'Neil JP, Jagust WJ (2012) Striatal dopamine influences the default mode network to affect shifting between object features. J Cogn Neurosci 24: 1960–1970.

55. Wiggett AJ, Downing PE (2011) Representation of action in occipito-temporal cortex. J Cogn Neurosci 23: 1765–1780.

56. Shulman GL, Fiez JA, Corbetta M, Buckner RL, Miezin FM, et al. (1997) Common Blood Flow Changes across Visual Tasks: II. Decreases in Cerebral Cortex. J Cogn Neurosci 9: 648–663.

57. Mazoyer B, Zago L, Mellet E, Bricogne S, Etard O, et al. (2001) Cortical networks for working memory and executive functions sustain the conscious resting state in man. Brain Research Bulletin 54: 287–298.

58. Murray JP, Liotti M, Ingmundson PT, Mayberg HS, Pu Y, Zamarripu F, et al. (2006) Children's brain activations while viewing televised violence revealed by fMRI. Media Psychology 8: 25–37.

59. Mathiak K, Weber R (2006) Toward brain correlates of natural behavior: fMRI during violent video games. Hum Brain Mapp 27: 948–956.

60. Bechara A, Damasio AR, Damasio H, Anderson SW (1994) Insensitivity to future consequences following damage to human prefrontal cortex. Cognition 50: 7–15.

61. Bechara A, Damasio H, Tranel D, Damasio AR (1997) Deciding advantageously before knowing the advantageous strategy. Science 275: 1293–1295.

62. Rudebeck PH, Bannerman DM, Rushworth MF (2008) The contribution of distinct subregions of the ventromedial frontal cortex to emotion, social behavior, and decision making. Cogn Affect Behav Neurosci 8: 485–497.

63. Davidson RJ, Putnam KM, Larson CL. (2000) Dysfunction in the neural circuitry of emotion regulation-A possible prelude to violence. Science 289: 591–572.

64. Izquierdo A, Suda RK, Murray EA (2005) Comparison of the effects of bilateral orbital prefrontal cortex lesions and amygdala lesions on emotional responses in rhesus monkeys. J Neurosci 25: 8534–8542.

65. Bechara A (2004) The role of emotion in decision-making: evidence from neurological patients with orbitofrontal damage. Brain Cogn 55: 30–40.

66. New AS, Hazlett EA, Buchsbaum MS, Goodman M, Reynolds D, et al. (2002) Blunted prefrontal cortical fluorodeoxyglucose Positron Emission Tomography Response to Meta-Chlorophenylpiperazine in impulsive aggression. Archives of General Psychiatry 59: 621–629.

67. Raine A, Meloy RJ, Bihrle S, Stoddard J, LaCasse L, et al. (1998) Reduced prefrontal and increased subcortical brain functioning assessed using positron emission tomography in predatory and affective murderers. Behavioral Sciences and the Law 16: 319–332.

68. Siever LJ, Buchsbaum MS, New AS, Spiegel-Cohen J, Wei T, et al. (1999) d,l-fenfluramine Response in Impulsive Personality Disorder Assessed with [18F]fluorodeoxyglucose Positron Emission Tomography. Neuropsychopharmacology 20: 413–423.

69. Funk JB (2005) Children's exposure to violent video games and desensitization to violence. Child Adolesc Psychiatr Clin N Am 14: 387–404, vii–viii.

70. Huesmann LR, Kriwil L (2007) Why observing violence increases the risk of violent behavior in the observer; (Ed.) DF, editor. Cambridge, UK: Cambridge University Press.

71. Fanti KA, Vanman E, Henrich CC, Avraamides MN (2009) Desensitization to media violence over a short period of time. Aggress Behav 35: 179–187.

72. Bailey K, West R, Anderson CA (2011) The association between chronic exposure to video game violence and affective picture processing: an ERP study. Cogn Affect Behav Neurosci 11: 259–276.

73. Kelly CR, Grinband J, Hirsch J (2007) Repeated exposure to media violence is associated with diminished response in an inhibitory frontolimbic network. PLoS One 2: e1268.

74. Raine A (1996) Autonomic nervous system factors underlying disinhibited antisocial and violent behavior. Annals New York Academy of Sciences: 46–60.

75. Hokanson JE, Burgess M (1962) The effects of status, type of frustration, and aggression on vascular processes. J Abnorm Soc Psychol 65: 232–237.

76. Hokanson JE, Burgess M (1962) The effects of three types of aggression on vascular processes. J Abnorm Soc Psychol 64: 446–449.

77. Critchley HD (2005) Neural mechanisms of autonomic, affective, and cognitive integration. J Comp Neurol 493: 154–166.

78. Mujica-Parodi LR, Korgaonkar M, Ravindranath B, Greenberg T, Tomasi D, et al. (2009) Limbic dysregulation is associated with lowered heart rate variability and increased trait anxiety in healthy adults. Hum Brain Mapp 30: 47–58.

79. Gianaros PJ, Sheu L (2009) A review of neuroimaging studies of stressor-evoked blood pressure reactivity: Emerging evidence for a brain-body pathway to coronary heart disease risk. NeuoImage 47.

80. Damasio A (1994) Descartes' Error: Emotion, Reason, and the Human Brain. New York: HarperCollins.

81. Chou YH, Yang BH, Hsu JW, Wang SJ, Lin CL, et al. (2013) Effects of video game playing on cerebral blood flow in young adults: a SPECT study. Psychiatry Res 212: 65–72.

82. Carnagey NL, Anderson CA (2007) Changes in attitudes towards war and violence after September 11, 2001. Aggress Behav 33: 118–129.

4

The Correlation between Lung Sound Distribution and Pulmonary Function in COPD Patients

Masamichi Mineshita[1]*, **Hirotaka Kida**[1], **Hiroshi Handa**[1], **Hiroki Nishine**[1], **Naoki Furuya**[1], **Seiichi Nobuyama**[1], **Takeo Inoue**[1], **Shin Matsuoka**[2], **Teruomi Miyazawa**[1]

1 Division of Respiratory and Infectious Diseases, Department of Internal Medicine, St. Marianna University School of Medicine, Kawasaki, Japan, 2 Department of Radiology, St. Marianna University School of Medicine, Kawasaki, Japan

Abstract

Background: Regional lung sound intensity in chronic obstructive pulmonary disease (COPD) patients is influenced by the severity and distribution of emphysema, obstructed peripheral airways, and altered ribcage and diaphragm configurations and movements due to hyperinflation. Changes in the lung sound distribution accompanied by pulmonary function improvements in COPD patients were observed after bronchodilator inhalation. We investigated the association of lung sound distribution with pulmonary functions, and the effects of emphysematous lesions on this association. These studies were designed to acquire the basic knowledge necessary for the application of lung sound analysis in the physiological evaluation of COPD patients.

Methods: Pulmonary function tests and the percentage of upper- and lower-lung sound intensity (quantitative lung data [QLD]) were evaluated in 47 stable male COPD patients (54 - 82 years of age). In 39 patients, computed tomography taken within 6 months of the study was available and analyzed.

Results: The ratio of lower QLD to upper QLD showed significant positive correlations with FEV_1 %predicted (%FEV_1; $\rho = 0.45$, $p < 0.005$) and MEF_{50} %predicted (%MEF_{50}; $\rho = 0.46$, $p < 0.005$). These correlations were not observed in COPD patients with dominant emphysema (% low attenuation area >40%, $n = 20$) and were stronger in less emphysematous patients ($n = 19$, %FEV_1; $\rho = 0.64$, $p < 0.005$, %MEF_{50}; $\rho = 0.71$, $p < 0.001$).

Conclusions: In COPD patients, the ratio of lower- to upper-lung sound intensities decreased according to the severity of obstructive changes, although emphysematous lesions considerably affected lung sound distribution.

Editor: Marco Gemma, Scientific Inst. S. Raffaele Hosp., Italy

Funding: This work was supported by the Japan Society for the Promotion of Science Grant-in-Aid for Scientific Research (C) Grant number (24591143). The funders had no role in study design, data collection and analysis, decision to publish, or preparation of the manuscript.

Competing Interests: The authors have declared that no competing interests exist.

* Email: m-mine@marianna-u.ac.jp

Introduction

Chronic obstructive pulmonary disease (COPD) is characterized by progressive airflow limitation. Because airflow in the lung produces sound, a generalized reduction in apparent lung sound is one of the indicators of COPD. A correlation between the perceived lung sound intensity and the percent-predicted forced expiratory volume over one second (FEV_1) has been reported [1]. Although lung sounds are reported to be generated primarily within the lobar to segmental airways [2], Ploysongsang compared Xenon ventilation scans with the distribution of lung sound intensities and reported that regional lung sound intensity could be used to quantify regional ventilation in subjects with emphysema in whom the physiological deficits are mainly caused by small airway obstruction [3].

Regional lung ventilation in COPD patients seems to be influenced by altered ribcage and diaphragm configurations and movement due to hyperinflation. In severe COPD patients, the

movements of the diaphragm are restricted, and accessory respiratory muscles, such as sternocleidomastoid and scalene muscles, are recruited during tidal breathing [4,5]. In these circumstances, it seems that regional ventilation may shift from the lower- to upper-lung field, according to the degree of hyperinflation. Therapeutic interventions that improve hyperinflation in COPD are thought to modulate regional airflow in the lung, which is reflected by the changes in regional lung sound distribution.

Recently, improvements in computer technology have provided new insights into acoustic analysis and have been introduced in clinical studies as a surrogate marker of regional ventilation [6–12]. In a previous study, we observed changes in the lung sound distribution that was accompanied by pulmonary function improvements in COPD patients after inhalation of a short-acting bronchodilator [13]. In seven patients with homogeneous emphysema, the relative regional lung sound intensity decreased in the upper-lung field and increased in the lower-lung field after bronchodilator inhalation. We hypothesized that this result was caused by an increase in lower lung airflow, which might reflect an improvement in diaphragm movement. However, we also found that the bronchodilator-induced relative increase in the lower lung sound intensity was not observed in one patient with heterogeneous emphysema or in one non-emphysematous patient. The distribution of emphysematous lesions and the bronchial reactivity appeared to influence regional lung ventilation and the distribution of lung sounds after bronchodilator use.

Although the distribution of emphysematous lesions was thought to influence the lung sound distribution, the assessment of regional lung sound might be applicable as a non-invasive tool for evaluating the regional physiological characteristics of COPD patients. In this study, we investigated the association of lung sound distribution with pulmonary function in COPD patients and healthy subjects, with the goal of acquiring basic knowledge regarding the association of lung sound distribution with pulmonary function. Furthermore, we analyzed the influence of emphysematous lesions on the lung sound distribution in COPD patients.

Methods

This study was performed at St. Marianna University Hospital (Kanagawa, Japan). The ethics committee of St. Marianna University Hospital (No1230) approved this study. Written informed consent was obtained from all of the participants.

Study population

Forty-seven clinically stable male COPD patients, each with a smoking history of more than 20 pack-years, were recruited. Patients were excluded from the study if they had received clinical diagnoses of asthma or bronchiectasis. The patients were permitted to continue using their medications for COPD. We were unable to recruit any female COPD patients due to the small number of female COPD patients at our hospital.

Forty healthy male smokers were recruited for comparison. Volunteers were deemed healthy on the basis of their clinical history, a physical examination and spirometric findings. Because all subjects underwent annual health checks, including chest X-rays, chest X-rays were not performed to avoid extra irradiation exposure. Subjects whose history included abnormal chest X-ray findings from the previous year were excluded. Individuals with a history of chronic cardiopulmonary disease, surgical chest procedures or recent (within 6 months) respiratory tract infections were excluded.

Pulmonary function tests

Spirometry was performed using a calibrated spirometer according to the American Thoracic Society guidelines. The forced vital capacity (FVC), FEV_1, maximum expiratory flow (MEF) at 50% of FVC (MEF_{50}) and MEF at 25% of FVC (MEF_{25}) were recorded. The predicted values for spirometric measurements were derived from the guidelines of the Japanese Respiratory Society [14]. The predicted values for the single-breath nitrogen washout test and the single-breath total lung diffusion capacity (DLco) were derived from Buist et al. [15] and Roca et al. [16].

Lung sound recording

The breath sounds were recorded using the VRIxp System (Deep Breeze, Ltd., Or-Akiva, Israel) during deep and regular breaths, and the percentage of regional lung sound energy

(quantitative lung data [QLD]) was calculated as previously described [6,7,9,13]. Just prior to breath sound recordings, a physician examined the patients using a stethoscope. VRI recordings were performed with 7-row arrays (40 active sensors in total) when the subjects' height was 165 cm or higher. We used 6-row arrays (34 active sensors in total) when the subjects' height was below 165 cm (26 COPD patients and 7 healthy volunteers). After recording, data were divided into upper (rows 1–2), middle (rows 3–4 in the 6-row arrays and rows 3–5 in the 7-row arrays) and lower (rows 5–6 in the 6-row arrays and rows 6–7 in the 7-row arrays) zones, and the QLD for each of these six zones was generated [17]. The signal data were band-pass filtered (100–250 Hz) to reduce interference generated by chest wall movement and heart sounds. At least three lung sound recordings from each subject were produced, and one acceptable VRI recording with the highest technical quality was chosen by a single investigator (M.M.) before QLD evaluation using the following criteria: (1) the recordings were free of artifacts; (2) the patient maintained a proper breathing cycle (3–4/12seconds); and (3) the recording reflected an adequate breathing intensity with the most consistent breathing pattern [17]. VRI measurements from 40 healthy male volunteers were also recorded for comparison.

Multi-detector computed tomography

In 39 patients, multi-detector computed tomography (Aquilion 64, Toshiba Medical Systems, Otawara, Japan) taken within 6 months was available and used for analysis. The CT parameters for inspiratory scans were as follows: collimation, 0.5 mm; 120 kVp; 200 mA; gantry rotation time, 0.5 sec; and beam pitch, 0.83 (table feed per gantry, 53; collimation beam width, 64). All images were reconstructed using a standard algorithm, with a slice thickness of 1 mm and a reconstruction interval of 0.5 mm. Three CT slices were selected for each subject; the upper cranial slice was obtained 1 cm above the upper margin of the aortic arch, the middle slice was obtained 1 cm below the carina, and the lower caudal slice was obtained 1 cm below the right inferior pulmonary vein. These CT images were then analyzed using a semiautomatic image processing program (Image J version 1.40 g, a public domain Java image-processing program available at http://rsb.info.nih.gov/ij/) as previously described [13]. Low-attenuation areas (LAA) between −950 to −1024 HU were identified as emphysema, and the percentage of the LAA for the entire lung area (%LAA) was calculated for both right and left sides of the upper, middle, and lower lung fields. In this study we defined emphysema-dominant COPD as an average regional %LAA of more than 40%.

Statistical analysis

The data are reported as the mean ± standard deviation unless otherwise indicated. All of the analyses were performed using SPSS software (ver19; IBM, Armonk, NY, USA). The upper, middle, and lower QLD of COPD patients and healthy subjects were compared using a Mann-Whitney U test. The correlations between the lower QLD/upper QLD ratio and the spirometric measurements were evaluated using Spearman's rank correlation coefficient. A p-value of <0.05 was considered to be statistically significant.

Results

Between April 2007 and March 2013, acceptable VRI recording data were obtained for 47 COPD patients. Recruited patients were free of respiratory infection and COPD exacerbation for at least 4 weeks prior to VRI recordings. Neither the radiograms nor the CT scans showed central airway obstructive lesions in these patients. A stethoscope examination performed before breath sound recordings revealed no wheezing for patients. The demographics, anthropometric values, and lung function test results of recruited COPD patients and healthy smokers are shown in Table 1. One patient was classified as GOLD I, 17 patients as GOLD II, 23 patients as GOLD III, and 6 patients as GOLD IV.

In the COPD patients, the upper QLD was significantly higher and the lower QLD was significantly lower than the corresponding values in healthy male smokers. As a result, the ratio of the lower QLD to upper QLD (Lower QLD/Upper QLD) in COPD patients was approximately 60% of the ratio for the healthy male smokers (Table 2). Receiver-operating characteristics (ROC) validation of Lower QLD/Upper QLD revealed that using a cut-off point of 2.5 yielded 72.3% sensitivity, 70% specificity, and 71.3% accuracy in the differentiation of COPD patients and healthy smokers (Figure 1). According to the effect of age on Lower QLD/Upper QLD in healthy subjects, there was no significant difference in Lower QLD/Upper QLD between younger subjects (<40 years old, n = 24, mean age; 30.5±5.1 years, mean pack-years; 8.8±7.7, Lower QLD/Upper QLD; 2.9±1.1) and older subjects (≥40 years old, n = 16, mean age; 54.1±14.2 years, mean pack-years; 33.4±19.5, Lower QLD/Upper QLD; 3.52±1.33).

The relationship between Lower QLD/Upper QLD and obstructive changes in the pulmonary function tests measurements were studied in COPD patients and healthy subjects (Table 3). Although there were no significant correlations between Lower QLD/Upper QLD and pulmonary functions in healthy subjects (Table 3), there were significant positive correlations for FEV_1 %predicted (%FEV_1), FEV_1/FVC, and MEF_{50} %predicted (%MEF_{50}) in COPD patients (Table 3). In 32 COPD patients for whom the results of the single-breath nitrogen washout test and DLco were obtained, Lower QLD/Upper QLD showed a

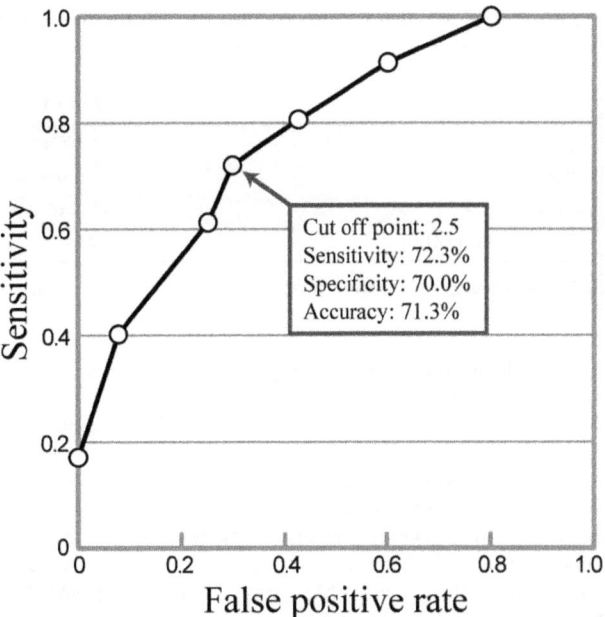

Figure 1. Receiver operating characteristic (ROC) validation of Lower QLD/Upper QLD. ROC validation of Lower QLD/Upper QLD revealed that a cut-off point of 2.5 yielded 72.3% sensitivity, 70% specificity, and 71.3% accuracy in the differentiation of COPD patients and healthy smokers.

significant negative correlation with the phase III slope of the single-breath nitrogen washout test%predicted (deltaN_2 %predicted), although there was no significant correlation between this ratio and DLco %predicted (Table 3).

Table 1. Characteristics of subjects.

	COPD	Healthy smokers
Subjects	47 (Male)	40 (Male)
Mean age (y)	71.6±6.3***	40.0±15.1
Pack-Years	81.9±36.5***	18.3±18.0
Duration of exposition to smoke (y)	47.1±6.0***	15.8±9.8
BMI	22.6±3.4	23.7±2.4
Pulmonary function tests		
FVC %predicted	88.1±18.2%	104.3±10.2%
FEV_1 %predicted	48.2±17.2%***	99.1±11.5%
FEV_1/FVC (%)	43.7±11.0%***	82.2±4.7%
MEF_{50} %predicted	17.3±10.0%***	96.1±27.3%
MEF_{25} %predicted	20.4±8.2%***	75.2±22.4%
deltaN_2 %predicted	556.4±274.4% (n = 32)	
DLco %predicted	37.4±13.6% (n = 32)	
GOLD I	1	
GOLD II	17	
GOLD III	23	
GOLD IV	6	

Definition of abbreviations: BMI = body mass index, FVC = forced vital capacity, FEV_1 = forced expiratory volume in 1 second, MEF_{50} and MEF_{25} = maximum expiratory flow at 50% and 25% of FVC, deltaN_2 = the phase III slope of the single-breath nitrogen washout test, DLco = the single-breath total lung diffusion capacity. Values are represented as mean ± standard deviation. ***; P<0.001 compared with healthy smokers.

Table 2. Quantitative lung data (QLD) in COPD patients and healthy smokers.

	COPD (n = 47)	Healthy smokers (n = 40)
Upper	22.55±6.80%***	15.92±4.18%
Middle	39.75±8.30%	38.15±5.94%
Lower	37.70±10.24%***	45.92±8.02%
Lower QLD/Upper QLD	1.91±0.94***	3.18±1.24

Values are represented as mean ± standard deviation. ***; P<0.001 compared with healthy smokers.

To evaluate the effect of emphysematous lesions on the relationships between lung sound distribution and obstructive changes, we analyzed CT images for 39 COPD patients. The mean value for the %LAA was 36.7% (4.3% to 65.2%), and there were 20 emphysema-dominant COPD patients (%LAA>40%) and 19 less emphysematous COPD patients (%LAA<40%). In the less emphysematous group, the relationship between Lower QLD/Upper QLD and obstructive changes was stronger (%FEV$_1$; $\rho = 0.65$ [p<0.005], FVC/FEV$_1$; $\rho = 0.74$ [p<0.001],%MEF$_{50}$; $\rho = 0.71$ [p<0.001]). However, these correlations were not observed in the emphysema-dominant group (Table 3, Figure 2).

The effect of emphysematous lesions on lung sound distribution was different in each patient. Figure 3 shows CT findings of two representative patients with upper-lung-dominant emphysema. One patient (Figure 3A–C) was an 80-year-old male with GOLD III airflow limitation (predicted FEV$_1$ = 46.6%, predicted FVC = 110.1%) and an average %LAA of 47.6%. The inspiration CT (Figure 3A) showed upper-lung-dominant centrilobular emphysema (%LAA of upper lung field; Right = 58.75%, Left = 59.22, %LAA of lower lung field: Right = 33.74%, Left = 32.68%). After expiration, the lower-lung volume tended to decrease to a greater extent than the upper-lung volume (Figure 3B). In this case, the lung sound intensity was lower-lung-dominant and Lower QLD/Upper QLD was similar to the average values of healthy subjects (Figure 3C; Upper QLD = 14.15%, Lower QLD = 44.82%, Lower QLD/Upper QLD = 3.17).

Figure 3D–F shows the CT and QLD findings of a subject with upper-lung-dominant emphysema. This subject was a 72-year-old male with GOLD II airflow limitation (predicted FEV$_1$ = 61.4%, predicted FVC = 106.4%) and an average %LAA of 44.1%. The inspiration CT showed upper-lung-dominant centrilobular em-physema (%LAA of upper lung field; Right = 64.11%, Left = 54.88, %LAA of lower lung field: Right = 35.27%, Left = 29.42%). After expiration, the decreases in upper- and lower-lung volumes were nearly equal (Figure 3E). In this case, Lower QLD/Upper QLD was lower than the average of COPD patients (Figure 3F; Upper QLD = 27.32%, Lower QLD = 40.77%, Lower QLD/Upper QLD = 1.49).

Discussion

In this study, we found that Lower QLD/Upper QLD in COPD patients was significantly lower than in healthy subjects. We also found that significant correlations between obstructive changes and the upper-lung-dominant distribution of lung sound intensities were present in the COPD patients. These correlations, however, were not observed in emphysematous patients whose%-LAA was over 40%. To the best of our knowledge, this is the first study to demonstrate that the correlation between lung sound distribution and the obstructive changes in pulmonary function was considerably affected by the presence of emphysematous lesions.

In severe COPD patients, movement of the abdominal ribcage and diaphragm are restricted by hyperinflation. A weak correlation between FEV$_1$ and the displacement of the lateral rib margin has been observed in severe COPD patients [18]. Furthermore, accessory respiratory muscles, such as the sternocleidomastoid and scalene muscles, are recruited to raise the rib cage during tidal breathing in patients with severe obstructive pulmonary function. Under these circumstances, the regional ventilation may shift from the lower- to the upper-lung field as a function of the degree of hyperinflation, and the lung sound intensity may reflect these changes. Shi et al. reported that lung sound analysis using VRI

Table 3. Relationship between Lower QLD/Upper QLD and pulmonary function tests.

	Lower QLD/Upper QLD			
	Normal (n = 40)	COPD (n = 47)	COPD %LAA <40% (n = 19)	COPD %LAA >40% (n = 20)
FVC %predicted	$\rho = 0.11$ (NS)	$\rho = 0.25$ (NS)	$\rho = 0.27$ (NS)	$\rho = 0.36$ (NS)
FEV$_1$ %predicted	$\rho = -0.06$ (NS)	$\rho = 0.45$ (p<0.005)	$\rho = 0.65$ (P<0.005)	$\rho = 0.24$ (NS)
FEV$_1$/FVC	$\rho = -0.03$ (NS)	$\rho = 0.42$ (p<0.005)	$\rho = 0.74$ (p<0.001)	$\rho = -0.21$ (NS)
MEF$_{50}$ %predicted	$\rho = -0.07$ (NS)	$\rho = 0.46$ (p<0.005)	$\rho = 0.71$ (p<0.001)	$\rho = 0.19$ (NS)
MEF$_{25}$ %predicted	$\rho = -0.13$ (NS)	$\rho = 0.19$ (NS)	$\rho = 0.36$ (NS)	$\rho = 0.07$ (NS)
delta N$_2$ %predicted	-	$\rho = -0.52$ (p<0.005, n = 32)	-	-
Dlco %predicted	-	$\rho = -0.11$ (NS, n = 32)	-	-

Definition of abbreviations: FVC = forced vital capacity, FEV1 = forced expiratory volume in 1 second, MEF$_{50}$ and MEF$_{25}$ = maximum expiratory flow at 50% and 25% of FVC, deltaN$_2$ = the phase III slope of the single-breath nitrogen washout test, DLco = the single-breath total lung diffusion capacity, %LAA = the percentage of the Low-attenuation areas for the entire lung, NS = not significant.

Correlation of PFTs and lung sound distribution in COPD patients
Effect of emphysematous lesion

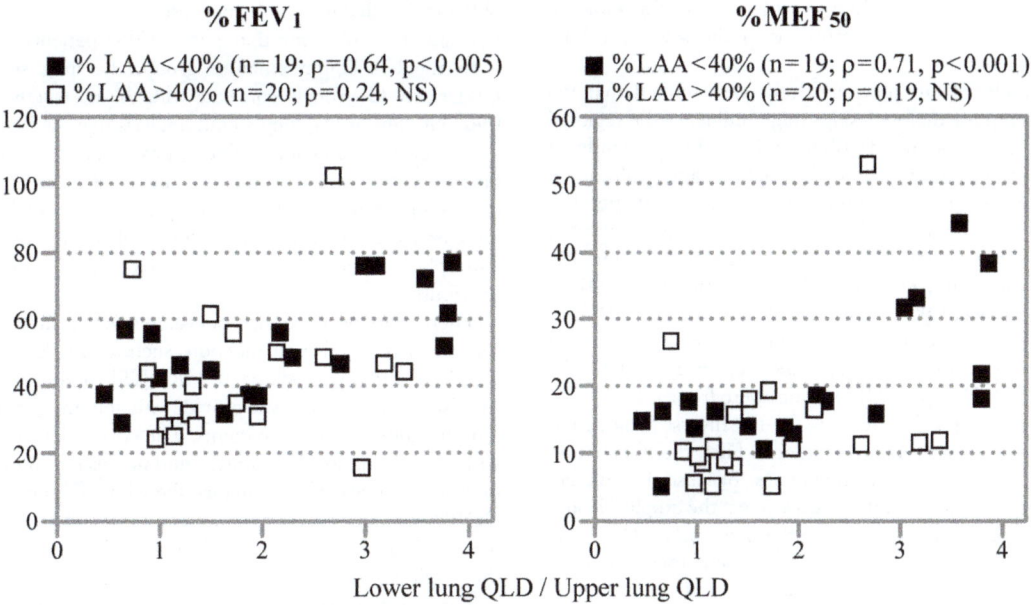

%FEV₁

■ % LAA<40% (n=19; ρ=0.64, p<0.005)
□ %LAA>40% (n=20; ρ=0.24, NS)

%MEF₅₀

■ %LAA<40% (n=19; ρ=0.71, p<0.001)
□ %LAA>40% (n=20; ρ=0.19, NS)

Lower lung QLD / Upper lung QLD

Figure 2. Correlation between PFTs and lung sound distribution in COPD patients and the effects of emphysematous lesions. In the less emphysematous group (%LAA <40%, n = 19), the relationship between Lower QLD/Upper QLD and obstructive changes (%FEV₁; r = 0.64 [p< 0.005], %MEF₅₀; r = 0.71 [p<0.001]) were stronger than in the emphysema-dominant group (%LAA >40%, n = 20), in which these correlations were not observed.

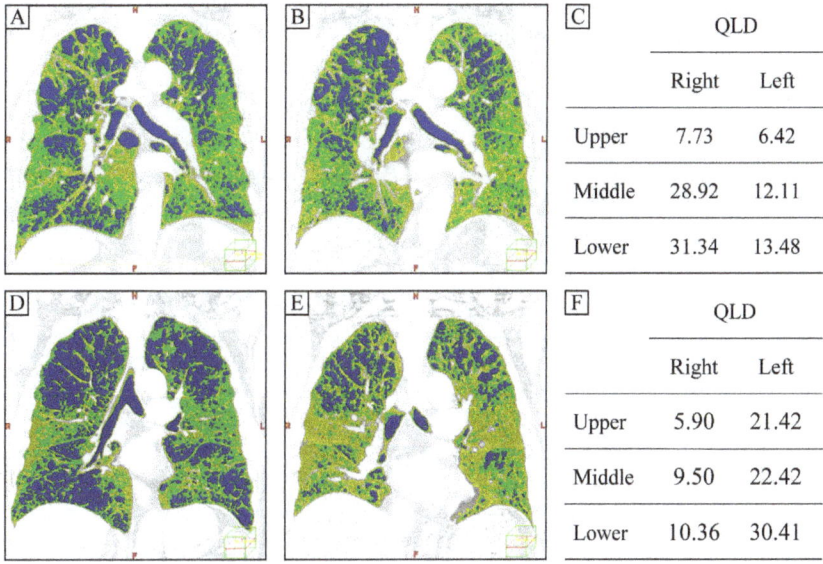

C	QLD	
	Right	Left
Upper	7.73	6.42
Middle	28.92	12.11
Lower	31.34	13.48

F	QLD	
	Right	Left
Upper	5.90	21.42
Middle	9.50	22.42
Lower	10.36	30.41

Figure 3. CT and lung sound distribution findings for 2 representative cases of upper-lung-dominant emphysema. Figure 3A to C: This subject was an 80-year-old male with GOLD III airflow limitation and an average %LAA of 47.6%. The inspiration CT showed upper-lung-dominant centrilobular emphysema (Figure 3A). After expiration, lower-lung volume tended to decrease more than upper-lung volume (Figure 3B). In this case, the lung sound intensity was lower-lung-dominant, and Lower QLD/Upper QLD was similar to the average value of healthy subjects (Figure 3C; Lower QLD/Upper QLD = 3.17). Figure 3D to F: This subject was a 72-year-old male with GOLD II airflow limitation and an average %LAA of 44.1%. Inspiration CT showed upper-lung-dominant centrilobular emphysema (Figure 3D). After expiration, the decreases in the upper- and lower-lung volumes were almost equal (Figure 3E). In this case Lower QLD/Upper QLD was lower than average values in the COPD patients (Figure 3F; Lower QLD/Upper QLD = 1.49).

was capable of detecting regional ventilation distribution under carefully controlled laboratory conditions [12]. In this study, we found that the ratio of lower- to upper-lung sound intensity in COPD patients was significantly lower than in healthy subjects, and that this ratio decreased according to the severity of the obstructive changes.

From the results of our previous study, we assumed that the distribution of emphysematous lesions might influence the regional lung ventilation and sound distribution [13]. In this study, a correlation between lung sound distribution and pulmonary function was not observed in emphysema-dominant patients. We found that lung sound distribution in emphysema-dominant patients varied. For example, in 8 upper-lung-dominant emphysema patients who had averaged %LAA values that were >40%, the range of the Lower QLD/Upper QLD values was from 0.73 to 3.17. On the other hand, in 3 lower-lung-dominant emphysema patients who had averaged %LAA values that were >40%, the range of Lower QLD/Upper QLD values were from 1.33 to 3.35.

There are several possible reasons for the diverse lung sound distribution in the emphysematous patients. First, the distribution of emphysematous lesions is heterogeneous. Because the changes in lung structure that occur in this disease affect the amplitude and sound transmission from the airways to the chest surface [19], lung sound intensity in the region of the emphysematous and non-emphysematous lesions is thought to be quite different. Second, the regional ventilation of each emphysematous lesion also differs. Using Dual Xenon CT, Park et al demonstrated that emphysematous lesions show different ventilation patterns, even in the same patients [20]. Emphysematous lesions with no or little regional ventilation may create a very weak lung sound and may even block sound transmission. On the other hand, ventilated emphysematous lesions may create respiratory sounds proportional to the level of ventilation. If the relationship between the regional lung sound intensity and ventilation in emphysematous lesions was determined, lung sound analysis could be used as a non-invasive bed-side physiological assessment tool for detection of emphysematous lesions in interventional treatments such as bronchoscopic lung volume reduction [21–23]. There is a possibility that a strong lung sound in the presence of emphysematous lesions might represent abundant collateral ventilation, which is a diagnostic criterion for the exclusion of patients from bronchoscopic lung volume reduction using one-way valves [23,24]. Since we could recruit only a few patients who had been examined by both inspiratory and expiratory CT, further study to evaluate the relationship between regional ventilation and lung sound intensity in emphysematous lesions is required. Third, the severity of small airway obstruction may vary within each patient. In some cases of heterogeneous emphysema, small airway disease seems to contribute to an obstructive change similar to that of the emphysematous lesions. Research on airway properties (i.e. airway

dimensions and airway wall thickness) and lung sound distribution will provide valuable insights in this field. For these aforementioned reasons, it may be difficult to find a correlation between obstructive changes and the distribution of the lung sound intensity in emphysema-dominant COPD patients.

In the less emphysematous group, the lung sound intensity moderately to strongly correlate with the obstructive changes. In these circumstances, lung sound analysis may be beneficial to the assessment of outcome after intervention. COPD treatment targeting the amelioration of hyperinflation may improve diaphragm movement by deflating the lungs, which may lead to increased ventilation and an airflow shift to the lower lung field. This phenomenon is reflected by a change in the lung sound distribution.

There have been extensive developments in functional imaging related to regional lung function, such as the Xenon ventilation CT [20] and hyperpolarized MRI [25]. These innovative and sophisticated methods will provide valuable insights into regional lung function in COPD patients. The correlation of these insights with the evaluation of acoustic findings using computer assisted lung sound analysis will enhance the value of lung auscultation in COPD management. Lung auscultation is still an essential part of the physical examination, which brings clinical information about the respiratory system quickly, easily, and cost-effectively [26].

There were some limitations to this study. First, the attachment of sensor to the bony posterior chest wall was difficult, which resulted in the exclusion of patients with a BMI of 19 or less. Low body weight is common in Japanese COPD patients, and further improvements in sensor attachment technology are expected. Second was the absence of female COPD patients in this study due to the low number of female COPD patients at our institution. Because there are differences in lung sound distribution between males and females in healthy subjects [17], further study including female COPD patients is needed. Third, we were unable to recruit a sufficient number of age-matched healthy smokers. Since we could not find an effect of age on Lower QLD/Upper QLD in healthy subjects, we believe the difference in age between healthy subjects and COPD patients did not influence the results of Lower QLD/Upper QLD analysis of this study.

Acknowledgments

The authors thank Mr. Jason Tonge for his assistance in manuscript preparation.

Author Contributions

Conceived and designed the experiments: MM. Performed the experiments: MM HK HH HN NF SN TI. Analyzed the data: MM SM. Wrote the paper: MM TM.

References

1. Pardee NE, Martin CJ, Morgan EH (1976) A test of the practical value of estimating breath sound intensity. Breath sounds related to measured ventilatory function. Chest 70: 341–344.
2. Kraman SS (1980) Determination of the site of production of respiratory sounds by subtraction phonopneumography. Am Rev Respir Dis 122: 303–309.
3. Ploysongsang Y, Paré JA, Macklem PT (1982) Correlation of regional breath sound with regional ventilation in emphysema. Am Rev Respir Dis 126: 526–9.
4. Martinez FJ, Couser JI, Celli BR (1990) Factors influencing ventilatory muscle recruitment in patients with chronic airflow obstruction. Am Rev Respir Dis 142: 276–82.
5. Levine S, Gillen M, Weiser P, Feiss G, Goldman M, et al. (1988) Inspiratory pressure generation: comparison of subjects with COPD and age-matched normals. J Appl Physiol 65: 888–99.
6. Dellinger RP, Parrillo JE, Kushnir A, Rossi M, Kushnir I (2008) Dynamic visualization of lung sounds with a vibration response device: a case series. Respiration 75: 60–72.
7. Maher TM, Gat M, Allen D, Devaraj A, Wells AU, et al. (2008) Reproducibility of dynamically represented acoustic lung images from healthy individuals. Thorax 63: 542–8.
8. Dellinger RP, Jean S, Cinel I, Tay C, Rajanala S, et al. (2007) Regional distribution of acoustic-based lung vibration as a function of mechanical ventilation mode. Crit Care 11: R26.
9. Becker HD, Slawik M, Miyazawa T, Gat M (2009) Vibration response imaging as a new tool for interventional-bronchoscopy outcome assessment: A prospective pilot study. Respiration 77: 179–94.
10. Wang Z, Bartter T, Baumann BM, Abouzgheib W, Chansky ME, et al. (2008) Asynchrony between left and right lung in acute asthma. J Asthma 45: 575–8.

11. Detterbeck F, Gat M, Miller D, Force S, Chin C, et al. (2013) A new method to predict postoperative lung function: quantitative breath sound measurements. Ann Thorac Surg 95: 968–75.

12. Shi C, Boehme S, Bentley AH, Hartmann EK, Klein KU, et al. (2014) Assessment of Regional Ventilation Distribution: Comparison of Vibration Response Imaging (VRI) with Electrical Impedance Tomography (EIT). PLoS One 9: e86638. doi: 10.1371.

13. Mineshita M, Matsuoka S, Miyazawa T (2014) The effects of bronchodilators on regional lung sound distribution in patients with COPD. Respiration 87: 45–53.

14. The Committee of Pulmonary Physiology, the Japanese Respiratory Society (2004) Guidelines for pulmonary Function Tests: spirometry, flow-volume curve, diffusion capacity of the lung. The Japanese Respiratory Society; Tokyo (in Japanese)

15. Buist AS, Ross BB (1973) Quantitative analysis of the alveolar plateau in the diagnosis of early airway obstruction. Am Rev Respir Dis 108: 1078–87.

16. Roca J1, Rodriguez-Roisin R, Cobo E, Burgos F, Perez J, et al. (1990) Single-breath carbon monoxide diffusing capacity prediction equations from a Mediterranean population. Am Rev Respir Dis 141(4 Pt 1): 1026–32.

17. Mineshita M, Shirakawa T, Saji J, Handa H, Furuya N, et al. (2014) Vibration Response Imaging in Healthy Japanese Subjects. Respir Investig 52: 28–35.

18. Gilmartin JJ, Gibson GJ (1984) Abnormalities of chest wall motion in patients with chronic airflow obstruction. Thorax 39: 264–71.

19. Pasterkamp H, Kraman SS, Wodicka G (1997) Respiratory sounds. Advances beyond the stethoscope. Am J Respir Crit Care Med 156: 974–987.

20. Park E, Goo J, Park S, Lee H, Lee C, et al. (2010) Chronic obstructive pulmonary disease: Quantitative and visual ventilation pattern analysis at Xenon ventilation CT performed by using a dual-energy technique. Radiology 256: 985–997.

21. Ingenito EP, Reilly JJ, Mentzer SJ, Swanson SJ, Vin R, et al. (2001) Bronchoscopic volume reduction: a safe and effective alternative to surgical therapy for emphysema. Am J Respir Crit Care Med 164: 295–301.

22. Gasparini S, Zuccatosta L, Bonifazi M, Bolliger CT (2012) Bronchoscopic treatment of emphysema: state of the art. Respiration 84: 250–63.

23. Shah P, Herth FJF (2014) Current status of bronchoscopic lung volume reduction with endobronchial valves. Thorax 69: 280–6.

24. Herth FJ, Eberhardt R, Gompelmann D, Ficker JH, Wagner M, et al. (2013) Radiological and clinical outcomes of using Chartis to plan endobronchial valve treatment. Eur Respir J 41: 302–308.

25. Fain S, Schiebler M, McCormack DG, Parraga G (2010) Imaging of lung function using hyperpolarized Helium-3 magnetic resonance imaging: Review of current and emerging translational methods and applications. J Magn Reson Imaging 32: 1398–1408.

26. Bohadana A, Izbicki G, Kraman SS (2014) Fundamentals of lung auscultation. N Engl J Med 370: 744–51.

5

Assessing Regional Cerebral Blood Flow in Depression Using 320-Slice Computed Tomography

Yiming Wang[1]*[⑨], **Hongming Zhang**[2⑨], **Songlin Tang**[1,3], **Xingde Liu**[4]*, **Adrienne O'Neil**[5,6], **Alyna Turner**[5,7,8], **Fangxian Chai**[1], **Fanying Chen**[9], **Michael Berk**[5,6,7,10,11]

1 Department of Psychiatry, Hospital Affiliated to Guiyang Medical University, Guiyang, Guizhou, China, 2 Department of Cardiology, The General Hospital of Jinan Military Region, Jinan, China, 3 Department of Neurology, First People's Hospital of Shaoyang, Shaoyang, Hunan, China, 4 Department of Cardiology, Hospital Affiliated to Guiyang Medical University, Guiyang City, Guizhou, China, 5 IMPACT Strategic Research Centre, School of Medicine, Deakin University, Geelong, Australia, 6 School of Public Health and Preventive Medicine, Monash University, Melbourne, Australia, 7 Department of Psychiatry, The University of Melbourne, Parkville, Victoria, Australia, 8 School of Medicine and Public Health, The University of Newcastle, Callaghan, New South Wales, Australia, 9 Mental Health Education And Counseling Center, Guiyang Medical University, Guiyang City, Guizhou, China, 10 Department of Psychiatry, Orygen Youth Health Research Centre, The University of Melbourne, Parkville, Victoria, Australia, 11 Florey Institute of Neuroscience and Mental Health, University of Melbourne, Parkville, Victoria, Australia

Abstract

While there is evidence that the development and course of major depressive disorder (MDD) symptomatology is associated with vascular disease, and that there are changes in energy utilization in the disorder, the extent to which cerebral blood flow is changed in this condition is not clear. This study utilized a novel imaging technique previously used in coronary and stroke patients, 320-slice Computed-Tomography (CT), to assess regional cerebral blood flow (rCBF) in those with MDD and examine the pattern of regional cerebral perfusion. Thirty nine participants with depressive symptoms (Hamilton Depression Rating Scale 24 (HAMD24) score >20, and Self-Rating Depression Scale (SDS) score >53) and 41 healthy volunteers were studied. For all subjects, 3 ml of venous blood was collected to assess hematological parameters. Trancranial Doppler (TCD) ultrasound was utilized to measure parameters of cerebral artery rCBFV and analyse the Pulsatility Index (PI). 16 subjects (8 = MDD; 8 = healthy) also had rCBF measured in different cerebral artery regions using 320-slice CT. Differences among groups were analyzed using ANOVA and Pearson's tests were employed in our statistical analyses. Compared with the control group, whole blood viscosity (including high\middle\low shear rate)and hematocrit (HCT) were significantly increased in the MDD group. PI values in different cerebral artery regions and parameters of rCBFV in the cerebral arteries were decreased in depressive participants, and there was a positive relationship between rCBFV and the corresponding vascular rCBF in both gray and white matter. rCBF of the left gray matter was lower than that of the right in MDD. Major depression is characterized by a wide range of CBF impairments and prominent changes in gray matter blood flow. 320-slice CT appears to be a valid and promising tool for measuring rCBF, and could thus be employed in psychiatric settings for biomarker and treatment response purposes.

Editor: Huafu Chen, University of Electronic Science and Technology of China, China

Funding: This study was supported by a Grant for YW from National Natural Science Foundation of China, (Project Grant 2012 31260237), YW has received Grant/Research Support from the Science and Technology Fund of Guizhou Province, China, Qiankehe Diquhe (2012) 7001, Qiankehe (LG, 2011, 005, J, 2006, 2065, SY, 2008, 3063), which was supported by High-Level Personnel Research Conditions, Special Assistant Funding (TZJF-2008 55), Guizhou Province Special Fund for Outstanding Scientific and Technology Education Talents 2012, 35, Guizhou Province Overseas Students studying science and technology activities funded projects 0011 006 and Scientific and Technology Projects in Guiyang City, China, 2009, Zhu subjects agriculture in Contract 3-008 for study design, the collection, analysis, and interpretation of data and the writing of the manuscript. MB is supported by a NHMRC Senior Principal Research Fellowship 1059660.

Competing Interests: The authors have declared that no competing interests exist.

* Email: yimingw66@yahoo.com (YW); lxd@gmc.edu.cn (XL)

⑨ These authors contributed equally to this work.

Introduction

In major depressive disorder (MDD), symptom development and course are influenced by brain circuits associated with vascular disease [1]. Studies conducted in depressed populations suggest that patients may exhibit impairments in regional cerebral blood flow (rCBF) and dysfunction in cortical and subcortical brain structures [2]; a close relationship has been observed between mild cognitive impairment and brain hypoperfusion [3]. rCBF is improved by treatment including cognitive-behavioral and electroconvulsive therapy (ECT) in MDD [4–5], suggesting a state

related change. This may be linked to reduced mitochondrial energy generation and dysfunction in the disorder [6–7]. In parallel, there is a large literature showing alterations in brain glucose utilization in depression [8]. Therefore, monitoring rCBF in psychiatric populations and settings may be useful in the context of monitoring treatment response.

Imaging studies have previously utilized techniques such as functional magnetic resonance imaging (fMRI) and have demonstrated changes in hemodynamics of the limbic system and subcortical regions in those with depression [9]. Single-photon

Table 1. The comparison of demographic data between control and depression groups (Mean ± SEM).

Items	control (n = 41)	depression (n = 39)
Ages(years)	46.22±11.68	46.74±11.42
(Ranges)	18–60	18–60
Sex(M/F)(n)	9/32	8/31
Resting SBP (mm Hg)	120±25	125±27
Resting DBP (mm Hg)	80±10	76±8
Smokers/non-smokers (n)	20/21(49%/51%)	21/18 (54%/46%)

Note: no significant differences in the demographic variables (age, sex, blood pressure, smoking) between two groups, SBP: systolic blood pressure, DBP: diastolic blood pressure.

emission computed tomography (SPECT) has also been employed to document hypoperfusion of the frontal and prefrontal regions in late-life depressed patients [10–13], as well as improvements in rCBF following treatment with antidepressants [14] and ECT [15]. Similarly, MRI with arterial spin labeling has demonstrated significant CBF elevation in white matter in those for whom depression remits following antidepressant use [16].

The use of heterogeneous imaging techniques has, in some instances, yielded inconsistent results. For example, studies of depressed patients using positron emission tomography (PET) have indicated decreased glucose utilization in temporal lobe cortex [17], while others have found increased cerebral glucose metabolism in older patient populations [18]. While these studies suggest that there is a potential relationship between cognitive impairment and altered rCBF, most studies are subject to limitations including their use of semi-quantitative measurement that do not objectively reflect rCBF changes.

In contrast, the Toshiba Aquilion ONE 320 slice dynamic volume CT [19] is a refined diagnostic imaging test which utilizes dynamic volume Computed Tomography (CT) technology. It has the capacity to display soft tissue, bones and blood vessels in a singular, high resolution image and can also capture dynamic processes including blood flow and organ function, in three-dimensional real-time. This technology has advanced patient care in a range of medical settings by reducing time to diagnosis in heart disease and stroke populations. If applied in psychiatry, this technique allows for the acquisition of data pertaining to brain blood circulation and perfusion maps, including unenhanced, enhanced, delayed patterns, and assessment of arterial and venous diagrams in the same phase. It uses relatively low radiation doses and could quickly and accurately determine changes in cerebral hemodynamics as well as quantitative examination of cerebral

perfusion. To date, several studies have been conducted using One 320 slice CT in coronary artery and pulmonary vascular populations [20–21]. While the advantages of employing whole brain CT perfusion in acute stroke, ahronic ischemia and arteriovenous malformation have been acknowledged [22], no publications investigating its utility in psychiatric populations were found at the time of writing. To our knowledge, this study will be the first to utilize 320-slice CT imaging previously used in coronary and stroke patients to assess rCBF in those with MDD and analyze the extent which it corresponds with regional cerebral blood flow velocity (rCBFV) as measured by Trancranial Doppler (TCD) ultrasound. We also aimed to compare rCBF in depressed patients to healthy control subjects to clarify regional cerebral perfusion patterns in the cerebral hemispheres, in order to explore its potential utility in psychiatric settings for possible diagnostic and treatment response purposes.

Materials and Methods

Subjects

The sample comprised patients (n = 39, 8 men and 31 women, aged 18–60 years, mean ages 46.74±11.42). They were hospitalized patients or outpatients with major depression seen in the Psychiatry Department of the affiliated hospital of Guiyang Medical University between April and December, 2009. Patients who met diagnostic criteria for a depressive disorder as defined by the Diagnostic and Statistical Manual of Mental Disorders-IV (DSM-IV) (diagnosed by two clinicians), had a Hamilton Depression Rating Scale 24 (HAMD24) score of >20 points, and a Self-Rating Depression Scale (SDS) score >53 were included in this study. Exclusion criteria included taking psychotropic substances or drugs influencing vessel compliance function

Table 2. The comparison of demographic data between control and depression groups using the 320 slice CT (Mean ±SEM).

Items	control (n = 8)	depression (n = 8)
Ages(years)	44.13±10.37	43.12±12.09
(Ranges)	18–60	18–60
Sex(M/F)(n)	1/8	1/8
Resting SBP (mm Hg)	118±22	120±27
Resting DBP (mm Hg)	75±10	78±8
Smokers/non-smokers (n)	1/7(13%/87%)	1/7 (13%/87%)

Note: no significant differences in the demographic variables (age, sex, blood pressure, smoking) between two groups, SBP: systolic blood pressure, DBP: diastolic blood pressure.

Table 3. The comparison of hemorheological parameters between depression and control groups (Mean ±SEM).

Items	Control (n = 41)	Depression(n = 39)
High shear rate (mPa.s/150S^{-1})	3.92±0.31	4.63±0.39*
Middle shear rate (mPa.s/60S^{-1})	4.38±0.36	5.72±0.47**
Low shear rate (mPa.s/10S^{-})	6.43±0.70	7.75±1.10**
Hematocrit	41.32±2.91	43.34±4.68*
Red blood cell sedimentation (mm/h)	39.34±6.62	38.07±8.90

Note: Compared with control group *$P<0.05$, **$P<0.01$.

upon enrollment (such as stimulants, hypnotics or sedatives), diseases of the nervous system (Aneurysms involving the supra-aortic vessels, chronic cerebral venous insufficiency), somatic diseases (e.g. diabetes, hypertension, coronary heart disease, atherosclerosis), or other mental disorders.

Forty one healthy volunteers, who were healthy and underwent physical examination in the physical examination center of the affiliated hospital of Guiyang Medical University between April and December 2009 were recruited concurrently as a control group. They were matched for age and gender (9 men and 32 women, aged 18–60 years, Mean age 46.22±11.68), with a

Table 4. The comparison of parameters of rCBFV between control and depression groups (Mean ± SEM, cm/s).

Items	Control (n = 41)	Depression(n = 39)
ACA-R-Vs	96.31±11.76	79.85±20.41**
ACA-R-Vm	63.95±8.15	54.44±14.80**
ACA-R-Vd	40.67±6.93	37.00±11.40
ACA-L-Vs	96.64±12.21	77.31±14.26**
ACA-L-Vm	64.10±7.82	52.90±11.17**
ACA-L-Vd	41.64±5.98	36.54±8.70**
TICA-R-Vs	114.03±13.44	95.87±17.40**
TICA-R-Vm	76.85±9.69	69.11±21.98*
TICA-R-Vd	51.28±7.18	46.46±10.30*
TICA-L-Vs	112.54±12.32	97.69±20.41**
TICA-L-Vm	75.28±9.16	67.90±15.47*
TICA-L-Vd	50.46±7.22	47.85±12.17
MCA-R-Vs	117.05±13.87	98.15±17.60**
MCA-R-Vm	78.97±10.24	68.62±12.39**
MCA-R-Vd	52.95±7.46	47.87±10.15*
MCA-L-Vs	114.59±12.94	98.10±20.17**
MCA-L-Vm	77.31±9.51	68.72±14.69**
MCA-L-Vd	51.72±7.70	48.46±11.41
VA-R-Vs	71.85±10.06	61.87±11.68**
VA-R-Vm	48.49±6.55	43.87±8.42**
VA-R-Vd	32.62±4.42	30.64±6.82
VA-L-Vs	72.59±8.93	62.79±10.77**
VA-L-Vm	49.67±6.04	45.08±7.56**
VA-L-Vd	33.49±4.18	32.08±5.56
BA-Vs	71.85±10.06	67.82±11.68**
BA-Vm	52.59±6.57	48.21±9.06*
BA-Vd	35.38±4.97	34.12±7.23

Note: compared to the control group, *$P<0.05$, **$P<0.01$.
rCBFV: regional cerebral blood flow velocity.
MCA: middle cerebral artery, ACA: anterior cerebral artery.
PCA: posterior cerebral artery, TICA: the tip of internal carotid artery.
VA: vertebral artery, BA: basilar artery, L: Left, R: Right,
Vs: systolic peak velocity, Vm: mean flow velocity, Vd: diastolic velocity.

Table 5. The comparison of the values of PI between control and depression groups (Mean±SEM).

Items	Control (n = 41)	Depression(n = 39)
ACA-R	0.89±0.10	0.80±0.18*
ACA-L	0.86±0.79	0.78±0.15*
TICA-R	0.88±0.08	0.76±0.12**
TICA-L	0.87±0.09	0.75±0.12**
MCA-R	0.82±0.08	0.74±0.11*
MCA-L	0.82±0.09	0.73±0.11*
VA-R	0.83±0.11	0.72±0.10**
VA-L	0.79±0.09	0.68±0.09**
BA	0.77±0.10	0.70±0.11*

Note: Compared with control group *P<0.05, ** P<0.01.
PI: Pulsatility index, ACA: anterior cerebral artery,
TICA: the tip of internal carotid artery, MCA: middle cerebral artery,
VA: vertebral artery, BA: basilar artery, L: Left, R: Right.

HAMD24 score <20 and Hamilton Anxiety score <8, and had no history of depression, anxiety or somatic disorders.

Ethics statement and consent

The study was approved by the Ethics of Human Investigation Committee at Guiyang Medical University (NO: 20090016) and all experiments were performed in accordance with relevant guidelines and regulations. The participants themselves or a legally authorized representative gave written informed consent to participate in the study and obtained safeguards in this study. The procedures followed were in accordance with the revised Declaration of Helsinki [23].

Hemorheologic measures

All subjects had 3 ml of venous blood collected in the early morning (07:00–08:00) to assess blood rheology parameters (blood viscosity and hemoconcentration). Heparin was used as an anticoagulant; whole blood viscosity (including high\middle\low shear rates), hematocrit (HCT) and red blood cell sedimentation were checked [24] by an automatic blood rheometer (LBY-N6B, Beijing Precil Instrument Co. Ltd.).

TCD screening methods

In a quiescent condition, all participants were assessed using the 2 MHz probe transcranial color-coded Doppler (TCD) sonography (Germany, DWL-X type), in accordance with Hua-Yang TCD ultrasound practices and diagnostic criteria guidelines [25]. The middle cerebral artery (MCA) and the anterior cerebral artery (ACA) were insonated through the temporal bone acoustic windows while the participant was in the conventional supine position. The vertebral artery (VA) and basilar artery (BA) were insonated through the occipital acoustic window while the participant was in the sitting position. Data were generated via the trace envelope of the measured arterial spectrum and a series

Table 6. The comparison of rCBF between control and depression groups (Mean ±SEM, ml·min-1·100 g-1, n = 8).

Items	Control	Depression
ACA-R-GM	46.11±12.41	36.96±10.20*
ACA-L-GM	44.72±10.95	36.45±11.67*
ACA-R-WM	23.74±6.74	20.20±5.71*
ACA-L-WM	25.21±6.63	21.67±6.68*
MCA-R-GM	49.63±10.78	44.09±12.76*
MCA-L-GM	49.71±15.61	41.19±13.77**
MCA-R-WM	25.05±6.94	21.97±5.71
MCA-L-WM	26.17±6.91	22.52±5.75*
PCA-R-GM	46.63±10.06	39.02±10.92*
PCA-L-GM	45.76±11.91	34.32±12.21**
PCA-R-WM	27.73±11.44	24.73±8.61
PCA-L-WM	28.33±10.85	25.65±8.45

Note: Compared with control group * P<0.05, ** P<0.01.
rCBF: regional cerebral blood flow, ACA: anterior.
cerebral artery, MCA: middle cerebral artery.
PCA: posterior cerebral artery, L: Left, R: Right.
GM: gray matter, WM: white matter.

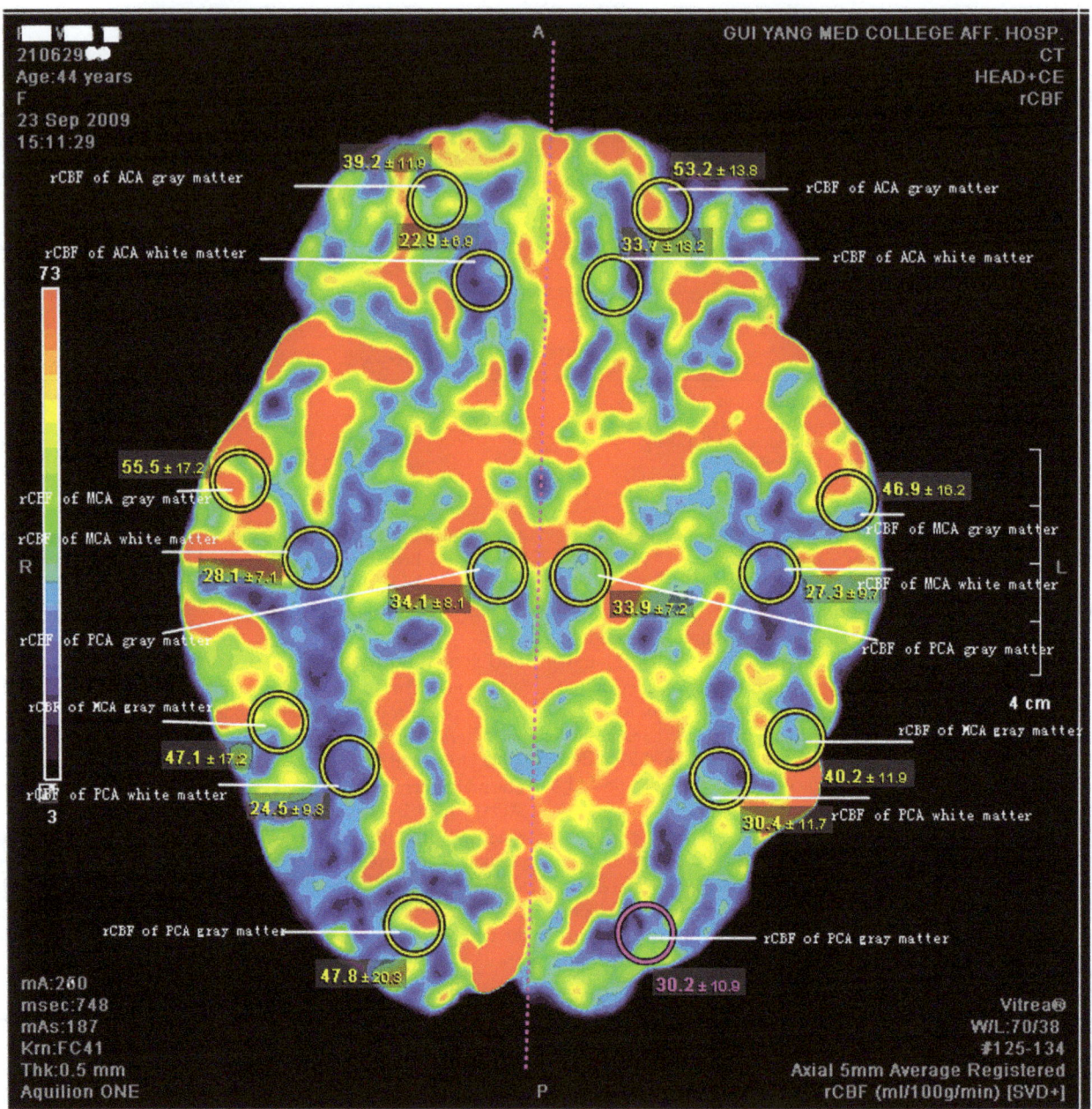

Figure 1. Case example: Coronal slices from dynamic CT angiography taken from a 44-year-old woman with depression. Circles represent regions of interest, with the mean ± SEM from 19 volume data presented. In MCA (middle cerebral artery) regions, the values of rCBF (regional cerebral blood flow) in left gray matter were lower than in the right [Left: 46.9 and 40.2 ml/(min·100 g),Right: 55.5 and 47.1 ml/(min·100 g)]. In PCA (posterior cerebral artery) regions, the values of rCBF in left gray matter were lower than in the right [Left: 30.2 ml/(min·100 g), Right: 47.8 ml/(min·100 g)].

of blood flow parameter values by the machine's software analyzer system. The Pulsatility Index (PI) was calculated as $PI = (peak systolic velocity–end diastolic velocity)/mean blood flow velocity.

rCBF measurement methods

Sixteen subjects (8 = depressed, 1 men and 7 women, mean ages 43.12±12.09; 8 = healthy, 1 men and 7 women, mean ages 44.13±10.37) were randomly selected to undergo rCBF assessment using the 320 slice CT [26] (Japan's Toshiba Aquilion ONE; non-helical scan mode, 912-channel, 16 cm coverage, lap rotation time 0.5 s, slice thickness 0.5 mm, vision 240 mm), After iodine

allergy testing, participants were asked to lie in the supine position, where a 20 th catheter tube was placed in the cubital vein before the scan. A plastic tube was connected to the Empower 9900P type binocular high-pressure syringe, and participants were injected with a nonionic contrast agent (iodine Pa Alcohol Injection 37 g(I)/100 ml/bottle, Shanghai Bracco Xinyi Pharmaceutical Co. Ltd.). 50 ml and 20 ml saline was administered intravenously in the cubital fossa with an injection rate of 6 ml/s. Scan parameters were as follows: 80 kv, 100 mA. Next, brain volumes were acquired after the injection of contrast medium, scan parameters as follows: 120 kv, 200 mA, dynamic volume scanning

Table 7. The comparison of rCBF between the left and right cerebral hemispheres in depression group (Mean ±SEM, ml·min-1·100 g-1, n = 8).

Items	Left	Right
ACA -GM	36.45±11.67	36.96±10.20
ACA -WM	21.67±6.67	20.21±5.71
MCA-GM	41.49±13.77*	44.09±12.77
MCA-WM	22.52±5.75	21.97±5.71
PCA-GM	34.32±12.21*	39.02±10.92
PCA-WM	25.64±8.45	24.73±8.61

Note: Compared with Right * P<0.05.
rCBF: region cerebral blood flow, ACA: anterior cerebral artery.
MCA: middle cerebral artery, PCA: posterior cerebral artery.
L: Left, R: Right, GM: gray matter, WM: white matter.

was delayed 5 s. The time series was as follows: volume scanning was delayed 7 s, during scan across the artery was 11 s, the scan interval was 1 s, 35 s to 60 s venous and delayed scans, during every other scan interval was 5 s. A total of 19 volume data were obtained, each consisting of 320 images. Each inspection obtained a total of 6080 images (each volume data = 0.5 min, total time = 9.5 min). Concordant with the national standard, the total radiation dose of CT plain scan and perfusion scan was approximately 4.6 mSv.

Perfusion image analysis methods

Nineteen volume data were imported into the perfusion fx special package for processing. The right ACA was selected as the input artery and superior sagittal sinus as an output vein. The time-density curves of the dynamic region of interest were automatically analyzed by the software. Perfusion parameters, including cerebral blood volume (CBV), CBF, mean transit time (MTT) and the time to peak (TTP), were generated using the deconvolution mathematical model. The CBV, CBF, MTT, TTP of CT perfusion images in the cross-section, sagittal and coronal plane in the whole brain were obtained by the computer pseudo-color processing. The specific hemodynamic portion of the brain in depression was obtained by drawing various regions of interests (ROIs) encompassing the regions of gray and white matter which were perfused by blood supply at every level of the ACA, MCA, and PCA, and then comparing them with the ROIs of the normal brain. The ROIs (100±5 Pix) were distributed in gray and white matter of regions of blood supply at every level of the ACA, MCA and PCA.

Statistical analyses

Data were analyzed using SPSS Version 22.0. All measurement indicators were expressed as Means ± SEM with independent samples t-tests used to determine significant differences between the depression and control groups, where P<0.05 was considered statistically significant. Differences among groups were analyzed using one-way ANOVA. Stepwise linear regression was conducted to calculate the regression equation. A series of Pearson's correlations were undertaken to observe the strength and direction of the relationship between rCBF and rCBFV parameters. 95% confidence intervals were used in the study.

Results

Demographic features

No significant differences between the control and depression groups were observed for demographic variables (age, sex, blood pressure, smoking), (Table 1, 2).

Comparison of hematological parameters between the depression and control groups

Compared with the control group, whole blood viscosity (including high\middle\low shear rate) and hematocrit were significantly increased in those with depression, however no significant difference was observed between the groups for red blood cell sedimentation (Table 3).

Comparison of parameters of rCBFV between the depression and control groups

Compared with the control group, selected rCBFV parameters in the majority of cerebral arteries were decreased for those with depressive disorder (Table 4). For example, peak systolic flow velocity (Vs) and mean flow velocity (Vm) in bilateral ACA and MCA regions, and in TICA, VA and BA regions were statistically different. Further, statistically significant between group-differences showing decreased end-diastolic flow velocity (Vd) in the left ACA and the right TICA were observed. PI values were significantly lower for the depressed group in all the cerebral artery regions when compared with the control group (Table 5).

Comparison of rCBF between the depression and control group

Compared with the control group, the values of rCBF in bilateral gray and white matter of the cerebral hemispheres were lower for those with a depressive disorder; with the exception of white matter in the left and right PCA region and white matter of the right MCA region (Table 6).

Comparison of rCBF between left and right cerebral hemisphere in depression

Compared with the right cerebral hemisphere, rCBF values in left gray matter in MCA and PCA regions were significantly lower in those with depressive disorder (Table 7, Figure 1).

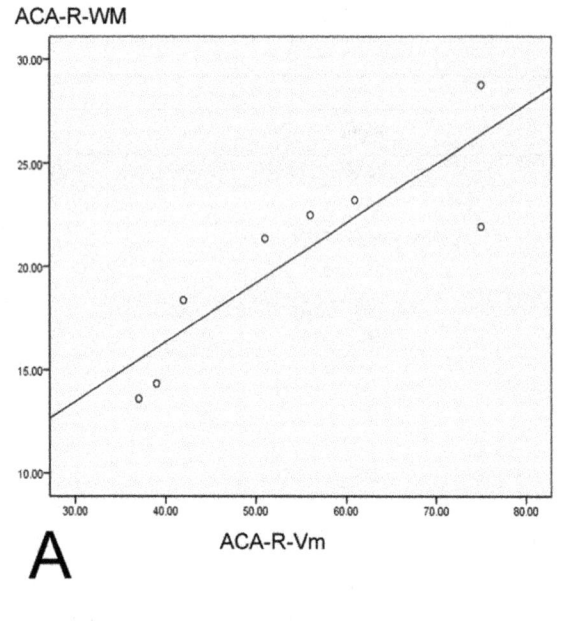

A

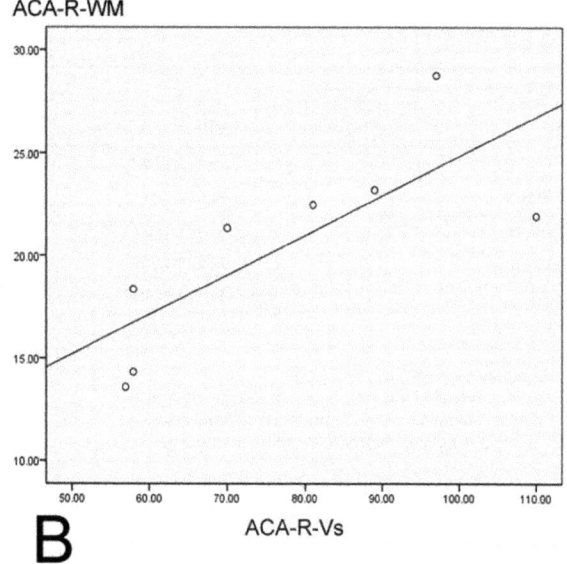

B

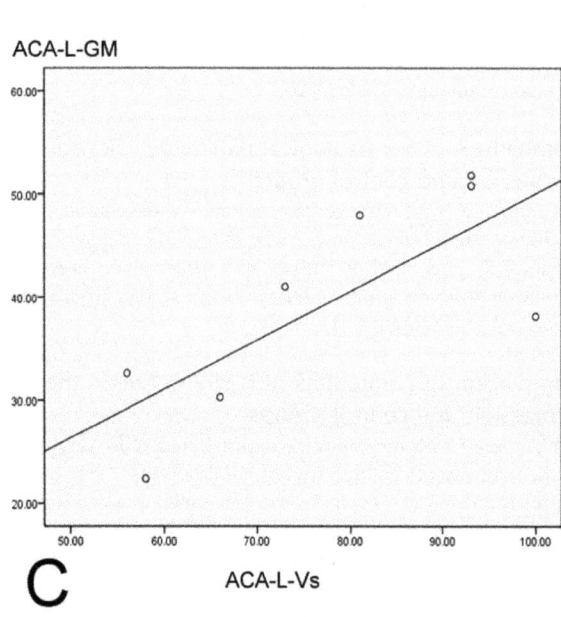

C

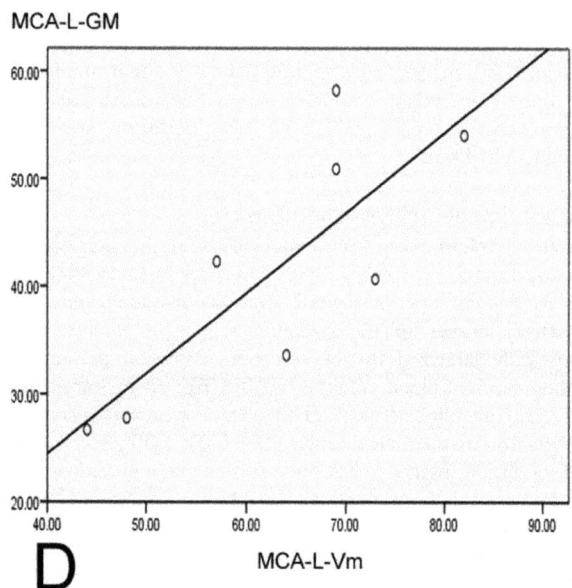

D

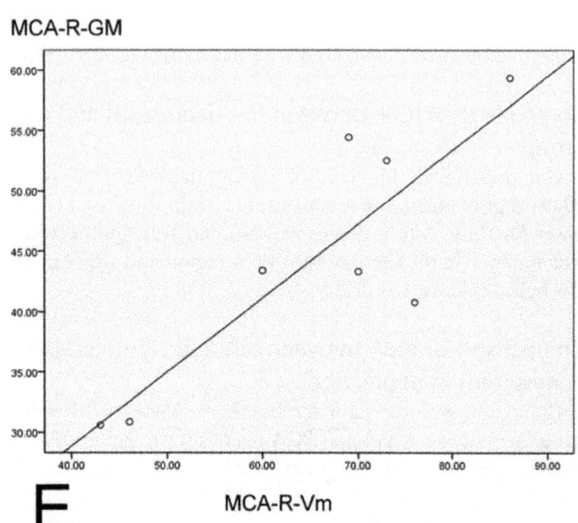

E

Figure 2. The correlation between rCBFV and rCBF in cerebral artery regions. A: A positive correlation between mean flow velocity (Vm) and rCBF in white matter (WM) of right ACA (anterior cerebral artery) (P<0.01; r = 0.874). B: A positive correlation between systolic peak velocity (Vs) and rCBF in WM of right ACA (P<0.01; r = 0.778). C: A positive correlation between Vs and rCBF in gray matter (GM) of left ACA (P<0.05; r = 0.758). D: A positive correlation between Vm and rCBF in GM of left MCA (middle cerebral artery) (P<0.05; r = 0.802). E: A positive correlation between Vm and rCBF in GM of right MCA (P<0.01; r = 0.859). rCBFV: regional cerebral blood flow velocity, rCBF: region cerebral blood flow.

The relationship between rCBF and rCBFV in MDD group

When exploring the strength and direction of the association between rCBF and rCBFV in the MDD group, we found a positive correlation for gray matter of the bilateral ACA and MCA regions, except for the right ACA (Vs, Vm, Vd) and left ACA (Vd); and in white matter of the right ACA (Vs, Vm, Vd) and right MCA (Vm). The strongest correlation coefficients were produced for right ACA (Vm r = 0.874, Vd r = 0.839 for white matter) and right MCA Vm (r = 0.859 for gray matter), left MCA (Vs r = 0.760, Vm r = 0.802, Vd r = 0.748 for gray matter). Overall, the strength of the relationships were most consistent for gray matter. The correlation coefficients are displayed in Table 8, the regression equation between rCBFV and rCBF in Table 9 and illustrated in Figures 2.

Discussion

For the first time to our knowledge, we have provided data on the potential utility and novel application of the 320 slice Dynamic volumes CT in a clinically depressed population, a tool validated in coronary and stroke populations. These data demonstrate that patients with depression are characterized by a wide range of CBF impairments, in particular prominent changes in gray matter, when compared with healthy controls. rCBF data generated using this technology in a sub-sample of MDD patients was shown to correlate well with those generated by other measures (TCD ultrasound), suggesting that it could be employed in psychiatric settings for potential diagnostic and treatment response purposes.

Previous studies have suggested reduced rCBF in MDD, illustrated by hypoperfusion in the frontal lobe, temporal lobe, and in the limbic system [27–28]. Indeed, our results are consistent with other functional imaging studies conducted in this area using SPECT imaging [29,12] and a range of other techniques. As these

techniques are often hampered by limitations including accessibility, poor resolution and subjectivity, this study provides some support for the use of CT perfusion imaging for rapid imaging and assessment to determine the CBF dynamics quickly, accurately and in 3 dimensional high resolution in a psychiatric setting [30–31]. The resulting image aligns with real data [32]. Therefore, the use of 320-slice CT for the objective study of cerebral perfusion appears to have clinical value potentially supplanting older techniques.

We found that there was decreased rCBFV in the majority of cerebral arteries in depressive patients, for example, Vs and Vm differed in the bilateral ACA, CA, TICA, VA and BA regions, while Vd differed in the left ACA and right TICA regions. Furthermore, in patients with depression, there was a positive relationship between the rCBFV and the corresponding vascular rCBF in the gray matter of bilateral ACA and MCA regions (with the exception of right ACA (Vs, Vm, Vd) and left ACA (Vd)), and the white matter of the right ACA (Vs, Vm, Vd) and MCA (Vm) regions. We also demonstrated that the rCBF values of left gray matter in MCA and PCA regions were lower than that of right in those with depressive disorder. Hardoy's results [33], in MDD showing hypoperfusion in the left frontal and temporal areas and perfusion asymmetry, was consistent with the findings in our cohort.

A reduction in blood flow could be due to either functional or structural deficiencies. TCD PI reflects cerebrovascular resistance by the flow velocity waveform [34]. Kwater et al. [35] reported a strong association between higher PI and systemic arterial stiffness in patients with atherosclerosis, however atherosclerosis reduces cerebrovascular reactivity, leading to higher PI values. In our study, however, PI was decreased in the depressive group compared with controls, suggesting that the reason for the reduced

Table 8. The correlation coefficients between rCBF and rCBFV in depression group (n = 8).

rCBFV items	rCBF of Gray matter	rCBF of White matter
ACA-R-Vs	0.599	0.778*
ACA-R-Vm	0.674	0.874**
ACA-R-Vd	0.624	0.839**
ACA-L-Vs	0.758*	0.607
ACA-L-Vm	0.720*	0.568
ACA-L-Vd	0.575	0.569
MCA-R-Vs	0.706*	0.520
MCA-R-Vm	0.859**	0.718*
MCA-R-Vd	0.748*	0.683
MCA-L-Vs	0.760**	0.426
MCA-L-Vm	0.802**	0.535
MCA-L-Vd	0.748**	0.538

Note: The correlation coefficient t test * P<0.05. ** P<0.01.
rCBFV: regional cerebral blood flow velocity, rCBF: region cerebral blood flow.
ACA: anterior cerebral artery, MCA: middle cerebral artery, L: Left, R: Right.
Vs: systolic peak velocity, Vm: mean flow velocity, Vd: diastolic velocity.

Table 9. Regression equation between rCBFV and rCBF in depression group (n = 8).

Regression equation	P value
ACA-L-GM-rCBF = 2.636+0.474(ACA-L-Vs)	0.029
ACA-R-WM-rCBF = 4.852+0.287(ACA-R-Vm)	0.005
ACA-R-WM-rCBF = 7.831+0.86(ACA-R-Vm)-0.441(ACA-R-Vs)	0.003
MCA-L-GM-rCBF = 0.745(MCA-L-Vm)-5.333	0.017
MCA-R-GM-rCBF = 4.420+0.612(MCA-R-Vm)	0.006

rCBFV: regional cerebral blood flow velocity, rCBF: region cerebral blood flow.
ACA: anterior cerebral artery, MCA: middle cerebral artery, L: Left, R: Right.
GM: gray matter, WM: white matter, Vs: systolic peak velocity, Vm: mean flow velocity.

blood flow in the depressive group may be functional rather than structural.

We also observed that the whole blood viscosity and hematocrit were significantly increased in the depressed patients. Blood viscosity is a measure of the thickness and stickiness of blood, and increased levels of blood viscosity has been associated with arterial disease including myocardial infarction and stroke [36–37]. It has been suggested that stress is associated with hemoconcentration of the cerebral hemispheres in patients with MDD [38]. Lechin [39] argued that blood viscosity is positively involved with the levels of neural sympathetic and cholinergic activity in MDD, while Wong et at. found that decreased blood viscosity is correlated with the improvement of depressive symptoms after antidepressant treatment in MDD.

There is evidence of significant hypoperfusion in the gray matter of the cerebral hemispheres in people with depression [40]. The reason for this may be concordant with the proximal relationship between the dominant hemisphere cortex and human cognition, emotion and related functions, while its relationship to deep white matter appears more peripheral. Botteron [41] reported that elderly depressed people with memory impairment showed changes in the medial temporal lobe and its adjacent structures.

Su liang et al [42] proposed that elderly depressive patients with cognitive impairment exhibited decreased local glucose metabolism in the caudate nucleus bilaterally, the inferior frontal gyrus, left cingulate and anterior central gyrus regions, and the decline in both executive function and memory function was related to low local glucose metabolism in the caudate nucleus bilaterally, the frontal lobe, temporal lobe, the left central gyrus and limbic brain regions of deep white matter. Indeed, our results were concordant with this study.

Limitations of both the technique and of the study

The specific hemodynamic regions of the brain in depression was obtained by drawing various regions of interests encompassing the regions of gray and white matter which were perfused by ACA, MCA, and PCA blood supply, and then comparing them with the ROIs of the normal brain. This captured representative regional cerebral blood flow, but not the actual value of the lobes of the brain. Secondly, because relatively few subjects had rCBF assessment, this could result in possible bias. While changes in rCBF were seen, potential clinical applications require further study. Lastly a multivariate ANOVA analysis testing multiple correlations was not performed, and differences between groups were analyzed using one-way ANOVA.

Conclusions

These data suggest that people with depression are characterized by a wide range of cerebral blood flow impairments and there appear to be more prominent changes in left gray matter. The 320 slice Dynamic volumes CT appears to be a potentially useful tool for measuring rCBF, with advantages over existing instruments. This technique could be employed in psychiatric settings for biomarker, diagnostic and treatment response purposes. Future studies should replicate this study in a larger sample, acquiring additional data to determine the factors influencing blood supply to the region of the brain of patients affected in those with depression. The relationship to treatment response in particular needs to be explored.

Acknowledgments

The manuscript is original, Data has not previously published, including in an abstract or poster, the figures, tables, and/or data that haven't been published elsewhere, and are also not under concurrent consideration elsewhere. The authors YW, HZ, ST, FC, AO, AT, XL, MB have personally reviewed and given final approval of the version submitted, and all authors have declared that there are no biomedical financial interest or potential conflicts of interest.

Author Contributions

Conceived and designed the experiments: YW XL ST. Performed the experiments: ST FC FC. Analyzed the data: YW ST FC FC. Contributed reagents/materials/analysis tools: YW ST MB. Wrote the paper: YW HZ ST FC AO AT XL FC MB.

References

1. Taylor WD, Aizenstein HJ, Alexopoulos GS (2013) The vascular depression hypothesis: mechanisms linking vascular disease with depression. Mol Psychiatry. 18: 964–974.
2. Oda K, Okubo Y, Ishida R, Murata Y, Ohta K, et al. (2003) Regional cerebral blood flow in depressed patients with white matter magnetic resonance hyperintensity. Biol Psychiatry 53: 150–156.
3. Kume K, Hanyu H, Murakami M, Sato T, Hirao K, et al. (2011) Frontal Assessment Battery and brain perfusion images in amnestic mild cognitive impairment. Geriatr Gerontol Int. 11: 77–82.
4. Aihua N, Yanzhu B, Chunying J, Shumiao G, Xiufen W (2007) Study of Regional Cerebral Blood Flow in the Patients with Depression Treated by Cognitive Behavioral Therapy or Citalopram. Chin Gen Prac (Chin) 10: 1944–1945.
5. Takano H, Kato M, Inagaki A, Watanabe K, Kashima H (2006) Time course of cerebral blood flow changes following electroconvulsive therapy in depressive patients–measured at 3 time points using single photon emission computed tomography. Keio J Med 55: 153–160.
6. Hroudová J, Fišar Z, Kitzlerová E, Zvěřová M, Raboch J (2013) Mitochondrial respiration in blood platelets of depressive patients. Mitochondrion 13: 795–800.

7. Manji H, Kato T, Di Prospero NA, Ness S, Beal MF, et al. (2012) Impaired mitochondrial function in psychiatric disorders. Nat Rev Neurosci 13: 293–307.
8. Sacher J, Neumann J, Fünfstück T, Soliman A, Villringer A, et al. (2012) Mapping the depressed brain: a meta-analysis of structural and functional alterations in major depressive disorder. J Affect Disord 140: 142–148.
9. Kessler H, Taubner S, Buchheim A, Münte TF, Stasch M, et al. (2011) Individualized and Clinically Derived Stimuli Activate Limbic Structures in Depression: An fMRI Study. PLoS One 6: e15712.
10. Awata S, Ito H, Konno M, Ono S, Kawashima R, et al. (1998) Regional cerebral blood flow abnormalities in late-life depression: relation to refractoriness and chronification. Psychiatry Clin Neurosci 52: 97–105.
11. Ishizaki J, Yamamoto H, Takahashi T, Takeda M, Yano M, et al. (2008) Changes in regional cerebral blood flow following antidepressant treatment in late-life depression. Int J Geriatr Psychiatry 23: 805–811.
12. Navarro V, Gastó C, Lomeña F, Mateos JJ, Marcos T (2001) Frontal cerebral perfusion dysfunction in elderly late-onset major depression assessed by 99MTC-HMPAO SPECT. Neuroimage 14: 202–205.
13. Nobler MS, Roose SP, Prohovnik I, Moeller JR, Louie J, et al. (2000) Sackeim HA. Regional cerebral blood flow in mood disorders, V: Effects of antidepressant medication in late-life depression. Am J Geriatr Psychiatry 8: 289–296.
14. Davies J, Lloyd KR, Jones IK, Barnes A, Pilowsky LS (2003) Changes in regional cerebral blood flow With Venlafaxine in the Treatment of Major Depression. Am J Psychiatry 160: 374–376.
15. Milo TJ, Kaufman GE, Barnes WE, Konopka LM, Crayton JW, et al. (2001) Changes in RCBF After Electroconvulsive Therapy for Depression. J ECT 17: 15–21.
16. Colloby SJ, Firbank MJ, He J, Thomas AJ, Vasudev A, et al. (2012) Regional cerebral blood flow in late-life depression: arterial spin labelling magnetic resonance study. Br J Psychiatry 200: 150–155.
17. Post RM, DeLisi LE, Holcomb HH, Uhde TW, Cohen R, et al. (1987) Glucose utilization in the temporal cortex of affectively ill patients: positron emission tomography. Biol Psychiatry 22: 545–553.
18. Smith GS, Kramer E, Ma Y, Kingsley P, Dhawan V, et al (2009) The functional neuroanatomy of geriatric depression. Int J Geriatr Psychiatry 24: 798–808.
19. Coolens C, Breen S, Purdie TG, Owrangi A, Publicover J, et al. (2009) Implementation and characterization of a 320-slice volumetric CT scanner for simulation in radiation oncology. Med Phys 36: 5120–5127.
20. Evangelista A, Pelliccia F, Arrivi A, Gaudio C (2011) Images in 320-slice CT and myocardial bridge. BMJ Case Rep doi:10.1136/bcr.05.2011.4200
21. Song ZJ, Chen GF, Lin Jia CY, Cao JX, Ao GK (2013) The ultra-early protective effect of ulinastatin on rabbit acute lung injury induced by paraquat. BMC Emerg Med. (suppl 1): S7.
22. Shankar JJ, Lum C (2011) Whole brain CT perfusion on a 320-slice CT scanner. Indian J Radiol Imaging 21: 209–214.
23. Rickham PP (1964) Human Experimentation: code of ethics of the World Medical Association. Br Med J 18, 2: 177.
24. Baskurt OK, Boynard M, Cokelet GC, Connes P, Cooke BM, et al. (2009) New guidelines for hemorheological laboratory techniques. Clin Hemorheol Microcirc 42: 75–97.
25. Guideline developed in conjunction with the American College of Radiology (ACR), the Society for Pediatric Radiology (SPR), and the Society of Radiologists in Ultrasound (SRU) (2012) AIUM Practice Guideline for the Performance of a Transcranial Doppler Ultrasound Examination for Adults and Children, 2 th ed. American Institute of Ultrasound in Medicine Press.
26. Siebert E, Bohner G, Dewey M, Masuhr F, Hoffmann KT, et al. (2009) 320-slice CT neuroimaging: initial clinical experience and image quality evaluation. Br J Radiol. 82: 561–70.
27. Vangu MDT, Esser JD, Boyd IH, Berk M (2003) Effects of electroconvulsive therapy on regional cerebral blood flow measured by 99mtechnetium HMPAO SPECT. Progr Neuro-Psychoph 27: 15–19.
28. Kawakatsu S, Komatani A (1994) Xe-133 inhalation single photon emission computerized tomography in manic-depressive illness. Nippon Rinsho 52: 1180–1184.
29. Brockmann H, Zobel A, Joe A, Biermann K, Scheef L, et al. (2009) The value of HMPAO SPECT in predicting treatment response to citalopram in patients with major depression. Psychiatry Res 173: 107–112.
30. Cenic A, Nabavi DG, Craen RA, Gelb AW, Lee TY (1999) Dynamic CT measurement of cerebral blood flow: A validation study. AJNR Am J Neuroradiol 20: 63–73.
31. Koenig M, Kraus M, Theek C, Klotz E, Gehlen W, et al. (2001) Quantitative assessment of the ischemic brain by means of perfusion-related parameters derived from perfusion CT. Stroke 32: 431–437.
32. Cody DD, Mahesh M (2007) AAPM/RSNA physics tutorial for residents: technologic advances in multidetector CT with a focus on cardiac imaging. RadioGraphics 27: 1829–1837.
33. Hardoy MC, Cadeddu M, Serra A, Moro MF, Mura G, et al. (2011) A pattern of cerebral perfusion anomalies between major depressive disorder and Hashimoto thyroiditis. BMC Psychiatry 11: 148.
34. Gosling RG, King DH (1974) Arterial assessment by Doppler shift ultrasound. Proc R Soc Med 67: 447–449.
35. Kwater A, Gsowski J, Gryglewska B, Wizner B, Grodzicki T (2009) Is blood flow in the middle cerebral artery determined by systemic arterial stiffness? Blood Pressure 18: 130–134.
36. Lowe GD (1986) Blood rheology in arterial disease. Clin Sci 71: 137–146.
37. Jan KM, Chien S, Bigger JT Jr (1975) Observations on blood viscosity changes after acute myocardial infarction. Circulation 51: 1079–1084.
38. Wong ML, Dong C, Esposito K, Thakur S, Liu W, et al. (2008) Elevated stress-hemoconcentration in major depression is normalized by antidepressant treatment: secondary analysis from a randomized, double-blind clinical trial and relevance to cardiovascular disease risk. PLoS One 3: e2350-2355. http://dx.doi.org/doi:10.1080/08037050902975114.
39. Lechin F, van der Dijs B, Orozco B, Lechin ME, Báez S, et al. (1995) Plasma neurotransmitters, blood pressure, and heart rate during supine-resting, orthostasis, and moderate exercise conditions in major depressed patients. Biol Psychiatry 38: 166–173.
40. Orosz A, Jann K, Federspiel A, Horn H, Höfle O, et al. (2012) Reduced cerebral blood flow within the default-mode network and within total gray matter in major depression. Brain Connect 2: 303–310.
41. Botteron KN, Raichle ME, Drevets WC, Heath AC, Todd RD (2002) Volumetric reduction in left subgenual prefrontal cortex in early onset depression. Biol Psychiatry 51: 342–344.
42. Liang S. Shenxun S, Yihui G, Chuantao Z, Mingyuan Z (2006) Depression in the elderly patients with brain positron emission tomography. Chin J Psychia 39: 81–84. http://dx.doi.org/doi:10.1080/08037050902975114.

6

A Recommendation for Revised Dose Calibrator Measurement Procedures for ^{89}Zr and ^{124}I

Bradley J. Beattie*, Keith S. Pentlow, Joseph O'Donoghue, John L. Humm

Medical Physics, Memorial Sloan Kettering Cancer Center, New York, New York, United States of America

Abstract

Because of their chemical properties and multiday half lives, iodine-124 and zirconium-89 are being used in a growing number of PET imaging studies. Some aspects of their quantitation, however, still need attention. For ^{89}Zr the PET images should, in principle, be as quantitatively accurate as similarly reconstructed ^{18}F measurements. We found, however, that images of a 20 cm well calibration phantom containing ^{89}Zr underestimated the activity by approximately 10% relative to a dose calibrator measurement (Capintec CRC-15R) using a published calibration setting number of 465. PET images of ^{124}I, in contrast, are complicated by the contribution of decays in cascade that add spurious coincident events to the PET data. When these cascade coincidences are properly accounted for, quantitatively accurate images should be possible. We found, however, that even with this correction we still encountered what appeared to be a large variability in the accuracy of the PET images when compared to dose calibrator measurements made using the calibration setting number, 570, recommended by Capintec. We derive new calibration setting numbers for ^{89}Zr and ^{124}I based on their 511 keV photon peaks as measured on an HPGe detector. The peaks were calibrated relative to an ^{18}F standard, the activity level of which was precisely measured in a dose calibrator under well-defined measurement conditions. When measuring ^{89}Zr on a Capintec CRC-15R we propose the use of calibration setting number 517. And for ^{124}I, we recommend the use of a copper filter surrounding the sample and the use of calibration setting number 494. The new dose calibrator measurement procedures we propose will result in more consistent and accurate radioactivity measurements of ^{89}Zr and ^{124}I. These and other positron emitting radionuclides can be accurately calibrated relative to ^{18}F based on measurements of their 511 keV peaks and knowledge of their relative positron abundances.

Editor: C. Andrew Boswell, Genentech, United States of America

Funding: Support was provided by the National Cancer Institute P30 CA08748 [http://www.cancer.gov/] and National Cancer Institute P50 CA086438-12 [http://www.cancer.gov/] to BJB and JLH. The funder had no role in study design, data collection and analysis, decision to publish, or preparation of the manuscript.

Competing Interests: The authors have declared that no competing interests exist.

* Email: beattieb@mskcc.org

Introduction

Zirconium-89

Zirconium-89 is a positron emitting radiometal with a 3.27 day half-life and a mean positron energy of 396 keV. It also emits 909 keV cascade gamma rays but with sufficient delay that they do not cause spurious coincidences [1]. These properties, along with its tendency to residualize in cells, make ^{89}Zr an increasingly popular choice as a radiolabel for PET imaging studies of in vivo antibody distribution.

In a conference proceedings in 2006 [2], Avila-Rodriguez et al. described using a calibration setting number of 465 for the Capintec CRC-15R. However, when we applied this calibration setting number in phantom measurements seeking to verify the quantitative accuracy of the PET scanning procedures, discrepancies between the observed activity concentration derived from the PET data and the expected values based on dose calibrator measurements were noted.

Earlier work by Verel et al. in 2003 [3] proposed a dose calibrator measurement for ^{89}Zr that involved using the setting for ^{54}Mn and multiplying the displayed activity by 0.67. This procedure is independent of the dose calibrator model used but

because it involves two steps, may be overlooked by many investigators and radiopharmacists in deference to the more recent value proposed by Avila-Rodriguez. The manufacturer of the dose calibrator used in our studies, Capintec, does not make a recommendation for ^{89}Zr but based on Capintec's recommendation for ^{54}Mn and their description of the relationship between calibration setting numbers and the dose calibrator response (see equation 1 derived from the CRC-15R Owner's Manual [4]), the procedure described by Verel corresponds to the use of a calibration setting number of 504 on the CRC-15R.

$$ c' = 1076 \cdot \left(\frac{(c/1076) + 0.08}{t/m} - 0.08 \right) \quad (1) $$

where: c' is the corrected calibration setting number, c is the calibration setting number that was used (e.g. the one for ^{54}Mn), t is the true activity and m is the activity measured using calibration setting number c (note: t/m is 0.67 in the above).

Neither Verel nor Avila-Rodriguez, however, described in detail how the values they recommend were determined.

Iodine-124

Iodine-124 is a radionuclide with a complex decay scheme including a 22.9% positron abundance and a 58% abundance of x-rays in the 20 to 40 keV range. Approximately half of its positrons are followed by prompt cascade 602 keV gamma-rays [5]. These cascades add spurious coincident events to the PET projection data, which if not properly corrected for, can lead to errors in the PET quantitation. The positrons and its 4.18 day half-life, make ^{124}I an appealing isotope for use as a radiolabel in PET antibody studies and, in its iodide form, for PET-based dose estimates of radiotherapies involving [^{131}I]-iodide.

In phantom studies involving ^{124}I, we frequently noted discrepancies between PET derived activity concentrations and dose calibrator data, even though a correction for cascade coincidences was being used. Similar discrepancies were noted previously by Jentzen [6]. The problem appears to result from a combination of an inappropriate calibration setting number and the aforementioned x-rays. The x-rays may or may not be attenuated significantly depending upon the volume of the sample and what material the container is made of (this combination of properties here onward will be referred to as the measurement "geometry") thereby affecting the radioactivity measurement.

Capintec recommends using a calibration setting number of 570 for ^{124}I on the CRC-15R [4] assuming a 5 mL solution in a 0.6 mm thick borosilicate glass vial. They warn, however, of an uncertainty of about +/-5% if a plastic or glass syringe, respectively, is used when measuring the activity. To avoid this uncertainty, we make use of the recommendation described by Wiarda in 1984 [7] to use a copper filter in order to remove the contribution of the $\sim$30 keV K x-rays from the dose calibrator measurement.

Calibration

In the work we describe here, we utilize a dose calibrator measurement of an ^{18}F sample made under precisely defined conditions as a reference standard against which we calibrate both our PET camera and our HPGe measurements. Our HPGe measurements of ^{89}Zr and ^{124}I, calibrated based on the 511 keV peak of the ^{18}F reference, allowed us to determine precise calibration setting numbers to be used on the CRC-15R when measuring these radionuclides under various defined geometries. The dose calibrator we used was checked using a NIST traceable, ^{18}F cross referenced, ^{68}Ge/^{68}Ga calibration standard (Radqual Model BM06S-681, serial # BM06068S14104102). This standard mimics a 5 mL syringe and can be hung from the dose calibrator's dipper. Daily accuracy tests of the dose calibrator established its stability over the time-course of all our measurements. PET measurements of phantoms containing ^{89}Zr or ^{124}I also served to cross-validate the new calibration setting numbers.

Materials and Methods

Radionuclides

The ^{89}Zr and ^{124}I sources used in these experiments were produced by the MSKCC Radiochemistry Core via the ^{89}Y$(p,n)^{89}$Zr and ^{124}Te$(p,n)^{124}$I reactions, respectively. Irradiations were conducted using an EBCO TR19/9 cyclotron (Ebco Industries Inc., Richmond, British Columbia, Canada). All measurements were conducted at least 5 days post end-of-bombardment. Radionuclidic purity was always greater than 99.98% as determined by gamma-spectroscopy using an HPGe detector (Canberra model GC2018) coupled to a calibrated multichannel analyzer (MCA, Canberra Inspector 2000, Canberra Industries, Oak Ridge, TN, USA). The MCA was calibrated by

using ^{133}Ba (81.0, 302.8 and 356.0 keV), ^{109}Cd (88.0 keV), ^{57}Co (122.1 keV), $^{6°}$Co (1173.2 and 1332.5 keV), ^{137}Cs (661.6 keV) and ^{22}Na (1274.5 keV) standard sources from Canberra Industries, Oak Ridge, TN, USA, and data were processed using the Genie-2000 software [8]. All ^{18}F samples were purchased as clinical grade [^{18}F]-FDG from IBA Molecular (Dulles, VA). Table 1 provides a summary of the properties of these three radionuclides, pertinent to the calculations in this paper.

Dose Calibrator

All dose calibrator measurements were made on a Capintec CRC-15R supplemented with a 4 cm lead Environmental Shield (item number 7300-2450, Capintec, Inc., Pittsburgh, PA) immediately surrounding the chamber. Backscatter from this shield while measuring ^{18}F, ^{89}Zr or ^{124}I was determined to have negligible effect on the activity measurements by comparing shielded and unshielded measurements once for each radionuclide. Measurements were made with either the plastic dipper provided by the manufacturer or instead within a cylinder, 20 cm long and having a 4.1 cm outside diameter with 1.52 mm walls, of Type L rigid copper water pipe. The bottom half of the pipe was stuffed loosely with foam rubber to support the source at a location in the center of the measurement chamber. Foam extending out the bottom, centered the pipe within the well.

HPGe Detector Setup

All calibration HPGe measurements were made with a Canberra HPGe detector (model GC2020, Canberra Industries, Inc. Meriden, CT) coupled to a calibrated multichannel analyzer (Canberra Inspector 2000). The GC2020 is a liquid nitrogen cooled Standard Electrode Coaxial Ge detector with a vertical slimline dipstick, 30 liter Dewar and endcap diameter of 7.6 cm. Its energy resolution (full width half max) at 122 and 1300 keV are 1.10 and 2.0 keV, respectively.

In all cases the source, consisting of a 10 mL solution in a 20 mL vial made of 1.13 mm thick borosilicate glass (typically used for liquid-scintillation counting and made by Kimble Chase, part #74504-20) surrounded by a 5mm thick polymethyl methacrylate cylinder, was suspended from the ceiling at a height of 1.68 m above the surface of the HPGe detector (oriented vertically). This large working distance was used for three reasons: 1) to maintain a low dead-time ($<$ 10%); 2) to minimize the impact of small changes in this distance from sample placement to sample placement (variability judged to be less than 5 mm) and 3) to minimize pileup. The software controlling the Canberra HPGe detector measures counts as a function of a calibrated energy (i.e. a spectrum) and adjusts the actual time of the sampling to account for dead time.

HPGe Data Processing

Immediately prior to and following the HPGe sample measurements on any given day, 5 minute background spectral measurements were made. For these measurements, all sources were removed from the room. The two background measures were compared to one another and examined for unexpected or interfering peaks caused by unseen sources introduced in the vicinity (e.g. on an adjacent floor). In all cases they were judged acceptable and averaged together to form a single background spectrum.

The HPGe spectral measurement of each ^{18}F, ^{89}Zr or ^{124}I sample, was also acquired for 5 minutes. The averaged background spectrum was subtracted from each. The tails surrounding the 511 keV peak, 506-507 keV and 515-516 keV, in each background corrected spectral measurement were fitted with a

Table 1. Radionuclide Properties.

Radionuclide	Half-life (hours)	Positron abundance (%)	Mean positron energy (keV)	Max positron energy (keV)	(20-200 keV) x-ray abundance (%)
^{18}F	1.8	96.7	250	634	0
^{89}Zr	78.4	22.7	396	902	0
^{124}I	100.2	22.9	819	2140	58

Data in this table was taken from ICRP Publication 107 [11].

ramp which was then subtracted from the peak. Note the full width half max resolution of the Doppler-broadened annihilation photopeak is about 2.6 keV. The remaining count data between 506.5 and 515.5 keV was numerically integrated and divided by the 5 minute target measurement time (thereby accounting for the dead time).

^{18}F Reference Standard

Our calibration reference consisted of a 1 mL [^{18}F]-FDG water solution in a 3 mL Beckton Dickinson plastic syringe (cat# 309657) with attached 19 gauge needle (Beckton Dickinson cat# 395186), suspended from the plastic dipper so as to be placed near the center of the chamber of a Capintec CRC-15R dose calibrator set on calibration setting number 484. In 2008, the US National Institute of Standards and Technology (NIST), in concert with Capintec, issued a recommendation to use a calibration setting number of 484 on the CRC-15R for this geometry in order to improve the accuracy of the ^{18}F activity measurement [9]. After measurement on the dose calibrator, the contents of the syringe were transferred to a liquid scintillation vial (previously described) and the volume of the solution increased to 10 mL, rinsing the syringe into the vial in the process. Residuals were generally negligible but in any case measured and applied prior to the measurements designed to calibrate the HPGe detector setup. The HPGe measurements were made as described above. Factoring in the appropriate corrections for decay and positron abundance, the sensitivity of the HPGe detector setup, in units of integrated counts per positron, was determined.

Sample Measurements

In total we measured 5 samples of ^{89}Zr, 4 samples of ^{124}I and for calibration purposes 6 samples of ^{18}F in both the dose calibrator and on the HPGe detector. Measurements were made over a period of several weeks. On any given day in which a ^{89}Zr or ^{124}I measurement was made on the HPGe, a reference pair of calibration measurements using an ^{18}F sample were made on the dose calibrator and on the HPGe to test for potential day-to-day differences in detector sensitivity.

The accuracy of the Capintec dose calibrator was evaluated using a NIST traceable ^{68}Ge/^{68}Ga positron standard that has been cross referenced to ^{18}F. At the time of first measurement, this source contained 35.594 MBq ± 0.53% (95% confidence interval) of ^{18}F equivalent radioactivity. Several measurements over a period of two weeks were made. Each of these measurements was found to be within 0.6% of the standard's nominal radioactivity level.

For most of the samples, only the liquid scintillation vial geometry was used. Measures of radioactivity using this geometry were calibrated based on a measurement at a single calibration setting number that was subsequently adjusted using equation 1. For a subset of the samples (one ^{124}I and two ^{89}Zr), dose calibrator

measurements were made at each of six different geometries, a small volume in a 5 mL syringe (Beckton Dickinson cat# 309646) with attached needle (Beckton Dickinson cat# 395186), 3 mL in a 5 mL syringe with needle, and 10 mL in a glass liquid scintillation vial (Kimble Chase, part #74504-20), each with and without the copper filter. For each geometry five calibration setting numbers (-60, -30, +0, +30 and +60) bracketing what was thought to be approximately the correct number were used. In addition, for ^{89}Zr the calibration setting numbers of 465 and 309 (the calibration setting number for ^{54}Mn) were used. The activity measured at the 309 setting was subsequently multiplied by 0.67 as per Verel's recommendation. For ^{124}I, a calibration setting number of 570 was also used.

The full bracketed measurements generally proceeded as follows. A small volume (typically below 0.1 mL depending on the stock concentration) of ^{89}Zr or ^{124}I was drawn into a 5 mL syringe. The activity of this sample varied between 10 and 40 MBq. The sample was then measured at each of the aforementioned calibration setting number settings with the syringe suspended from the ring on the plastic dipper. The time-of-day of each measurement was recorded. All measurements were then repeated, this time with the syringe centered within the copper filter (replacing the plastic dipper) at the center of the dose calibrator's chamber. Tap water was then drawn into the syringe to bring the volume up to 3 mL. Measurements with the plastic dipper and within the copper filter were once again repeated, each time incorporating adjustments to the central bracketed calibration setting number. Finally, the contents of the syringe were transferred to a Kimble Chase KG-33 borosilicate glass 20 mL scintillation vial (cat# 03-340-4C) and the volume of the solution brought up to 10 mL. Residual activity in the syringe was generally negligible but nevertheless was measured using the copper filter at one of the calibration setting number settings used previously. All radioactivity measurements were decay corrected to a single reference time. The residual, was expressed as a fraction of the total (determined at the same calibration setting number used in the copper filter measurement) and each of the activity measures was adjusted accordingly.

Plots of activity versus bracketed calibration setting number for each sample geometry were generated and least-squares fitted to a quadratic curve. The presumed "true" activity of each sample was determined by applying the HPGe sensitivity factor to the sample's integrated counts per second and accounting for positron abundance, decay and any residual losses. Using this activity, the quadratic associated with each measurement geometry was solved to determine the calibration setting number. The calibration setting numbers for the liquid scintillation vial, with and without the copper filter, were then used in a pair of additional cross-checking dose calibrator measurements. In all cases these measures confirmed the interpolated calibration setting number.

PET Measurements

One of the ^{89}Zr samples and one of the ^{124}I samples, thus calibrated and residing in a liquid scintillation vial, was transferred (separately) to a water filled 20 cm diameter by 19 cm polymethyl methacrylate PET phantom. This phantom was then imaged on a General Electric Discovery STE PET/CT scanner. The ^{89}Zr phantom was imaged while positioned in the center of the field of view while the ^{124}I phantom was imaged both at the center and also displaced 9.3 cm vertically off-center.

This scanner uses BGO detectors and is capable of both 2D (with septa) and 3D (without septa) mode acquisitions. Its sensitivity at the center of the field of view was measured to be 2.2 cps/kBq in 2D and 8.6 cps/kBq in 3D. Its resolution in 2D is 5.4×5.4×5.4 mm at 1 cm from the central axis, falling off to 5.7×5.7×6.1 at 10 cm. In 3D at 1 cm it is 5.5×5.5×6.1 mm and at 10 cm it is 5.8×5.8×6.1 mm. The scatter fraction for the described 20 cm phantom when uniformly filled with ^{18}F is estimated to be 18% in 2D mode, while in 3D it is 26%. The measurement of the ^{89}Zr containing phantom was made in 3D mode while the measurements of ^{124}I were made in 2D. The ^{124}I raw data were corrected for cascade coincidences prior to image reconstruction using the convolution subtraction method described by Beattie et al. [10]. Volumes of interest were defined on each of the reconstructed images covering almost the entire interior volume of the phantom, but extending no closer than 1 cm to any surface. The mean activity concentration within this region, adjusted for decay and multiplied by the phantom volume, provided the PET estimate of the total radioactivity which was cross-checked against the HPGe and dose calibrator measurements.

It should be noted that particularly on some of the older PET scanners, it is wise to check that the positron abundance and decay rates entered into the scanner for ^{89}Zr and ^{124}I are indeed correct.

Results

Plots of background spectra measured on the HPGe showed negligible signal above baseline within the 511 keV window, 506-516 keV (see Figure 1A). The spectra for ^{18}F, ^{89}Zr and ^{124}I (see Figure 1B, C and D, respectively) contained no significant peaks corresponding to radioactive impurities that might contribute to the signal measured at or near to the 511 keV peak.

The measures of the six ^{18}F standards established the sensitivity of our HPGe setup to be 3.544e-05 integrated counts per positron. The coefficient of variation was 0.27%. No trend in this sensitivity was seen over time and no outliers were seen on any given day.

Plots of activity versus calibration setting number for selected samples of ^{89}Zr and ^{124}I measured in various geometries are shown in Figures 2A and B, respectively. Groups of points corresponding to a given geometry are fitted with the quadratic curve shown. The vertical bars indicate the correct activity as determined by the HPGe measurement. The height at which this bar intersects the fitted curves describes the correct calibration setting number to use for the corresponding geometry and radionuclide.

As can be appreciated from the range of calibration setting numbers needed to correctly measure ^{124}I when the copper filter is *not* used, the ^{124}I measurements are very geometry sensitive. Conversely, use of the copper filter greatly reduces the range of calibration setting numbers needed to the point where a single average calibration setting number could be used without significant error, especially if the measurement of very small volumes is avoided.

The calibration setting numbers for the syringe measurements (columns 2 and 3) in Table 2 have been interpolated from the fitted curves shown in Figure 2. The calibration setting numbers for the liquid scintillation vial (column 4) have been averaged over all calibrations. The coefficient of variation is also shown. When bracketed measures were made, the calibrated calibration setting number was determined by interpolation of the fitted quadratic. When a single measure using a single calibration setting number was made, the corrected calibration setting number was arrived at using equation 1. Our recommendation of 517 as the calibration setting number to use for ^{89}Zr is the average of the 3 ml in a 5 mL syringe and liquid scintillation vial calibration setting numbers.

Table 3 shows the errors that would have been encountered if we had assumed that the standard calibration setting numbers for ^{89}Zr and ^{124}I were correct. For ^{89}Zr, these results corroborate the procedure proposed by Verel and suggest a small but significant improvement over using a calibration setting number of 465. In general we found activity measurements of very small volumes to be relatively inaccurate. We speculate that for these small volumes, a relatively large fraction of the volume is within or near to the metal syringe needle and thus subject to different photon attenuation and positron stopping potential.

The PET measurements of ^{89}Zr confirm the HPGe calibrations to within 1.11%. For ^{124}I, the PET measurements agreed with the HPGe to within 0.43% when the phantom was centered in the field of view and to within 1.05% when the phantom was off-center.

Discussion

The absolute accuracy of the calibration setting numbers we propose for ^{89}Zr and ^{124}I are ultimately dependent upon the accuracy of our dose calibrator measurement of ^{18}F. To guard against the potential that our absolute quantitation was off, we used a well-defined geometry when making the ^{18}F activity measurements, one that precisely mimicked the measurement conditions that were used by NIST in 2009. We guarded against the potential that our dose calibrator was miscalibrated by calibrating it against a NIST traceable, ^{18}F cross referenced, ^{68}Ge/^{68}Ga dose calibrator reference standard.

The remaining potential source of error in our calibration measurements is related to the difference in the positron energies of ^{18}F, ^{89}Zr and ^{124}I. Higher energy positrons are more likely to escape the liquid scintillation vial, annihilate and produce 511 keV photons remote from the vial. The positrons of ^{18}F have a mean energy of 250 keV and max of 634 keV, ^{89}Zr has a mean of 396 keV and max of 902 keV, while ^{124}I has positrons with a mean energy of 819 keV and max of 2.14 MeV [11].

We minimized the impact of these positron energy differences by ensuring that the overwhelming majority of the positrons would annihilate within or very near to the container holding the radioactive sample. The relatively large (10 mL) volume of the radioactive solution has a small surface area to volume ratio. The glass of the liquid scintillation vial and the thick additional surrounding plastic, further ensure that the positrons are stopped locally. Based on the NIST ESTAR Stopping Power and Range Tables for Electrons [12] and on the positron energy spectra available through the DECDATA software [13], we calculated that, of the positrons at the interior surface of the glass vial emitted outward perpendicular to the surface, just 4.5% of the ^{124}I, 0.2% of the ^{89}Zr and 0.007% of the ^{18}F escape past the cylinder. Considering the small fraction of positrons at the glass surface and directed outward, the overall fraction of lost positrons is negligibly small.

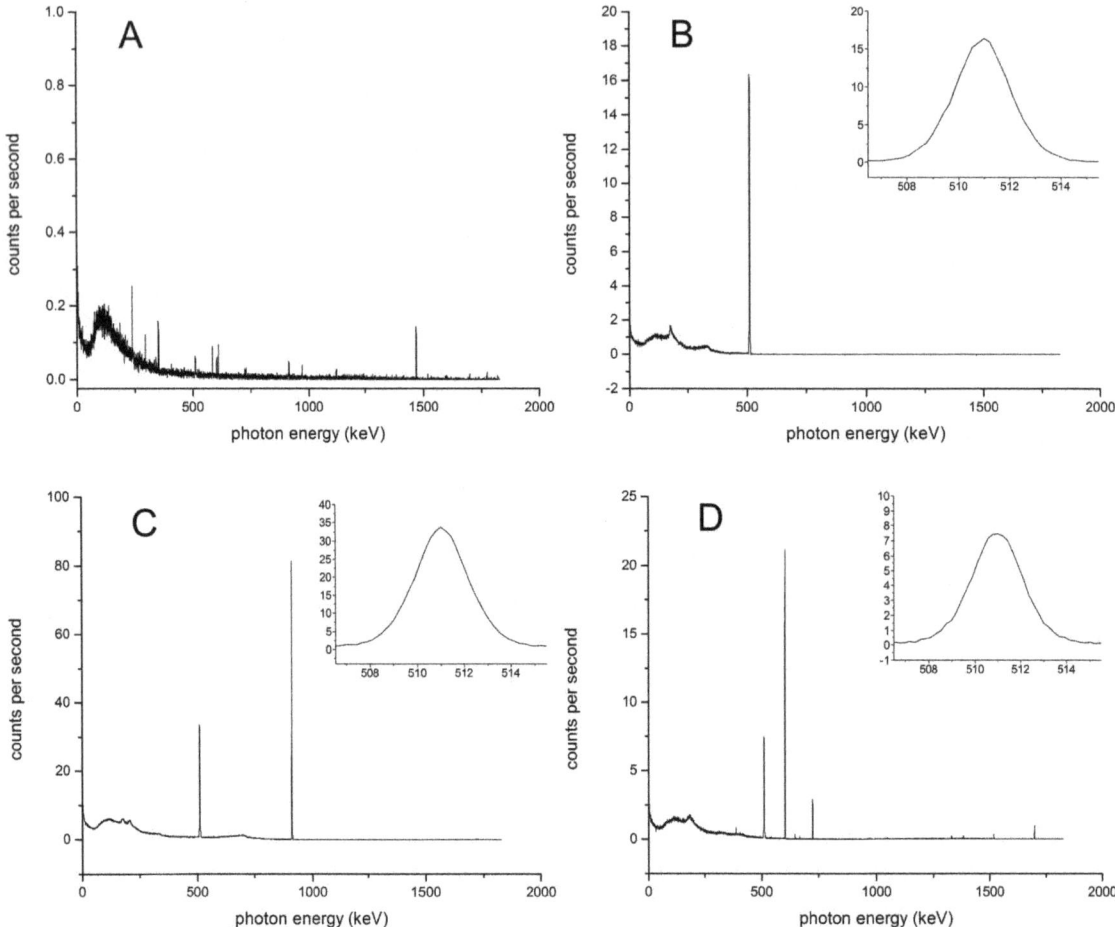

Figure 1. Photon energy spectra as measured by the Canberra HPGe detector for A) background, B) F-18, C) Zr-89 and D) I-124. Insets show close-up of 511 keV annihilation photon peak upon which calibrations were based.

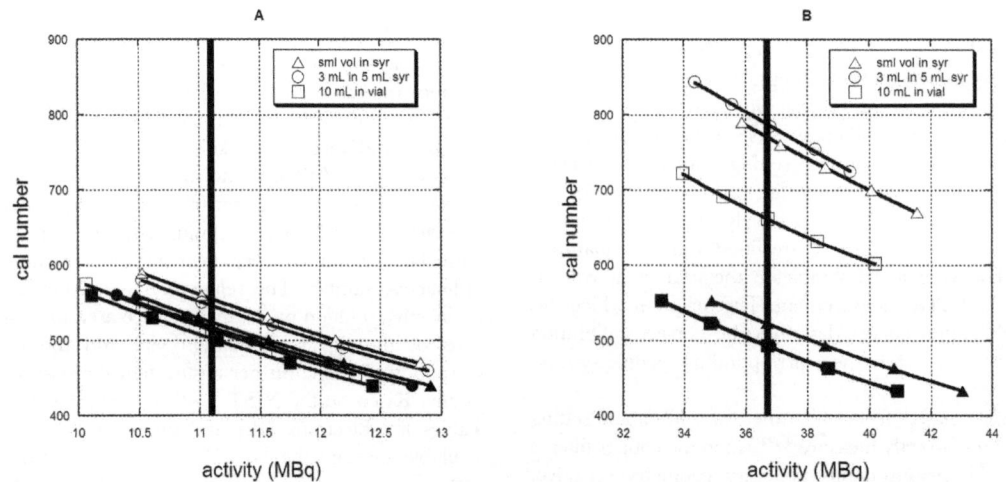

Figure 2. Activity versus calibration setting number as measured on a Capintec CRC-15R dose calibrator for A) Zr-89 and B) I-124, measured in different geometries. Filled symbols identify the curves corresponding to the measurements with the copper filter; open symbols without the filter. Triangles correspond to the small volume in the 5 mL syringe, circles to the 3 mL volume in the 5 mL syringe and squares to the 10 mL volume in the liquid scintillation vial. Note that for I-124 the filled squares almost completely obscure the filled circles.

Table 2. Recommended Calibration setting Numbers.

	Small vol 5 mL syringe calibration setting number	3 mL in 5 mL syringe calibration setting number	10 mL in liq scint vial calibration setting number +/- coef_of_var
^{89}Zr	529	524	510 +/- 0.3%
^{89}Zr in Cu filter	500	497	498 +/- 0.2%
^{124}I	749	788	664 +/- 0.5%
^{124}I in Cu filter	507	494	494 +/- 0.9%

In theory, a similar positron energy dependent difference exists for the PET measurements as well, but here with a PET phantom volume over 500 times larger, the effect is clearly negligible. That the PET measures corroborate the HPGe measurements is a further indication that the effect is indeed negligible in both circumstances.

The confidence in the corroboration between the PET and HPGe measurements is strongest between ^{89}Zr and ^{18}F, both because the positron energy distributions are more similar, but also because the PET measures are more similar in that neither ^{89}Zr nor ^{18}F require a correction for cascade coincidences. Although ^{89}Zr does indeed have 909 keV gamma-ray emissions that are in cascade with its positron, the half-time of the intermediate state (16 seconds) is longer than the timing window defining coincidences in PET.

^{124}I, on the other hand, does suffer from spurious cascade coincidences. We chose to acquire our ^{124}I PET data in 2D mode so as to minimize the magnitude of this confound, however high quantitative accuracy still requires the application of a cascade coincidence correction. The correction procedure we chose to apply is based on first principles, not a heuristic designed to produce an expected (and potentially erroneous) quantitative outcome.

The net result of our work with regard to ^{89}Zr is a recommendation to use a calibration setting number that more closely agrees with measurement procedure published by Verel. Our one-step measurement is slightly easier than Verel's but more importantly our results select between the two published (and significantly different) calibrations, the second being the 465 calibration setting number recommended by Avila-Rodriguez. Our work also shows the degree to which a single calibration setting number is accurate for ^{89}Zr over a range of geometries.

In the case of ^{124}I, we show that using the Capintec recommended calibration setting number results in large errors. There is also great variability depending on the volume and container material used in the measurement. As a means of avoiding these errors, we recommend the use of a copper filter and a calibration setting number of 494 regardless of the container and volume. The reason the copper filter has this effect is because it removes the contribution of the x-rays emitted by ^{124}I in the 20-40 keV range from the dose calibrator measurement. The x-rays in this range (in total) are 58% abundant [11] but in terms of total energy output from ^{124}I, their contribution is very small. However, for many dose calibrators the contribution of a 40 keV photon can be as great or greater than a photon with 10 times that energy (see Figure 3). Without the copper filter, the attenuation of the 20-40 keV x-rays is very variable, depending on the path length through water, plastic and glass in the sample. The photoelectric plus Compton scattering attenuation coefficient for a 40 keV photon is just 0.24 cm^{-1} in water, 0.25 cm^{-1} in plastic and 0.88 cm^{-1} in glass, whereas the attenuation coefficient in copper is 43 cm^{-1} [14]. Thus even a small amount of copper removes virtually all of these photons (the 1.52 mm copper filter we used removes 99.9%) while allowing most of the higher energy gamma-rays to still pass through. The net result is a more robust but somewhat less sensitive measurement of ^{124}I activity.

^{89}Zr also has a significant abundance of x-rays at energies that could conceivably cause geometry dependent variability in a dose calibrator measurement. These photons, in fact, likely explain the slightly reduced variability in our copper filtered measurements relative to the unfiltered. These x-rays however are in the 13 to 15 keV range which although technically above Capintec's stated 13 keV threshold, contribute much less to the radioactivity measurement compared to the 20 to 40 keV x-rays of ^{124}I. For most purposes, measurements of ^{89}Zr without a copper filter should be sufficiently accurate. However, investigators seeking greater accuracy are urged to use the copper filter with ^{89}Zr at a calibration number of 498.

Our goal in proposing these new calibration number settings and measurement procedures for ^{89}Zr and ^{124}I is to improve the accuracy of radioactivity measurements involving these radionuclides sufficient for their predominant use, in PET imaging studies. We urge others to make more careful measurements and propose calibration number settings for specific geometries to be used in applications requiring greater accuracy and precision.

Conclusion

Based on this work, we propose a new calibration setting number, 517, to be used on a Capintec CRC-15R dose calibrator

Table 3. Error in Radioactivity when Standard Calibration Setting Numbers are Used.

	Small vol 5 mL syringe (% error)	3 mL in 5 mL syringe (% error)	10 mL in liq scint vial (% error)
^{89}Zr at 465	+12.0	+11.0	+8.00
^{89}Zr at 309 × 0.67	+5.1	+3.7	+1.1
^{124}I at 570	+28.0	+33.6	+14.9

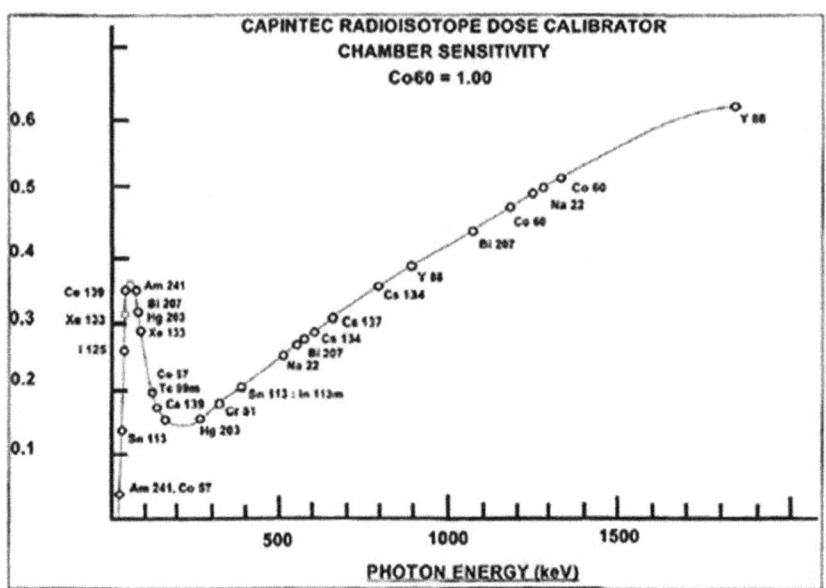

Figure 3. Plot of photon energy versus sensitivity for a Capintec CRC-15R dose calibrator. (Reprinted with permission of Capintec Inc. from the CRC-15R Owner's Manual).

when measuring samples of ^{89}Zr. Use of this number will result in approximately a 10% change in the activity measurement compared to measurements made with another published and widely used calibration setting number of 465. Our value is relatively close to an alternate two-step procedure, confirming the accuracy of that work.

We also propose the use of a copper filter and corresponding new calibration setting number, 494, to be used in activity measurements of ^{124}I. Use of this filter will avoid geometry dependent errors in the ^{124}I activity measurement. Continued use of the Capintec recommended setting of 570 can result in overestimates of the radioactivity as high as 33%. Errors of this magnitude may have serious consequences for patients if the information is used to determine the activity to be administered for therapeutic purposes and may need to be reported as misadministrations in some jurisdictions.

For each of the radionuclides, ^{18}F, ^{89}Zr and ^{124}I, with or without the copper filter, we found that very small volumes in the 5 mL syringe were measured less accurately in the dose calibrator at the recommended settings. Therefore we suggest either avoiding this geometry when accurate radioactivity measurements are needed, or that individual users derive their own calibration number settings for this geometry.

Acknowledgments

The authors wish to thank Dr. Serge Lyashchenko, Charles Davis and Yiauchung Sheh for providing us with radionuclide and access to their facilities. We further acknowledge the Radiochemistry & Molecular Imaging Probes Core of MSKCC. We wish to thank Capintec Inc. for allowing us to reprint the graph in Figure 3. And finally we wish to make note that CRC is a registered trade name of Capintec.

Supporting Information

Table S1   Zr-89 Bracketed dose calibrator measurements.

Table S2   I-124 Bracketed dose calibrator measurements.

Table S3   HPGe spectra and PET measurements.

Author Contributions

Conceived and designed the experiments: BJB KSP. Performed the experiments: BJB. Analyzed the data: BJB. Contributed reagents/materials/analysis tools: BJB JLH. Contributed to the writing of the manuscript: BJB KSP JO JLH.

References

1. Hinrichsen P (1968) Decay of 78.4 h Zr-89. Nuclear Physics A 118: 538-544.
2. Avila-Rodriguez M, Selwyn R, Converse A, Nickles R (2006) Y-86 and Zr-89 as PET Imaging Surrogates for Y-90: A Comparative Study. Medical Physics: Ninth Mexican Symposium on Medical Physics 854: 45-47.
3. Verel I, Visser GWM, Boellaard R, Stigter-van Walsum M, Snow GB, et al. (2003) Zr-89 immuno-PET: Comprehensive procedures for the production of Zr-89-labeled monoclonal antibodies. Journal of Nuclear Medicine 44: 1271-1281.
4. Capintec (2001) CRC-15R Radioisotope Dose Calibrator Owner's Manual. Ramsey, NJ: Capintec, Inc. A1-9.

5. Pentlow KS, Graham MC, Lambrecht RM, Daghighian F, Bacharach SL, et al. (1996) Quantitative imaging of iodine-124 with PET. Journal of Nuclear Medicine 37: 1557-1562.
6. Jentzen W (2010) Experimental investigation of factors affecting the absolute recovery coefficients in iodine-124 PET lesion imaging. Physics in Medicine and Biology 55: 2365-2398.
7. Wiarda K (1984) Use of a Copper Filter for Dose-Calibrator Measurements of Nuclides Emitting K X-Rays. Journal of Nuclear Medicine 25: 633-634.
8. Holland JP, Sheh YC, Lewis JS (2009) Standardized methods for the production of high specific-activity zirconium-89. Nuclear medicine and biology 36: 729-739.

9. Cessna JT, Schultz MK, Leslie T, Bores N (2008) Radionuclide calibrator measurements of F-18 in a 3 ml plastic syringe. Applied Radiation and Isotopes 66: 988-993.

10. Beattie B, Finn R, Rowland D, Pentlow K (2003) Quantitative imaging of bromine-76 and yttrium-86 with PET: A method for removal of spurious activity introduced by cascade gamma rays. Medical Physics 30: 2410-2423.

11. Eckerman K, Endo A (2008) ICRP Publication 107. Nuclear decay data for dosimetric calculations. Annals of the ICRP 38: 7-96.

12. ESTAR: Stopping Power and Range Tables for Electrons. Available: http://physics.nist.gov/PhysRefData/Star/Text/ESTAR.html. Accessed 2014 Jun 1.

13. Eckerman K, Endo A (2008) User guide to the ICRP CD and the DECDATA software. Annals of the ICRP 38: e1-e25.

14. XCOM: Photon Cross Sections Database. Available: http://www.nist.gov/pml/data/xcom/index.cfm. Accessed 2014 Jun 1.

7

Validation of a Low Dose Simulation Technique for Computed Tomography Images

Daniela Muenzel[1]*, Thomas Koehler[2], Kevin Brown[3], Stanislav Žabić[3], Alexander A. Fingerle[1], Simone Waldt[1], Edgar Bendik[1], Tina Zahel[1], Armin Schneider[4], Martin Dobritz[1], Ernst J. Rummeny[1], Peter B. Noël[1]

1 Department of Radiology, Technische Universitaet Muenchen, Munich, Germany, 2 Philips Technologie GmbH, Innovative Technologies, Hamburg, Germany, 3 Philips Healthcare, Cleveland, Ohio, United States of America, 4 MITI - Minimal-invasive Interdisciplinary therapeutic intervention research group, Technische Universitaet Muenchen, Munich, Germany

Abstract

Purpose: Evaluation of a new software tool for generation of simulated low-dose computed tomography (CT) images from an original higher dose scan.

Materials and Methods: Original CT scan data (100 mAs, 80 mAs, 60 mAs, 40 mAs, 20 mAs, 10 mAs; 100 kV) of a swine were acquired (approved by the regional governmental commission for animal protection). Simulations of CT acquisition with a lower dose (simulated 10–80 mAs) were calculated using a low-dose simulation algorithm. The simulations were compared to the originals of the same dose level with regard to density values and image noise. Four radiologists assessed the realistic visual appearance of the simulated images.

Results: Image characteristics of simulated low dose scans were similar to the originals. Mean overall discrepancy of image noise and CT values was -1.2% (range -9% to 3.2%) and -0.2% (range -8.2% to 3.2%), respectively, $p > 0.05$. Confidence intervals of discrepancies ranged between 0.9–10.2 HU (noise) and 1.9–13.4 HU (CT values), without significant differences ($p > 0.05$). Subjective observer evaluation of image appearance showed no visually detectable difference.

Conclusion: Simulated low dose images showed excellent agreement with the originals concerning image noise, CT density values, and subjective assessment of the visual appearance of the simulated images. An authentic low-dose simulation opens up opportunity with regard to staff education, protocol optimization and introduction of new techniques.

Editor: Peter M. A. van Ooijen, University of Groningen, University Medical Center Groningen, Netherlands

Funding: This work is supported by Philips Healthcare. The funder provided support in the form of salaries for authors (TK, KB, SZ), but did not have any additional role in the study design, data collection and analysis, decision to publish, or preparation of the manuscript.

Competing Interests: TK is an employee of Philips Technologie GmbH; KB and SZ are employees of Philips Healthcare. The remaining authors have no financial disclosures and had complete, unrestricted access to the study data at all stages of the study.

* Email: muenzel@tum.de

Introduction

Computed tomography (CT) examination plays a fundamental role in an all-day radiological work-up of patients in hospitals with modern healthcare equipment all around the world. Its excellent diagnostic value combined with a very short image acquisition time makes it a basic and essential diagnostic imaging tool. During the last decade there were a lot of discussions concerning an increased risk of cancer caused by the use of ionizing radiation in medicine [1,2]. On the other hand, Hendee and O'Connor recently warned against an anxiety and fear of patients sensationalized by public media with the risk of delayed or refused medical imaging and, as a consequence, delayed or missed diagnosis [3]. A clinically justified CT examination and its benefit of an accurate diagnostic work-up always outweigh its associated individual risks like e.g. stochastically induced risk of cancer [4,5]. However, these considerations encourage the demand for establishment of CT examination protocols according to the "as low as reasonably achievable" (ALARA) principle. This means an image acquisition at a radiation dose as low as possible while still maintaining a diagnostic image quality. A valid determination of the optimized dose levels for all specific CT examination protocols would demand a comparison of images of patients obtained at different dose levels. However, this would require repeated scans of the patients resulting in a significant increase of radiation exposure to these patients or probands. Therefore, it is desirable to have a computer simulation tool for reconstructing images from one original data set simulating images were acquired at lower dose levels.

The aim of this study was to evaluate and validate the software tool described in [6] for simulation of a lower dose CT acquisition from an original higher dose scan, using an animal model for non-contrast and contrast enhanced CT scans.

Methods

Animal experiment

A female landrace pig was examined with a bodyweight of 49 kg. CT image acquisition was performed with the animal under deep general anaesthesia with endotracheal intubation and controlled ventilation. All animal procedures were performed in strict accordance with the German animal protection law and were approved by the Regierung von Oberbayern; 209.1/211-2531.3-5/03.

The animal received regular feeding until 24 h before the procedure. Subsequently, it had a liquid diet until 12 h before the intervention and was kept off food for the remaining time. An 18 G venous access was placed in an ear vein for the administration of iodinated contrast. Pre-anaesthesia sedation was performed with an intramuscular injection of Azaperon (2.0 mg/kg), Atropin (0.02 mg/kg) and Ketamin (15 mg/kg). General anaesthesia was initiated by the injection of Propofol (1%) by effect. After endotracheal intubation maintenance of anaesthesia was achieved by continuous injection of propofol 2% with bolus application of Fentanyl. Oxygenation, temperature, and heart rate were continuously monitored and anaesthetic medication adapted if necessary. After completion of the CT scans, the pig was euthanized using a lethal dose of pentobarbitone and potassium chloride.

CT image acquisition

CT examinations were performed using a wide coverage 256-slice multidetector CT scanner (Brilliance iCT, Philips Healthcare, Cleveland, OH, USA). The animal was positioned in the center of the gantry. Spiral data acquisition was performed using 64×0.625 mm collimation, a pitch factor of 0.985, and a gantry rotation time of 0.4 s. Tube settings were 100 kV in all studies and 100 mAs, 80 mAs, 60 mAs, 40 mAs, 20 mAs, and 10 mAs, respectively.

Native and contrast enhanced CT examination of the chest and abdomen in arterial contrast phase were performed during end-expiratory breath-hold with the pig in supine position. For the contrast enhanced scans, a fixed volume of 50 ml of contrast agent (Imeron 400 MCT, Bracco Imaging Deutschland GmbH, Konstanz, Germany) was injected at a flow of 4 ml/s into an ear vein via an 18-gauge catheter using a dual syringe injection system (Stellant, MEDRAD, Inc., Indianola, Pennsylvania). The contrast bolus was followed by 40 mL saline solution. The scanner started data acquisition by bolus tracking. The contrast agent was washed out between the contrast-enhanced CT examinations by saline flushing for 30 minutes. However, there was an accumulation of contrast load over time, with a subsequent increase of HU of the liver parenchyma from 68 HU to 141 HU (100 mAs: 68 HU, 60 mAs: 82 HU, 20 mAs: 90 HU, 100 mAs: 116 HU, 10 mAs: 113 HU, 80 mAs: 125 HU, 40 mAs: 142 HU). To avoid any unblinding due to insufficient contrast wash-out or accumulation of contrast material in the urinary tract and the organs, CT scans of different dose levels were performed in a random order. In addition, 100 mAs data set (base of all simulations) was scanned twice, once at the beginning and once in the middle of the study protocol, in order to create simulations with more and less contrast material in the urinary tract. The time flow of image acquisition is illustrated in Figure 1.

Standard image reconstructions (filtered back projection) were obtained with 3 mm slice thickness using the CA (smooth) kernel. The reconstruction field of view was 380 mm and matrix size was 512×512.

CT low dose simulation

The CT raw data of the 100 mAs scans were retrieved from the scanner and used as input for the low dose simulation tool, which takes in account both photonic and electronic noise. Details of the low dose simulation algorithm are given in reference [6]. The resulting simulated scans at target mAs ranging from 80 mAs down to 10 mAs were reconstructed off-line with the same reconstruction parameters as the original scans.

CT values and image noise

Hounsfield units (HU) of defined regions of interest (ROI) were determined and compared for original and simulated data. Image noise was defined as the standard deviation of a 50 mm^2 ROI. Therefore, 10 representative ROIs were defined for the following material: back muscles, subcutaneous fat tissue of the ventral abdominal wall, lung tissue, fluid content of the gallbladder, and the lumbar vertebral bodies of the spine. For comparison of noise levels in different anatomical regions, image noise was defined of the shoulder girdle, dorsum, abdominal wall, and pelvis. Results of image noise were statistically analyzed for original and simulated data at corresponding radiation dose levels. Confidence intervals of mean discrepancies between the originals and simulations were calculated for all tissue and dose levels, respectively.

Observer discrimination of simulated versus original images

For a qualitative assessment of the simulated images and to approve a realistic appearance of the images, observer evaluation was performed for the contrast- enhanced images of the swine. Therefore, transverse and coronal slices (slice thickness 3 mm) were formatted for the original and simulated data sets for all dose levels. Selection of imaging features and parameters are shown in Table 1. Therefore, multiplanar reformations with different windows settings were created. In total, 160 images (5 dose levels, 16 reconstructions, original and simulation) were evaluated. 2D images were randomly arranged one by one for subjective image evaluation. Four experienced radiologists (mean clinical experience 7 years, range 3–15 years) were instructed to rate each image with regard to originality (1 = original scan or 2 = simulated one).

Statistical Analysis

Continuous data are expressed as arithmetic mean ± SD. Differences of the mean are displayed with confidence intervals. A two-tailed paired Student t-test was performed for comparison of image noise and Hounsfield units of original and simulated images for different regions of interest. Cohen kappa statistic was used for evaluation of interobserver agreement. A p-value ≤0.05 was considered to indicate statistical significance. All statistics were computed with Microsoft Excel and SPSS.

Results

CT values and image noise

CTDI values of all scan data (100 kV; 100 mAs, 80 mAs, 60 mAs, 40 mAs, 20 mAs, and 10 mAs, respectively) ranged from 4.4 mGy to 0.44 mGy.

Mean density values of different tissues such as soft tissue, bone, lung, fluid, and fat were determined in characteristic slices of the non-enhanced CT examination of the animal study. Corresponding mean HU values are shown in Figure 2.

Mean discrepancy of image noise between original and simulated CT images calculated for all tissues and all dose levels was −1.2% (range −9% to 3.2%; p>0.05). The differences in CT

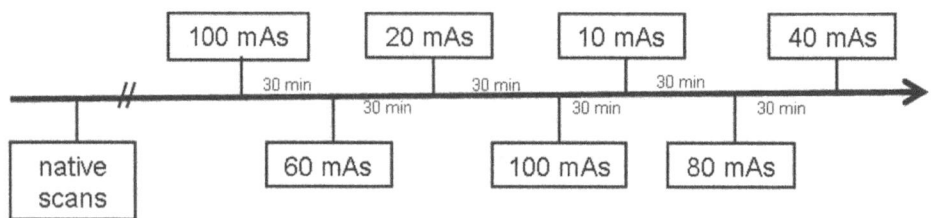

Figure 1. Time flow of CT scans at different dose levels. First, all native scans were performed. Afterwards, contrast enhanced scans were acquired, in a random order of the different dose levels. There was a gap of 30 minutes between the scans. 100 mAs scan (= base of the simulations) was achieved twice in order to minimize discrepancies between originals and simulations caused by differences in contrast accumulation.

values between original and simulated data ranged between −8.2% and 3.2%, with a mean of −0.2% (p>0.05). Image noise and CT values of characteristic tissue at different dose levels are presented in Figure 2. Similar noise was obtained for all dose levels in original and simulated images, with mean values of 21.0 vs. 20.8 (80 mAs), 24.2 vs. 23.9 (60 mAs), 29.0 vs. 28.3 (40 mAs), 42.9 vs. 42.5 (20 mAs), and 68.4 vs. 68.7 (10 mAs), p>0.05, respectively. Image noise in different anatomical regions is shown in Table 2.

Differences of the mean of noise and CT value measurements for original and simulated images were calculated for each tissue at all dose levels (Figure 3). Confidence intervals for all tissues and dose levels ranged between 0.9–10.2 HU (noise) and 1.9–13.4 HU (CT values). The value of 0 was included in all confidence intervals, and there were no significant differences between the original and simulations for all tissue and all dose levels (p>0.05).

Observer discrimination of simulated versus original images

Four radiologists rated a total of 640 images to be original or simulated. Figure 4 illustrates several examples of simulated and original images, presented for different tissue windows settings, and slice orientation. There is no visible difference between the originals and simulation. The total of 323 images (50.5%) were detected correctly as original (n = 160, 25%) or simulated (n = 163, 25.5%), p>0.05 respectively. The total of 317 images (49.5%) were mistaken to be an original (but simulated, n = 157, 24.5%) and to be a simulation (but original, n = 160, 25%). The detailed results for each observer are shown in Table 3. Comparing the results of all 4 observers, a total of 83 images were rated equally by at least 3 radiologists. In this regard, the group of radiologists consistently categorized 25 (29.1%) of the original images correctly as originals and 22 (25.6%) of the simulated images correctly as simulations. Beyond that, 45.3% (n = 39) of the images were congruently misclassified (original but simulation 24.4%, simulation but original 20.9%).

The four possible combinations of image type (original or simulation) and image rating (original and simulation) showed similar percentages of about 25% (range 24.5%–28.8%), without an observable discrimination between original and simulated images above chance level. Kappa values for all observer pairs were 0.06, −0.02, 0.09, 0.1, −0.08, and −0.09, respectively, which represents a poor interobserver agreement suggesting a subjective rating by random.

Table 1. Synopsis of the images created for individual image assessment (original versus simulated).

No.	Slice orientation	Location	Main tissue
1	transverse	Aortic arch	Vessel, lung
2	transverse	mediastinum	heart
3	transverse	hilus	Mediastinum, vessel, lung
4	transverse	abdomen	liver, stomach, spleen
5	transverse	abdomen	gallbladder, liver
6	transverse	abdomen	small bowel
7	transverse	abdomen	kidneys, small bowel
8	transverse	pelvis	bladder, bowel, soft tissue
9	transverse	pelvis	bone
10	transverse	chest	lung
11	coronal	chest	lung
12	coronal	mediastinum	Mediastinum, vessel, lung
13	coronal	abdomen	Liver, spleen, bowel, kidneys
14	coronal	abdomen	Aorta, retroperitoneum
15	coronal	chest	ribs
16	Sagittal	spine	bone

Typical clinical reformations of characteristic anatomic regions with appropriate windows settings were created, with a total of 16 images prepared for all dose levels.

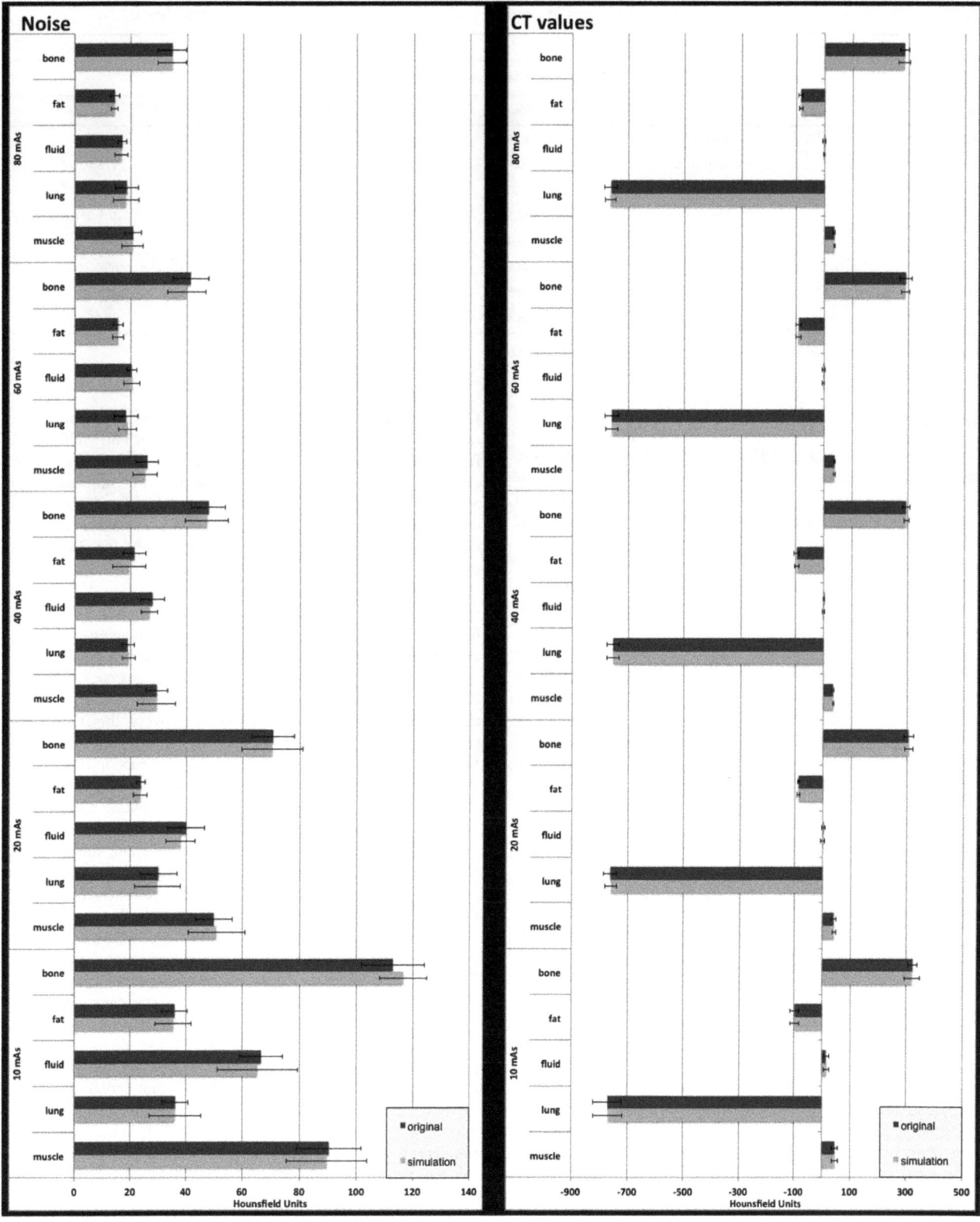

Figure 2. Mean values of image noise (left side) and CT values (right side) of characteristic tissues (bone, fat, fluid, lung, and muscle) for original (black bars) and simulated (grey bars) transverse slice images (3 mm slice thickness) at different dose levels (10, 20, 40, 60, and 80 mAs). There were no significant differences with mean discrepancies of −1.2% in image noise and −0.2% in CT values between simulated and original images. Error bars indicate standard deviation.

Table 2. Image noise for different anatomical regions in original and simulated images at different dose levels.

		dose level (mAs)				
anatomy		80	60	40	20	10
shoulder girdle	original	36.4	38.2	68.7	117.6	174.3
	simulation	38.7	40.2	68.7	115.0	173.2
dorsum	original	27.0	27.9	36.6	57.2	108.3
	simulation	27.1	28.8	33.7	58.8	109.9
abdominal wall	original	20.4	24.2	29.5	32.2	66.3
	simulation	20.5	25.5	28.7	36.2	65.3
pelvis	original	70.3	76.7	94.1	134.0	206.3
	simulation	68.7	77.5	98.5	130.4	204.5

There were no significant differences between originals and simulations (p>0.05).

Discussion

We showed in our study that it is possible to accurately simulate, based on a single acquired scan, another scan with lower dose than the actually acquired one. This technique offers the possibility to calculate lower dose images when only one examination was performed.

We approved congruent objective image parameters (noise level and HU-values) for a non-contrast CT examination of a swine. Prior studies concerning low dose computer simulation assessed metric parameters as noise and density values for comparison of original and calculated low dose images in digital chest radiography [7], tomosynthesis [8], and CT images [9–11]. Mayo et al. presented a computer modification tool for simulation images with increased image noise already in 1997 [12]. Prior simulation techniques mainly focused on the addition of image noise for simulation of lower dose images [10,12,13]. In our study, we evaluated a new technique [6], which makes use of the conditional variance identity to properly account for the variance of the input high-dose data, and allows for the inclusion of real samples of detector noise, properly scaled according to the level of the simulated x-ray signals. Phantom measurements using this technique and noise power spectrum analysis were described previously by Zabić et al. [6].

The major difference of our model compared the other models that we know of are the following: First, all other models make an approximation at some point in their derivation that a noisy signal from the high dose scan can be assumed noiseless. We use conditional variance identity to avoid that approximation which ultimately results in a method which does not depend on the noise variance in the original data set. We can start from any tube current and simulate any lower dose tube current without making that key approximation (described in detail in [6]). Another big step is that we use electronic noise samples from the real scanner, rather than simulating them as zero-mean Gaussian distribution. As discussed in [6] we conclude that if one wants to simulate contributions of the electronic noise correctly, then one has to take in account that the statistical distribution of the noise is strictly non-Gaussian.

We also included subjective evaluation of simulated images for contrast-enhanced CT in order to evaluate the potential of acquisition simulation in an examination setting closely adapted to the clinical examination of patients. This additional analysis was performed by a subjective image assessment by four experienced radiologists. They were not able do distinguish the original from simulated images above chance level, as the visual impact of original and simulated images was equivalent. This is of fundamental importance for the validation of a low dose simulator, as a final objective low dose simulation should be implemented in a clinical investigation setting. Here, radiologists will be able to determine the specific radiation dose that is necessary to achieve diagnostic quality of CT images by a minimized radiation exposure according to the ALARA principle.

CT is an essential imaging tool for the clinical day-to-day routine, as e.g. tumor follow-up in malignancy, trauma emergency department, or new techniques like perfusion imaging of the brain and the myocardium. There are a lot of CT examination protocols with different scan parameters (mAs, kVp, filters etc.) adapted to the individual clinical symptoms and specific diseases. On this note, with additional capabilities CT overs the number of protocols has significantly increased over the last years [14]. Especially the introduction of iterative reconstruction methods has widened the number of parameters possible for each protocol [15–20]. For each CT protocol, the optimal combination of required dose and imaging parameters has to be defined. However, this is problematic: systematic analysis of dose level and image quality would require repetitive scan of the patients, resulting in an inadequate high effective dose for those volunteers. Still, it is important to adjust the scan protocols to the standards of diagnostic imaging, while lowering the effective dose as far as possible. Adequate parameters for tube current and tube output have do be defined for each examination setting, but also for different scanners and different patient characteristics e.g. body weight. This topic is of special interest in pediatric radiology. Here, it is of special importance to define CT examination protocols providing diagnostic image quality by using preferably low radiation dose. Frush et al. presented a simulation technology for systematic evaluation of radiation dose reduction for abdominal multidetector CT of pediatric patients [21]. Thus, a valid dose simulation technique offers the possibility to perform dose calculation and optimization for CT examinations of each part of the body without repetitive scans of a group of test subjects.

In addition, low dose simulations can be used for education for medical technical assistants and the radiologists to depict the potential differences or equivalency of the same examination in the same patient at different dose levels. Training programs for radiological departments can help to substantially reduce radiation dose [22]. Therefore, CT simulation tools may visualize and facilitate the comprehension of potential dose saving strategies. Thus, the approach of dose reduction in routine clinical

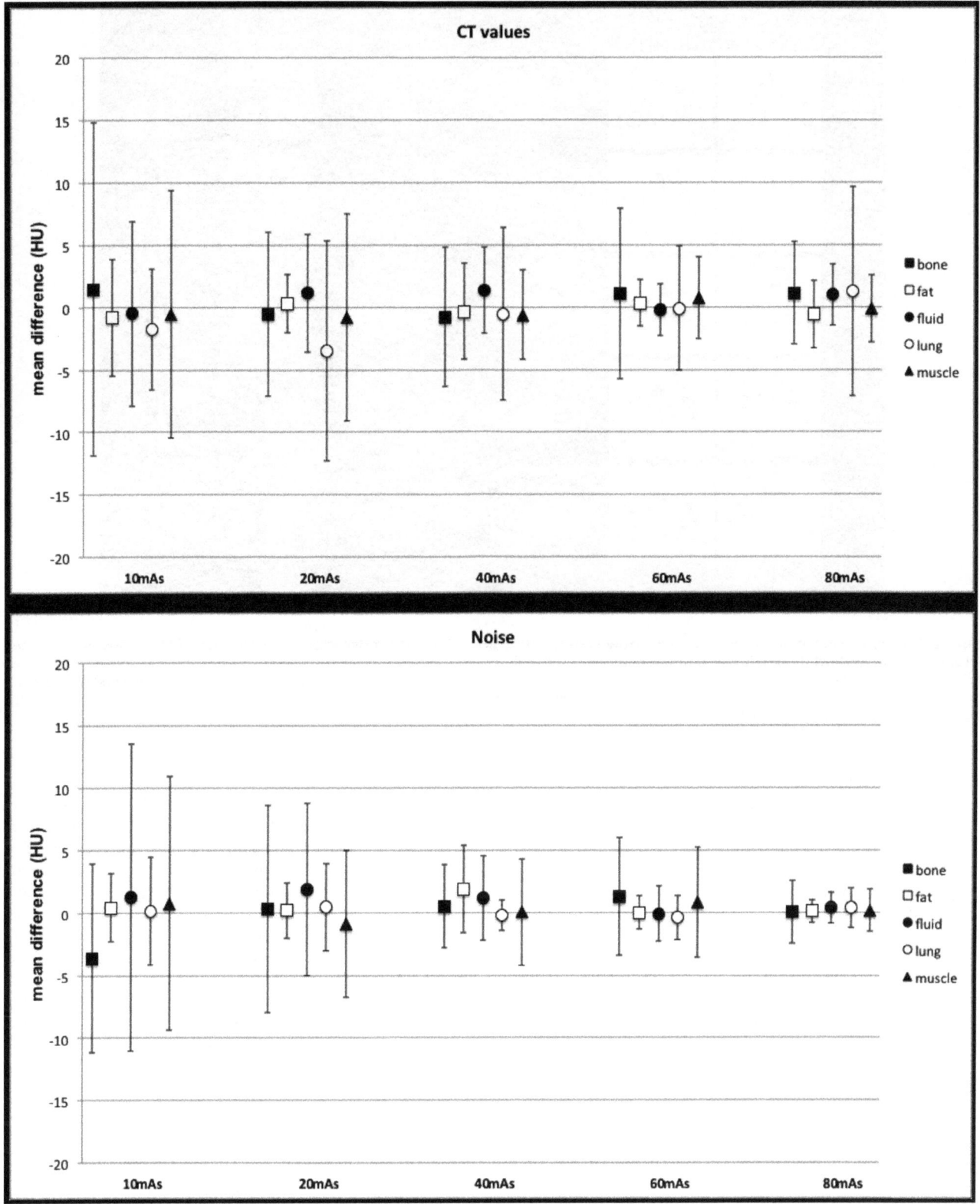

Figure 3. Differences of the mean and confidence interval for noise (a) and CT values (b) for bone, fat, fluid, lung, and muscle at different dose levels.

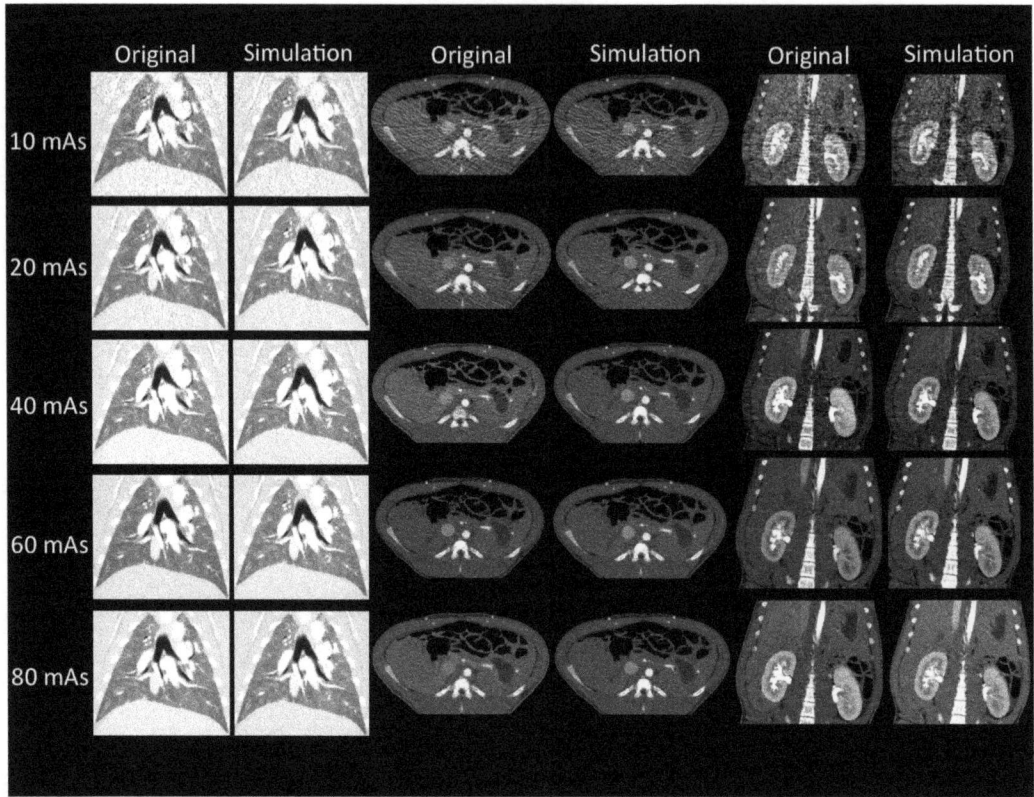

Figure 4. Coronal reformations with lung window settings (left side) showed similar image appearance of the lungs in simulated (right column) and original (left column) images. Simulated (right column) versus original (left column) images of the abdomen in transverse orientation are shown in the middle part. Image noise and streak artifacts are increased in lower dose images without visually detectable differences between original and simulated images. Also the simulated (right column) and original (left column) reformations of the abdomen including the kidneys in coronal orientation matched closely (right side).

radiological examinations will attract increased interest, providing a concrete and demonstrative view on the resulting image quality and diagnostic value.

Lowering radiation dose is the hot topic of CT imaging techniques today. During the last ten years, several techniques for adapting of radiation dose to the patient physiognomy and the individual examination procedures were implemented to routine CT protocols [23–26]. In addition, there are several new approaches such as noise reduction techniques, iterative reconstruction or postprocessing techniques [15,23,27–29]. All these methods target a substantial decrease in radiation dose while maintaining diagnostic image quality. So routine CT examinations with effective radiation dose less than 1 mSv seem to be realistic in

the near future. As a consequence, J. Thrall raised the question of considerations on radiation dose in clinical CT examinations should change from ALARA principle to AHARA (as high as reasonably achievable), pointing out the importance of a maximum benefit of diagnostic imaging using ionizing radiation dose [14]. So it will remain a challenge to optimize the balance between lowest radiation dose and highest diagnostic value. In this discussion, lower dose simulation techniques may help for visualization and determination of adequate dose settings in clinical CT.

There are some limitations of our study. First, the contrast enhancement of simulated and original images was not identical, because of slightly different contrast enhancement of the vessels

Table 3. Subjective image evaluation.

observer 1	rated original	rated simulated	observer 2	rated original	rated simulated
Original	37 (23.1%)	43 (26.9%)	Original	35 (21.9%)	45 (28.1%)
Simulation	42 (26.3%)	38 (23.8%)	Simulation	38 (23.8%)	42 (26.2%)
observer 3	rated original	rated simulated	observer 4	rated original	rated simulated
Original	42 (26.3%)	38 (23.8%)	Original	46 (28.8%)	34 (21.3%)
Simulation	39 (24.4%)	41 (25.6%)	Simulation	38 (23.8%)	42 (26.3%)

The total of 160 images (80 original and 80 simulated) were presented to four radiologists. The four possible combinations of image type (original or simulation) and image rating (original and simulation) showed similar percentages of about 25% (range 24.5%–28.8%), suggesting a subjective rating by random.

and an accumulation of contrast material due to repetitive examinations; therefore, quantitative measurements have been performed on non contrast-enhanced scans. In addition, we did not use topogram-based tube current modulation in our study. However, as shown by Zabic et al., this simulation method is also compatible with tube modulation.

In conclusion, we showed that CT low dose simulation is a feasible and valid method for definition of adequate dose levels in CT. Thus, computer simulation of different dose levels provides an excellent base for future radiation dose optimization of diverse CT examination protocols for improved patient care.

Author Contributions

Conceived and designed the experiments: DM TK KB SZ EJR PBN. Performed the experiments: DM AS PBN MD. Analyzed the data: DM TK AAF SW EB TZ. Contributed reagents/materials/analysis tools: DM AS TK KB SZ PBN EJR. Wrote the paper: DM TK KB SZ PBN.

References

1. Amis ES Jr, Butler PF, Applegate KE, Birnbaum SB, Brateman LF, et al. (2007) American College of Radiology white paper on radiation dose in medicine. J Am Coll Radiol 4: 272–284.
2. McCollough C, Cody D, Edyvean S, Geise R, Gould B, et al. (2008) The measurement, reporting, and management of radiation dose in CT. College Park, MD: American Association of Physicists in Medicine, AAPM report no.96.
3. Hendee WR, O'Connor MK (2012) Radiation risks of medical imaging: separating fact from fantasy. Radiology 264: 312–321.
4. Brenner DJ, Doll R, Goodhead DT, Hall EJ, Land CE, et al. (2003) Cancer risks attributable to low doses of ionizing radiation: assessing what we really know. Proc Natl Acad Sci U S A 100: 13761–13766.
5. Schmidt CW (2012) CT scans: balancing health risks and medical benefits. Environ Health Perspect 120: A118–121.
6. Žabić S, Wang Q, Morton T, Brown KM (2013) A low dose simulation tool for CT systems with energy integrating detectors. Medical physics 40: 1–14.
7. Veldkamp WJ, Kroft LJ, van Delft JP, Geleijns J (2009) A technique for simulating the effect of dose reduction on image quality in digital chest radiography. J Digit Imaging 22: 114–125.
8. Svalkvist A, Båth M (2010) Simulation of dose reduction in tomosynthesis. Med Phys 37: 258–269.
9. Joemai RM, Geleijns J, Veldkamp WJ (2010) Development and validation of a low dose simulator for computed tomography. Eur Radiol 20: 958–966.
10. Söderberg M, Gunnarsson M, Nilsson M (2010) Simulated dose reduction by adding artificial noise to measured raw data: a validation study. Radiat Prot Dosimetry 139: 71–77.
11. Wang AS, Pelc NJ (2011) Synthetic CT: simulating low dose single and dual energy protocols from a dual energy scan. Med Phys 38: 5551–5562.
12. Mayo JR, Whittall KP, Leung AN, Hartman TE, Park CS, et al. (1997) Simulated dose reduction in conventional chest CT: validation study. Radiology 202: 453–457.
13. Britten AJ, Crotty M, Kiremidjian H, Grundy A, Adam EJ (2004) The addition of computer simulated noise to investigate radiation dose and image quality in images with spatial correlation of statistical noise: an example application to X-ray CT of the brain. Br J Radiol 77: 323–328.
14. Thrall JH (2012) Radiation Exposure in CT Scanning and Risk: Where Are We? Radiology 264: 325–328.
15. Noël PB, Fingerle AA, Renger B, Münzel D, Rummeny EJ, et al. (2011) Initial performance characterization of a clinical noise-suppressing reconstruction algorithm for MDCT. AJR Am J Roentgenol 197: 1404–1409.
16. Winklehner A, Karlo C, Puippe G, Schmidt B, Flohr T, et al. (2011) Raw data-based iterative reconstruction in body CTA: evaluation of radiation dose saving potential. Eur Radiol 21: 2521–2526.
17. Becker HC, Augart D, Karpitschka M, Ulzheimer S, Bamberg F, et al. (2012) Radiation exposure and image quality of normal computed tomography brain images acquired with automated and organ-based tube current modulation multiband filtering and iterative reconstruction. Invest Radiol 47: 202–207.
18. Gramer BM, Muenzel D, Leber V, von Thaden AK, Feussner H, et al. (2012) Impact of iterative reconstruction on CNR and SNR in dynamic myocardial perfusion imaging in an animal model. Eur Radiol 22: 2654–2661.
19. Han BK, Grant KL, Garberich R, Sedlmair M, Lindberg J, et al. (2012) Assessment of an iterative reconstruction algorithm (SAFIRE) on image quality in pediatric cardiac CT datasets. J Cardiovasc Comput Tomogr 6: 200–204.
20. Nakaura T, Nakamura S, Maruyama N, Funama Y, Awai K, et al. (2012) Low contrast agent and radiation dose protocol for hepatic dynamic CT of thin adults at 256-detector row CT: effect of low tube voltage and hybrid iterative reconstruction algorithm on image quality. Radiology 264: 445–454.
21. Frush DP, Slack CC, Hollingsworth CL, Bisset GS, Donnelly LF, et al. (2002) Computer-simulated radiation dose reduction for abdominal multidetector CT of pediatric patients. AJR Am J Roentgenol 179: 1107–1113.
22. Schindera ST, Treier R, von Allmen G, Nauer C, Trueb PR, et al. (2011) An education and training programme for radiological institutes: impact on the reduction of the CT radiation dose. Eur Radiol 21: 2039–2045.
23. McCollough CH, Chen GH, Kalender W, Leng S, Samei E, et al. (2012) Achieving routine submillisievert CT scanning: report from the summit on management of radiation dose in CT. Radiology 264: 567–580.
24. Mulkens TH, Bellinck P, Baeyaert M, Ghysen D, Van Dijck X, et al. (2005) Use of an automatic exposure control mechanism for dose optimization in multi-detector row CT examinations: clinical evaluation. Radiology 237: 213–223.
25. Gies M, Kalender WA, Wolf H, Suess C (1999) Dose reduction in CT by anatomically adapted tube current modulation. I. Simulation studies. Med Phys 26: 2235–2247.
26. McCollough CH, Bruesewitz MR, Kofler JM (2006) CT dose reduction and dose management tools: overview of available options. RadioGraphics 26: 503–512.
27. Thibault JB, Sauer KD, Bouman CA, Hsieh J (2007) A three-dimensional statistical approach to improved image quality for multislice helical CT. Med Phys 34: 4526–4544.
28. Deák Z, Grimm JM, Treitl M, Geyer LL, Linsenmaier U, et al. (2013) Filtered back projection, adaptive statistical iterative reconstruction, and a model-based iterative reconstruction in abdominal CT: an experimental clinical study. Radiology 266: 197–206.
29. Beister M, Kolditz D, Kalender WA (2012) Iterative reconstruction methods in X-ray CT. Phys Med 28: 94–108.

8

A Comparison of Micro-CT and Dental CT in Assessing Cortical Bone Morphology and Trabecular Bone Microarchitecture

Jui-Ting Hsu[1], Ying-Ju Chen[2], Jung-Ting Ho[1], Heng-Li Huang[1], Shun-Ping Wang[3], Fu-Chou Cheng[2], Jay Wu[4], Ming-Tzu Tsai[5]*

1 School of Dentistry, College of Medicine, China Medical University, Taichung, Taiwan, 2 Stem Cell Medical Research Center, Department of Medical Research, Taichung Veterans General Hospital, Taichung, Taiwan, 3 Department of Orthopaedics, Taichung Veterans General Hospital, Taichung, Taiwan, 4 Department of Biomedical Imaging and Radiological Science, China Medical University, Taichung, Taiwan, 5 Department of Biomedical Engineering, Hungkuang University, Taichung, Taiwan

Abstract

Objective: The objective of this study was to evaluate the relationship between the trabecular bone microarchitecture and cortical bone morphology by using micro-computed tomography (micro-CT) and dental cone-beam computed tomography (dental CT).

Materials and Methods: Sixteen femurs and eight fifth lumbar vertebrae were collected from eight male Sprague Dawley rats. Four trabecular bone microarchitecture parameters related to the fifth lumbar vertebral body (percent bone volume [BV/TV], trabecular thickness [TbTh], trabecular separation [TbSp], and trabecular number [TbN]) were calculated using micro-CT. In addition, the volumetric cancellous bone grayscale value (vCanGrayscale) of the fifth lumbar vertebral body was measured using dental CT. Furthermore, four cortical bone morphology parameters of the femoral diaphysis (total cross-sectional area [TtAr], cortical area [CtAr], cortical bone area fraction [CtAr/TtAr], and cortical thickness [CtTh]) were calculated using both micro-CT and dental CT. Pearson analysis was conducted to calculate the correlation coefficients (r) of the micro-CT and dental CT measurements. Paired-sample t tests were used to compare the differences between the measurements of the four cortical bone morphology parameters obtained using micro-CT and dental CT.

Results: High correlations between the vCanGrayscale measured using dental CT and the trabecular bone microarchitecture parameters (BV/TV [$r = 0.84$] and TbTh [$r = 0.84$]) measured using micro-CT were observed. The absolute value of the four cortical bone morphology parameters may be different between the dental CT and micro-CT approaches. However, high correlations (r ranged from 0.71 to 0.90) among these four cortical bone morphology parameters measured using the two approaches were obtained.

Conclusion: We observed high correlations between the vCanGrayscale measured using dental CT and the trabecular bone microarchitecture parameters (BV/TV and TbTh) measured using micro-CT, in addition to high correlations between the cortical bone morphology measured using micro-CT and dental CT. Further experiments are necessary to validate the use of dental CT on human bone.

Editor: Luc Malaval, Université Jean Monnet, France

Funding: This study was supported by China Medical University, Taiwan (Grant number: CMU102-S-23) and the National Science Council, Taiwan (Grant number: NSC 102-2221-E-039-011). The funders had no role in study design, data collection and analysis, decision to publish, or preparation of the manuscript.

Competing Interests: The authors have declared that no competing interests exist.

* Email: anniemtt@gmail.com

Introduction

Human bones are generally classified into cortical bone (synonymous with compact bone) and cancellous bone (synonymous with trabecular bone or spongy bone). The two types are classified based on porosity and the unit microstructure. Cortical bone is much denser than cancellous bone with a porosity ranging between 5% and 30% [1]. Cortical bone is primarily located in the shaft of long bones and forms the outer shell around cancellous bone (vertebrae or pelvis). Cancellous bone is considerably more porous than cortical bone with a porosity ranging between 30%

and 90% [1]. It is located at the end of long bones and vertebrae, and in flat bones such as the pelvis.

Bone quality and quantity are affected by numerous factors, such as age, hormones, arthritis, and exercise. Clinically, orthopedic physicians commonly use dual energy X-ray absorptiometry (DXA) to measure the bone mineral density (BMD) of the femoral neck or spine for determining patients' bone strength [2]. Bone strength is affected by both geometric parameters and densitometric parameters. However, DXA provides only areal BMD information [3,4], and does not include geometric parameters, such as size and shape. Although quantitative computed tomography (QCT) can provide both geometric and densitometric parameters [2,5], the clinical application of this technique is not extensive because of the cost and high radiation dosage.

In the past two decades, microcomputed tomography (micro-CT) has been extensively used in the study of bone tissue [6–14]. Except for the densitometric parameters (volumetric BMD), the geometric parameters of bone can be precisely detected using micro-CT; for example, total cross-sectional area (TtAr), cortical area (CtAr), cortical bone area fraction (CtAr/TtAr), and cortical thickness (CtTh) can be detected [15]. Furthermore, micro-CT can provide detailed information on the trabecular bone, such as percent bone volume (BV/TV), bone specific surface (BS/BV), trabecular thickness (TbTh), trabecular bone separation (TbSp), and mean trabecular bone number (TbN) [15]. Therefore, micro-CT can be considered the gold standard for evaluating trabecular bone structure. However, micro-CT cannot be applied on humans because of the small scanning range [16].

Recently, dental cone-beam computed tomography (dental CT) has been widely used to evaluate alveolar bone density prior to dental implant placement [17–23]. Nomura et al. [24] indicated that dental CT could be used to evaluate bone mineral content based on the voxel values. In addition, numerous researchers have used the grayscale of dental CT to represent bone density (bone density in grayscale value), which is also called radiographic bone density [20–23]. However, most of these researchers have used dental CT in dental-related research or clinical trials. In our previous study [16], we indicated that dental CT is superior to DXA for predicting cortical bone fracture loads in rat femurs and tibias. Nevertheless, the relation between the bone density in grayscale measured using dental CT and trabecular bone microarchitectures is still unclear. Therefore, the purpose of this study was to evaluate the relationship between cortical bone morphology and trabecular bone microarchitecture by using micro-CT and dental CT.

Materials and Methods

Specimen preparation

Sixteen femurs and eight fifth lumbar vertebrae were collected from eight 4-month-old healthy male Sprague Dawley rats. All rats were killed by carbon dioxide asphyxiation, the entirety of the femurs and fifth lumbar vertebrae were harvested from every rat within 20 min. The bone specimens were wrapped with gauze soaked in saline and stored in a −20°C freezer. The study procedures were conducted in strict accordance with the recommendations provided in the Guide for the Care and Use of Laboratory Animals of the National Institutes of Health. We obtained animal research ethics approval from the Research Ethics Committee of the Taichung Veterans General Hospital (Permit Number: La-1021069).

Micro-CT measurement

The micro-CT images of each femur and fifth lumbar vertebrae were obtained using a Skyscan 1076 micro-CT device (Skyscan, Aartselaar, Belgium) (Fig. 1a). The scanning parameters were set at 49 kV, 200 μA, 500 ms, and a voxel resolution of 18.27 μm. The micro-CT images were imported into CTAn software (Skyscan) to measure the four parameters of trabecular bone microarchitecture: BV/TV, TbTh, TbSp, and TbN of the cancellous bone in the fifth lumbar vertebral body (Fig. 1b). Furthermore, four parameters of cortical bone morphology, TtAr, CtAr, CtAr/TtAr, and CtTh of the femoral diaphysis, were

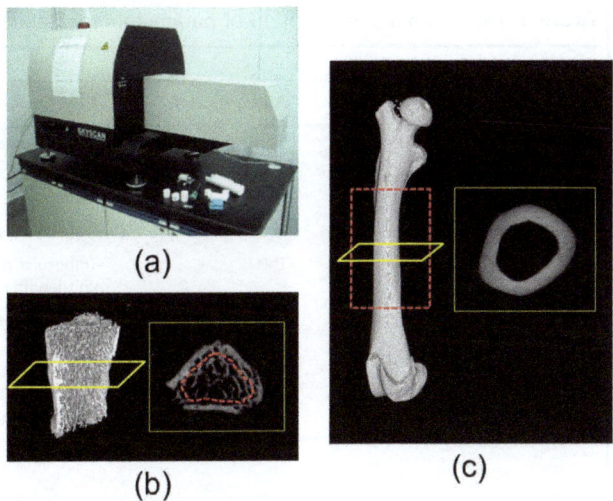

Figure 1. Micro-CT machine, images and 3D renderings. (a) Micro-CT machine (Skyscan 1076), (b) hemi 5th lumbar vertebral body (excluded the posterior element) in left, the section of the micro-CT image in right (the region of interest for trabecular bone calculated also shown in dotted red line), and (c) intact femur (the region of interest for cortical bone calculated also shown in dotted red line) in left, the section of the micro-CT image in right.

calculated (Fig. 1c) using ImageJ (Rasband, W.S., ImageJ, U.S. National Institutes of Health, Bethesda, MD, USA). The parameters of trabecular bone microarchitecture and cortical bone morphology measured in this study are listed in Table 1.

Dental CT measurement

A dental CT device (AZ 3000, Asahi Roentgen, Japan) was used to obtain dental CT images of each femur (Fig. 2a). The scanning parameters were set at 85 kV, 3 mA, and a voxel resolution of 100 μm. In the dental CT approach, we used only one grayscale value (volumetric cancellous bone grayscale value, vCanGrayscale) to represent the cancellous bone of the fifth lumbar vertebral body because the resolution of dental CT is not sufficiently high for detecting the trabecular bone structure of rats. In addition, because identifying the border between the cortical and cancellous bone of a vertebral body is difficult, we first segmented the vertebral body (including the inner cancellous bone and outer cortical layer) and then eroded the segments using 3 voxel (0.3 mm) to exclude the cortical bone. Finally, the vCanGrayscale of the fifth lumbar vertebral body could be obtained (Fig. 2b). In addition, using a similar micro-CT approach, the TtAr, CtAr, CtAr/TtAr, and CtTh of the midshaft of the femurs (in the same region as that used for the micro-CT scans) were calculated (Fig. 2c). All measurements obtained in the dental CT approach were calculated using ImageJ.

Statistical analysis

The mean, standard deviation, and coefficient of variation (CV) were calculated for all measurements. The Shapiro-Wilk test was used to determine if the measurements conformed to a normal distribution. The Pearson correlation coefficients (r values) between the vCanGrayscale measurements obtained using dental CT and the four trabecular bone microarchitecture parameters (BV/TV, TbN, TbTh, and TbSp) were calculated. Paired-sample t tests were used to compare the differences between the measurements of the four cortical bone morphology parameters

Table 1. Definition and description of parameters for trabecular bone microarchitecture and cortical bone morphology.

Bone type	Abbreviation	Description	Unit
Trabecular bone (5th lumbar vertebral body)	BV/TV	Bone volume fraction: Ratio of the segmented bone volume to the total volume of the region of interest	%
	TbTh	Trabecular thickness: Mean thickness of trabeculae	mm
	TbSp	Trabecular separation: Mean distance between trabeculae	mm
	TbN	Trabecular number: Measure of the average number of trabeculae per unit length	1/mm
Cortical bone (femoral diaphysis)	TtAr	Total cross-sectional area inside the periosteal envelope	mm^2
	CtAr	Cortical bone area	mm^2
	CtAr/TtAr	Cortical area fraction	%
	CtTh	Average cortical thickness	mm

(TbAr, CtAr, CtAr/TbAr, and CtTh) measured using micro-CT and the dental CT measurements. In addition, the Pearson correlation coefficients (r values) between these parameters measured using the two approaches were calculated. All statistical analyses of the data were performed using OriginPro software (version 8, OriginLab, Northampton, MA, USA). The level of statistical significance was set as $p < 0.05$.

Results

Relation between the trabecular bone microarchitecture parameters measured using micro-CT and dental CT

The trabecular bone parameters of the fifth vertebral body measured using micro-CT and dental CT are listed in Table 2. All of the experimental data were normally distributed based on the Shapiro-Wilk test analysis. In the dental CT approach, the CV of the vCanGrayscale was 32.112%, which is higher than the CV of the four trabecular bone microarchitecture parameters (24.509%,

6.974%, 19.088%, and 20.769 for BV/TV, TbTh, TbSp, and TbN, respectively.) The correlation coefficient between the grayscale measured using dental CT and the BV/TV measured using micro-CT was 0.84 ($p < 0.01$), which is slightly higher than the value of 0.84 ($p < 0.01$), which was the correlation coefficient between the grayscale measured using dental CT and the TbTh measured using micro-CT (Fig. 3ab). These two coefficient values (both equal to 0.84) are all highly positive correlations. In addition, the correlation coefficients between the grayscale measured using dental CT and the TbN and TbSp measured using micro-CT were 0.67 ($p = 0.07$) and -0.38 ($p = 0.36$), respectively. However, both correlation coefficient values were nonsignificant ($p > 0.05$) (Fig. 3cd).

Relation between the cortical bone morphology parameters measured using micro-CT and dental CT

The cortical bone morphology parameters of the femoral diaphysis measured using micro-CT and dental CT are listed in Table 3. All of the experimental data were normally distributed based on the Shapiro-Wilk test analysis. The TtAr parameter, which was measured using micro-CT (9.22 ± 0.47 mm^2), was significantly ($p < 0.01$) larger than that measured using dental CT (8.82 ± 0.59 mm^2). However, the CtAr/TtAr and CtTh parameters, both measured using dental CT (0.71 ± 0.05 for CtAr/TtAr, 0.87 ± 0.07 for CtTh), were significantly ($p < 0.01$) larger than that measured using micro-CT (0.66 ± 0.04 for CtAr/TtAr, 0.71 ± 0.03 for CtTh). For the CtAr parameter, no significant difference between the two approaches was observed (6.28 ± 0.61 for dental CT and 6.11 ± 0.34 for micro-CT). The correlation coefficient between the TtAr, CtAr, CtAr/TtAr, and CtTh measured using micro-CT and dental CT was 0.90 ($p < 0.01$), 0.76 ($p < 0.01$), 0.79 ($p < 0.01$), and 0.71 ($p < 0.01$), respectively (Fig. 4). All of these values indicated highly positive correlations.

Discussion

Measuring bone quality, quantity, and strength is a clinically crucial topic. Although micro-CT can be used to obtain trabecular bone microarchitectures and cortical bone morphology, this technology cannot be employed in measuring human bones because of the size limitations of such devices. Dental CT is becoming widely used in recent years. However, most previous studies on adopting dental CT to assess bone quality and bone quantity have been mainly concerned with presurgical dental implant assessments. According to our extensive research, no

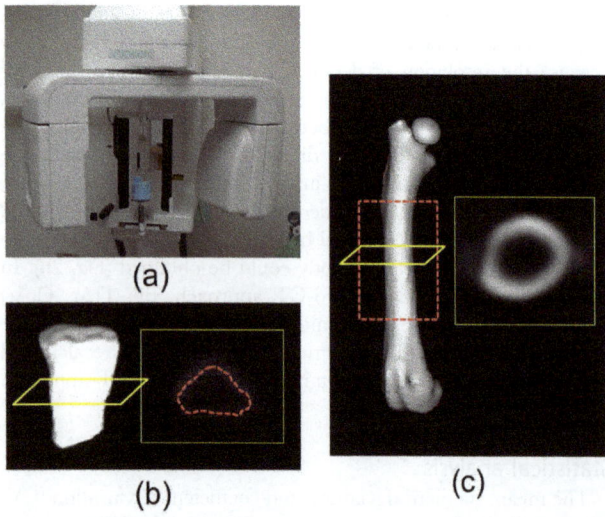

(a)

(b)

(c)

Figure 2. Dental CT machine, images and 3D renderings. (a) Dental CT machine (Asahi AZ 3000), (b) hemi 5th lumbar vertebral body (excluded the posterior element) in left, the section of the dental CT image in right (the region of interest for trabecular bone calculated also shown in dotted red line), and (c) intact femur (the region of interest for cortical bone calculated also shown in dotted red line) in left, the section of the dental CT image in right.

Table 2. Trabecular bone parameters of the 5th vertebral body: the four trabecular bone microarchitecture parameter (BV/TV, TbN, TbTh, TbSp) measured by micro-CT and the grayscale measured by dental CT.

Scanning type	Parameter	Unit	Mean±SD	CV (%)	Max	Min
Micro-CT	BV/TV	%	22.95±5.63	24.51	32.40	16.16
	TbTh	mm	0.10±0.01	6.974	0.12	0.09
	TbSp	mm	0.31±0.06	19.09	0.43	0.23
	TbN	1/mm	2.20±0.46	20.77	2.95	1.53
dental CT	vCanGrayscale		603.57±193.82	32.11	931.28	299.33

SD = standard deviation; CV = coefficient of variation (100×SD/mean); BV/TV = percent bone volume [bone volume (BV)/total volume (TV)]; TbTh = trabecular thickness; TbSp = trabecular separation; TbN = trabecular number; vCanGrayscale = volumetric cancellous bone grayscale value.

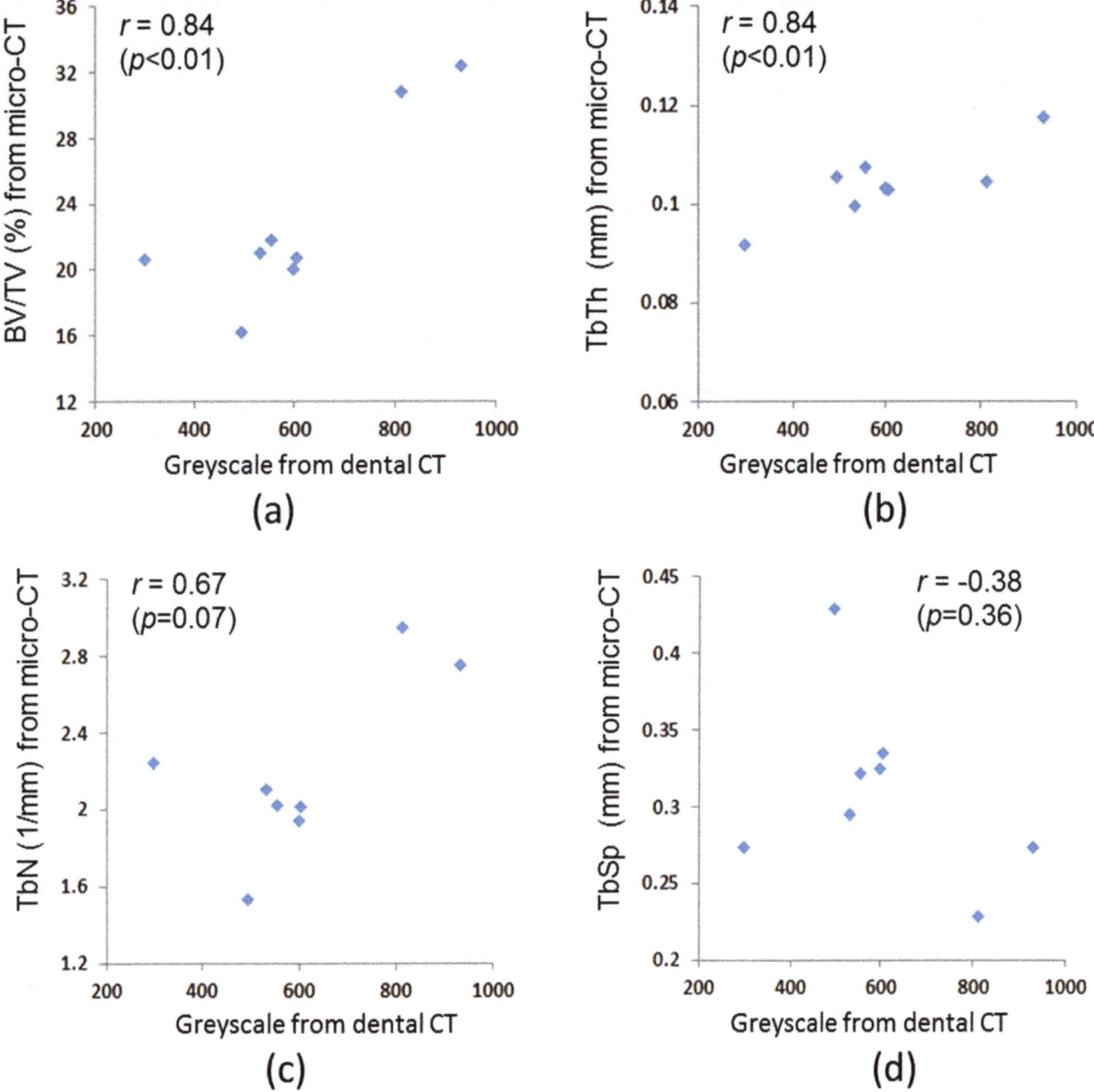

Figure 3. Correlations of the vCanGrayscale (grayscale value of the cancellous bone of 5th vertebral body) measured using dental CT and micro-CT with BV/TV (a), (b) TbTh, (c) TbN, (d) TbSp.

Table 3. Cortical bone parameters of the femoral diaphysis: the four cortical bone morphology parameters (TbAr,CtAr, CtAr/TbAr, and CtTh) measured by micro-CT and dental CT.

	Parameter	Unit	Mean±SD	CV (%)	Max	Min
Micro-CT	TtAr	mm^2	9.22±0.47	5.13	9.70	8.31
	CtAr	mm^2	6.11±0.34	5.62	6.72	5.55
	CtAr/TtAr		0.66±0.04	5.51	0.71	0.58
	CtTh	mm	0.71±0.03	6.09	0.76	0.62
Dental CT	TtAr	mm^2	8.82±0.59	6.70	9.64	7.79
	CtAr	mm^2	6.28±0.61	9.74	7.29	5.38
	CtAr/TtAr		0.71±0.05	7.03	0.78	0.59
	CtTh	mm	0.87±0.07	8.42	0.96	0.71

SD = standard deviation; CV = coefficient of variation (100×SD/mean); TtAr = total cross-sectional area; CtAr = cortical area; CtAr/TtAr = cortical bone area fraction; CtTh = cortical thickness.

previous study has focused on the relationship between cortical bone morphology and trabecular bone microarchitecture by using both micro-CT and dental CT. The experiment conducted in this study revealed that, in measuring the four trabecular microarchitecture parameters of the cancellous bone of fifth lumbar vertebrae in rats, high correlations existed between the BV/TV [$r = 0.84$] and TbTh [$r = 0.84$] values measured using micro-CT and the vCanGrayscale values measured using dental CT. Similarly, the assessments of the four cortical bone morphology parameters of the femoral diaphysis in rats conducted using micro-CT and dental CT were highly correlated (r ranged from 0.71 to 0.90).

In laboratory experiments, the femoral diaphysis is one of the most frequently examined regions for measuring cortical bone strength because the region can be used to conduct three-point and four-point bending tests to measure the structural stiffness of the cortical bone [16,25]. In addition, the femoral head and spinal vertebral body are generally selected to represent cancellous bone tissue [6,8,10,11,13]. This study adopted the fifth vertebral body of rats instead of the femoral head mainly because a rat's femur is small and contains insufficient cancellous bone. To prevent the image quality from being affected by the partial volume effects of dental CT, the fifth vertebral body of rats was used in this study as the sample of cancellous bone tissue. However, because the exterior of a vertebral body is covered by a thin cortical layer and the interior is covered by the cancellous bone tissue (Fig. 1b), dental CT with limited resolution cannot be used to accurately determine the trabecular bone microarchitecture in cancellous bone. Therefore, we first segmented the entire vertebral body, and then eroded the segments by 0.3 mm to represent the cancellous tissue inside the vertebral body.

Since Layton et al. [26] pioneered the use of micro-CT in analyzing the bone morphology of guinea pigs in 1988, micro-CT has been considered the gold standard for assessing bone morphology and microstructures [15]. Numerous bone parameters can be measured using micro-CT. In 2010, Bouxsein et al. [15] indicated that BV/TV, TbTh, TbSp, and TbN are the most crucial indices of trabecular bone microarchitecture parameters, and TtAr, CtAr, CtAr/TtAr, and CtTh are the most critical indices of cortical bone morphology parameters. Therefore, these eight parameters were adopted as the indices for assessing trabecular bone microarchitecture and cortical bone morphology parameters. According to a previous study, a rat's trabecular bone thickness and trabecular bone separation are approximately

50 μm and 150 μm, respectively [27]. The resolution of the micro-CT used in this study was 18.3 μm, which was sufficient for measuring trabecular bone microarchitectures. However, the resolution of the dental CT employed in this study was 100 μm, by which the trabecular bone microarchitectures could not be determined. Therefore, we adopted the vCanGrayscale to represent the cancellous bone tissue of the fifth vertebral body in rats.

Regarding the trabecular bone microarchitecture parameters of the cancellous bone, previous studies have used the femoral head of a rat as the typical region of interest [6,10]. Because of the limited resolution of dental CT, the fifth lumbar vertebral body of rats was used in the experiment. In a comparison between this study and previous studies in which the third to fifth lumbar vertebral bodies of rats were measured, the BV/TV values (22.95%±5.63%) of the rats' fifth lumbar vertebral body scanned using micro-CT in this study were lower than those (29.18%±3.6%) measured by Ito et al. [8] or those (37.6%±5.0%) measured by Yao et al. [13]. This difference existed mainly because the 4-month-old rats used in this study were younger than the 10- and 6-month-old rats selected in the studies of Ito et al. [8] and Yao et al. [13], respectively. In addition, although the ratio of TbSp to TbTh in this study was fairly close to that reported in Ma et al. [11], the ratio of TbTh to TbSp in this study was greater than those obtained in previous research [8,11,13]. These value variations may have resulted from differences in the rat species used, rat age, and experimental design.

Regarding the cortical bone morphology parameters, micro-CT has been rarely applied to measure the four cortical bone morphology parameters (TtAr, CtAr, CtAr/TtAr, and CtTh) of a rat's femoral diaphysis. In this experiment, the TtAr and CtAr values of a the femoral diaphysis of rats measured using micro-CT were 9.22±0.47 mm^2 and 6.11±0.34 mm^2, respectively, which were only approximately half of the values (18.64±0.45 mm^2 and 11.67±0.21 mm^2, respectively) obtained by Sibilia et al. [28]. However, this study and the study of Sibilia et al. reported similar CtAr/TtAr values. In addition, the CtTh values (0.71±0.03 mm) obtained in this study were lower than those (1.095±0.03 mm) of Sibilia et al. In addition to the aforementioned differences in rat age, rat species, and experimental design, the partial volume effects of peripheral quantitative computed tomography (pQCT; resolution = 70 μm) used by Sibilia et al. [28] may have caused

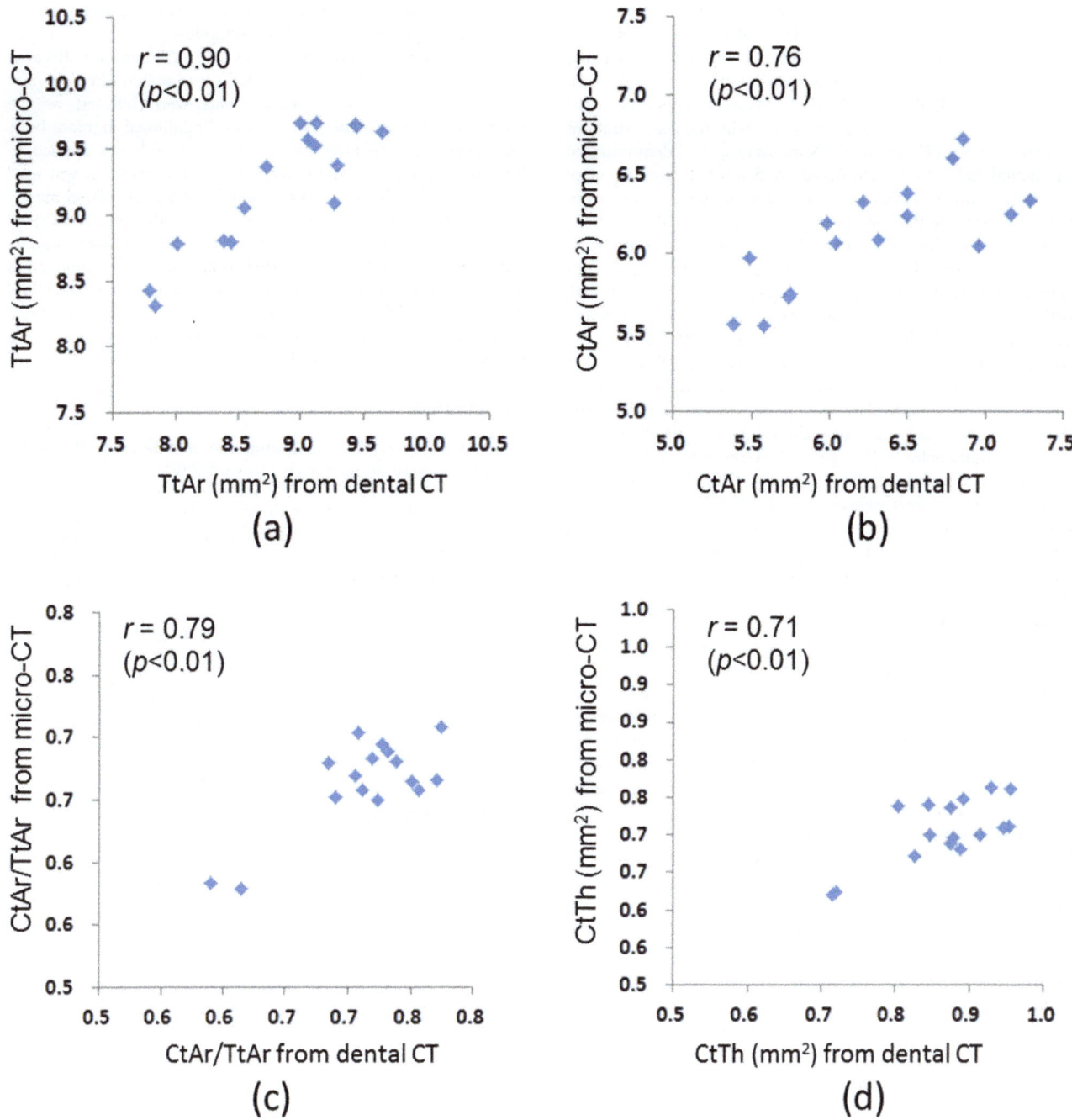

Figure 4. Correlations of the (a)TtAr, (b)CtAr, (c)CtAr/TtAr, (d)CtTh measured by micro-CT and dental CT.

measurement errors, which could have resulted in the differences in the absolute values.

In recent years, dental CT has been widely used in dental clinical practices mainly because dental CT is not only inexpensive and involves low radiation doses [18,29,30], but it also possesses higher spatial resolutions for precisely measuring bone shapes and contours than traditional computed tomography does. Hashimoto et al. [31] indicated that both the magnification and distortion of dental CT are extremely small (error < 0.1 mm). In addition to employing dental CT to observe tissue shapes and contours, several recent studies on the application of grayscale values measured using dental CT for determining bone density have

demonstrated that bone quality and quantity have a specific relationship with grayscale values [22,23]. However, because dental CT is generally used in dental clinics and by dentists or dental radiologists, most studies have been restricted to the dental field, which consequently reduced the applicability of dental CT to other orthopedic fields. Therefore, this study aimed to adopt dental CT to measure the cortical bone morphology parameters of a rat's femoral diaphysis and the grayscale values of the cancellous bone density of a rat's fifth vertebral body.

Previous studies have indicated that the image quality of dental CT is less stable than that of traditional computed tomography, and that the Hounsfield unit scale is not a suitable image unit in dental CT. Moreover, the image quality can be affected by the scanning position [19,32]. Nevertheless, flat panel detectors have been used in most dental CT devices recently, which has substantially improved the image quality of dental CT [24]. Nomura et al. [33] also proved that the grayscale values measured using dental CT have a strong correlation with the concentrations of iodine solutions. Furthermore, Nomura et al. [24] demonstrated that dental CT can be employed to determine bone mineral content. In addition, dental CT has been adopted in numerous studies for assessing the bone quality and quantity of alveolar bone before dental implant placements. In this study, the vCanGrayscale values measured using dental CT represented the cancellous bone density of the fifth vertebral body, and exhibited high correlations (r) with the trabecular bone microarchitecture parameters, specifically BV/TV (0.84) and TbTh (0.84), measured using micro-CT. Therefore, dental CT can be clinically applied to scan patients' bones and indirectly estimate the trabecular bone microarchitecture (particularly the parameters of BV/TV and TbTh) by calculating the grayscale values of cancellous bone density. Additionally, although vCanGrayscale values were moderately correlated with TbN values ($r = 0.67$), the correlation exhibited no statistical significance ($p = 0.070$). Moreover, no correlations existed between the vCanGrayscale and TbSp values.

Several scholars have adopted QCT or pQCT to measure the morphology parameters of the femur [2,3,5,34], and proved that QCT and pQCT can provide not only bone densitometric parameters as DXA does, but also bone geometric parameters for accurately predicting bone strength. However, scant studies have involved the use of dental CT for measuring the cortical bone morphology parameters of long bone diaphysis. In this experiment, the TtAr values (8.82 ± 0.59 mm^2) measured using dental CT were smaller than those (9.22 ± 0.47 mm^2) measured using micro-CT and, conversely, the CtAr/TtAr and CtTh values (0.71 ± 0.05 mm and 0.87 ± 0.07 mm, respectively) measured using dental CT were greater than those (0.66 ± 0.04 mm and 0.71 ± 0.01 mm, respectively) measured using micro-CT. Although differences existed in the absolute values measured using micro-CT and dental CT, the absolute values obtained using the two methods exhibited strong correlations. These absolute values should considerably decrease when the methods are applied in human clinical trials (thicker bones). However, further experiments are required to verify this assumption.

In this study, the experiment has several limitations. Because fresh human cadaver bones were difficult to obtain, the rat bones most commonly used in experiments were selected as the experimental specimens. Nevertheless, additional human bone experiments are required before these methods are applied to human bodies. In this study, only the femoral diaphysis was used to assess cortical bone, and cancellous bone was evaluated merely based on the fifth vertebral body. Consequently, the effectiveness of using other bone regions to test cortical and cancellous bone by using dental CT still requires further evaluation. In addition, all of the bone specimens were scanned in vitro by using micro-CT and dental CT, which generated clearer images than in vivo bone scanning did. Nonetheless, further experimental investigations are required for analyzing such differences.

Conclusion

Based on the experimental setup and limitations, the following conclusions were derived from this study:

1. High correlations between the vCanGrayscale (grayscale value of the cancellous bone of the fifth vertebral body) measured using dental CT and the trabecular bone microarchitecture parameters (BV/TV and TbTh) measured using micro-CT were observed.

2. The absolute value of the cortical bone morphology parameters (TtAr, CtAr/TtAr, and CtTh) may be different between the measurements obtained using the dental CT and micro-CT approaches. However, high correlations between these four parameter measured using micro-CT and dental CT were demonstrated.

Author Contributions

Conceived and designed the experiments: J.-T. Hsu MTT HLH JW. Performed the experiments: J.-T. Hsu YJC J.-T. Ho SPW FCC. Analyzed the data: J.-T. Hsu J.-T. Ho MTT YJC SPW FCC. Contributed reagents/materials/analysis tools: J.-T. Hsu YJC J.-T. Ho HLH JW. Contributed to the writing of the manuscript: J.-T. Hsu HLH MTT.

References

1. Zioupos P, Cook RB, Hutchinson JR (2008) Some basic relationships between density values in cancellous and cortical bone. J Biomech 41: 1961–1968.
2. Link TM (2012) Osteoporosis Imaging: State of the Art and Advanced Imaging. Radiology 263: 3–17.
3. Siu WS, Qin L, Leung KS (2003) pQCT bone strength index may serve as a better predictor than bone mineral density for long bone breaking strength. J Bone Miner Metab 21: 316–322.
4. Genant HK, Engelke K, Fuerst T, Glüer CC, Grampp S, et al. (1996) Noninvasive assessment of bone mineral and structure: state of the art. J Bone Miner Res 11: 707–730.
5. Genant H, Engelke K, Prevrhal S (2008) Advanced CT bone imaging in osteoporosis. Rheumatology 47: iv9–iv16.
6. Bagi CM, Berryman E, Moalli MR (2011) Comparative bone anatomy of commonly used laboratory animals: implications for drug discovery. Comp Med 61: 76–85.
7. Heep H, Wedemeyer C, Wegner A, Hofmeister S, Von Knoch M (2008) Differences in trabecular bone of leptin-deficient ob/ob mice in response to biomechanical loading. Int J Biol Sci 4: 169–175.
8. Ito M, Nishida A, Koga A, Ikeda S, Shiraishi A, et al. (2002) Contribution of trabecular and cortical components to the mechanical properties of bone and their regulating parameters. Bone 31: 351–358.
9. Jiang S-D, Jiang L-S, Dai L-Y (2006) Spinal cord injury causes more damage to bone mass, bone structure, biomechanical properties and bone metabolism than sciatic neurectomy in young rats. Osteoporos Int 17: 1552–1561.
10. Lima I, Rocha M, Lopes R (2008) Ethanol bone evaluation using 3D microtomography. Micron 39: 617–622.
11. Ma L, Ji J, Ji H, Yu X, Ding L, et al. (2010) Telmisartan alleviates rosiglitazone-induced bone loss in ovariectomized spontaneous hypertensive rats. Bone 47: 5–11.
12. Medeiros DM, Stoecker B, Plattner A, Jennings D, Haub M (2004) Iron deficiency negatively affects vertebrae and femurs of rats independently of energy intake and body weight. J Nutr 134: 3061–3067.
13. Yao W, Hadi T, Jiang Y, Lotz J, Wronski TJ, et al. (2005) Basic fibroblast growth factor improves trabecular bone connectivity and bone strength in the lumbar vertebral body of osteopenic rats. Osteoporos Int 16: 1939–1947.
14. Hsu JT, Wang SP, Huang HL, Chen YJ, Wu J, et al. (2013) The assessment of trabecular bone parameters and cortical bone strength: A comparison of micro-CT and dental cone-beam CT. J Biomech 46: 2611–2618.
15. Bouxsein ML, Boyd SK, Christiansen BA, Guldberg RE, Jepsen KJ, et al. (2010) Guidelines for assessment of bone microstructure in rodents using micro-computed tomography. J Bone Miner Res 25: 1468–1486.
16. Hsu JT, Chen YJ, Tsai MT, Lan HHC, Cheng FC, et al. (2012) Predicting Cortical Bone Strength from DXA and Dental Cone-Beam CT. PLoS One 7: e50008.
17. Arisan V, Karabuda ZC, Avsever H, Özdemir T (2012) Conventional Multi-Slice Computed Tomography (CT) and Cone-Beam CT (CBCT) for Computer-Assisted Implant Placement. Part I: Relationship of Radiographic Gray Density and Implant Stability. Clin Implant Dent Relat Res 15: 893–906.
18. Benavides E, Rios HF, Ganz SD, An CH, Resnik R, et al. (2012) Use of Cone Beam Computed Tomography in Implant Dentistry: The International Congress of Oral Implantologists Consensus Report. Implant Dent 21: 78–86.
19. Nackaerts O, Maes F, Yan H, Couto Souza P, Pauwels R, et al. (2011) Analysis of intensity variability in multislice and cone beam computed tomography. Clin Oral Implants Res 22: 873–879.

20. González-García R, Monje F (2013) The reliability of cone-beam computed tomography to assess bone density at dental implant recipient sites: a histomorphometric analysis by micro-CT. Clin Oral Implants Res 24:871–879.

21. Hasan I, Dominiak M, Blaszczyszyn A, Bourauel C, Gedrange T, et al. (2014) Radiographic evaluation of bone density around immediately loaded implants. Ann Anat S0940-9602(14)00027-2.

22. Monje A, Monje F, González-García R, Galindo-Moreno P, Rodriguez-Salvanes F, et al. (2014) Comparison between microcomputed tomography and cone-beam computed tomography radiologic bone to assess atrophic posterior maxilla density and microarchitecture. Clin Oral Implants Res 25: 723–728.

23. Parsa A, Ibrahim N, Hassan B, Stelt P, Wismeijer D (2013) Bone quality evaluation at dental implant site using multislice CT, micro-CT, and cone beam CT. Clin Oral Implants Res doi: 10.1111/clr.12315. [Epub ahead of print]

24. Nomura Y, Watanabe H, Shirotsu K, Honda E, Sumi Y, et al. (2013) Stability of voxel values from cone-beam computed tomography for dental use in evaluating bone mineral content. Clin Oral Implants Res 24: 543–548.

25. Leppänen OV, Sievänen H, Järvinen TLN (2008) Biomechanical testing in experimental bone interventions—May the power be with you. J Biomech 41: 1623–1631.

26. Layton MW, Goldstein SA, Goulet RW, Feldkamp LA, Kubinski DJ, et al. (1988) Examination of subchondral bone architecture in experimental osteoarthritis by microscopic computed axial tomography. Arthritis Rheum 31: 1400–1405.

27. Jiang Y, Zhao J, White D, Genant H (2000) Micro CT and Micro MR imaging of 3D architecture of animal skeleton. J Musculoskelet Neuronal Interact 1: 45–51.

28. Sibilia V, Pagani F, Dieci E, Mrak E, Marchese M, et al. (2013) Dietary tryptophan manipulation reveals a central role for serotonin in the anabolic response of appendicular skeleton to physical activity in rats. Endocrine 44: 790–802.

29. Dawood A, Brown J, Sauret-Jackson V, Purkayastha S (2012) Optimization of cone beam CT exposure for pre-surgical evaluation of the implant site. Dentomaxillofac Radiol 41: 70–74.

30. Fanning B (2011) CBCT–the justification process, audit and review of the recent literature. J Ir Dent Assoc 57: 256–261.

31. Hashimoto K, Kawashima S, Araki M, Iwai K, Sawada K, et al. (2006) Comparison of image performance between cone-beam computed tomography for dental use and four-row multidetector helical CT. J Oral Sci 48: 27–34.

32. Katsumata A, Hirukawa A, Okumura S, Naitoh M, Fujishita M, et al. (2007) Effects of image artifacts on gray-value density in limited-volume cone-beam computerized tomography. Oral Surg Oral Med Oral Pathol Oral Radiol Endod 104: 829–836.

33. Nomura Y, Watanabe H, Honda E, Kurabayashi T (2010) Reliability of voxel values from cone-beam computed tomography for dental use in evaluating bone mineral density. Clin Oral Implants Res 21: 558–562.

34. Moisio K, Podolskaya G, Barnhart B, Berzins A, Sumner D (2003) pQCT provides better prediction of canine femur breaking load than does DXA. J Musculoskelet Neuronal Interact 3: 240–245.

The Strong *In Vivo* Anti-Tumor Effect of the UIC2 Monoclonal Antibody Is the Combined Result of Pgp Inhibition and Antibody Dependent Cell-Mediated Cytotoxicity

Gábor Szalóki[1], Zoárd T. Krasznai[2], Ágnes Tóth[1], Laura Vízkeleti[3], Attila G. Szöllősi[4], György Trencsényi[5], Imre Lajtos[5], István Juhász[6,7], Zoltán Krasznai[1], Teréz Márián[5], Margit Balázs[3], Gábor Szabó[1¶], Katalin Goda[1*¶]

1 Department of Biophysics and Cell Biology, Faculty of Medicine, University of Debrecen, Debrecen, Hungary, 2 Department of Obstetrics and Gynecology, Faculty of Medicine, University of Debrecen, Debrecen, Hungary, 3 Department of Preventive Medicine, Faculty of Medicine, University of Debrecen, Debrecen, Hungary, 4 Department of Physiology, Faculty of Medicine, University of Debrecen, Debrecen, Hungary, 5 Department of Nuclear Medicine, Faculty of Medicine, University of Debrecen, Debrecen, Hungary, 6 Department of Dermatology, Faculty of Medicine, University of Debrecen, Debrecen, Hungary, 7 Department of Surgery and Operative Techniques, Faculty of Medicine, University of Debrecen, Debrecen, Hungary

Abstract

P-glycoprotein (Pgp) extrudes a large variety of chemotherapeutic drugs from the cells, causing multidrug resistance (MDR). The UIC2 monoclonal antibody recognizes human Pgp and inhibits its drug transport activity. However, this inhibition is partial, since UIC2 binds only to 10–40% of cell surface Pgps, while the rest becomes accessible to this antibody only in the presence of certain substrates or modulators (e.g. cyclosporine A (CsA)). The combined addition of UIC2 and 10 times lower concentrations of CsA than what is necessary for Pgp inhibition when the modulator is applied alone, decreased the EC_{50} of doxorubicin (DOX) in KB-V1 (Pgp^+) cells *in vitro* almost to the level of KB-3-1 (Pgp^-) cells. At the same time, UIC2 alone did not affect the EC_{50} value of DOX significantly. In xenotransplanted severe combined immunodeficient (SCID) mice co-treated with DOX, UIC2 and CsA, the average weight of Pgp^+ tumors was only ~10% of the untreated control and in 52% of these animals we could not detect tumors at all, while DOX treatment alone did not decrease the weight of Pgp^+ tumors. These data were confirmed by visualizing the tumors *in vivo* by positron emission tomography (PET) based on their increased ^{18}FDG accumulation. Unexpectedly, UIC2+DOX treatment also decreased the size of tumors compared to the DOX only treated animals, as opposed to the results of our *in vitro* cytotoxicity assays, suggesting that immunological factors are also involved in the antitumor effect of *in vivo* UIC2 treatment. Since UIC2 binding itself did not affect the viability of Pgp expressing cells, but it triggered *in vitro* cell killing by peripheral blood mononuclear cells (PBMCs), it is concluded that the impressive *in vivo* anti-tumor effect of the DOX-UIC2-CsA treatment is the combined result of Pgp inhibition and antibody dependent cell-mediated cytotoxicity (ADCC).

Editor: Mária A. Deli, Hungarian Academy of Sciences, Hungary

Funding: This work was supported by Szodoray Grant from the University of Debrecen (recipients are Katalin Goda and Zoárd T. Krasznai) and Astellas Pharma Kft and Libra Foundation (recipient is Gábor Szalóki). The work was also supported by Hungarian National Science and Research Foundation (OTKA) grants PD75994, K72762, NK101337 and by TÁMOP grants: TÁMOP 4.2.2-08/1-2008-0015, TÁMOP 4.2.1/B-09/1/KONV-2010-0007 and TÁMOP 4.2.2.A-11/1/KONV-2012-0023 "VÉD-ELEM" project. Gábor Szalóki's research was realized in the frames of TÁMOP 4.2.4. A/2-11-1-2012-0001 "National Excellence Program – Elaborating and operating an inland student and researcher personal support system convergence program." The funders had no role in study design, data collection and analysis, decision to publish, or preparation of the manuscript.

Competing Interests: The authors have declared that no competing interests exist.

* Email: goda@med.unideb.hu

¶ These authors are shared last authors on this work.

Introduction

One of the most common causes of cancer chemotherapy failure is the development of resistance against chemotherapeutic agents. In most cases the tumor cells are either intrinsically resistant, or become resistant in the course of chemotherapy, to a broad spectrum of chemotherapeutic agents, including compounds they have never met before [1]. This phenomenon is called multidrug resistance (MDR) and it is often associated with high-level expression of active transporter proteins belonging to the ATP Binding Cassette (ABC) super-family, such as ABCB1 (MDR1, P-glycoprotein, Pgp), ABCC1 (MRP1, multidrug resistance protein 1) or ABCG2 (BCRP, breast cancer resistance protein)[2,3]. Pgp was the first transporter described in connection with multidrug resistance, and it seems to have the most significant role in clinical cases [3].

The Pgp molecule consists of two almost identical halves connected by a 75 amino acid long intracellular linker region. Both halves comprise six membrane spanning α-helices forming a transmembrane domain (TMD) and a nucleotide binding domain

(NBD). The two TMDs define the substrate binding sites and the translocation pathway, allowing the protein to transport various hydrophobic compounds out of the cells [4]. The overall energy requirement of drug efflux is covered by ATP hydrolysis conducted by the two NBDs (for possible models, see e.g. Senior [5], Ambudkar et al. [6]).

Pgp is generally expressed in tissues having barrier functions (e.g., in endothelial cells of the blood-brain barrier, in hepatocytes, in epithelial cells of the kidney and the intestines) and it is suggested to have an important role in protection of the body from toxic substances [2,3,7]. However, the loss of the *abcb1a/b* genes in mice (homologues of the human *ABCB1* gene) is not accompanied by major physiological consequences [8,9]; hence, inhibition of Pgp molecules may be a plausible strategy of overcoming drug resistance without serious side effects. The classical pharmacological approach involves co-administration of the cytotoxic compounds that are substrates of Pgp with pump inhibitors, to increase the accumulation of the former into the tumor cells. Unfortunately, Pgp inhibitors often induce unpredictable and intolerable pharmacokinetic interactions and toxicity through inhibiting other drug transporters or cytochrome P450, by changing the clearance and metabolism of the co-administered chemotherapeutic agents [10–12]

Several monoclonal antibodies (mAb) recognizing extracellular epitopes have been developed against Pgp. A few of them (e.g., MRK16, MRK17, MC57, HYB-241, and UIC2) are thought to recognize discontinuous conformation sensitive epitopes. Upon binding, these antibodies can partially inhibit Pgp mediated drug transport *in vivo* and *in vitro* [13–16]. However, this inhibitory effect is often weak [13–18], its extent may depend on the transported substrate [15,17,18], and it is variable even in the case of the same substrate according to general experience.

UIC2 is an IgG2a isotype mouse monoclonal antibody raised against human Pgp. It recognizes a complex epitope involving at least the first [19] and the third extracellular loops of the protein [20]. In the absence of Pgp substrates and modulators UIC2 can bind only to 10–40% of cell surface Pgps, while the rest adopts the UIC2 binding conformation only in the presence of a distinct group of substrates or modulators (e.g., cyclosporine A (CsA), SDZ PSC 833, vinblastine and paclitaxel [21–23]. In previous studies we have demonstrated that the UIC2 antibody itself completely inhibits Pgp function when it is applied together with any of the above Pgp modulators added at low, sub-inhibitory concentrations [22]. The above phenomenon was also confirmed *in vitro*, by measuring the cellular accumulation of various fluorescent Pgp substrates including DNR, R123, calcein and a radioactive tracer ^{99m}Tc-Mibi [22]. In line with the above, combined treatment with either CSA + UIC2 or paclitaxel + UIC2 specifically decreased the rate of glucose metabolism in Pgp$^+$ cells, as measured in 2-[^{18}F]fluoro-2-deoxy-D-glucose (^{18}FDG) accumulation experiments, also suggesting that Pgp inhibition with concomitant decrease of energy consumption has occurred [23]. On the other hand, we also demonstrated in xenotransplanted severe combined immunodeficient (SCID) mice that UIC2 could readily penetrate into the compact solid tumors, intensively staining cell surface Pgps and increasing daunorubicin accumulation in the Pgp$^+$ tumors to the level of the Pgp$^-$ ones [22].

In the present study we tested whether the combined treatment with CsA and UIC2 mAb can potentiate the anti-tumor effect of doxorubicin (DOX) in Pgp$^+$ tumors to achieve clinically relevant reduction in tumor size, applying the above experimental model [22]. Tumor growth was followed by weighing the mass of the tumors in sacrificed animals and also *in vivo* on the basis of ^{18}FDG accumulation. In the latter case a small-animal Positron Emission

Tomography (PET) camera was applied to visualize tumors on the basis of their increased rate of glucose metabolism [24–26]. Our data demonstrate that the combined application of a class of modulators (including CsA) used at sub-inhibitory concentrations and of the UIC2 antibody may serve as an effective tool for blocking the growth of Pgp expressing tumors.

Materials and Methods

Ethics Statement

The experiments using human blood were done with the approval of the Scientific and Research Ethics Committee of the Medical Research Council (ETT TUKEB, permission number: 25364-1/2012/EKU (449/P1/12.)). Written informed consent was obtained from donors prior to blood donation, and their data were processed and stored according to the principles expressed in the Declaration of Helsinki.

In animal experiments the *Principles of Laboratory Animal Care* (National Institute of Health) was strictly followed, and the experimental protocol was approved by the Laboratory Animal Care and Use Committee of the University of Debrecen (Permission Numbers: 26/2006/DE-MAB and 122/2009/DE-MAB).

Cell Lines

KB-3-1 human epidermoid carcinoma cell line and KB-V1, its Pgp positive counterpart were used in the experiments (obtained from Michael Gottesman's lab, NIH, Bethesda) [27,28]. The cells were grown as monolayer cultures at 37°C in Dulbecco's modified Eagle's medium (DMEM) containing 4.5 g/l glucose and supplemented with 10% heat-inactivated fetal bovine serum (FBS), 2 mM L-glutamine and 25 μM/ml gentamycin. The KB-V1 cells were cultured in the presence of 180 nM vinblastine until 3 days before their use. The viability of the cells in our experiments was always higher than 90%, as assessed by the trypan blue exclusion test. The cells were regularly checked for mycoplasma by the Plasmo Test mycoplasma detection kit (San Diego, CA) and found to be negative.

Chemicals

All the Pgp substrates, modulators, cell culture media and supplements were from Sigma–Aldrich (Budapest, Hungary). The UIC2, 15D3, 5D3 and QCRL-3 mAbs were purified from the supernatants of hybridoma cell lines using affinity chromatography. The hybridoma cell lines were purchased from the American Type Culture Collections, Manassas, VA, USA), except the 5D3 hybridoma cell line, which was a kind gift from Brain P. Sorrentino (Division of Experimental Hematology, Department of Hematology/Oncology, St. Jude Children's Research Hospital, Memphis, Tennessee). The mAb preparations were>97% pure by SDS/PAGE. The glucose analogue 2-[^{18}F]fluoro-2-deoxy-D-glucose (^{18}FDG) was synthesized and labeled with the positron-decaying isotope ^{18}F according to Hamacher et al. [29].

Indirect immunofluorescence

For detection of Pgp and ABCG2 living cells (10^6 cells/ml) were incubated in the presence of 30 μg/ml 15D3 anti- Pgp mAb or 2 μg/ml 5D3 anti-ABCG2 mAb for 30 min at 37°C. For measurement of MRP1 (ABCC1) expression cells were fixed and permeabilised with 1% para-formaldehyde and 0.1% TritonX-100 in PBS (15 min; 4°C) and then labeled with 2 μg/ml QCRL-3 mAb (30 min; 4°C). After two washes with ice-cold PBS containing 1% bovine serum albumin (BSA-PBS), cells were incubated with goat anti-mouse IgG (0.5 μg/ml CruzFluor 647

(CFL647-GaMIgG), Santa Cruz Biotechnology, Inc., Texas) for 30 min at 4°C. Fluorescence intensities were detected using a Becton Dickinson FACSAria III Cell Sorter (Becton Dickinson) measuring the 633 nm/660±20 nm fluorescence intensities. Fluorescence signals were collected in logarithmic mode and the cytofluorimetric data were analyzed by the BDIS CELLQUEST (Becton Dickinson) software.

To detect Pgp expression in tumors 5-μm-thick cryosections were prepared, dried at room temperature and fixed in pre-cooled acetone (-20°C) for 10 min. Sections were then washed with PBS and blocked with 1% BSA-PBS for 20 minutes to avoid non-specific labeling and further incubated at room temperature with the UIC2 (10 μg/ml) mouse mAb for 60 min. To visualize the binding of the primary antibody an Alexa-488 conjugated goat anti-mouse IgG (A488-GaMIgG, Invitrogen) was used at 1:1000 dilution. Negative controls were obtained by omitting the primary antibody.

A Zeiss LSM 510 confocal laser-scanning microscope was used for the measurements. Alexa-488 was excited at the 488 nm line of an argon-ion laser. Fluorescence was detected through a 505–550 nm band pass filter. Images of 512×512 pixels were obtained in extended focus mode, through a 63× (numerical aperture = 1.4) Plan-Apochromat oil immersion objective.

In vitro cytotoxicity tests

Cells were seeded in 96-well plates at a cell density of 5×10^3 cells/well. 24 hours later DOX was added at different concentrations with CsA and/or UIC2 mAb or the modulator alone, and the plates were further incubated for 72 h at 37°C. The cell viability was determined using the AlamarBlue assay (Serotec, UK) measuring the 530/590 nm fluorescence intensity of the dye in an automated microplate reader (BioTec Synergy HT, US). The fluorescence intensities of the samples were normalized to the fluorescence of the untreated (DOX, antibody and CsA free) control sample, and plotted as a function of DOX concentration. Dose-response curves were fitted, and EC_{50} values were calculated by SigmaPlot 12.0 programme (Systat Software, Inc., USA).

In vitro antibody-dependent cell-mediated cytotoxicity (ADCC) assay

ADCC experiments were performed as described previously [30] with minor modifications. Human peripheral blood mononuclear cells (PBMCs) were prepared from the blood of healthy donors by Ficoll (Histopaque-1077, Sigma-Aldrich, Budapest) density gradient centrifugation. The PBMC rich fraction (effector cells) was washed three times and re-suspended in DMEM containing 10% FCS. After trypsinization, KB-V1 and KB-3-1 (target cells) cells were labeled with 5(6)-carboxyfluorescein diacetate N-succinimidyl ester (CFDA-SE) at a concentration of 10 μM at 37°C for 10 min. Then, the cells were washed thrice with DMEM containing 10% FCS and 1% BSA to remove unbound CFDA-SE and finally re-suspended in DMEM containing 10% FCS. 1.5×10^5 target cells were mixed with effector cells at target/effector cell ratios of 1:5, 1:10, 1:50 and 1:100 in a final volume of 1 ml. Samples were incubated in the absence or presence of 0.1 μM CsA and/or 20 μg/ml UIC2 at 37°C for 8 hours in CO_2 incubator. After incubation the cells were washed and then re-suspended in ice cold phosphate-buffered saline (PBS), containing 8 mM glucose and 5 μg/ml propidium iodide (PI) and were analyzed using a Becton Dickinson FACScan flow cytometer (Mountain View, CA). The labeling distinguishes four populations of cells as it is demonstrated in Fig. S1: **1**. living target cells in green (CFDA-SE positive cells); **2**. dead target cells in green and red (CFDA-SE and PI double positive cells); **3**. dead effector cells

in red (PI positive cells), and **4**. live effector cells, which remain unstained. The negative control sample did not contain PBMCs, while tumor cells killed by 4% para-formaldehyde served as the positive control. The percentage of killed target cells was calculated dividing the number of PI and CFDA-SE double positive cells (dead cells) by the number of the CFDA-SE positive cells.

In vitro complement-dependent cytotoxicity (CDC) assay

Samples containing 2.5×10^5 KB-V1 or KB-3-1 cells and 20 μg/ml UIC2 mAb in the presence or absence of 0.1 μM CsA were treated with freshly prepared human serum at different dilutions in DMEM medium. The samples were incubated for 4 hours in CO_2 incubator at 37°C and then stained with 5 μg/ml PI. The percentage of the PI positive dead cell was determined by a Becton Dickinson FACScan flow cytometer (Mountain View, CA).

The hemolytic complement activity of the human serum samples was determined applying sheep red blood cells sensitized with a rabbit stroma antibody (SSRBC) kindly provided by Attila Bácsi (Inst. of Immunology, University of Debrecen, Faculty of Medicine). 50 μl of 1% SSRBC was mixed with different dilutions of human serum or heat inactivated human serum (inactivated at 56°C for 30 min) and incubated for 30 min at 37°C. After centrifugation the absorbance of the supernatants was measured at 541 nm by BioTek Synergy HT plate reader. The HC_{50} value where 50% of the RBCs were lysed was determined for the human sera and found to be normal.

Animal model and study design

Adult (10 to 12 week-old), pathogen-free B-17 severe combined immunodeficiency (SCID) mice were used in this study [31]. Animals were housed under pathogen free circumstances at a temperature of 26±2°C, with 50±10% humidity and artificial lighting with a circadian cycle of 12 h. The food and drinking water (sterilized by autoclaving) were available ad-libitum to all animals.

SCID mice were injected subcutaneously with KB-3-1 (Pgp⁻; 1.5×10^6 cells in 150 μl sterile phosphate-buffered saline (PBS)) on the left and KB-V1 (Pgp⁺; 3×10^6 cells in 150 μl sterile PBS) cells on the right thighs. To obtain approximately similar tumor sizes in case of KB-V1 and KB-3-1 cells we had to inject double number of KB-V1 cells, because of their slower cell proliferation rate. In another experiment we grafted four tumors per animal in order to limit the number of animals and to maximize the number of tumors imaged. In this case each animal received two injections in the shoulders and two in the upper part of the thighs. Tumors were grown for 4 days and then the mice were treated with DOX alone (5 mg/kg, i.v.), or DOX combined with either UIC2 mAb (5 mg/kg, i.v.) or CsA (Sandimmun, Novartis, Basel, Switzerland; 10 mg/kg i.p.) or both. The animals were killed 8 days after treatment with chemotherapy by cervical dislocation and the tumors were removed to weigh them and then they were snap frozen in liquid nitrogen and stored at -70°C till mRNA expression analysis.

mRNA expression analysis

The frozen tumor sections were equilibrated in 10 volumes pre-chilled RNAlater-ICE solution (Applied Biosystem, CA) at -20°C overnight to protect RNA from degradation and then total RNA was isolated using the RNeasy Mini kit (Qiagen Inc., CA) according to the protocol. RNA quantity was determined by NanoDrop ND-1000 UV-Vis Spectrophotometer (NanoDrop Technologies, Wilmington, DE). RNA was then subjected to reverse transcription-real time quantitative polymerase chain reaction (RT-qPCR) using the Taqman assay with stocked primers and probes (Applied Biosystem, CA). Pgp mRNA expression was normalized to the human glyceraldehyde-3-phosphate dehydrogenase (GAPDH) expression.

Small-animal PET imaging using ^{18}FDG

After the implantation of tumor cells ^{18}FDG PET scans were repeated at different time points. Prior to PET measurements, mice were fasted overnight. On the day of PET imaging mice were pre-warmed to a body temperature of $37°C$ and this temperature was maintained throughout the uptake and scanning period to minimize the visualization of brown fat. Mice were injected via the tail vein with $5.5±0.2$ MBq of ^{18}FDG. 40 min after tracer injection animal were anaesthetized by 3% isoflurane with a dedicated small animal anesthesia device and then 20 min long static single-frame PET scans were acquired using a small-animal PET scanner (MiniPET-II, Department of Nuclear Medicine, Faculty of Medicine, University of Debrecen) to visualize the tumors.

The MiniPET-II system is a dedicated small animal PET scanner developed with the help of a Hungarian project. The MiniPET-II scanner consists of 12 detector modules including LYSO (Cerium Doped Lutetium Yttrium Orthosilicate) scintillation crystal blocks and position sensitive photo multiplier tubes. Each crystal block comprises $35×35$ pins of $1.27×1.27×12$ mm size. Scanner normalization and random correction were applied on the data and the images were reconstructed with the standard maximum likelihood expectation maximization iterative algorithm. The pixel size was $0.27×0.27×1.35$ mm and the spatial resolution varies between 1.4 to 2.1 mm from central to 25 mm radial distances. The system sensitivity is 11.4%.

^{18}FDG-PET data analysis

The ^{18}FDG uptake was expressed in terms of standardized uptake values (SUVs) and tumor to muscle (T/M) ratios. Ellipsoidal 3-dimensional regions of interest (ROI) were manually drawn around the edges of the tumor xenografts by visual inspection using BrainCad software (Institute of Nuclear Medicine, University of Debrecen). The standardized uptake value (SUV) was calculated as follows: SUV = [ROI activity (Bq/ml)]/[injected activity (Bq)/animal weight (g)], assuming a density of 1 g/cm^3. The T/M ratios were computed as the ratio of the mean activity in the tumor volume of interest (VOI) and the background (muscle) VOI.

Statistical analysis

The displayed data are the means ± SD of the results of at least three independent experiments. Data have been analyzed using SigmaPlot 12.0 programme (Systat Software, Inc., USA) and IBM SPSS Statistics 20 (IBM Corp., USA). Statistical significance was assessed using analysis of variance (ANOVA), applying Holm-Sidak method for post hoc pair-wise comparison of the different samples. In the case of unequal variances Dunnett T3 post hoc pair-wise comparison method was used. Differences were considered to be significant at $P<0.05$.

Results

In vitro cytotoxicity measurements

KB-V1 cells express Pgp at high level, while other drug transporting ABC proteins ABCG2 and ABCC1 were not detectable by means of indirect immunofluorescence and flow cytometry (Fig. S2). KB-3-1 cells do not express any of the above

ABC transporters at measurable level (Fig. S2). In accordance with the high Pgp expression level of KB-V1 cells the EC$_{50}$ value of DOX was $2.19±0.39$ μM in these cells, while it was only $44±3$ nM in KB-3-1 (Pgp$^-$) cells (Fig. 1). In KB-V1 cells CsA co-treatment decreased the EC$_{50}$ value of DOX in a dose dependent manner, while UIC2 had only a weak, statistically not significant effect. Interestingly, the combined treatment of KB-V1 cells with 1 μM CsA and a saturating concentration of UIC2 mAb decreased the EC$_{50}$ value to $33±19.7$ nM, which could be achieved by 10 times higher CsA concentration when it was applied alone (Fig. 1). In contrast, administration of the UIC2 mAb and 1 μM CsA to cultures of KB-3-1 cells, simultaneously or alone, had no significant effects on their DOX sensitivity.

mRNA expression analysis of Pgp in the tumor xenografts and cells used for grafting the tumors

Based on the above in vitro results, we have designed in vivo experiments to test the effectiveness of the combined treatment with low dose of CsA, UIC2 and DOX. SCID mice were inoculated with KB-V1 and KB-3-1 cells, respectively. Palpable subcutaneous tumors developed in 10–12 days. Their Pgp expression was compared to that of the tumor cells used for grafting the tumors. Since the immunofluorescence intensities in frozen tissue sections and cell monolayers are not directly comparable, Pgp expression was examined at the mRNA level. In the KB-3-1 tumors a well detectable ~60-fold increment of Pgp mRNA levels occurred compared to the inoculated cells, while the Pgp mRNA level of the KB-V1 tumors did not change upon proliferation of the inoculated cells (Fig. 2). The Pgp mRNA levels proved to be at least three orders of magnitude higher in the KB-V1 tumors compared to the KB-3-1 xenografts (see Fig. 2). Thus, the KB-V1 tumor xenografts retained their MDR phenotype as it was also proved by indirect immunofluorescent labeling (see Fig. S3), while the KB-3-1 cells continued to express Pgp at very low levels (not detectable by immunofluorescence, Fig. S3) in the developed tumors on the time scale of the in vivo experiments.

^{18}FDG accumulation in xenotransplanted tumors

Grafted tumors were grown for 4 days, then the mice were treated with DOX alone (5 mg/kg, i.v.) or DOX combined with either the UIC2 mAb (5 mg/kg, i.v.) or CsA (10 mg/kg, i.p.), or

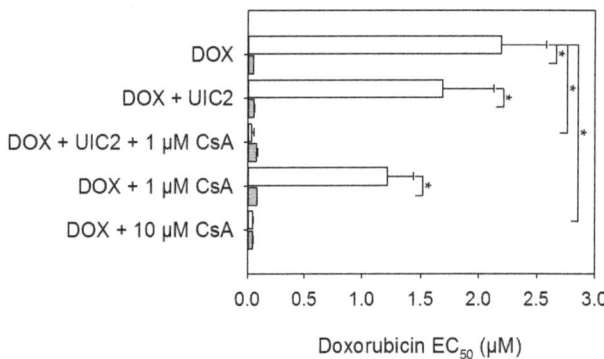

Figure 1. Cytotoxic effect of DOX in KB-3-1 (Pgp⁻; grey bars) and KB-V1 (Pgp⁺; empty bars) cells and its potentiation by treatments with CsA (used at the indicated concentrations) and/or UIC2 mAb (20 μg/ml). EC$_{50}$ values were calculated by fitting the dose-response curves. Values are means (± SD) of 3 independent experiments. Statistically significant differences are shown by * (P< 0.05).

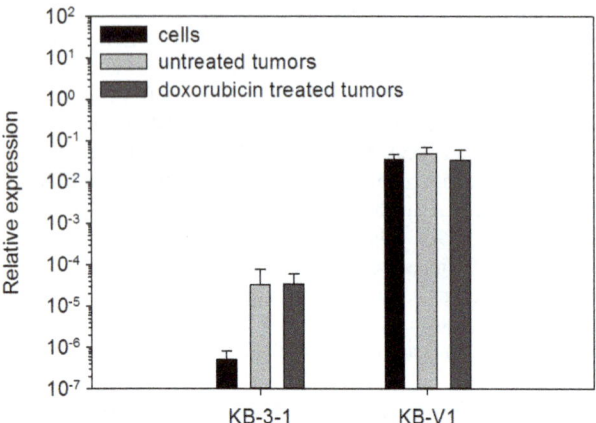

Figure 2. Relative Pgp mRNA expression levels of the KB-V1 and KB-3-1 tumors and the cells applied for grafting the tumors. Pgp expression levels are normalized to the expression level of GAPDH mRNA (mean ± SD, n = 5). The Pgp expression levels of inoculated KB-V1 cells and tumors were significantly different from those of the KB-3-1 cells and tumors (P<0.01), while the Pgp expression levels of tumors were not statistically different from those of the cells they originated from.

both. For an *in vivo* visualization of their effects, miniPET-^{18}FDG accumulation measurements were performed, carrying out the scans 6–8 days after the above treatments. Fig. 3 shows representative ^{18}FDG accumulation scans and the anatomical pictures of untreated (Fig. 3*A and C*) and DOX-UIC2-CsA treated (Fig. 3*B and D*) SCID mice bearing Pgp⁺ (KB-V1, right shoulder and thigh) and Pgp⁻ (KB-3-1, left shoulder and thigh) tumor xenografts. At the time of the measurements the tumors of untreated mice were 5–8 mm in diameter (6.43±1.13 mm mean ± SD, KB-3-1; 6.0±1.15 mm mean ± SD, KB-V1), and well-detectable on the basis of their increased rate of glucose metabolism.

The tumor (T) to skeletal muscle (M) ^{18}FDG accumulation ratio (T/M) was 4.2±0.6 in the case of Pgp⁻ and 4.8±0.7 for the Pgp⁺ tissues (n = 7, ± SD), indicating significantly higher rate of glucose consumption in tumors compared to the muscle cells in both cases.

No visible or palpable tumors developed in 20% of the animals treated with the combination of DOX-UIC2-CsA. This observation was confirmed by the mini-PET scans, since no significant ^{18}FDG accumulation was observed at the sites of tumor cell inoculation in these animals, as reflected by the T/M ^{18}FDG accumulation ratios being close to 1 (T/M = 1.1±0.2 for Pgp⁺ and T/M = 0.97±0.1 for Pgp⁻ tumors; (n = 4)).

Effect of DOX treatment combined with UIC2 and/or a low dose of CsA on the weights of grafted tumors

Eight days after chemotherapy, the animals were sacrificed by cervical dislocation and the tumors were removed to weigh them. As it is shown in Fig. 4*A*, DOX treatment alone was almost ineffective in the case of KB-V1 tumors, while the weight of the KB-3-1 tumors decreased considerably. Co-administration of 10 mg/kg CsA decreased the size of the KB-V1 tumors only mildly and did not affect the KB-3-1 tumors. Combined treatment with DOX-CsA-UIC2 decreased the mean weight of the KB-V1 tumors 9 fold compared to the animals treated with DOX alone. The combined treatment also decreased the mean weight of the KB-3-1 tumors, but not in a statistically significant extent. Importantly, only 52% of the grafted Pgp⁺ or Pgp⁻ tumors

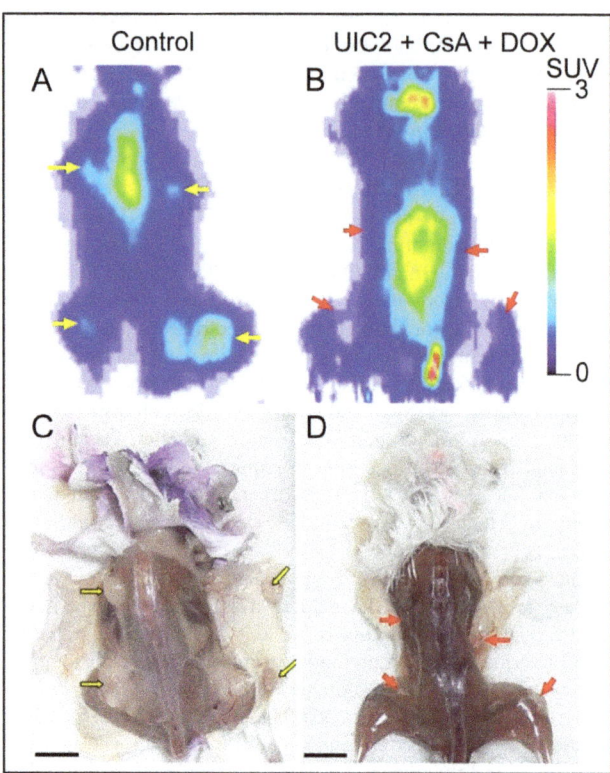

Figure 3. Effect of combined treatment with DOX+CsA+UIC2 on the KB-V1 and KB-3-1 tumors visualized *in vivo* by ^{18}FDG-miniPET. Coronal section of ^{18}FDG-miniPET image of a representative control (*A*) and a DOX-CsA-UIC2-treated tumor bearing mouse (*B*). Standardized uptake values (SUV) are calculated as described in Materials and Methods. The sites of tumor cell inoculation are shown by arrows (KB-V1 tumors, right side arrows; KB-3-1 tumors, left side arrows). Below: autopsies of the same control (*C*) and treated (*D*) animals. Bar: 10 mm.

developed into detectable tumors in the DOX-CSA-UIC2 treated animals (see Fig. 4*B*), and 20% of the animals remained completely tumor-free. In contrast, we always detected tumors in the other treatment groups. Co-administration of UIC2 and DOX also decreased tumor size significantly compared to DOX alone in the case of KB-V1 tumors. This finding, in view of the fact that UIC2 treatment alone does not affect the EC$_{50}$ value of DOX in *in vitro* cytotoxicity tests (Fig. 1), suggested to us that the growth inhibitory effect of the antibody is not exclusively due to Pgp inhibition. UIC2 binding did not affect the *in vitro* cell viability significantly (Fig. 5); therefore, the contribution of the immune system, that is partly functional in the SCID mice, was tested.

In vitro ADCC and CDC measurements

Fig. 6 shows the effect of human peripheral blood mononuclear cells (PBMCs), and of human serum samples, on UIC2 mAb treated KB-V1 and KB-3-1 cells, *in vitro*. PBMCs killed about 70-80% of the UIC2 treated KB-V1 cells both in the presence and absence of CsA, at target to effector cell ratios of 1:50 and 1:100, respectively (Fig. 6*A*), in contrast with the UIC2 treated KB-3-1 cells that exhibited a survival rate similar to that of the untreated control (Fig. 6*B*). In the absence of UIC2, the percentages of dead target cells were low (see Fig. 6*A and B*).

In order to assess the possible role of CDC in UIC2 mediated *in vivo* tumor cell killing, the cytotoxicity of human serum samples

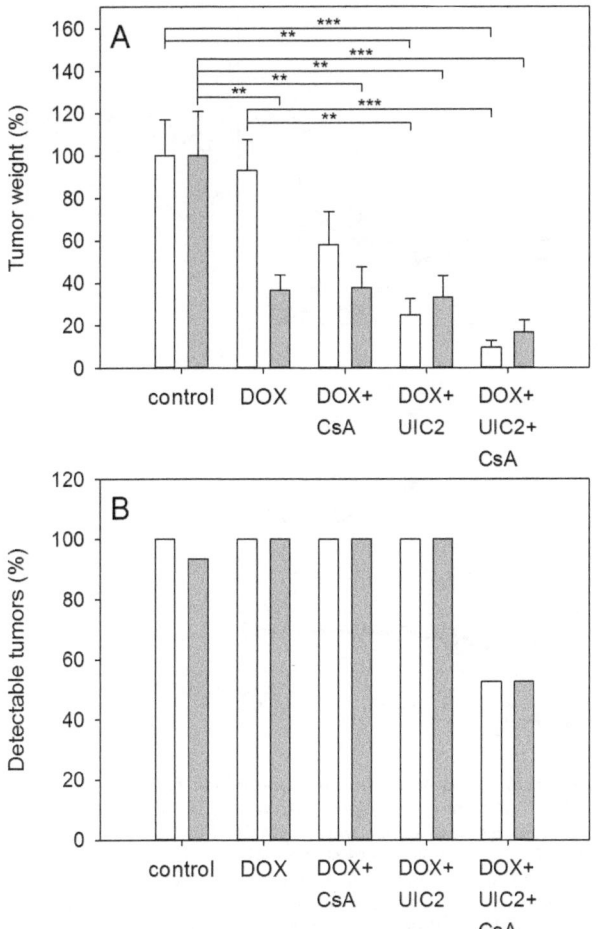

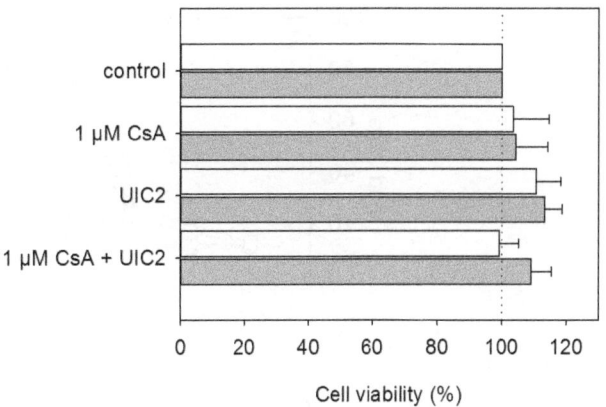

Figure 5. Effect of the UIC2 mAb treatment on the *in vitro* viability of KB-3-1 (Pgp⁻; grey bars) and KB-V1 cells (Pgp⁺; empty bars) in the presence or absence of 1 μM CsA. Cell viability was expressed as percentage of the untreated control. Values are means (± SD) of three independent experiments.

Figure 4. Effect of treatment with DOX combined with UIC2 and/or a low dose of CsA on the weights of the grafted tumors (*A*) and on the percentage of the detectable tumors in the different treatment groups (*B*). Tumor weights were expressed as a percentage of the average weight of the tumors of untreated animals measured at the time of the termination of the experiment (mean values ± SEM, n = 8). Statistically significant differences relative to the untreated control and the DOX-only treated groups are marked with *: P<0.05; **: P<0.01; ***: P<0.001). Grey bars: KB-3-1 (Pgp⁻) and empty bars: KB-V1 (Pgp⁺) tumors.

was measured *in vitro*. Cell killing did not increase in the UIC2 treated KB-V1 (Fig. 6*C*) and KB-3-1 (Fig. 6*D*) samples despite the strong hemolytic activity of the applied sera (Fig. 6*D, inset*).

Discussion

In the present experiments SCID mice xenotransplanted with Pgp⁺ and Pgp⁻ tumors were used to study the efficacy of an antibody-based multidrug resistance reversal strategy. The KB-V1/KB-3-1 cell pair does not express ABCG2 and MRP1 (ABCC1) at detectable levels, while the KB-V1 cells have high Pgp expression level (see Fig. S2 and Fig. 2). They are growing fast and develop into subcutaneous tumors of ~1 cm diameter in about 10–12 days after inoculation of $1-3 \times 10^6$ cells into the animals. An advantage of the fast tumor growth in this model system is that the Pgp expression level of the tumor cells does not decline in the absence of Pgp substrates (see Fig. 2) on the time scale of the *in vivo* experiments.

In the above model system, co-treatment with UIC2 + CsA potentiated the anti-tumor effect of DOX and inhibited or hindered the development of KB-V1 Pgp⁺ tumors *in vivo* (Fig. 4). At the same time, DOX treatment alone did not have a significant effect on the size of the KB-V1 tumors. These data are in line with the conclusions of our previously published *in vitro* and *in vivo* drug accumulation studies [22] and with the results of the *in vitro* cytotoxicity measurements shown in Fig. 1. Although these observations may suggest that the dramatic antitumor effect of the combined treatment is the result of increased antibody binding with consequential Pgp inhibition and DOX accumulation, the mechanism proved more complex.

SCID mice have intact complement system as well as functioning macrophages, natural killer cells and polymorphonu-clear cells [32]. Therefore, antibody binding to the tumor cells may elicit cytotoxicity directly through complement binding (complement-dependent cytotoxicity, CDC) or indirectly, via the recruitment of the above effector cells to the antibody covered tumor cells (antibody-dependent cell-mediated cytotoxicity, ADCC). The possibility, that immunological factors contribute to the cytotoxic effect of our treatment protocol is strongly supported by the difference between the outcomes of *in vitro* cytotoxicity measurements and of the *in vivo* experiments conducted in SCID mice (compare Fig. 1 and Fig. 4). In the *in vitro* cytotoxicity assay, UIC2 alone only mildly aggravated DOX cytotoxicity (see Fig. 1) what could be explained by the trapping and inhibition of only a small fraction of cell surface Pgps by UIC2 in the absence of CsA [22]. In contrast, we experienced *in vivo* a marked decrease of tumor size in response to the DOX+UIC2-only treatment, as the average weight of the KB-V1 tumors was approx. 4 fold smaller compared to the animals treated with DOX alone (Fig. 4*A*). These data are in line with the positive results of our *in vitro* ADCC assays (Fig. 6), supporting the notion that the UIC2 mAb also induces ADCC *in vivo* in the SCID mice.

The involvement of ADCC in the *in vivo* anti-tumor effect of UIC2 treatment is an unexpected finding of our experiments, since IgG₂ antibodies are mostly inefficient at supporting effector functions and are chosen for antibody therapy when effector functions are unnecessary or undesirable [33]. However, there is an example [34] when the antitumor and antimetastatic effects of two IgG₂ isotye anti-Pgp antibodies (the mouse-human chimeric Ab (MH162) and its mouse counterpart (MRK16)) was attributed

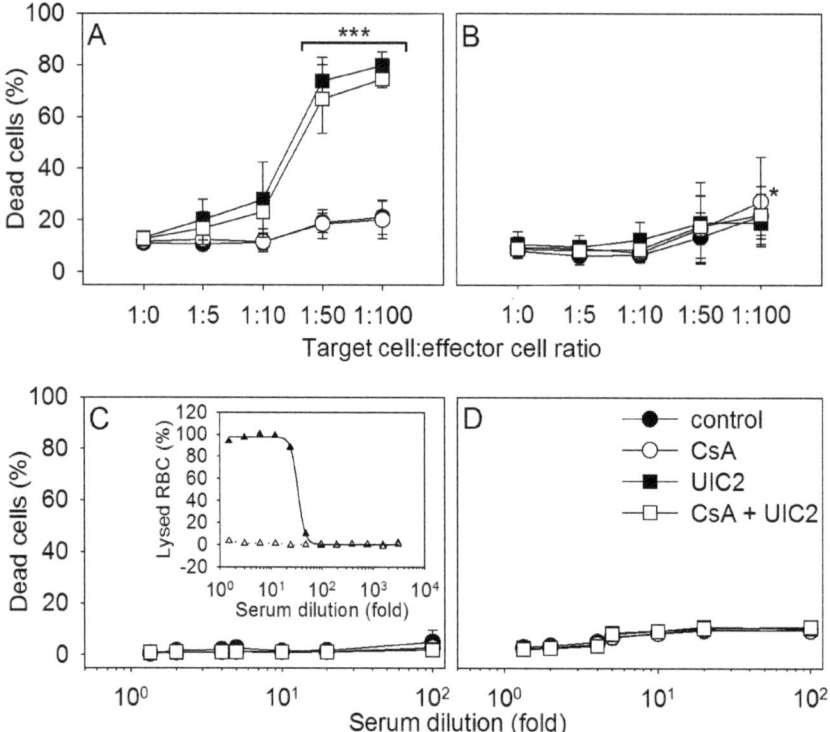

Figure 6. Antibody-dependent cell-mediated cytotoxicity (ADCC, *panels A* and *B*) and complement mediated lysis (CDC, *panels C* and *D*) induced by UIC2 mAb treatment *in vitro.* In the ADCC assay KB-V1 (*A*) and KB-3-1 (*B*) tumor cells were labeled with CFDA-SE then mixed with PBMCs freshly isolated from peripheral blood at different target to effector cell ratios. Samples were treated with 10 μM CsA (○), 20 μg/ml UIC2 mAb (■), 10 μM CsA and 20 μg/ml UIC2 mAb (□) or buffer (●). After 8 h incubation at 37°C, samples were stained with PI and analyzed by flow cytometry. In the CDC assay, cells were incubated with human serum at different dilutions for 4 h. *Inset of panel C*: Hemolytic effect of the serum (▲) and of heat inactivated serum (△) on sensitized sheep red blood cells served as positive and negative control, respectively. The percentages of killed cells were calculated as described in Materials and Methods. Values are means (± SD) of four independent experiments, ***P<0,001.

to ADCC. Similarly, it was proven in a recent study that a human IgG₂ isotype mAb specific for epidermal growth factor receptor effectively triggers ADCC by recruting monocytes and neutrophils [35] via FcγRIIa binding [36,37]. Since IgG₂ isotype antibodies do not trigger natural killer cell mediated ADCC [35], therefore in our *in vitro* ADCC experiments carried out with PBMCs cell killing was mediated by monocytes. Since SCID mice also have monocytes [32] the same mechanism is functional and probably explains our *in vivo* results.

The strong anti-tumor effect of the combined treatment might be attributed exclusively to ADCC triggered by the UIC2 mAb binding. However, the fact that the extents of the *in vitro* ADCC effects were indistinguishable in the presence of UIC2 or UIC2+ CsA suggests that binding of the antibody to a small fraction of the cell surface Pgps (20-40%) is sufficient to induce a maximal ADCC effect (Fig. 6*A*). Consequently, the differences in the size of the KB-V1 tumors between the UIC2 and UIC2+CsA treated animals and the lack of the KB-V1 tumors in 52% of these animals (Fig 4*A and B*) argue against the above assumption and suggests that the stronger Pgp inhibitory effect of the UIC2+CsA combination mediates the anti-tumor effect at least in part. Pgp inhibition by the antibody requires saturating antibody concentrations that seems to be reached in our experiments, since strong UIC2 staining and a two fold increase in the accumulation of a Pgp substrate daunorubicin was measured in the tumor sections prepared from the tumors 8 hours after the injection of UIC2 and CsA [22] added at similar conditions. Taken together, our *in vitro* and *in vivo* data suggest that strong anti-tumor effect can be

reached by the combinative treatment studied, as a joint result of Pgp inhibition and ADCC. However, the relative contribution of these mechanisms to the anti-tumor effect of the UIC2 mAb is not known.

ADCC can be triggered at relatively low receptor occupancy by the antibody or at low receptor abundance [35,38]. Thus, the 60 fold increased Pgp expression level of the KB-3-1 tumors compared to the KB-3-1 cells (see Fig. 2.) is probably sufficient to trigger ADCC effect, when the Pgp molecules are saturated by the antibody in the presence of CsA. In line with this assumption in 52% of the DOX-UIC2-CsA treated animals we could not detect KB-3-1 tumors, while they appeared in all of the DOX or DOX+UIC2 treated animals (see Fig. 4*B*).

It could be a limitation of our study that only one cell line pair was used in the experiments. However, the observed effects have been proven to be Pgp specific, since decreased tumor size was detected exclusively in those animal groups that received UIC2 mAb treatment. In addition, in our previous studies we compared the KB-V1 cell line with mdr1 transfected NIH 3T3 murine fibroblast cells [22], and Pgp⁺ A2780^AD ovarian carcinoma cells [23] and found them equivalent in every aspect of their multidrug resistant phenotype including the inhibition of Pgp-mediated drug transport by UIC2 mAb. On the other hand, ADCC effect is not dependent on the tissue origin of the target cells; rather it is determined by the interaction between the Fc part of the antibody and the Fc receptor of the effector cells.

Doubts about the possible clinical application of an anti-Pgp mAb based tumor therapy are related to the likely side effects that may arise as a result of either Pgp inhibition or ADCC, both exerted on cells expressing Pgp at physiological barriers of the body. For instance, inhibition of Pgp expressed in the blood-brain barrier may lead to increased accumulation of its substrates in the central nervous system leading to neurotoxicity, as it was experienced in mdr1a/b knock-out mice [8]. However, administration of Pgp modulators in clinical trials does not seem to cause toxicity to the central nervous system [39] probably because other ABC transporters (e.g. MRP1, BCRP1) may compensate for the loss off Pgp's gatekeeper function in the blood-brain barrier [40]. However, in contrast to Pgp inhibition, ADCC may damage the tissues at the physiological Pgp expression sites. Our *in vitro* assays using human PBMCs confirmed that UIC2 mAb effectively triggers ADCC. Since ADCC is mediated via the Fc portion of the antibody, to avoid this side-effect upon human applications the whole UIC2 antibody could be substituted for by its Fab fragments (that behave very similarly to whole antibodies *in vitro*; our unpublished data) or upon humanization of the antibody its effector functions may be fine-tuned by the design of the Fc part [33]. However, it remains to be studied if inhibition of Pgp function alone may augment DOX cytotoxicity sufficiently enough for a therapeutically significant anti-tumor effect.

The UIC2 mAb does not bind to mouse Pgp [14], therefore the SCID mouse model system is not applicable for studying the possible side effects brought about by antibody binding to physiological Pgp expression sites. Since the UIC2 mAb also recognizes primate [14] and sheep [41] Pgp, such animal models may be used for the evaluation of the feasibility of the strategy demonstrated herein. Direct injection of the antibody into the tumor tissue may also be tested for the purposes of reducing antibody dose and decrease systemic side effects.

In our model system, treatments were applied shortly (four days) after injection of the tumor cells, when the tumors were still rather small, a situation perhaps analogous to the clinical setting when systemic therapy is applied to prevent or hinder the development of multidrug resistant primary or metastatic tumors.

Each multidrug resistant tumor may have a unique signature of resistance mechanisms. Consequently, cancer therapy will need to be personalized, not only with respect to the mechanisms of malignant transformation but also regarding the mechanisms of resistance [42]. The strategy of Pgp inhibition demonstrated herein is offered to enrich the repertoir of possible protocols that can be considered for the treatment of multidrug resistant tumors, once humanized UIC2 becomes available.

Supporting Information

Figure S1   In the ADCC assay KB-V1 (panels *A*, *B*, *C*) and KB-3-1 (*D*, *E*, *F*) tumor cells were labeled with CFDA-SE, then mixed with PBMCs freshly isolated from peripheral blood at 1:5 (*B*, *E*) or 1:100 (*C*, *F*) target to effector cell ratios. Samples were treated with 20 µg/ml UIC2 mAb. After 8 h incubation at 37°C, samples were stained with PI and analyzed by flow cytometry. *Green gates* mark living target cells, while *red gates* show dead target cells.

Figure S2   Flow cytometric analysis of Pgp, ABCG2 and MRP1 expression in KB-V1 (*A*, *C*, *E*) and KB-3-1 (*B*, *D*, *F*) cell lines applying indirect immunofluorescence staining by CFL647-conjugated GaMIgG. Pgp was detected by 15D3 mAb, while ABCG2 and MRP1 (ABCC1) were labeled by 5D3 and QCRL-3 mAbs, respectively. Grey filled histograms show antibody untreated cells, while dashed lines represent samples treated with secondary antibody only. The ABCG2 positive MDCK ABCG2 cells (*G*) and the MRP1 (*I*) expressing GLC4-ADR cell line and their nonexpressing counterparts (*H* and *J*) were used as controls. The GLC4 human small cell lung carcinoma cell line pair was a kind gift from Pinedo HM (Department of Medical Oncology, Academic Hospital Vrije Universiteit, Amsterdam), while the MDCK (Madin-Darby canine kidney) cell line and its ABCG2 transfected counterpart was kindly provided by Sarkadi B (Biomembrane Institute of Molecular Pharmacology, Budapest)

Figure S3   Pgp expression of KB-V1 (*A*) and KB-3-1 (*C*) tumor xenografts visualized by indirect immunofluorescence. Panels (*B*) and (*D*) are phase contrast images of the same tumor slices. The 5 µm thick cryosections were fixed in acetone, labeled with UIC2 mAb followed by A488-GaMIgG at room temperature for 60 min.

Acknowledgments

We thank Anita Szabóné Jeney (Department of Biophysics and Cell Biology), Judit Pélyi and Tamás Nagy (Department of Nuclear Medicine) for their technical assistance.

Author Contributions

Conceived and designed the experiments: G. Szalóki KG G. Szabó ZK TM ZTK GT IL IJ. Performed the experiments: G. Szalóki ZTK LV AGS IL IJ GT ÁT ZK TM. Analyzed the data: G. Szalóki ZTK GT ZK TM MB. Wrote the paper: KG G. Szabó GT TM G. Szalóki.

References

1. Gottesman MM, Fojo T, Bates SE (2002) Multidrug resistance in cancer: role of ATP-dependent transporters. Nat Rev Cancer 2: 48–58.
2. Borst P, Elferink RO (2002) Mammalian ABC transporters in health and disease. Annu Rev Biochem 71: 537–592.
3. Glavinas H, Krajcsi P, Cserepes J, Sarkadi B (2004) The role of ABC transporters in drug resistance, metabolism and toxicity. Curr Drug Deliv 1: 27–42.
4. Rosenberg MF, Callaghan R, Ford RC, Higgins CF (1997) Structure of the multidrug resistance P-glycoprotein to 2.5 nm resolution determined by electron microscopy and image analysis. J Biol Chem 272: 10685–10694.
5. Senior AE (2012) Two ATPases. J Biol Chem 287: 30049–30062.
6. Ambudkar SV, Kim IW, Sauna ZE (2006) The power of the pump: mechanisms of action of P-glycoprotein (ABCB1). Eur J Pharm Sci 27: 392–400.
7. Leonard GD, Fojo T, Bates SE (2003) The role of ABC transporters in clinical practice. Oncologist 8: 411–424.
8. Schinkel AH, Smit JJ, van Tellingen O, Beijnen JH, Wagenaar E, et al. (1994) Disruption of the mouse mdr1a P-glycoprotein gene leads to a deficiency in the blood-brain barrier and to increased sensitivity to drugs. Cell 77: 491–502.
9. Schinkel AH, Mayer U, Wagenaar E, Mol CA, van Deemter L, et al. (1997) Normal viability and altered pharmacokinetics in mice lacking mdr1-type (drug-transporting) P-glycoproteins. Proc Natl Acad Sci U S A 94: 4028–4033.
10. Friedenberg WR, Rue M, Blood EA, Dalton WS, Shustik C, et al. (2006) Phase III study of PSC-833 (valspodar) in combination with vincristine, doxorubicin, and dexamethasone (valspodar/VAD) versus VAD alone in patients with recurring or refractory multiple myeloma (E1A95): a trial of the Eastern Cooperative Oncology Group. Cancer 106: 830–838.
11. Chico I, Kang MH, Bergan R, Abraham J, Bakke S, et al. (2001) Phase I study of infusional paclitaxel in combination with the P-glycoprotein antagonist PSC 833. J Clin Oncol 19: 832–842.
12. Szakacs G, Varadi A, Ozvegy-Laczka C, Sarkadi B (2008) The role of ABC transporters in drug absorption, distribution, metabolism, excretion and toxicity (ADME-Tox). Drug Discov Today 13: 379–393.
13. Chaudhary PM, Mechetner EB, Roninson IB (1992) Expression and activity of the multidrug resistance P-glycoprotein in human peripheral blood lymphocytes. Blood 80: 2735–2739.

14. Mechetner EB, Roninson IB (1992) Efficient inhibition of P-glycoprotein-mediated multidrug resistance with a monoclonal antibody. Proc Natl Acad Sci U S A 89: 5824–5828.

15. Rittmann-Grauer LS, Yong MA, Sanders V, Mackensen DG (1992) Reversal of Vinca alkaloid resistance by anti-P-glycoprotein monoclonal antibody HYB-241 in a human tumor xenograft. Cancer Res 52: 1810–1816.

16. Jachez B, Cianfriglia M, Loor F (1994) Modulation of human P-glycoprotein epitope expression by temperature and/or resistance-modulating agents. Anticancer Drugs 5: 655–665.

17. Watanabe T, Naito M, Kokubu N, Tsuruo T (1997) Regression of established tumors expressing P-glycoprotein by combinations of adriamycin, cyclosporin derivatives, and MRK-16 antibodies. J Natl Cancer Inst 89: 512–518.

18. Naito M, Watanabe T, Tsuge H, Koyama T, Oh-hara T, et al. (1996) Potentiation of the reversal activity of SDZ PSC833 on multi-drug resistance by an anti-P-glycoprotein monoclonal antibody MRK-16. Int J Cancer 67: 435–440.

19. Schinkel AH, Arceci RJ, Smit JJ, Wagenaar E, Baas F, et al. (1993) Binding properties of monoclonal antibodies recognizing external epitopes of the human MDR1 P-glycoprotein. Int J Cancer 55: 478–484.

20. Zhou Y, Gottesman MM, Pastan I (1999) The extracellular loop between TM5 and TM6 of P-glycoprotein is required for reactivity with monoclonal antibody UIC2. Arch Biochem Biophys 367: 74–80.

21. Nagy H, Goda K, Fenyvesi F, Bacsó Z, Szilasi M, et al. (2004) Distinct groups of multidrug resistance modulating agents are distinguished by competition of P-glycoprotein-specific antibodies. Biochem Biophys Res Commun 315: 942–949.

22. Goda K, Fenyvesi F, Bacsó Z, Nagy H, Márián T, et al. (2007) Complete inhibition of P-glycoprotein by simultaneous treatment with a distinct class of modulators and the UIC2 monoclonal antibody. J Pharmacol Exp Ther 320: 81–88.

23. Krasznai ZT, Tóth A, Mikecz P, Fodor Z, Szabó G, et al. (2010) Pgp inhibition by UIC2 antibody can be followed in vitro by using tumor-diagnostic radiotracers, 99mTc-MIBI and 18FDG. Eur J Pharm Sci 41: 665–669.

24. Pauwels EK, Ribeiro MJ, Stoot JH, McCready VR, Bourguignon M, et al. (1998) FDG accumulation and tumor biology. Nucl Med Biol 25: 317–322.

25. Wahl RL (1996) Targeting glucose transporters for tumor imaging: "sweet" idea, "sour" result. J Nucl Med 37: 1038–1041.

26. Mankoff DA, Bellon JR (2001) Positron-emission tomographic imaging of cancer: glucose metabolism and beyond. Semin Radiat Oncol 11: 16–27.

27. Shen DW, Cardarelli C, Hwang J, Cornwell M, Richert N, et al. (1986) Multiple drug-resistant human KB carcinoma cells independently selected for high-level resistance to colchicine, adriamycin, or vinblastine show changes in expression of specific proteins. J Biol Chem 261: 7762–7770.

28. Akiyama S, Fojo A, Hanover JA, Pastan I, Gottesman MM (1985) Isolation and genetic characterization of human KB cell lines resistant to multiple drugs. Somat Cell Mol Genet 11: 117–126.

29. Hamacher K, Coenen HH, Stocklin G (1986) Efficient stereospecific synthesis of no-carrier-added 2-[18F]-fluoro-2-deoxy-D-glucose using aminopolyether supported nucleophilic substitution. J Nucl Med 27: 235–238.

30. Barok M, Isola J, Pályi-Krekk Z, Nagy P, Juhász I, et al. (2007) Trastuzumab causes antibody-dependent cellular cytotoxicity-mediated growth inhibition of submacroscopic JIMT-1 breast cancer xenografts despite intrinsic drug resistance. Mol Cancer Ther 6: 2065–2072.

31. Márián T, Szabó G, Goda K, Nagy H, Szincsák N, et al. (2003) In vivo and in vitro multitracer analyses of P-glycoprotein expression-related multidrug resistance. Eur J Nucl Med Mol Imaging 30: 1147–1154.

32. Bosma MJ, Carroll AM (1991) The SCID mouse mutant: definition, characterization, and potential uses. Annu Rev Immunol 9: 323–350.

33. Carter PJ (2006) Potent antibody therapeutics by design. Nat Rev Immunol 6: 343–357.

34. Yano S, Hanibuchi M, Nishioka Y, Nokihara H, Nishimura N, et al. (1999) Combined therapy with anti-P-glycoprotein antibody and macrophage colony-stimulating factor gene transduction for multiorgan metastases of multidrug-resistant human small cell lung cancer in NK cell-depleted SCID mice. Int J Cancer 82: 105–111.

35. Schneider-Merck T, Lammerts van Bueren JJ, Berger S, Rossen K, van Berkel PH, et al. (2010) Human IgG2 antibodies against epidermal growth factor receptor effectively trigger antibody-dependent cellular cytotoxicity but, in contrast to IgG1, only by cells of myeloid lineage. J Immunol 184: 512–520.

36. van de Winkel JG, Anderson CL (1991) Biology of human immunoglobulin G Fc receptors. Journal of leukocyte biology 49: 511–524.

37. Ravetch JV, Bolland S (2001) IgG Fc receptors. Annu Rev Immunol 19: 275–290.

38. Bleeker WK, Lammerts van Bueren JJ, van Ojik HH, Gerritsen AF, Pluyter M, et al. (2004) Dual mode of action of a human anti-epidermal growth factor receptor monoclonal antibody for cancer therapy. J Immunol 173: 4699–4707.

39. Sikic BI, Fisher GA, Lum BL, Halsey J, Beketic-Oreskovic L, et al. (1997) Modulation and prevention of multidrug resistance by inhibitors of P-glycoprotein. Cancer Chemother Pharmacol 40 Suppl: S13–19.

40. Loscher W, Potschka H (2005) Blood-brain barrier active efflux transporters: ATP-binding cassette gene family. NeuroRx 2: 86–98.

41. Bougoin S, Lomet D, Kerboeuf D, Le Vern Y, Malpaux B, et al. (2008) Evidence that the choroids plexus in female sheep express P-glycoprotein. Neuro Endocrinol Lett 29: 438–442.

42. Gottesman MM, Ludwig J, Xia D, Szakacs G (2006) Defeating drug resistance in cancer. Discov Med 6: 18–23.

10

Retrocrural Space Involvement on Computed Tomography as a Predictor of Mortality and Disease Severity in Acute Pancreatitis

Haotong Xu[1,2]*, Lukas Ebner[3], Shiming Jiang[4], Yi Wu[5], Andreas Christe[3], Shaoxiang Zhang[5], Xiaoming Zhang[6], Zhulin Luo[1], Fuzhou Tian[1]*

1 Postdoctoral Workstation, the General Surgery Center of the Peoples' Liberation Army, Chengdu Army General Hospital, Chengdu, Sichuan, P. R. China, 2 Department of Radiology, Sichuan Provincial People's Hospital Supo, Chengdu, Sichuan, P. R. China, 3 Department of Radiology, Inselspital, University of Bern, Freiburgstrasse, Bern, Switzerland, 4 Department of Radiology, Nanchong Central Hospital of North Sichuan Medical College, Nanchong, Sichuan, P. R. China, 5 Institute of Computing Medicine, Third Military Medical University, Chongqing, P. R. China, 6 Sichuan Key Laboratory of Medical Imaging, Department of Radiology, Affiliated Hospital of North Sichuan Medical College, Nanchong, Sichuan, P. R. China

Abstract

Background: Because computed tomography (CT) has advantages for visualizing the manifestation of necrosis and local complications, a series of scoring systems based on CT manifestations have been developed for assessing the clinical outcomes of acute pancreatitis (AP), including the CT severity index (CTSI), modified CTSI, etc. Despite the internationally accepted CTSI having been successfully used to predict the overall mortality and disease severity of AP, recent literature has revealed the limitations of the CTSI. Using the Delphi method, we establish a new scoring system based on retrocrural space involvement (RCSI), and compared its effectiveness at evaluating the mortality and severity of AP with that of the CTSI.

Methods: We reviewed CT images of 257 patients with AP taken within 3–5 days of admission in 2012. The RCSI scoring system, which includes assessment of infectious conditions involving the retrocrural space and the adjacent pleural cavity, was established using the Delphi method. Two radiologists independently assessed the RCSI and CTSI scores. The predictive points of the RCSI and CTSI scoring systems in evaluating the mortality and severity of AP were estimated using receiver operating characteristic (ROC) curves.

Principal Findings: The RCSI score can accurately predict the mortality and disease severity. The area under the ROC curve for the RCSI versus CTSI score was 0.962 ± 0.011 versus 0.900 ± 0.021 for predicting the mortality, and 0.888 ± 0.025 versus 0.904 ± 0.020 for predicting the severity of AP. Applying ROC analysis to our data showed that a RCSI score of 4 was the best cutoff value, above which mortality could be identified.

Conclusion: The Delphi method was innovatively adopted to establish a scoring system to predict the clinical outcome of AP. The RCSI scoring system can predict the mortality of AP better than the CTSI system, and the severity of AP equally as well.

Editor: Henrik Einwaechter, Klinikum rechts der Isar der TU München, Germany

Funding: This work was supported by the National Science Foundation of China (No. 61190122 and 81100480) (http://www.nsfc.gov.cn). This work was also supported by the Military Twelfth-five Major Research Project of China (BWS12J020) (http://211.162.67.9/Depart/Desc/20). The funders had no role in study design, data collection and analysis, decision to publish, or preparation of the manuscript.

* Email: tfz3006@yahoo.com (FT); xuliangxman@hotmail.com (HX)

Introduction

In addition to the pathological changes of the pancreas itself from acute pancreatitis (AP), various local complications of AP may appear in the retroperitoneal space or the structures around the pancreas. These complications involve fluid collections, pseudocyst, peripancreatic abscess and vascular disorders, etc. The complications around the pancreas, especially those in the retroperitoneal space, will progress to severe AP, and can lead to a poor prognosis [1].

The diagnostic imaging modalities for AP have a significant role in confirming the diagnosis of the disease, helping detect the extent of pancreatic necrosis, and diagnosing local complications [2]. Because of their advantages for visualizing the manifestation of necrosis and local complications, CT and magnetic resonance imaging (MRI) have been used in assessing the clinical outcomes of patients with AP. A series of scoring systems and prediction methods based on imaging manifestations have been developed for this purpose, including the CT severity index (CTSI), modified CTSI, extrapancreatic inflammation on CT (EPIC), and MR severity index (MRSI) [3,4,5,6].

The CTSI, developed by Balthazar and colleagues in 1994 [3], was a significant advance in assessing the clinical outcomes of patients because it helped clinicians to discriminate among mild, moderate, and severe forms of pancreatitis. The CTSI focuses on the presence and degree of pancreatic inflammation and necrosis. On a 10-point severity scale, points are awarded for the presence or absence of fluid collections, in combination with an assessment of the presence and degree of pancreatic necrosis [3]. Although this system has been successfully used to predict overall morbidity and mortality in patients with AP, we found limitations in the application of the CTSI scoring system. Observers often diverged from each other in counting the locations for fluid collections due to the development of the radiological anatomy of the retroperitoneal space. Subsequently, the inter-rater agreement for scoring CT scans using the CTSI may be poor.

Mortelé et al. have indicated other shortcomings of the CTSI, such as no correlation with extrapancreatic parenchymal complications, and no significant difference in mortality between 30 and 50% and more than 50% necrosis [7,8]. Thus, researchers have attempted to establish a new scoring systems - the modified CTSI, which incorporates extrapancreatic complications into the CTSI, and the EPIC, which is based exclusively on the presence of systemic inflammation (including pleural effusion, ascites, and retroperitoneal inflammation) [4,5]. Although some comparative studies have confirmed that the predictive value of these new scoring systems was better than that of the CTSI, the effective forecasting method has not been applied in constructing these scoring systems.

Originally developed as a systematic, interactive forecasting method that relies on a panel of experts [9], the Delphi method is a structured communication technique based on the principle that forecasts from a structured group of individuals are more accurate than those from unstructured groups [10]. Experts answer questionnaires in two or more rounds. After each round, a facilitator provides an anonymous summary of the experts' forecasts from the previous round as well as the reasons they provided for their judgments. Thus, the experts are encouraged to revise their earlier answers in light of the replies from other members of their panel. It is believed that during this process, the range of the discrimination will decrease and the group will converge towards a consensus. The process is stopped after a pre-defined stop criterion (e.g. number of rounds, achievement of consensus); namely, the experts will agree with all items of the scoring system in the final round. In 1999, Ricke et al. used a Delphi consensus procedure to establish guidelines for standardized diagnostic imaging of neuroendocrine tumors [11].

Calculating the accuracy of a diagnostic test using standard definitions (such as CTSI) unavoidably includes the risk of bias in some circumstances. Receiver operating characteristic (ROC) analysis offers the possibility of bias-correction by which the most appropriate cutoff value can be determined [12]. Moreover, the area under the ROC curve is a reliable measure of overall predictive discrimination [13]. Thus, ROC analysis should be the preferred method for assessing the predictive value of imaging techniques [5].

In our previous research employing the Visible Human Project and CT images to study the draining pathways of peripancreatic fluid to the mediastinum in recurrent AP, we discovered that most of the pancreatic fluid might first enter the retrocrural space on its transdiaphragmatic passage into the mediastinum, except for the fluid in the right posterior mediastinum [14]. The retrocrural space is the sentinel mediastinal space involved in AP. Therefore, our purpose was the following: (1) to observe the CT manifestations of RCSI in AP, RCSI is the infectious conditions involving the bilateral crus of diaphragm, the mediastinal pleura, the retrocrural space itself and the adjacent pleural cavity; (2) to establish the RCSI scoring system based on the Delphi method; and (3) to use ROC analysis of the RCSI score in predicting the mortality and disease severity in patients with AP, and compare the RCSI score with the CTSI score.

Materials and Methods

1 Ethics statement

This study was approved by the Ethics Review Board of the Chengdu Army General Hospital. The second Chinese Visible Human (CVH2) dataset was from a voluntary donation and was approved for medical research [15]. Obtaining CT scans of patients with AP was approved by the Institutional Review Board of our Hospital. Written informed consent was obtained from the patients before CT scans, and no identifiable information (i.e., age and gender) was reported in this study.

2 Patients

Medical records and CT images were reviewed retrospectively for consecutive patients with AP admitted to our hospital between January and December 2012. Patients were diagnosed with AP using the International Classification of Diseases, Ninth Revision, Clinical Modification code for AP (577.0) [16]. Eligibility criteria for patients in this study were: (1) in-patient, (2) acute onset of symptoms, (3) pancreatitis at first onset, (4) abdominal CT scans, with scanned coverage from the diaphragmatic dome to the iliac crest, and (5) CT examinations obtained 3–5 days after admission. Exclusion criteria in this study were: (1) history of traumatic pancreatitis or postoperative pancreatitis, (2) history of laparotomy or a previous hospitalization for AP that might hinder the interpretation of the severity of AP, and (3) without contrast-enhanced CT scans because of contraindication to iodinated contrast medium and the potential risk of nephrotoxicity.

A total of 257 patients, including 196 men and 61 women, with a mean age of 51.2 ± 12.3 years (range 23–89 years), was recruited for this study. The etiologies of AP were gallstones in 92 patients, alcohol abuse in 71, gallstones and chronic alcohol abuse in 55, post-endoscopic retrograde cholangiopancreatography inflammation in 17, and miscellaneous or uncertain origin in 22.

3 Clinical observation

Clinical outcome was recorded as: (1) severe AP, diagnosed according to the Atlanta classification system [17]; and (2) systemic disease (intensive care unit admission [ICU] or mortality). Percutaneous CT-guided catheter drainage and/or surgical procedures were performed in patients who had pseudocysts at follow-up examinations, infected pancreatic necrosis and in those with abdominal compartment syndrome.

4 Abdominal CT scans

All patients underwent CT scans on a 64-slice scanner (GE Healthcare, Milwaukee, WI, USA) in our hospital. The CT parameters were 120 kVp, 260 mAs, 8×1.25-mm detector configuration, 10.0-mm beam collimation, 18.75 mm/rotation table speed, 5.0-mm section thickness, 0.5-s gantry rotation time, and standard reconstruction algorithm. Unenhanced CT scans were done first, then contrast material (Iopamiron 300, Schering, Berlin, Germany) was administered intravenously to all patients at a flow rate of 3–5 ml/s. The scans extended from the diaphragmatic dome to the iliac crest. If an abnormality was observed on the highest or lowest section, additional images were obtained after the enhanced scan; especially when the RCSI or the combined interfascial plane involved was shown on CT images.

5 Anatomic observation of the retrocrural space

The anatomic features of the retrocrural space were observed on thin-slice cross-sectional images derived from the CVH2 dataset [15]. In consecutive cross-sectional images, the retrocrural space can be defined as a triangular region that represents the most inferior portion of the posterior mediastinum, with no distinct border with the retrocardiac space of the posterior mediastinum in the cranial direction. We defined the appearance of the esophageal hiatus as the first section of the retrocrural space on consecutive cross sections. The point at which the right crura adheres to the lateral surface of the third lumber vertebral body is the inferior border of the retrocrural space. Except for the diaphragmatic hiatuses, the space is delineated anteriorly and laterally by the diaphragmatic crura in the anteroinferior direction, and the mediastinal pleura in the posterosuperior direction. Posteriorly, boundaries include the ventral aspect of the thoracolumbar vertebra (Fig. 1).

6 Establishment of RCSI scoring system based on the Delphi process

To begin, we clarify definitions in the RCSI scoring system. First, normal pleura cannot be imaged on CT scans. Mediastinal pleura that can be visualized indicates thickening of the pleura [18,19]. Second, hydropsia of the diaphragm indicates fluid distribution. Partial swelling in these areas attenuates the CT values [18,20]. Third, haziness and a streaky density in the retrocrural space indicate infectious conditions involving this space similar to the gastric bare area involved in AP [21]. Fourth, we have confirmed that the peripancreatic fluid might extend into the retrocrural space only via esophageal or aortic hiatus in AP [14]. Fifth, pleural effusions, which could be symptomatic in mediastinal fluid collections or result from the development of a fistulous tract into the pleural cavity, might be present during the second stage of the pulmonary complications of AP [22]. As an important item, the "pleural effusion" was adopted in the RCSI scoring system.

Sixth, if the single crura and/or the partial retrocrural space at the posterointernal direction of the homolateral crura are involved in AP, it means unilateral involvement. When both sides of the crura and/or the bilateral sides of the retrocrural space are involved simultaneously, it means bilateral involvement.

To date, the Delphi method has been used widely to establish index systems and to identify a specific index. A Delphi seminar aimed at establishing an RCSI scoring system in evaluating the mortality and disease severity in AP was held on November 5, 2011. A multidisciplinary panel of 12 medical experts was selected to take part in the Delphi process. The criteria for inclusion on the panel were radiological and clinical experts with at least 20 years of experience in AP, and anatomical experts with at least 15 years of experience in sectional anatomy. Prior to the conference, all the experts were provided with recent radiological research reports of pathologic conditions that involved or invaded the retrocrural space, and a radiological scoring system for evaluating the severity of AP, besides of the CTSI, the modified CTSI, the MRSI [3,4,6,23,24,25]. The updated results of the discussion were given to all experts during the initial two rounds of the Delphi procedure. The feedback served as a basis for discussion in the subsequent round. Finally, in the third round, all experts in the panel reached a consensus on a scoring system for RCSI.

7 Quantification of RCSI and CTSI scores on CT

All CT examinations were reviewed by two raters with 10 and 16 years of experience in interpreting abdominal CT images, who were blinded to the laboratory data and clinical outcome. CTSI scores were calculated for every patient (Tab. 1). RCSI scores were quantified for every patient, based on the presence of CT manifestations of RCSI (Tab. 2).

8 Statistical analysis

Results of the RCSI and CTSI scores were given as the mean of the two raters. Inter-rater agreement for the RCSI and CTSI scores was tested using the kappa statistic, which was used to estimate the proportion of inter-rater agreement above that expected by chance. A weighted kappa statistic of 0.41–0.60 was

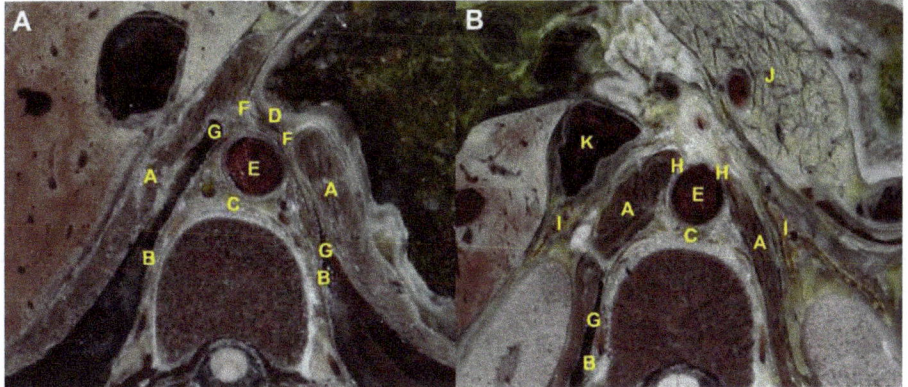

Figure 1. Visualization of the anatomic location of retrocrural space across diaphragmatic hiatuses section on CVH2. (A) On the upper section, the anterior margin of the retrocrural space (C) consists of the distal esophagus (D), the posterior border is thoracolumbar vertebra, both anterolateral borders are composed of the diaphragmatic crus (A), both posterolateral borders are made up of the mediastinal pleura (B). The aorta (E) is situated in the retrocrural space. The potential recess located between the diaphragmatic crura and the mediastinal pleura is the interior costophrenic sulcus (G). The peripancreatic fluid may drain into the retrocrural space via the esophageal hiatus (F). **(B)** On the lower section, the anterior border of the retrocrural space is open to the retroperotoneum, the posterior border is the lumbar vertebra, both lateral borders are made up of the diaphragmatic crus (A), the mediastinal pleura (B) constitutes the right posterolateral border. The inferior vena cava (K) and the both sides of adrenal glands (I) are distributed at the anterolateral direction of the retrocrural space. Furthermore, the peripancreatic fluid that originates from the pancreas (J) may drain into the retrocrural space across the aortic hiatus (H).

Table 1. CTSI scoring system on CT scans in AP.

Prognostic Indicator	Score
Pancreatic inflammation	
Normal pancreas	0
Focal or diffuse enlargement of the pancreas	1
Intrinsic pancreatic abnormalities with inflammatory changes in peripancreatic fat	2
Single, ill defined fluid colletion or phlegmon	3
Two or more poorly defined collections or presence of gas in or adjacent to pancreas	4
Pancreatic Necrosis	
None	0
≤30%	2
30–50%	4
>50%	6

considered moderate agreement, 0.61–0.80 good agreement, and 0.81–1.00 excellent agreement.

ROC analysis was also performed to examine the predictive effect of RCSI and CTSI scoring on the mortality and severity of AP, using mortality and severe AP as the dependent variables. The discriminative powers of the RCSI and CTSI scoring systems were visualized using ROC curves, including the area under the curve (AUC), with 95% confidence interval (CI). Additionally, the AUC values of the two scoring systems were compared using the z-test. The best cutoff values on the ROC curves of the RCSI and CTSI scores were calculated based on the maximum Youden index.

Statistical analysis was performed using commercially available software (SPSS 13.0 version, Chicago, IL, USA), except for the comparison of the AUC of the two scoring systems, which was done with MedCalc 11.6 (MedCalc Software, Mariakerke, Belgium).

Results

1 Patient Outcome

Of the 257 patients surveyed, 60 (23.3%) were admitted to the ICU. A total of 166 patients (64.6%) were diagnosed as having severe AP; 134 patients (52.1%) recovered with medical treatment alone and were discharged, while 123 patients (47.9%) underwent surgical and/or percutaneous interventions. Percutaneous CT-guided catheter drainage of peripancreatic fluid collections was performed in 68 patients (26.5%), local irrigation to the lesser sac in 52 patients and the drainage for a pseudocyst in 16 patients (6.2%). Twelve patients (4.7%) underwent surgical decompression for abdominal compartment syndrome. Moreover, 43 patients (16.7%) underwent a combination of procedures (necrosectomy and drainage) for the infected pancreatic necrosis. Fourteen patients (5.4%) with sepsis died. Eleven patients (4.3%) with alimentary tract hemorrhages died, and 48 patients (18.7%) died of multiple organ failure.

2 CTSI score

Pancreatic enlargement was seen in 12 patients (4.7%), pancreatic and/or peripancreatic fat inflammation was detected in 103 patients (40.1%), a single peripancreatic fluid collection was shown in 59 patients (23.0%), and two or more fluid collections and/or retroperitoneal air was imaged in 83 patients (32.3%); 73 patients (28.4%) did not have any necrosis; 87 patients (33.9%) exhibited imaging signs of necrosis in less than one-third of the pancreas; 58 patients (22.6%) demonstrated necrosis in one-third to one-half of the pancreas. Thirty-nine patients (15.2%) were diagnosed with necrosis in more than one-half of the pancreas.

Table 2. RCSI scoring system on CT scans in AP.

Prognostic indicator	Score[b]
Hydropsia and rough edge of the diaphragm outside the retrocrural space	1
Thickening of the mediastinal pleura outside the retrocrural space	1
Haziness and streaky density in the retrocrural space	1
Fluid extends into the retrocrural space across esophageal or aortic hiatus[a]	1
Pleural effusion	2

[a]If fluid extends into the retrocrural space across both hiatuses, the score should be 2. [b]If CT manifestations shows bilateral involvement, the score should be doubled.

3 RCSI score

On the CT scans, one side or both sides of the diaphragmatic crura had been involved in 194 patients (75.5%) (Fig. 2A, B and 3B). Hydropsia and the rough edge of the mediastinal pleura were present in 123 patients (47.9%) (Fig. 2A). Haziness and streaky density in the retrocrural space were manifested in 105 patients (40.9%) (Fig. 2B). Pancreatic fluid had drained into the retrocrural space via the esophageal hiatus in 127 patients (49.4%), and via the aortic hiatus in 71 patients (27.6%) (Fig. 3A, C). One hundred fifty-four patients (59.9%) developed pleural effusion (Fig. 3A).

4 Comparison between RCSI and CTSI scores

The kappa statistics for the RCSI and CTSI scores between the two raters were 0.735 ± 0.032 and 0.605 ± 0.035, respectively. These values indicate good agreement for RCSI scores, but moderate agreement for CTSI scores; indicating RCSI scores are superior to CTSI scores. The mean RCSI score was 4.22 ± 2.04

points (range 1–10) for all 257 patients, and the mean CTSI score was 5.26 ± 2.58 points (range 1–10).

5 Predictive value of RCSI and CTSI scores for mortality

The AUC for the RCSI score was 0.962 (95% CI 0.942–0.983), which shows the high accuracy of this index in predicting mortality (Fig. 4). An RCSI score of 4.0 was identified as the best cutoff value (maximum Youden index, YI = 0.854). The AUC for the CTSI score was 0.900 (0.859–0.940), with a best cutoff value of 2.0 (maximum YI = 0.727). The AUC of the RCSI score for the prediction of mortality was significantly higher than the AUC of the CTSI score ($P<0.05$, z-test). The sensitivity and specificity also showed that the RCSI score was superior to the CTSI score for predicting mortality (Tab. 3).

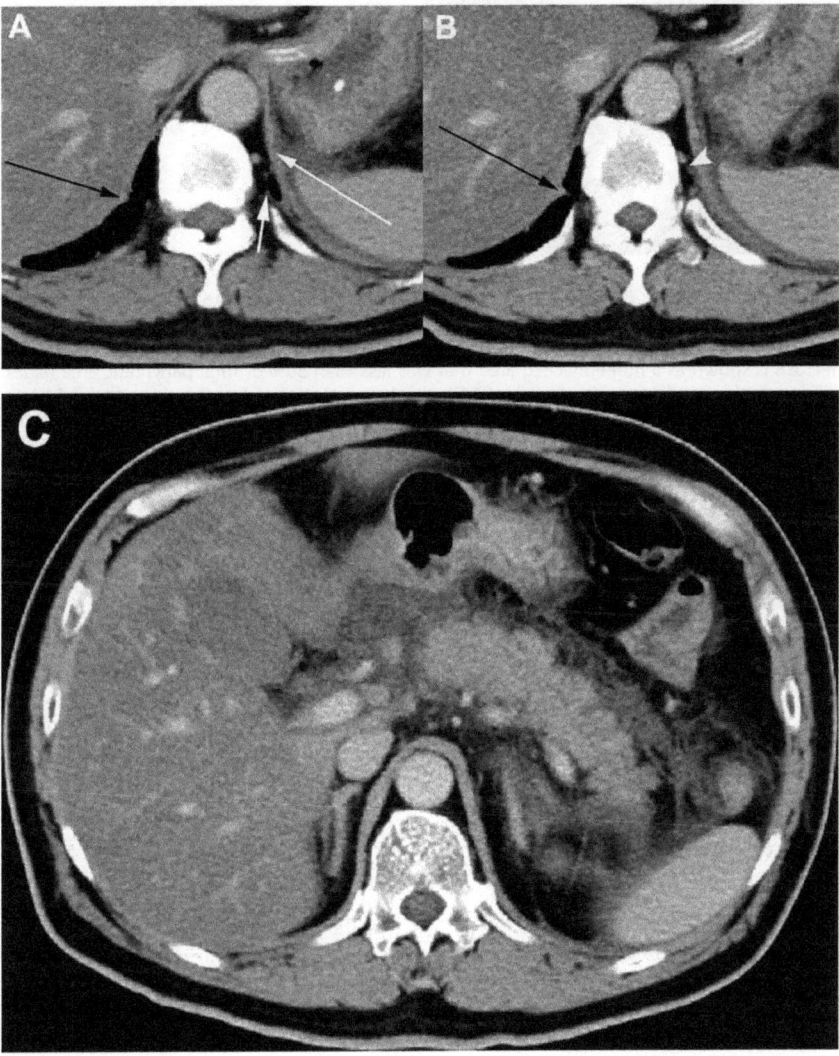

Figure 2. CT manifestations of the retrocrural space involvement in a 48-year-old man with AP. (A, B) CT scans obtained 3 days after admission showed acute fluid collections at the left subphrenic spaces. They resulted in the hydropsia of the left diaphragm (*long white arrow*), and the thickening of the left mediastinal pleura (*short white arrow*). In addition, a streaky density occurred at the left retrocrural space (*arrowhead*). On the opposite side, the right crus has a rough edge (*black arrow*). **(C)** CT scans displayed the peripancreatic fluid collections had extended into the left retroperitoneal space.

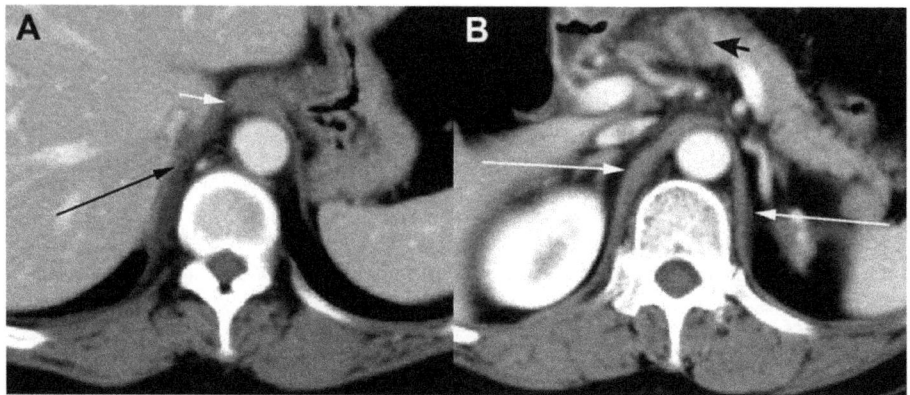

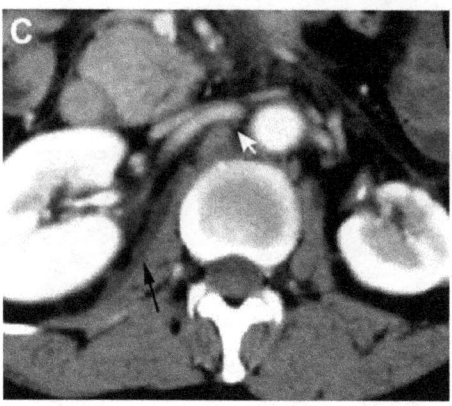

Figure 3. CT scans showing peripancreatic fluid draining into retrocrural space in a 46-year-old woman with AP. (A) On the upper section, CT scans obtained 4 days after admission showed the peripancreatic fluid had drained into the retrocrural space across the esophageal hiatus (*short white arrow*); then formed a fistulous tract into pleural cavity and developed into the pleural effusion (*long black arrow*). **(B)** On the middle section, pancreatic head necrosis is shown as a non-enhanced area that was less than 30% of total pancreatic area (*black arrowhead*). The bilateral diaphragmatic crus were shown hydropsia (*long white arrow*). **(C)** On the lower section, CT scans show the fluid had extended into the right retroperitoneal space (*short black arrow*) and further drained into the retrocrural space across the aortic hiatus (*white arrowhead*).

6 Predictive value of RCSI and CTSI scores for severity of AP

The AUC value for the CTSI score was 0.904 (0.864–0.944; Fig. 5). A CTSI score of 4.0 was identified as the best cutoff value (maximum YI = 0.744). The AUC value for the RCSI score was 0.888 (0.840–0.936) and the best cutoff value for the RCSI score was 3.0 (maximum YI = 0.736). There was no significant difference between the AUC of the CTSI score for predicting the severity of pancreatitis and the AUC of the RCSI score ($P >$ 0.001, z-test). The sensitivity and specificity, which were calculated to evaluate the diagnostic capacity of the two scoring systems for identifying the severity of pancreatitis, also indicated that there was no significant difference between the two scoring systems.

Discussion

The present study is a follow-up to our previous research about draining pathways from the peripancreatic space to mediastinum in patients with AP [14]. These two studies show that transformation of the radiological anatomy to consequent CT manifestations can be used to predict prognosis. We investigated the RCSI scoring system to predict the patients' prognosis and disease severity, and found that the RCSI score can accurately predict the mortality and disease severity in patients with AP. The RCSI score can substitute for the CTSI score to predict clinical outcomes of AP in some conditions; especially when the pelvis has not been

included in the scanned coverage, but we can deduce that the fluid collections may occur in the pelvic extraperitoneal space due to the combined interfascial plane involved on CT images. Simultaneously, we should pay attention to the rarely anatomic variants and anomalies of the retrocrural space, because these variants may be mistaken for the CT manifestations of the RCSI [24]. For instance, the duplicated accessory diaphragm will probably be regarded as the hydropsia of the diaphragm.

The introduction of the CTSI in 1994 was a significant advance in the assessment of patients with AP [3]. Despite the CTSI having been successfully used to predict overall mortality in patients with AP, Balthazar and others have confirmed that when using the CTSI there was no significant difference in mortality between patients who have 30–50% necrosis and patients who have more than 50% necrosis [7,26]. Recent publications have confirmed that the mediastinal acute fluid collection in patients with AP can result in increased morbidity and mortality [27]. Furthermore, as a risk factor for severe AP, pleural effusion was included in the RCSI scoring system [28]. We speculate that the presence of fluid drainage into the retrocrural space and pleural fluid may be responsible for the improved efficiency of prediction (Fig. 4), because they may be indicators of organ dysfunction. Our study also showed that an RCSI cutoff value of 4 was best for identifying the mortality rate. For an RCSI score higher than 4, clinicians should be alert to the possibility of further development of RCSI to

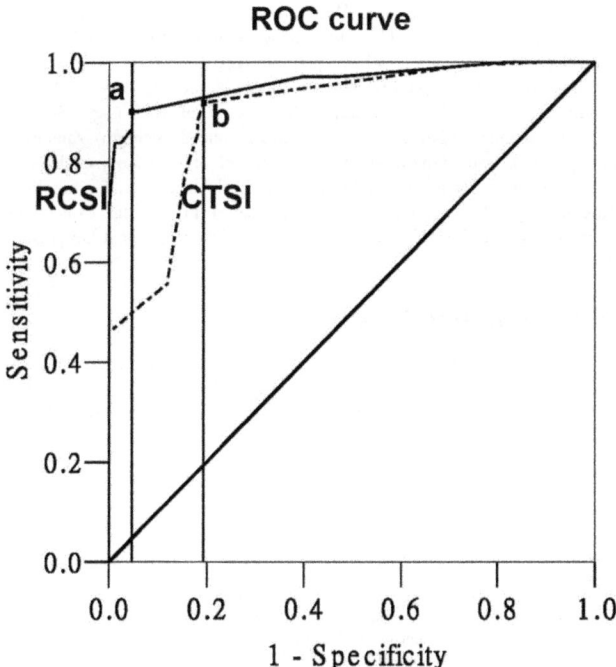
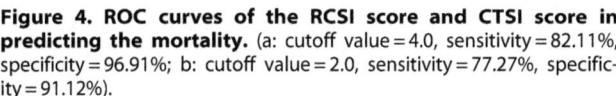
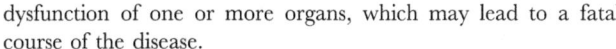

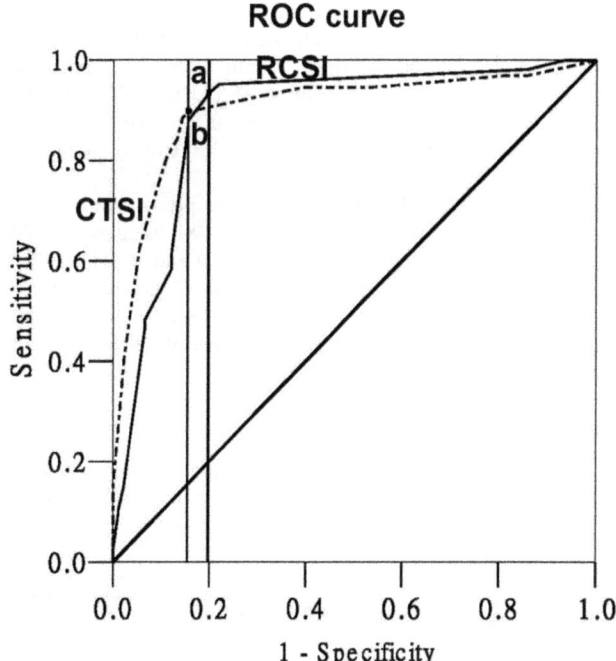

Figure 4. ROC curves of the RCSI score and CTSI score in predicting the mortality. (a: cutoff value = 4.0, sensitivity = 82.11%, specificity = 96.91%; b: cutoff value = 2.0, sensitivity = 77.27%, specificity = 91.12%).

Figure 5. ROC curves of the RCSI and CTSI score in distinguishing between mild and severe AP. (a: cutoff value = 3.0, sensitivity = 79.38%, specificity = 87.50%; b: cutoff value = 4.0, sensitivity = 81.91%, specificity = 91.41%).

dysfunction of one or more organs, which may lead to a fatal course of the disease.

An ideal prognostic method should have low inter-rater variability. The inter-rater variability of the RCSI score was lower than that of the CTSI score in our study (0.735 ± 0.032 vs. 0.605 ± 0.035). On the one hand, two observers often diverged from each other in counting the locations for fluid collections. Especially when the peripancreatic fluid involved both the left and right anterior pararenal space, or both the superior and inferior recess of the lesser sac in necrotizing pancreatitis, the two observers usually could not agree on whether to count it as one location or as two locations. It will influence the CTSI score. On the other hand, they are more familiar with the imaging of pathologic conditions that involve the retrocrural space than other radiologists because they have focused on the study of the radiological anatomy of the retroperitoneal space; they usually can reach an agreement on RCSI scores in a double-blinded condition.

Accompanied by the further study of the radiological anatomy of the retroperitoneal space [29], the concept of "interfascial

planes" of the retroperitoneal space was suggested by Molmenti et al. in 1996 [30]. The study by Gore et al. confirmed the ability of interfascial planes to serve as spaces that can decompress retroperitoneal fluid collections and infiltrating diseases, especially when large volumes of fluid develop rapidly in severe AP [31]. Based on this concept, we suggest that these fascial planes be regarded as the locations for fluid collections when calculating the score for the CTSI.

Our study had some limitations. The RCSI scoring system was established based on the experience of experts, two radiologists came from our institute that focused on the study to the radiological anatomy of the retroperitoneal space, so some confounders were unavoidable. To control the confounders as much as possible, a multidisciplinary and anonymous panel of 12 experts was recruited, with one panelist being a radiological expert in image processing. However, the selected panelists were all local experts from southwest China; no international experts were included. Thus, whether this scoring system can be implemented in areas outside China requires further study. In order to build a rational consensus, we took some measures to assure that the process of collecting expert assessments is subject to the following

Table 3. Value of RCSI and CTSI scoring systems for predicting the mortality and severity of AP.

Scoring system	Cutoff value	Sensitivity	Specificity	PPV	NPV
RCSI (for MOR prediction)	4.0	82.11%	96.91%	93.98%	90.23%
CTSI (for MOR prediction)	2.0	77.27%	91.12%	81.93%	88.51%
RCSI (for SAP prediction)	3.0	79.38%	87.50%	84.62%	87.95%
CTSI (for SAP prediction)	4.0	81.91%	91.41%	84.62%	89.76%

MOR: mortality, SAP: severe acute pancreatitis, PPV: positive predictive value, NPV: negative predictive value.

principles: accountability, empirical control, neutrality, and fairness [32]. Although our study suggests that the predictive value of the RCSI scoring system for the mortality (AUC = 0.962±0.011) and severity of AP (AUC = 0.888±0.025) is valid, with low inter-rater variability (0.735±0.032), further study on the validity and reliability of this scoring system is necessary.

In summary, the main contribution of the present study is the establishment of a new scoring system, the RCSI, using the Delphi method. The RCSI can predict the mortality and severity of AP from initial CT scans. In addition, the RCSI is recommended for use as a supplement to the CTSI when we encounter the difficulty in calculating the CTSI score, especially when the pelvis has not been included in the scanned coverage.

Acknowledgments

We thank the panelists for their work and input in establishing the scoring system of the RCSI. The experts in the panel were Ruifeng Wang, Yong Pang, Jiandong Ren and Tao Wang (General Surgery Center of the Peoples' Liberation Army, Chengdu Army General Hospital, Chengdu), Guoli Dong and Zhaohua Zhai (Sichuan Key Laboratory of Medical Imaging, Affiliated Hospital of North Sichuan Medical College, Sichuan), Jingchi Xiang and Fuzhou Zhang (Department of Radiology, Second Affiliated Hospital of North Sichuan Medical College, Sichuan), Zhengzhi Zhang, Kai Li, and Guangjiu Liu (Department of Anatomy, College of Basic Medical Sciences, Third Military Medical University, Chongqing), Mingguo Qiu (Department of Medical Images Processing, College of Bioengineering and Medical Imaging, Third Military Medical University, Chongqing).

Author Contributions

Conceived and designed the experiments: FT HX. Performed the experiments: ZL YW. Analyzed the data: HX XZ ZL. Contributed reagents/materials/analysis tools: SZ YW SJ. Wrote the paper: HX AC LE XZ.

References

1. Balthazar EJ (2002) Complications of acute pancreatitis: clinical and CT evaluation. Radiol Clin North Am 40: 1211–1227.
2. Lenhart DK, Balthazar EJ (2008) MDCT of acute mild (nonnecrotizing) pancreatitis: abdominal complications and fate of fluid collections. American Journal of Roentgenology 190: 643–649.
3. Balthazar EJ, Freeny PC, vanSonnenberg E (1994) Imaging and intervention in acute pancreatitis. Radiology 193: 297–306.
4. Mortele KJ, Wiesner W, Intriere L, Shankar S, Zou KH, et al. (2004) A modified CT severity index for evaluating acute pancreatitis: improved correlation with patient outcome. AJR Am J Roentgenol 183: 1261–1265.
5. De Waele JJ, Delrue L, Hoste EA, De Vos M, Duyck P, et al. (2007) Extrapancreatic inflammation on abdominal computed tomography as an early predictor of disease severity in acute pancreatitis: evaluation of a new scoring system. Pancreas 34: 185–190.
6. Tang W, Zhang XM, Xiao B, Zeng NL, Pan HS, et al. (2011) Magnetic resonance imaging versus Acute Physiology And Chronic Healthy Evaluation II score in predicting the severity of acute pancreatitis. European journal of radiology 80: 637–642.
7. Lecesne R, Taourel P, Bret PM, Atri M, Reinhold C (1999) Acute pancreatitis: interobserver agreement and correlation of CT and MR cholangiopancreatography with outcome. Radiology 211: 727–735.
8. Mortelé KJ, Mergo PJ, Taylor HM, Ernst MD, Ros PR (2000) Renal and perirenal space involvement in acute pancreatitis: spiral CT findings. Abdominal Imaging 25: 272–278.
9. Rowe G, Wright G (1999) The Delphi technique as a forecasting tool: issues and analysis. International Journal of Forecasting 15: 353–375.
10. Rowe G, Wright G (2001) Expert opinions in forecasting. role of the Delphi technique. In: Armstrong (Ed.). Principles of forecasting: a handbook of researchers and practitioners, Boston: Kluwer Academic Publishers.
11. Ricke J, Klose KJ, Mignon M, Öberg K, Wiedenmann B (2001) Standardisation of imaging in neuroendocrine tumours: results of a European delphi process. European Journal of Radiology 37: 8–17.
12. Zhou X-H (1998) Correcting for verification bias in studies of a diagnostic test's accuracy. Statistical Methods in Medical Research 7: 337–353.
13. Hanley JA, McNeil BJ (1982) The meaning and use of the area under a receiver operating characteristic (ROC) curve. Radiology 143: 29–36.
14. Xu H, Zhang X, Christe A, Ebner L, Zhang S, et al. (2013) Anatomic pathways of peripancreatic fluid draining to mediastinum in recurrent acute pancreatitis: Visible Human Project and CT Study. PLoS ONE 8: e62025.
15. Zhang SX, Heng PA, Liu ZJ, Tan LW, Qiu MG, et al. (2004) The Chinese Visible Human (CVH) datasets incorporate technical and imaging advances on earlier digital humans. J Anat 204: 165–173.
16. U.S. (2000) Department of Health and Human Services. International classification of diseases: ninth revision–clinical modification, 6th ed Washington, DC: US Department of Health and Human Services.
17. Bollen TL, van Santvoort HC, Besselink MG, van Leeuwen MS, Horvath KD, et al. (2008) The Atlanta Classification of acute pancreatitis revisited. Br J Surg 95: 6–21.
18. Im JG, Webb WR, Rosen A, Gamsu G (1989) Costal pleura: appearances at high-resolution CT. Radiology 171: 125–131.
19. Ishikawa K, Idoguchi K, Tanaka H, Tohma Y, Ukai I, et al. (2006) Classification of acute pancreatitis based on retroperitoneal extension: application of the concept of interfascial planes. Eur J Radiol 60: 445–452.
20. McLoud TC, Flower CD (1991) Imaging the pleura: sonography, CT, and MR imaging. American Journal of Roentgenology 156: 1145–1153.
21. Liu Z, Yan Z, Min P, Liang C, Wang Y (2008) Gastric bare area and left adrenal gland involvement on abdominal computed tomography and their prognostic value in acute pancreatitis. Eur Radiol 18: 1611–1616.
22. Browne GW, Pitchumoni CS (2006) Pathophysiology of pulmonary complications of acute pancreatitis. World J Gastroenterol 12: 7087–7096.
23. Becmeur F, Horta P, Donato L, Christmann D, Sauvage P (1995) Accessory diaphragm–review of 31 cases in the literature. Eur J Pediatr Surg 5: 43–47.
24. Restrepo CS, Eraso A, Ocazionez D, Lemos J, Martinez S, et al. (2008) The diaphragmatic crura and retrocrural space: normal imaging appearance, variants, and pathologic conditions. Radiographics 28: 1289–1305.
25. François C, Demos T, Iqbal N (2005) Pancreaticothoracic fistulas: imaging findings in five patients. Abdominal Imaging 30: 761–767.
26. Balthazar EJ, Robinson DL, Megibow AJ, Ranson JH (1990) Acute pancreatitis: value of CT in establishing prognosis. Radiology 174: 331–336.
27. Singh P, Holubka J, Patel S (1996) Acute mediastinal pancreatic fluid collection with pericardial and pleural effusion. complete resolution after treatment with octreotide acetate. Dig Dis Sci 41: 1966–1971.
28. Heller SJ, Noordhoek E, Tenner SM, Ramagopal V, Abramowitz M, et al. (1997) Pleural effusion as a predictor of severity in acute pancreatitis. Pancreas 15: 222–225.
29. Xu H, Li X, Zhang Z, Qiu M, Mu Q, et al. (2011) Visualization of the left extraperitoneal space and spatial relationships to its related spaces by the Visible Human Project. PLoS ONE 6: e27166.
30. Molmenti EP, Balfe DM, Kanterman RY, Bennett HF (1996) Anatomy of the retroperitoneum: observations of the distribution of pathologic fluid collections. Radiology 200: 95–103.
31. Gore RM, Balfe DM, Aizenstein RI, Silverman PM (2000) The great escape: interfascial decompression planes of the retroperitoneum. AJR Am J Roentgenol 175: 363–370.
32. Ouchi F, Bank W (2003) A literature review on the use of expert opinion in probabilistic risk analysis: World Bank.

11

Coordinate Based Meta-Analysis of Functional Neuroimaging Data Using Activation Likelihood Estimation; Full Width Half Max and Group Comparisons

Christopher R. Tench[1]*, **Radu Tanasescu[1,2]**, **Dorothee P. Auer[3,4]**, **William J. Cottam[3,4]**, **Cris S. Constantinescu[1]**

1 Division of Clinical Neurosciences, Clinical Neurology, University of Nottingham, Queen's Medical Centre, Nottingham, United Kingdom, 2 Department of Neurology, Neurosurgery, and Psychiatry, University of Medicine and Pharmacy Carol Davila Bucharest, Colentina Hospital, Bucharest, Romania, 3 Division of Clinical Neurosciences, Radiological and Imaging Sciences, University of Nottingham, Queen's Medical Centre, Nottingham, United Kingdom, 4 ARUK National Pain Centre, University of Nottingham, Queen's Medical Centre, Nottingham, United Kingdom

Abstract

Coordinate based meta-analysis (CBMA) is used to find regions of consistent activation across fMRI and PET studies selected for their functional relevance to a hypothesis. Results are clusters of foci where multiple studies report in the same spatial region, indicating functional relevance. Contrast meta-analysis finds regions where there are consistent differences in activation pattern between two groups. The activation likelihood estimate methods tackle these problems, but require a specification of uncertainty in foci location: the full width half max (FWHM). Results are sensitive to FWHM. Furthermore, contrast meta-analysis requires correction for multiple statistical tests. Consequently it is sensitive only to very significant localised differences that produce very small p-values, which remain significant after correction; subtle diffuse differences between the groups can be overlooked. In this report we redefine the FWHM parameter, by analogy with a density clustering algorithm, and provide a method to estimate it. The FWHM is modified to account for the number of studies in the analysis, and represents a substantial change to the CBMA philosophy that can be applied to the current algorithms. Consequently we observe more reliable detection of clusters when there are few studies in the CBMA, and a decreasing false positive rate with larger study numbers. By contrast the standard definition (FWHM independent of the number of studies) is demonstrated to paradoxically increase the false positive rate as the number of studies increases, while reducing ability to detect true clusters for small numbers of studies. We also provide an algorithm for contrast meta-analysis, which includes a correction for multiple correlated tests that controls for the proportion of false clusters expected under the null hypothesis. Furthermore, we detail an omnibus test of difference between groups that is more sensitive than contrast meta-analysis when differences are diffuse. This test is useful where contrast meta-analysis is unrevealing.

Editor: Satoru Hayasaka, Wake Forest School of Medicine, United States of America

Funding: The authors have no support or funding to report.

Competing Interests: The authors have declared that no competing interests exist.

* Email: Christopher.tench@nottingham.ac.uk

Introduction

A very popular method of performing a meta-analysis (MA) of functional magnetic resonance imaging (fMRI) and positron emission tomography (PET) data is coordinate based meta-analysis (CBMA). There are various approaches [1–10], but the common aim is to locate regions where different studies agree on the location of activation peaks (foci) better than expected by chance alone. Results are then thought to be of significance to the common functional aspect(s) of the studies included in the analysis. A further aim is to compare different groups, for example healthy control and patient groups, using contrast meta-analysis.

Here we focus on the activation likelihood estimate (ALE) based method, which is possibly the most widely known of the CBMA schemes. The ALE method models the uncertainty of the reported foci using a Gaussian function with specified full width half max (FWHM) [1]. It then estimates the likelihood, at each voxel, that there is consistent activation across multiple studies. Clusters of voxels with significantly high ALE are tested for by a permutation test. The ALE method is very popular, and has been, and is being, used to generate many publications. Despite this, there remain major problems.

The FWHM parameter, which is often set at ≈ 10 mm, has a major effect on the results [11]. In the similar kernel density analysis (KDA) method of CBMA, a FWHM of 10 mm or 15 mm is reported to produce the best results [7]. The signed differential mapping (SDM) uses 25 mm [5]. For the ALE methods, in an attempt to quantify the FWHM it has recently been estimated by fMRI experiment and a dependency on the number of subjects suggested [3]. Nevertheless, the lack of consensus on this parameter is one of the issues for CBMA. Indeed some CBMA methods remove the FWHM as a fixed parameter [9,10].

However, these methods are sensitive to the required prior knowledge elicited from experts, and in the case of the method of Yue et. al. has not been generalised, in a computationally practical sense, to three dimensions.

Here a new FWHM scheme is introduced. This is motivated by the reasonable requirement that CBMA of a small set of studies should ideally produce results commensurate with those produced if the number of studies were increased. It redefines the FWHM as a density clustering parameter, rather than a specification of the uncertainty of the reported foci used by current ALE algorithms.

The correction for many correlated statistical tests is a problem for contrast meta-analysis that has not yet been addressed [12]; indeed contrast meta-analysis has previously been performed without any correction [13], which will inevitably lead to false positive results. Several methods are used to impose voxel-level (since testing is performed at each voxel) control of the rate of falsely rejected null hypotheses in CBMA; for example false discovery rate (FDR) control [4,14]. The latest ALE algorithms have introduced cluster-level control to CBMA [2], which is preferred to voxel-level control since it directly relates to the results, by limiting cluster sizes to be larger than expected under the null hypothesis. CBMA is performed many ($\sim 10^3$) times using foci randomised throughout a brain mask and a user specified voxel-level threshold (for example $p < 0.001$ uncorrected). The distribution of the size of the resulting clusters is recorded, and a user specified quantile of this distribution (for example 95%) subsequently used as a lower permissible cluster size in the CBMA of the original foci. However, this scheme requires two independent user specified thresholds, so it is not clear exactly what this means for the proportion of falsely rejected null hypotheses. Furthermore, while this cluster-level control may be appropriate for CBMA where the null hypothesis is closely related to that obtained using random foci, it is not appropriate for contrast meta-analysis where the null hypothesis is obtained by permutation of the grouping variable.

We previously detailed a CBMA method that employed a false cluster discovery rate (FCDR) control scheme that has the particularly interpretable aim of limiting the proportion of the significant clusters expected under the null hypothesis. The control problem is further tackled by substantially reducing the number of statistical tests by testing only at the reported foci ($\sim 10^2$ tests), rather than at each voxel ($\sim 10^5$ tests). We showed that this leads to fewer false positive results than using FDR correction at the voxel level, or using cluster-level control via minimum cluster size thresholding, yet maintains sensitivity [15]. Here we extend FCDR to contrast meta-analysis. The proposed method requires specification of only one threshold, is interpretable, and does not assume independence of the many tests.

The contrast meta-analysis method can localise significant focal differences between groups, indicating brain structures where functional activation differs. However, due to the need to correct for multiple comparisons, this method lacks sensitivity for detecting more diffuse subtle differences between the groups; such differences do not produce the very small p-values required to survive the correction. Lack of significant results from contrast meta-analysis is not, therefore, a good indicator that the two groups do not differ in activation pattern. Here we introduce an omnibus test of difference between groups. Only one test is performed, so no correction is necessary; this is similar to Fisher's combined probability test [16], but without the assumption for independence of the probabilities. Consequently it is better able to detect diffuse differences than contrast meta-analysis. The test can provide evidence for difference between groups when the contrast meta-analysis is unrevealing.

In summary, this report describes new tools for ALE based experiments. Specifically: 1) a new definition and method for setting the FWHM parameter, 2) a description of the contrast meta-analysis algorithm and subsequent correction for multiple correlated comparisons at the cluster-level, and 3) an omnibus test of difference between groups.

Materials and Methods

Statistical significance in the ALE method is judged relative to a null distribution of ALEs, generated by permutation of the foci throughout a grey matter (GM) mask [2,7]. When many studies report activations in similar locations, the foci density is high so there is little distance between them. In regions reported as active by few studies, the foci are lower in density.

While our algorithm (LocalALE) has been detailed previously [15], some specifics are important to the methods presented in this report. The ALE method models the spatial distribution ($S_{ij}(r)$) of the ith reported foci in the jth study (r_{ij}) by a Gaussian distribution of specified standard deviation (σ) or FWHM. The Gaussians are truncated at $2.8 \times \sigma$, or equivalently $1.2 \times$ FWHM,

$$S_{ij}(r) = w(|r - r_{ij}|) \exp\left(-\frac{|r - r_{ij}|^2}{2\sigma^2}\right), \qquad (1)$$

where

$$w(|r - r_{ij}|) = \frac{1}{\sqrt{2\pi}^3 \sigma^3} \text{ if } |r - r_{ij}| < 2.8\sigma, \qquad (2)$$

and is zero otherwise. The truncation removes 5% of the 'mass' of the Gaussian, and is performed to reduce the influence of foci over long distance, and to make testing only at the foci possible [15]. It has previously been shown that with 5% truncation, the resulting clusters are similar to those obtained using the 'full' Gaussian [15]; clearly some truncation is always present even with the 'full' Gaussian, imposed by the brain volume. The spatial activation distribution for study j is

$$ma_j(r) = \max_i S_{ij}(r), \qquad (3)$$

from which the ALE is computed.

Foci separated by a distance $\leq 1.2 \times$ FWHM overlap (are separated by less than the truncation distance). Overlapping foci across studies form clusters, which, if significant, are the results of the CBMA.

The software is available to download and use freely from www.nottingham.ac.uk/research/groups/clinicalneurology/neuroi.aspx.

The FWHM in ALE based CBMA

The FWHM can affect the results of ALE based CBMA [11]. Often the FWHM is set to ≈ 10mm, but there is some variance on this. An empirical FWHM has been described [3], based on the idea that it measures the variance of activation peak position on repeating the same experiment in a group of volunteers. This suggests that the FWHM should depend on the number of subjects within a study; the larger the number, the smaller the uncertainty in the location of the peak of the activation, and so the smaller the FWHM. While this is intuitively reasonable, it does create some issues. Firstly, the suggested estimate is based on a specific functional experiment, and might not be generalizable. Secondly, ideally the results from a small CBMA study should agree with a larger CBMA performed if more studies were available. In this report a new definition and estimate for FWHM that depends on the number of studies in the CBMA is presented.

Each study in the CBMA reports foci of activation, some of which are common to a proportion of the studies, while others are due to some study specific aspect. Where there is better than chance agreement across studies about the activation peaks, the foci form clusters of higher than average density. Between the clusters, the study specific foci form a lower than average density noise. Identifying clusters of high density points in the presence of noise can be tackled using the density-based spatial clustering in applications with noise (DBSCAN) [17] algorithm. Clusters in DBSCAN are formed by points that are density reachable, such that any point in the cluster can be connected to any other within the cluster via a chain of points that are separated by a distance less than parameter 'Eps'. The problem is depicted in figures 1a and 1b; figure 1a shows a sparse set of points and figure 1b a larger set of points. If Eps is set too large, the clusters begin to merge, and the noise points are recruited to the clusters. If Eps is set too small, the clusters are missed. In figures 1c and 1d Eps is represented by the radius of the dotted circles. For the algorithm to succeed the Eps parameter must be set such that within-cluster the points fall within a distance Eps of other points in the cluster, while the noise must be beyond this distance. Consequently, for the sparse set of points (figures 1a and 1c), Eps is larger than for the larger set of points (figures 1b and 1d).

Since the density clustering problem is analogous to CBMA, it is proposed that the FWHM parameter be redefined to be analogous to the Eps parameter in density clustering. The aim is to increase

the FWHM for small numbers of studies such that the within-cluster foci can overlap, and reduce the FWHM for larger numbers of studies to prevent the study specific foci joining the clusters. To achieve this it is proposed that the characteristic volume occupied by each foci ($\sim \text{FWHM}^3$) is inversely proportional to the number of studies such that

$$\text{FWHM}_{\text{Eps}} = \frac{\alpha}{\sqrt[3]{N}} \qquad (4)$$

where N is the total number of studies, and α is a constant to be estimated. The proposed estimate of FWHM is now FWHM_{Eps} to signify its relationship to both the FWHM conventionally used in CBMA and the clustering parameter used by DBSCAN. The parameter α can be estimated under the null hypothesis (randomised foci) where the average density of the foci across studies is higher than the study specific foci, and lower than the clustered foci. It is hypothesised that this scheme will: 1) help to prevent incidental recruitment of study specific foci to the clusters, and 2) help with the detection of low density clusters when there is little data.

This constitutes a redefinition of the FWHM parameter. It no longer represents spatial uncertainty in the location of the foci, but rather it is a density parameter similar to Eps, used in the DBSCAN [17] algorithm.

FWHM Experiments. The effect of varying the FWHM between 6 mm and 18 mm is visually assessed, using LocalALE, in three sets of fMRI data: 1) the pain data (47 experiments) used in [15], 2) n-back data (61 experiments) used in [18] and downloaded using Sleuth (downloadable from www.BrainMap.org) from the BrainMap database [19], and 3) Stroop test data used in [20] and again downloaded using Sleuth; workspace files for downloading the data via Sleuth are available from the BrainMap website. It is expected that if the FWHM is too small, the clusters will be small, or even vanish. It is also expected that if the FWHM is too large, the clusters will merge and expand in spatial extent by including more nearby foci. In the case of the Stroop experiment, the data are separated into two groups: pooled studies requiring either a verbal response or a mechanical response (19 studies), and those specifically requiring mechanical response (6 studies). From the original meta-analysis it is expected that there is some similarity between these, and certainly this is expected on the grounds that one is a subset of the other. The difference in numbers of experiments in the two groups is used to demonstrate how FWHM must be modified to make the results commensurate.

The mean effect of FWHM on the clustering under the null hypothesis is also investigated; under the null hypothesis it is expected that large clusters do not form on average. Foci are randomised throughout a grey matter mask, as detailed in [15], 10 times. For each randomisation the number of clusters (sets of foci in different studies separated by a distance smaller than $1.2 \times \text{FWHM}$) is counted. The mean number of clusters, as a proportion of the total number of foci, is plotted against FWHM to see when the clusters begin to form. It is expected that for very small FWHM the foci in different studies do not overlap under the null hypothesis, so the number of clusters will be equal to the number of foci; each non-overlapping focus being considered a cluster of one focus. As the FWHM is increased, foci will start to overlap and form larger clusters. An empirical estimate for parameter α (equation (4)) is obtained by identifying the point where clusters just begin to form under the null hypothesis.

Two large data sets used previously [21] to examine the functional connectivity of two structures, the right amygdala (RA;

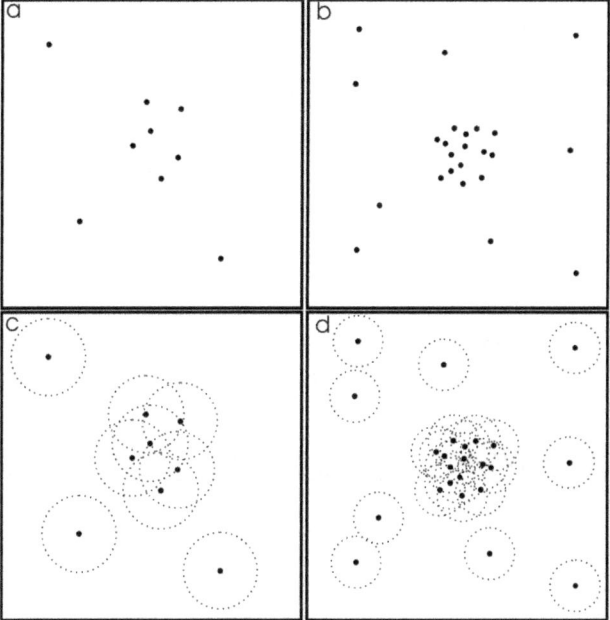

Figure 1. Depicts how the Eps parameter in the density clustering algorithm DBSCAN is modified as the size of the data set is changed. For sparse data sets (a) the Eps parameter is large (represented by the radius of the circles in (c)). For the larger data set, Eps is smaller. Eps is chosen so that the dense cluster of points and the noise are separate. This clustering algorithm is analogous to CBMA, and the Eps parameter analogous to the FWHM.

189 studies) and the orbitofrontal cortex (OFC; 142 studies), are explored. The data sets are available for download from www. BrainMap.org, and were originally created by searching the BrainMap database [22] for any studies that report at least one activation within a seed region of interest (ROI); the ROIs are depicted in [21]. These datasets are of interest since it is obvious that there are significant clusters where the seed ROIs are defined, and that those clusters should be similar in size to the seed ROIs because they determine where the foci are located. Coordinate based meta-analysis is performed on the full datasets, and also on smaller subsets of 25 (25 is arbitrary, but not an unusual size for a typical CBMA experiment) randomly selected studies from each full dataset. The proposed $FWHM_{Eps}$, and the FWHM specified in [3] and incorporated into GingerALE (a popular and freely available program used for ALE analysis; available from www. brainmap.org) are compared; GingerALE is used to demonstrate that the sensitivity to FWHM is not specific to our LocalALE method. It is expected that the clusters in the RA and OFC should be similar in the small and full datasets.

Finally a numerically generated pseudo experiment is created. Each pseudo study in the experiment has 10 foci (around 10 foci would not be unusual in a real study), which are placed either within one of three clusters, or at random with uniform probability within the GM mask but outside of the clusters. The experiment is performed twice: a) with the proportion of studies reporting in the three clusters being 40%, 50%, and 60%, to reflect the proportion ranges observed in most significant clusters from the pain, Stroop, and n-back experiments, and b) with the proportion of studies reporting in the three clusters being 20%, 30%, and 40%, to consider the impact of less consistent activations. Foci that are truly members of the ith cluster are placed at location $\{x_i + d_x, y_i + d_y, z_i + d_z\}$, where d are randomly generated from a truncated (at ± 2 standard deviations from the mean) Gaussian distribution with mean zero and FWHM = 10 mm. The results of CBMA on these experiments are depicted for: 1) $FWHM_{Eps}$ using α (equation (4)) estimated from the pain, n-back, and Stroop experiments, 2) FWHM = 10 mm, and 3) using the FWHM estimate detailed by [3] and employed in GingerALE.

True and false positive rates are explored quantitatively for this numerical experiment as a function of the number of studies (10 to 150 studies); 100 averages are performed for each number of studies. The true positive rates are the proportion of true cluster foci that are declared as cluster members, while the false positive rates are the non-cluster foci declared as members of a cluster. Both true and false rates are expressed as a proportion of the total number of true cluster foci to make them easy to compare. If the clustering analogy is valid for our CBMA experiment, it is expected that with FWHM = 10 mm there will be fewer true positive results for few studies compared to $FWHM_{Eps}$. Furthermore, it is expected that for large numbers of studies that the false positive rate will be higher for FWHM = 10 mm than for $FWHM_{Eps}$.

Contrast meta-analysis

Contrast meta-analysis attempts to find differences in activation pattern between two groups of studies. The results are clusters of foci where there is localised significant difference in ALE between the groups. The null hypothesis is that there is no difference between the groups, so a permutation (of the group variable) test is employed. Following on from our LocalALE algorithm, tests for differences are performed only at the foci in the method reported here; instead of at each voxel. It also employs the false cluster discovery rate (FCDR) control of false positive results, as detailed

previously in [15]. FCDR is particularly interpretable since it controls for the proportion of significant clusters expected under the null hypothesis. It also takes account of the correlated nature of the tests; the ALE values, and p-values, for each focus depends on the other foci and are therefore not independent. Contrast meta-analysis is useful when there are very significant localised differences between the groups that can survive the FCDR control.

Studies are separated into two groups, A & B, containing N_A and N_B studies, respectively. Of all the permutations, the ith is specified by

$$A_i = \{a_{i1}, a_{i2}, \ldots, a_{iN_A}\} \tag{5}$$

and

$$B_i = \{b_{i1}, b_{i2}, \ldots, b_{iN_B}\}, \tag{6}$$

where a_{ij} (b_{ij}) are the study numbers, and $a_{ij} < a_{ij+1}(b_{ij} < b_{ij+1})$ since order is not important. The ALE for group A, permutation i, at location r is

$$ALE_{A_i}(r) = 1 - \prod_{j=1}^{N_A} \left(1 - ma_{a_{ij}}(r)\right), \tag{7}$$

and similar for group B. The difference in ALE between the two groups is

$$\Delta_i(r) = ALE_{A_i}(r) - ALE_{B_i}(r). \tag{8}$$

For a particular permutation, k, and for a particular focus r_{ij}, the significance (p-value) of the difference in ALE between the groups is

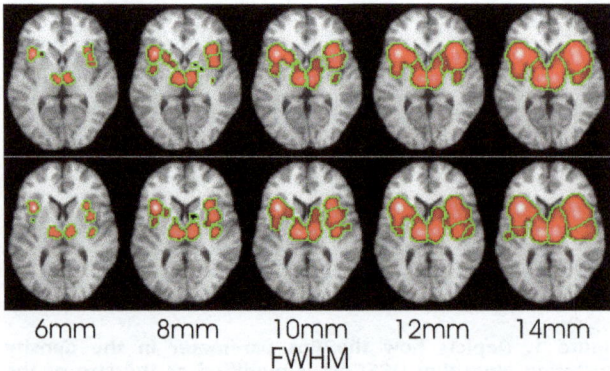

6mm   8mm   10mm   12mm   14mm
FWHM

Figure 2. CBMA results for the 47 studies included in the pain CBMA for a range of FWHM produced using LocalALE. With small FWHM, the clusters shrink, or vanish. With large FWHM, the clusters merge and expand.

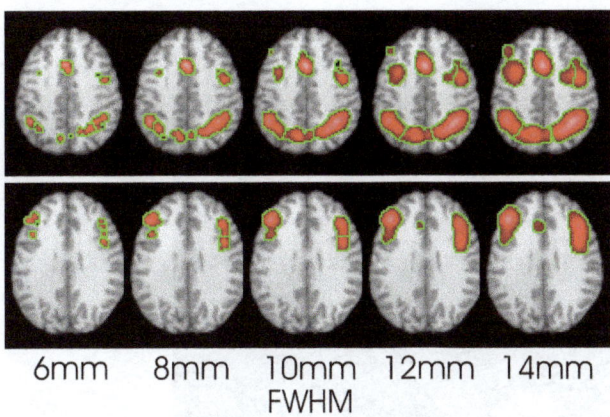

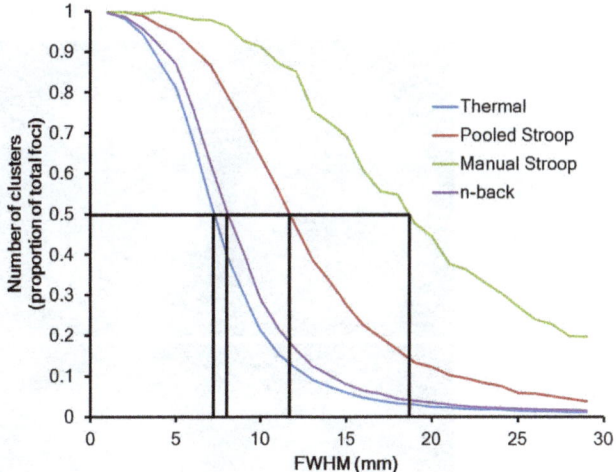

Figure 3. CBMA results for the 61 studies included in the n-back CBMA for a range of FWHM produced using LocalALE. With small FWHM, the clusters shrink, or vanish. With large FWHM, the clusters merge and expand.

Figure 5. Depiction of cluster forming under the null hypothesis (randomised foci) as a function of FWHM. For small FWHM, the foci do not overlap, so there are as many clusters as foci (single focus clusters). As the FWHM increases, larger clusters begin to form.

$$p_{kij} = \frac{\sum_{l\in\Omega} I\big(\Delta_l(r_{ij}) \leq \Delta_k(r_{ij})\big)}{\sum_{l\in\Omega} 1} \quad \text{if } j\in A_k \qquad (9)$$

or

$$p_{kij} = \frac{\sum_{l\in\Omega} I\big(\Delta_l(r_{ij}) \geq \Delta_k(r_{ij})\big)}{\sum_{l\in\Omega} 1} \quad \text{if } j\in B_k; \qquad (10)$$

$I(E)$ is an indicator function that equals 1 if E is true, and zero otherwise. A small value of p_{kij} indicates that the magnitude of the ALE difference for foci r_{ij} is particularly large for the kth permutation. The sums in these expressions are over the set (Ω) of all possible permutations of the grouping. However, since Ω is

typically very large, p-values are estimated using a random selection of 10×10^3 permutations. Here, as suggested previously [13], statistical tests are performed only for foci that are found to be significant by CBMA. This reduces the number of tests, and so increases the power, at the expense of testing for differences between the complete groups.

It is hypothesised that the groups A_0 and B_0, which might be patients and healthy controls for example, have localised differences in activation pattern. The p-values p_{0ij} measure the significance of that difference. Clusters of significant foci are found, and counted, using the clustering algorithm provided in the supplement (File S1); the algorithm finds the most significant foci first then uses Dijkstra's algorithm [23] to locate all other foci in the cluster, repeating the process to locate all clusters. The number of significant clusters is $N_0(\gamma)$, which is computed using only the foci with $p_{0ij} \leq \gamma$. To control the FCDR, an estimate of the number of clusters expected under the null hypothesis is needed. This is estimated using a randomly selected set of 2000 permutations $(K = \{k_1, k_2, \ldots, k_{2000}\})$, computing the number of clusters for each of these permutations $(N_i(\gamma)$ with $i\in K)$ and averaging; 2000 is considered sufficient as repeating the experiments gives similar estimates of FCDR. Controlling the FCDR at a level of 0.05 (for example) is then performed by maximising γ such that

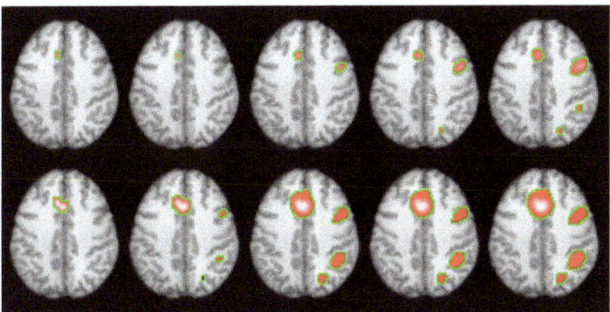

Figure 4. CBMA results for the Stroop experiment, for a range of FWHM produced using LocalALE. Top row shows the Stroop studies where manual response was required (6 studies). Bottom row shows the pooled Stroop studies (19 studies). The studies give similar activation patterns, but only if the FWHM is modified to account for the number of studies per experiment.

$$\frac{1}{2000} \frac{\sum_{k\in K} N_k(\gamma)}{N_0(\gamma)} \leq 0.05; \qquad (11)$$

the proportion of clusters expected under the null hypothesis is, at most, 0.05 with this γ. Further detail about the calculation of FCDR is given in [15].

An omnibus test for difference between groups. Contrast meta-analysis looks for differences in activation patterns, between groups, by location. But such analysis requires very significant differences; since the p-values need to be very small to remain significant after controlling for many statistical tests. An omnibus test can provide evidence of pattern differences when contrast meta-analysis produces no significant results. Such a test may be

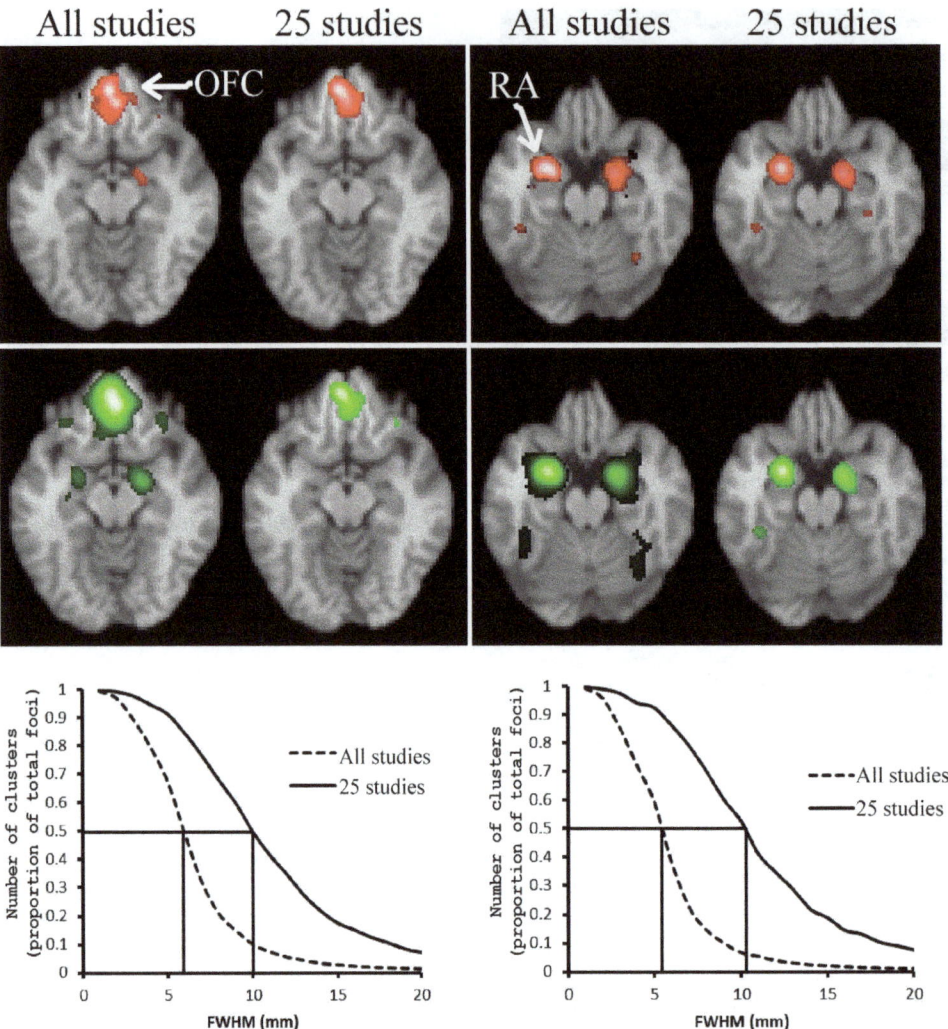

Figure 6. CBMA of the orbitofrontal cortex (OFC) and right amygdala (RA) studies, and smaller sub-studies. The top row depicts the results using $FWHM_{Eps}$, the middle row is the result from GingerALE, and the bottom row depicts the number of clusters, as a function of FWHM, counted under the null hypothesis.

useful for detecting differences that are subtle, but spread across substantial regions of the activation pattern.

A log likelihood value can be computed using the p-values from equations (9) and (10),

$$L_k = \sum_{ij} \log(p_{kij}), \qquad (12)$$

where the sum is over all foci in permutation k. The magnitude of this will be small under the null hypothesis and larger when the data are critical of the null hypothesis. The distribution of L_k is not known because the p-values are not independent (for independent p-values, Fisher's combined probability test can be used), but can be estimated using a random selection of permutations $K = \{k_1, k_2, \ldots, k_{1000}\}$. Only 1000 permutations are used, and found to be sufficient, to estimate the single p-value for the omnibus test

$$p_0 = \frac{\sum_{k \in K} I(L_k \leq L_0)}{\sum_{k \in K} 1}. \qquad (13)$$

This test is performed including all foci in the experiment.

Experiments for contrast analysis. To explore the two different scenarios considered above (highly significant local differences between groups, and more subtle wide spread differences) numerical experiments have been devised.

The first experiment involves two groups of studies with a cluster reported at $\{34, 10, 16\}$mm (Talairach coordinates) in group A and $\{-34, 10, 16\}$mm in group B. A further eight clusters are reported similarly by both groups. All foci that form part of a cluster have a random spatial perturbation as described for the FWHM numerical experiment. From the pain and n-back experiments, about 50% of studies report at the site of the most significant clusters. Therefore, each of the clusters in this

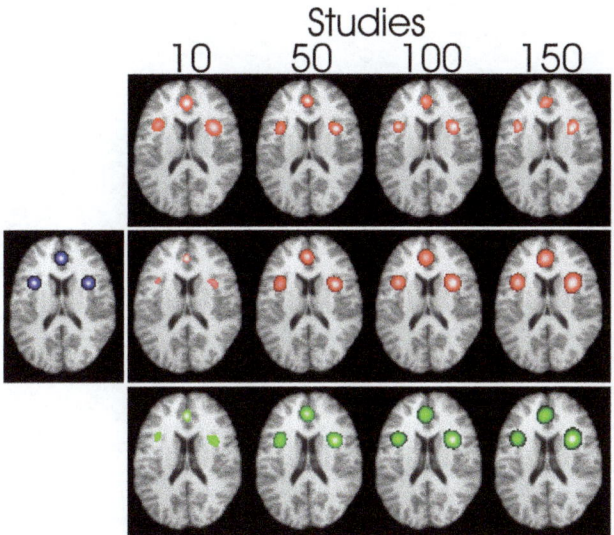

Figure 7. CBMA results for various numbers of studies, and using three definitions of the FWHM: top row uses FWHM$_{Eps}$, middle uses FWHM = 10 mm, and bottom uses the method reported by [3]; produced using GingerALE. The left-most image shows the distribution function of the foci as a blue overlay.

experiment contains foci from half of the studies, and half of the foci in each study are distributed randomly, and with uniform probability, throughout the GM mask.

The two clusters at $\{\pm 34,10,16\}$mm should be highly significant with sufficient studies in the experiment. The clusters that are reported similarly by both groups should not produce significant differences. Results are reported in a table indicating number of clusters reported by both groups, number of studies per group, and significances by contrast meta-analysis and the omnibus test.

The second experiment involves up-to sixteen clusters reported by both groups. In group A the clusters involve foci (with the random perturbation used in the first experiment) from 50% of the studies, and half of the foci in each study will be randomly distributed, with uniform probability, throughout the GM mask. Group B is similar, but the proportion of studies reporting at each cluster is lower. The differences between the studies are then subtle, and spread across the activation pattern. Results are reported in a table indicating number of studies, proportion of studies reporting at clusters, and significances by contrast meta-analysis and the omnibus test.

The contrast meta-analysis and omnibus tests are performed using FWHM$_{Eps}$.

Results

FWHM experiments
Assessment of the effect of the FWHM parameter on real data. Figure 2 shows the result of CBMA of 47 pain studies performed on healthy subjects. Result are shown for two different slices (top and bottom rows) using FWHM ranging from 6 mm to 14 mm. For very small FWHM the clusters (outlined in green) become fragmented and small. At larger FWHM the clusters begin to merge and grow.

Figure 3 shows the CBMA results for the 61 n-back studies. Two different slices are shown (top and bottom rows) using FWHM ranging from 6 mm to 14 mm. As expected, for very

small FWHM the clusters become fragmented and small. At larger FWHM the clusters begin to merge and grow.

Figure 4 shows the CBMA results for the 6 manual (top row) response and 19 pooled (bottom row) Stroop studies. The results are similar, but at different FWHM. Below 18 mm in the manual Stroop experiment, the clusters vanish or shrink. Above 12 mm in the pooled stroop experiment the clusters just increase in size.

Estimating the parameter α. Figure 5 depicts the number of clusters, under the null hypothesis (foci randomised), for each experiment as a function of FWHM. Also indicated are the FWHM where clustering just begins (number of clusters = 0.5) under the null hypothesis for the pain, n-back, and Stroop experiments. Higher FWHM generates larger clusters, which is not expected under the null hypothesis.

An estimate of α can be obtained from figure 5. If the FWHM$_{Eps}$ is the parameter value that just starts to form clusters under the null hypothesis, such that the foci overlap on average with one other, then the intercept of the curves with 0.5 on the y axis gives FWHM estimates of around 7 mm, 8 mm, 12 mm, and 18 mm for these experiments. Given the number of studies in the experiments, and using equation (4), yields an estimate for α of about 30 mm. The FWHM$_{Eps}$ estimates are then 8.3 mm, 7.6 mm, 11.2 mm, and 16.5 mm for the pain, n-back, pooled Stroop, and manual Stroop studies respectively.

Figure 6 shows the results from CBMA of the RA and OFC experiments. Using FWHM$_{Eps}$ (top row), with $\alpha = 30$mm, produces clusters that are quite independent of the number of studies. Furthermore, the clusters are of a reasonable size given the seed ROIs presented in [21]. When the FWHM is determined as detailed in [3] (middle row), the clusters are quite large for the complete data sets, particularly considering the seed ROIs. The cluster sizes are also quite dependent on the number of studies. The number of clusters expected under the null hypothesis, as a function of FWHM, is shown on the bottom row. Estimates of a obtained at the point where the foci just begin to cluster (intercepting the y axis at 0.5) are 29 mm, 29 mm, 29 mm, and 31 mm for these four experiments.

Numerical simulation experiments. Figure 7 shows the CBMA results for the simulated experiments; only the experiment with 40%, 50% and 60% of studies reporting in the clusters is shown as the lower proportion experiment is visually similar. The number of studies per experiment clearly has an impact on the results when using fixed FWHM; middle (FWHM = 10 mm) and bottom (FWHM as defined in [3] and produced using GingerALE) rows. When using FWHM$_{Eps}$ with $\alpha = 30$mm in equation (4) (top row) the results are not so dependent on the number of studies. Furthermore, the cluster size, using FWHM$_{Eps}$, is the most consistent with the foci distribution function, shown as a blue overlay on the left-most image; with the other FWHM estimates the clusters are small with just 10 studies, but expand in size beyond the boundary of the distribution function for large number of studies.

Figure 8a explores the true and false positive rates associated with the numerical experiment where the proportion of studies reporting at the clusters is in the range 40% to 60%; both rates expressed as a proportion of the true cluster members. True cluster rates were very high regardless of the FWHM estimate used, except for ten studies where the larger FWHM$_{Eps}$ estimate is able to detect a greater proportion of true cluster members. This, however, is associated with an increase in the false cluster rate, since the larger FWHM$_{Eps}$will also capture some of the study specific foci, which is noticeable in figure 7. More striking are the false cluster rate trends in this plot. For a FWHM of 10 mm, the false cluster rate is increasing with the number of experiments.

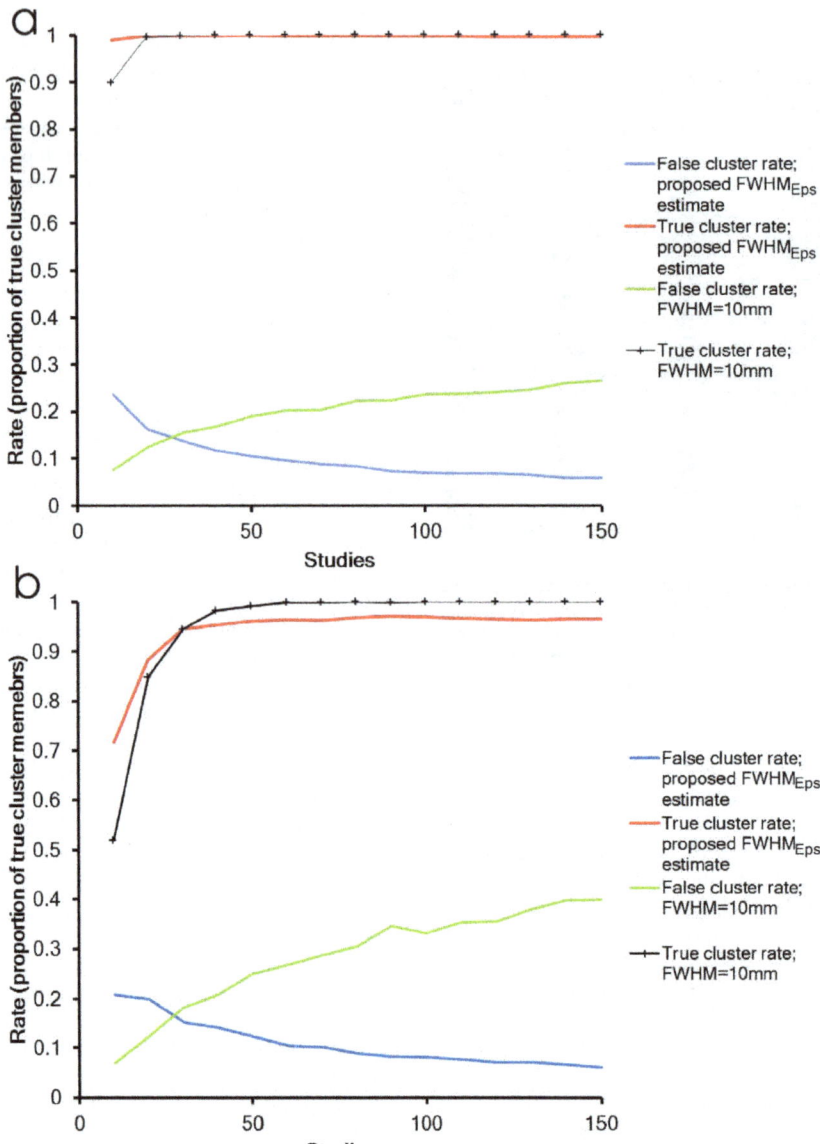

Figure 8. True and false cluster rates for FWHM_{Eps} **and for FWHM = 10 mm.** a) shows rates when the proportion of studies reporting in the clusters is 40%, 50%, and 60%. b) shows the rates when the proportion of studies reporting in the clusters is 20%, 30%, and 40%.

This leads to the paradoxical observation that increasing the number of studies included in the meta-analysis can be detrimental to the results. Using FWHM_{Eps} results in a reducing false cluster rate with increasing study numbers, which is sensible for a meta-analysis; a fit revealed that the false cluster rate was $\propto N^{-0.5}$ for this experiment.

Figure 8b explores the true and false positive rates associated with the numerical experiment where the proportion of studies reporting at the clusters is in the range 20% to 40%. In this case the true cluster rate is reduced when there are few studies because the FWHM is not large enough to cause clustering. The impact of this is reduced in the proposed method, which has a larger FWHM for fewer than 30 studies, but at the expense of higher false cluster rates. For larger numbers of studies the true cluster rate reaches 100% for FWHM = 10 mm, but is slightly lower (97%) for the proposed method due to its smaller FWHM. Once more the most striking trends are those of the false cluster rates. While using

FWHM_{Eps} reduces this as the number of studies increases (again the rate was $\propto N^{-0.5}$), it is increased when the FWHM is fixed at 10 mm.

These results are not specific to LocalALE, as we have shown in figure 7. Indeed the contribution list for each cluster provided by GingerALE confirmed that a very high proportion of studies were reported falsely. Adjustment of the FWHM to account for the number of studies is therefore suggested.

Contrast analysis experiments. Figure 9 shows the clusters used for the first contrast meta-analysis experiment. The eight clusters reported by both groups are seen in the left and middle image, along with the group specific clusters; highlighted by green ROIs. The rightmost image shows the contrast image, indicating where the activation patterns differ. In both groups 50% of studies report in each cluster.

Table 1 shows that the results of contrast meta-analysis are not significant (FCDR>0.05) for 10 or 14 studies per group, and just

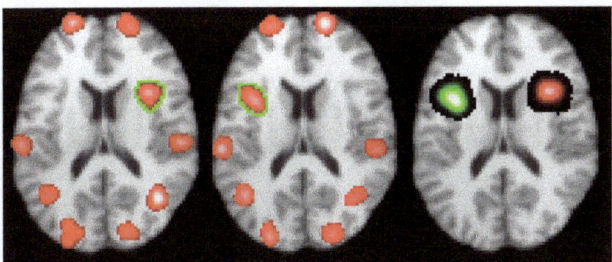

Figure 9. CBMA results of the first contrast meta-analysis experiment. The left and middle images show groups A & B, which have eight clusters in common, and two (one each) group specific clusters. The right image shows the difference between the groups found using contrast meta-analysis. This experiment tests the ability of contrast meta-analysis and the omnibus test to detect very significant differences between groups in the presence of an otherwise similar activation pattern. Note that while an intensity threshold (the lowest significant ALE value) is applied the leftmost and middle images, no such threshold is applied to the ALE difference image (right).

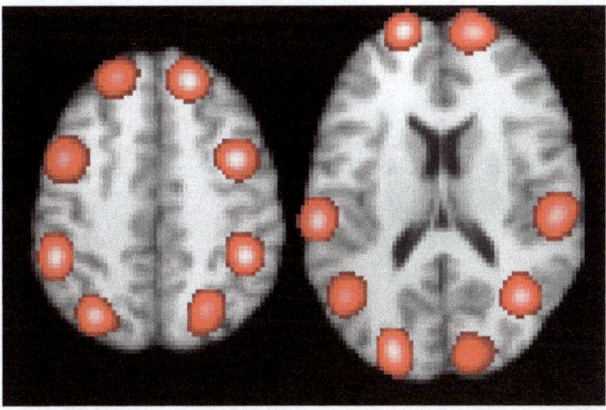

Figure 10. CBMA results of the second contrast meta-analysis experiment. Each group reports the same number of clusters (up-to 16, as shown), but with different frequencies. This experiment tests the ability of contrast meta-analysis and the omnibus test to detect subtle differences spread across the activation pattern.

about significant with 16 studies per group. When contrast meta-analysis was significant, it managed to find both group specific clusters, as expected. The omnibus test is significant in all of the experiments, indicating greater sensitivity. This is because the omnibus test needs no correction for the multiple tests. It should be noted that the p-values and FCDR values reported in table 1 are approximate; partly because they are estimated by permutation test, but mostly because the experiments include random foci, which would be different if the experiment were re-generated. Experiments were therefore repeated several times to check that the results presented were representative.

Figure 10 shows the 16 clusters used for the second contrast meta-analysis experiment. Both group A and group B report some, or all, of these clusters. In group A 50% of studies report in each cluster, while a smaller percentage of studies in group B report at each cluster (see table 2).

Table 2 shows the results of contrast meta-analysis and the omnibus test when differences between groups are spread over the activation pattern. As the differences between the studies increase, either per cluster or as the number of clusters that are different increases, the tests become more sensitive as expected. However, contrast meta-analysis is not completely successful in finding all differences between the two groups, as indicated by the range of clusters found on repeating the experiment; with different random foci. The omnibus test is certainly more sensitive, able to detect differences between even small groups of studies. It should be noted that the smallest p-value reported for the omnibus test is

0.001; since only 1000 permutations are used to compute the p-value, 0.001 is the smallest non-zero value possible.

Discussion

We have detailed three tools for use with coordinate based meta-analysis. By analogy with density clustering, we have redefined the FWHM parameter used in CBMA as a cluster density parameter, which depends on the cube root number of studies in the analysis, and is based on the idea that the results of CBMA should be commensurate when performed with different numbers of studies. We have also detailed an algorithm for comparing activation patterns between groups, contrast meta-analysis, using similar methods to our previously described LocalALE algorithm. Statistical testing is performed only at the foci, rather than at each voxel, and our FCDR method of false positive control is employed. Such contrast meta-analyses are only sensitive to very significant localised differences in activation, so we also detail an omnibus test of difference between groups. The omnibus test is sensitive even to subtle diffuse differences between activation patterns, and can provide evidence for a difference where contrast meta-analysis is unrevealing.

By visually inspecting the resulting clusters for several CBMAs, it becomes clear that the FWHM parameter has a major effect on the results. To preserve the cluster characteristics we proposed, by analogy with the density clustering algorithm DBSCAN, that the characteristic volume of each foci ($\sim$ FWHM^3) should be adjusted for the number of studies included in the analysis. This

Table 1. Results for the first group comparison experiment.

Number of studies per group	Results of contrast meta-analysis	Omnibus test using all foci (p-value)
10	0.4	0.04
14	0.1	0.02
16	0.05	0.01
20	0.02	0.002

The omnibus test is able to find differences between the two activation patterns (see figure 9), even when the contrast meta-analysis test is unrevealing. The two tests are more sensitive for larger numbers of studies.

Table 2. Results for the second group comparison experiment (see figure 10).

Number of studies per group	Number of clusters in experiment	Number of foci per group	Number (%) of studies reporting at clusters in group A	Number (%) of studies reporting at clusters in group B	Number of clusters found by contrast meta-analysis with FCDR≤0.05	Omnibus test using all foci (p-value)
6	8	48	3 (50%)	1 (17%)	0	0.03
6	16	96	3 (50%)	1 (17%)	0	0.03
10	8	80	5 (50%)	2 (20%)	0	0.01
10	8	80	5 (50%)	1 (10%)	0–6	0.004
10	16	160	5 (50%)	2 (20%)	0–1	0.02
20	8	160	10 (50%)	4 (20%)	0	0.001
20	8	160	10 (50%)	2 (10%)	5–8	0.001
20	16	320	10 (50%)	4 (20%)	0–4	0.001
40	8	320	20 (50%)	8 (20%)	0	0.001
40	8	320	20 (50%)	4 (10%)	7–8	0.001
40	16	640	20 (50%)	8 (20%)	4–16	0.001

The omnibus test is able to find differences between the two activation patterns, even when the contrast meta-analysis test is unrevealing. The two tests are more sensitive for larger numbers of studies, larger differences per cluster, or more clusters that are different.

method of specifying FWHM completely changes the original meaning that the FWHM represented the spatial uncertainty in the reported foci, for example due to registration error.

Using a typical (10 mm) FWHM, or the FWHM suggested by Eickhoff et. al. [3], results in diminishing or vanishing clusters as the number of studies is reduced, and expanding and merging clusters as the number of studies is increased. This was demonstrated using numerically generated experiments, and by using small selections of studies from real CBMAs. It is clear from the experiments that using a FWHM that is independent of the number of studies could easily lead to the incorrect conclusion that groups with different numbers of studies have different activation patterns; consider the Stroop experiments (figure 4). Figure 7 demonstrates that for increasing study numbers, the cluster sizes increase if the FWHM parameter is not adjusted. This is counter intuitive, as the cluster size and location should be convergent as the experiment size increases. Taking this to its limit of very large numbers of studies, clusters will merge, and study specific foci recruited to them, which is incorrect.

Our proposed method of estimating the FWHM aims to allow overlapping of the high density foci that form clusters, but prevent overlapping of the low density study-specific foci between the clusters. We use an empirical estimate of FWHM based on that which just starts to cause overlapping of foci between different studies under the null hypothesis (figure 5). This is commensurate with the DBSCAN analogy, since at that FWHM the densely packed within-cluster foci overlap, while the between-cluster foci do not. This leads to an estimate of the parameter α ($\alpha \approx 30$mm) in equation (4).

The experiments depicted in figure 6 are of particular interest because for these we know where the clusters are located, and their approximate size, since this was predefined as part of the experimental procedure [21]. Using $FWHM_{Eps}$ gives results that are reasonable given the original seed ROIs, independent of the number of studies included. Using the FWHM specified in [3], on the other hand, produces rather large clusters for the full dataset. Using these experiments, another estimate of the parameter α is obtained ($\alpha \approx 29.5$mm).

We have quantitatively analysed the true and false positive rates associated with FWHM estimates using numerical simulation (figures 7 and 8). Three clusters were defined and foci generated to be either true or false cluster members. The results are in keeping with the proposed idea that the FWHM must be adjusted for the number of studies. For very few studies FWHM needs to be increased to allow the foci to overlap and form clusters, albeit with an associated increase in the false cluster rate. Failing to do this could result in missed clusters, as shown by the Stroop experiment. On the other hand, the FWHM must be reduced as the number of studies increases to prevent recruitment of non-cluster foci into the clusters. Indeed the striking observation from figure 8 is that increasing the number of studies in the meta-analysis can be detrimental if the FWHM is fixed due to increased false positives. This is entirely contrary to the aim of meta-analysis, which attempts to reduce uncertainty in estimates.

We have estimated the parameter α in equation (4) to be ≈ 30mm, using multiple independent observations; giving the typically used ~ 10mm FWHM for an experiment including 30 studies. However, there is some variance on this estimate, and some minor adjustment might be necessary if the clusters are visually fragmented or merging.

Control of false positives in our contrast meta-analysis algorithm is achieved using FCDR; a cluster-level control scheme. Cluster-level schemes have been incorporated into CBMA algorithms previously, and are preferred since they control at the level of interest (clusters) rather than at the voxel-level, but not into algorithms performing contrast of the ALE; indeed no method of control, other than conservative p-value threshold, has previously been described [12].

The contrast meta-analysis and omnibus test for differences between two groups were demonstrated using numerically generated experiments. The first experiment showed the ability of contrast meta-analysis to find local differences, if those differences were very significant. The omnibus test was also able to detect such differences, and with greater sensitivity, but without specifying where the differences are. A second experiment showed that when there are multiple subtle differences between groups, the omnibus test again had more power to detect it than contrast meta-analysis; as expected. Both methods are more sensitive with higher numbers of studies, more significant local differences, or more widespread subtle differences.

Lack of spatial difference in contrast meta-analysis experiments is not a good indicator that there is no difference between the groups being compared because the test is not sensitive to diffuse subtle differences. The omnibus test is more powerful, and should be used where the contrast meta-analysis produces no results. If the omnibus test is not significant, it is more likely that any real difference between groups is small. If it is significant, it can indicate widespread subtle differences between the groups that are undetectable by contrast meta-analysis.

Conclusions

The FWHM parameter used in ALE coordinate based meta-analysis algorithms is a source of heterogeneity between CBMA results. The meaning of the parameter has been redefined here from being the spatial uncertainty of the reported foci, to a parameter similar to that employed in a density clustering algorithm that works analogously to CBMA. This definition helps reduce the observed heterogeneity. More importantly, fixing the FWHM can paradoxically result in increased false positives as the number of studies increases, while the proposed $FWHM_{Eps}$

estimate can reduce the false positive rates in the meta-analysis with increasing study numbers.

The many tests used to compare the activation patterns between two groups necessitate a correction for multiple comparisons. We have detailed a contrast meta-analysis algorithm and correction for multiple tests that controls for the proportion of clusters expected under the null hypothesis, the false cluster discovery rate, and takes explicit account of the correlated tests. However, the contrast meta-analysis is not sensitive to diffuse differences between groups. We have therefore detailed an omnibus test that can provide evidence of differences in activation pattern between two groups even when contrast meta-analysis is unrevealing.

Supporting Information

File S1   Cluster finding algorithm.

Author Contributions

Conceived and designed the experiments: CRT RT. Performed the experiments: CRT. Analyzed the data: CRT. Contributed reagents/materials/analysis tools: CRT. Contributed to the writing of the manuscript: CRT RT DPA WC CSC.

References

1. Turkeltaub PE, Eden GF, Jones KM, Zeffiro TA (2002) Meta-analysis of the functional neuroanatomy of single-word reading: method and validation. Neuroimage 16: 765–80.
2. Eickhoff SB, Bzdok D, Laird AR, Kurth F, Fox PT (2012) Activation likelihood estimation meta-analysis revisited. Neuroimage 59: 2349–61.
3. Eickhoff SB, Laird AR, Grefkes C, Wang LE, Zilles K, et al. (2009) Coordinate-based activation likelihood estimation meta-analysis of neuroimaging data: a random-effects approach based on empirical estimates of spatial uncertainty. Hum Brain Mapp 30: 2907–26.
4. Laird AR, Fox PM, Price CJ, Glahn DC, Uecker AM, et al. (2005) ALE meta-analysis: controlling the false discovery rate and performing statistical contrasts. Hum Brain Mapp 25: 155–64.
5. Radua J, Mataix-Cols D (2009) Voxel-wise meta-analysis of grey matter changes in obsessive-compulsive disorder. Br J Psychiatry 195: 393–402.
6. Turkeltaub PE, Eickhoff SB, Laird AR, Fox M, Wiener M, et al. (2012) Minimizing within-experiment and within-group effects in Activation Likelihood Estimation meta-analyses. Hum Brain Mapp 33: 1–13.
7. Wager TD, Lindquist M, Kaplan L (2007) Meta-analysis of functional neuroimaging data: current and future directions. Soc Cogn Affect Neurosci 2: 150–8.
8. Wager TD, Phan KL, Liberzon I, Taylor SF (2003) Valence, gender, and lateralization of functional brain anatomy in emotion: a meta-analysis of findings from neuroimaging. Neuroimage 19: 513–31.
9. Yue YR, Lindquist MA, Loh JM (2012) Meta-analysis of functional neuroimaging data using Bayesian nonparametric binary regression. Ann. of Appl. Stat. 6:
10. Kang J, Johnson TD, Nichols TE, Wager TD (2011) Meta Analysis of Functional Neuroimaging Data via Bayesian Spatial Point Processes. J Am Stat Assoc 106: 124–134.
11. Ferreira LK, Busatto GF (2010) Heterogeneity of coordinate-based meta-analyses of neuroimaging data: an example from studies in OCD. Br J Psychiatry 197: 76–7; author reply 77.
12. Eickhoff SB, Bzdok D, Laird AR, Roski C, Caspers S, et al. (2011) Co-activation patterns distinguish cortical modules, their connectivity and functional differentiation. Neuroimage 57: 938–49.
13. Friebel U, Eickhoff SB, Lotze M (2011) Coordinate-based meta-analysis of experimentally induced and chronic persistent neuropathic pain. Neuroimage 58: 1070–80.
14. Benjamini Y, Hochberg Y (1995) Controlling the False Discovery Rate: A Practical and Powerful Approach to Multiple Testing. Journal of the Royal Statistical Society. Series B (Methodological) 57: 289–300.
15. Tench CR, Tanasescu R, Auer DP, Constantinescu CS (2013) Coordinate based meta-analysis of functional neuroimaging data; false discovery control and diagnostics. PLoS One 8: e70143.
16. RAF Statistical Methods For Research Workers (1925) Oliver and Boyd. Edinburgh.
17. Ester M, Kriegel H, Sander J, Xu X (1996) A Density-Based Algorithm for Discovering Clusters in Large Spatial Databases with Noise. In: E Simoudis, J Han and U Fayyad, editors. AAAI Press. pp. 226–231.
18. Owen AM, McMillan KM, Laird AR, Bullmore E (2005) N-back working memory paradigm: a meta-analysis of normative functional neuroimaging studies. Hum Brain Mapp 25: 46–59.
19. Laird AR, Lancaster JL, Fox PT (2005) BrainMap: the social evolution of a human brain mapping database. Neuroinformatics 3: 65–78.
20. Laird AR, McMillan KM, Lancaster JL, Kochunov P, Turkeltaub PE, et al. (2005) A comparison of label-based review and ALE meta-analysis in the Stroop task. Hum Brain Mapp 25: 6–21.
21. Kellermann TS, Caspers S, Fox PT, Zilles K, Roski C, et al. (2013) Task- and resting-state functional connectivity of brain regions related to affection and susceptible to concurrent cognitive demand. Neuroimage 72: 69–82.
22. Fox PT, Lancaster JL (2002) Opinion: Mapping context and content: the BrainMap model. Nat Rev Neurosci 3: 319–21.
23. Dijkstra EW (1959) A note on two problems in connexion with graphs. Numerische Mathematik 1: 269–271.

12

Analysis of Fundus Shape in Highly Myopic Eyes by Using Curvature Maps Constructed from Optical Coherence Tomography

Masahiro Miyake, Kenji Yamashiro*, Yumiko Akagi-Kurashige, Akio Oishi, Akitaka Tsujikawa, Masanori Hangai, Nagahisa Yoshimura

Department of Ophthalmology and Visual Sciences, Kyoto University Graduate School of Medicine, Kyoto, Japan

Abstract

Purpose: To evaluate fundus shape in highly myopic eyes using color maps created through optical coherence tomography (OCT) image analysis.

Methods: We retrospectively evaluated 182 highly myopic eyes from 113 patients. After obtaining 12 lines of 9-mm radial OCT scans with the fovea at the center, the Bruch's membrane line was plotted and its curvature was measured at 1-μm intervals in each image, which was reflected as a color topography map. For the quantitative analysis of the eye shape, mean absolute curvature and variance of curvature were calculated.

Results: The color maps allowed staphyloma visualization as a ring of green color at the edge and as that of orange-red color at the bottom. Analyses of mean and variance of curvature revealed that eyes with myopic choroidal neovascularization tended to have relatively flat posterior poles with smooth surfaces, while eyes with chorioretinal atrophy exhibited a steep, curved shape with an undulated surface ($P<0.001$). Furthermore, eyes with staphylomas and those without clearly differed in terms of mean curvature and the variance of curvature: 98.4% of eyes with staphylomas had mean curvature $\geq 7.8 \times 10^{-5}$ [1/μm] and variance of curvature $\geq 0.26 \times 10^{-8}$ [1/μm].

Conclusions: We established a novel method to analyze posterior pole shape by using OCT images to construct curvature maps. Our quantitative analysis revealed that fundus shape is associated with myopic complications. These values were also effective in distinguishing eyes with staphylomas from those without. This tool for the quantitative evaluation of eye shape should facilitate future research of myopic complications.

Editor: Bang V. Bui, University of Melbourne, Australia

Funding: This study was supported in part by grants-in-aid for scientific research (Nos. 21249084 and 200791294) from the Japan Society for the Promotion of Science, Tokyo, Japan, and the Japan National Society for the Prevention of Blindness, Tokyo, Japan. The funders had no role in study design, data collection and analysis, decision to publish, or preparation of the manuscript. Financial Disclosures: Nagahisa Yoshimura: Canon (Financial support), Topcon (Financial support); Masanori Hangai: Canon (Financial support), Topcon (Financial support).

Competing Interests: The authors have read the journal's policy and have the following conflicts: Nagahisa Yoshimura: Canon (Financial support), Topcon (Financial support); Masanori Hangai: Canon (Financial support), Topcon (Financial support).

* Email: yamashro@kuhp.kyoto-u.ac.jp

Introduction

Myopia is one of the most common visual disorders worldwide, representing a major public health concern among East Asian populations. [1–4] Myopic eyes with very long axial lengths ($\geq$ 26.0 mm, $\geq$26.5 mm, or $\geq$28.0 mm) or a high degree of myopic refractive error (≤-5D, ≤-6D, or ≤-8D) are classified as highly myopic. [5–11] High myopia is typically associated with excessive elongation of the globe and, in middle-aged individuals, often leads to pathological changes such as posterior staphyloma. [12,13] Moriyama et al. analyzed the shapes of eyes with pathologic myopia using three-dimensional magnetic resonance imaging (MRI). The results demonstrated a clear association between eye shape and the likelihood of optic neuropathy. [14] However, eyeball shape as classified by MRI was not associated

with myopic complications at the posterior pole such as myopic choroidal neovascularization (mCNV), chorioretinal atrophy (CRA), or myopic tractional maculopathy. Owing to the resolutional limitations of MRI, this technique cannot be used for detailed morphological investigations of the posterior pole, where most major myopic complications develop.

Today, optical coherence tomography (OCT) is emerging as a popular modality by which we can obtain precise cross-sectional images of retina and fundus, though its scan width is limited. While MRI is a very useful device with which to macroscopically evaluate eyeball shape, [14–16] OCT is more suitable for microscopic evaluation owing to its high resolution. The rapid scanning speed utilized for spectral-domain OCT can minimize the effects of ocular movement, allowing for a more precise analysis of retinal structure. [17] To date, several studies have examined staphylomas using OCT. [18,19] Notably, the height of a posterior staphyloma affects the development of mCNV. Previous reports investigated this phenomenon using several narrow 6-mm scans, which collectively captured only a small portion of the entire staphyloma. [18] In the current study, we evaluated twelve 9-mm radial OCT scans in each highly myopic eye studied. This information was used to create a curvature map for the nearly entirety of Bruch's membrane; the staphyloma edge and degree of staphyloma were clearly visualized with the aid of this map. Subsequent analyses revealed associations between posterior pole shape and myopic complications.

Materials and Methods

We examined 192 eyes respectively, having axial length $\geq$ 26 mm from 120 consecutive patients who underwent the analysis below during the period from April 2010 to March 2012. All procedures in this study adhered to the tenets of the Declaration of Helsinki. The ethics committee (Ethics Committee of Kyoto University Graduate School and Faculty of Medicine, Japan) approved the study protocol. All of the patients were fully informed about the purpose and procedures of this study, and written consent was obtained from each. Patient records/ information was anonymized and de-identified prior to analysis.

Data collection

Of the 192 eyes, 10 eyes from 7 patients were excluded either because the OCT images and/or color fundus photographs were of poor quality or because they had a history of ocular surgery other than cataract surgery. A total of 182 highly myopic eyes from 113 patients were analyzed. Each subject underwent a complete ophthalmic examination, including axial length measurement using an IOL master (Carl Zeiss Meditec, Dublin, CA), indirect ophthalmoscopy and slit-lamp biomicroscopy, and optical coherence tomography (RS-3000, Nidek, Tokyo, Japan). Fluorescein angiography was performed if mCNV was suspected.

Mapping fundus curvature

In this analysis, we used Burch's membrane lines as representative lines of the fundus shape instead of the retina or RPE lines, which allowed us to overcome the drawbacks of previous method using retinal topography [20,21]; retinal or RPE topography can be easily biased by complications such as CNV, schisis, and MHRD.

We built new software to calculate the eye curvatures from their OCT images and construct a color curvature map. This software presents a measure of retinal shape with distribution of local curvature. By calculating the local curvature, it was possible to detect small unevenness of the retina. After obtaining 12 lines of a 9-mm radial OCT scan at center of the fovea, Bruch's membrane line was plotted (Figure 1A). The size of each OCT image was adjusted to correct for the difference in pixel resolution in the transverse and longitudinal directions. A case in which a curvature of the Bruch's membrane was used as shape analysis is described below using the OCT image shown in Figure 1. The curvature of the Bruch's membrane line as an analysis target was calculated. The curvature κ can be obtained by calculating, at respective points at the Bruch's membrane line:

$$\kappa = \frac{\frac{d^2 z}{dx^2}}{\left(1 + \left(\frac{dz}{dx}\right)^2\right)^{\frac{3}{2}}} \tag{1}$$

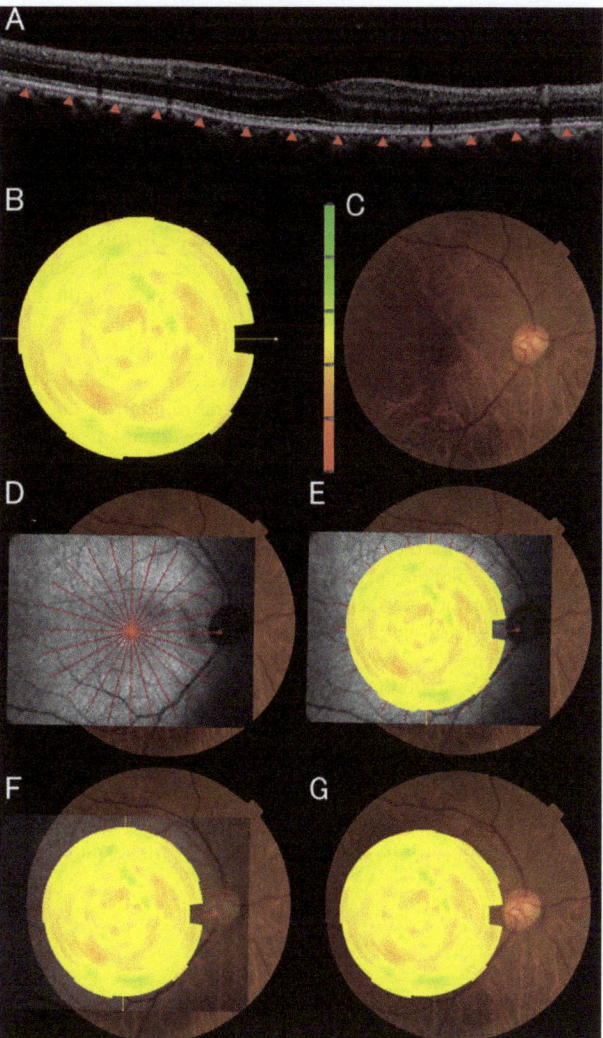

Figure 1. Construction of the curvature map for a normal eye. A, Bruch's membrane was plotted in each of 12 radial OCT scans with the fovea at the center. Local curvature was measured from 3 sequential points (sampled at 500-µm intervals). The sine of curvature was defined as positive when the membrane was convex upward. **B,** The value of curvature was mapped using yellow (RGB(255, 255, 0)) to represent zero curvature (flat), green (gradient from RGB(255, 255, 0) to RGB(0, 192, 32) according to curvature [1/µm]) for positive curvature (convex-upward), and red (gradient from RGB(255, 255, 0) to RGB(255, 0, 0) according to curvature [1/µm]) for negative curvature (convex-downward). **C,** Color fundus photograph on which the topographic maps will be overlaid. **D,** Scanning Laser Ophthalmoscope (SLO) images are overlaid on the fundus photographs. **E,** Topographic maps are overlaid on the SLO images. **F and G,** SLO image transparency was increased for an accurate superimposition.

The differentials in equation (1) were calculated by central difference. These equations are represented by:

$$\frac{dz}{dx} = \frac{f(x+h) - f(x-h)}{2h} \tag{2}$$

$$\frac{d^2 z}{dx^2} = \frac{f(x+h) - 2f(x) + f(x-h)}{h^2} \tag{3}$$

where f(x) is the Bruch's membrane line, and h is the spacing between two adjacent A-scans (500-μm apart). The curvature κ was measured using 3 sequential A-scans. Therefore, it represents local shape in the range of 1,000-μm (Local curvature). The values of the local curvature were calculated using all A-scans except in regions within 500-μm from right and left boundaries of an image. The unit of curvature κ was inverse micrometer. Positive, negative, or zero value of the curvature κ represents upward concave, downward convex, or flat respectively. In this study, the curvature was calculated with three points on the Bruch's membrane line. Because distance from the first point to the third point was 1000-μm, this localized curvature was allowed to be zero.

The degree of curvature was measured for the radial OCT scans with the fovea at the center. The distribution of the local curvature was presented as a color map overlaid on a c-scan retinal image: yellow (RGB(255, 255, 0)) for the local curvature value of 0.0 (1/infinity) [1/μm], green (RGB(0, 192, 32)) for the local curvature value of +0.0005 (1/2000) [1/μm], and red (RGB(255, 0, 0)) for the local curvature value of −0.0005 (1/2000) [1/μm]. The color of curvature map was limited to 1/2000 [1/μm]. The curvature map set a color to show a gradient from green to yellow as a local curvature value changes from 0.0005 to 0.0, and a gradient from red to yellow as a local curvature value changes from −0.0005 to 0.0. Examples of correspondence between fundus shape, curvature, and color were presented in Figure 2. Generated color map was then superimposed on a fundus photo, being intermediated by a Scanning Laser Ophthalmoscope (SLO) image (Figure 1B–1F). Figure 1G depicts a normal eye. Considering the spherical shape of a normal eye, the curvature of its posterior pole should be negative. However, its

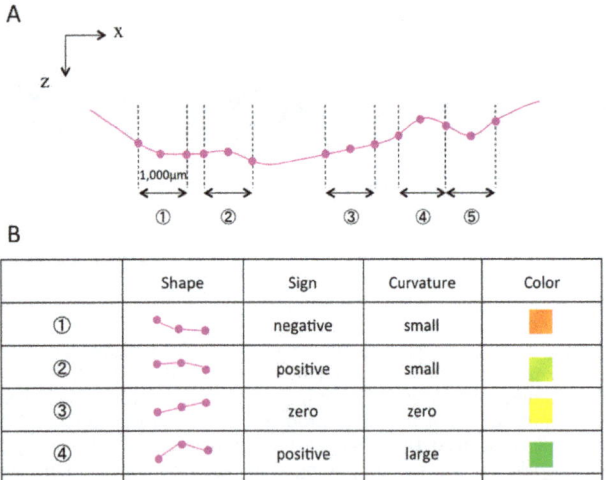

Figure 2. Image of correspondence between fundus shape, curvature, and color. A, An imaginary Bruch's membrane line to exemplify the correspondence. The curvature of one point was measured using 3 sequential A-scans (500-μm apart) so that it represented local shape in the range of 1,000-μm (Local curvature). Five points are exemplified in this figure. **B,** Corresponding curvature [1/μm] and color image for each 5 point. Positive, negative, or zero value of the curvature κ represents upward concave, downward convex, or flat, respectively. The color of curvature map showed a gradient from green (RGB(0, 192, 32)) to yellow (RGB(255, 255, 0)) as a local curvature value changes from 0.0005 to 0.0, and a gradient from red (RGB(255, 0, 0)) to yellow (RGB(255, 255, 0)) as a local curvature value changes from −0.0005 to 0.0.

curvature is very low so that the map shows an overall yellow appearance.

Segmentation Method

A smoothing filter (Median filter) was applied to OCT images to remove noise components. Layer boundary extraction could be implemented by edge detection filter (Sobel filter) and the layer structure-emphasized filter (Hessian filter).

As for the inner limiting membrane, a peak of the layer structure emphasizing filter was searched for in the depth direction of fundus from the vitreum side, and a first peak position equal to or larger than a threshold was detected as an initial value of the inner limiting membrane and nerve fiber layer boundary. From that initial value, a gradient feature was searched for toward the vitreum side, and a gradient peak position was detected as the inner limiting membrane.

Likewise, as for the nerve fiber layer boundary, a gradient feature was searched for from that initial value in the depth direction of the fundus, and a gradient peak position was detected as the nerve fiber layer boundary.

As for the Bruch's membrane line, a peak of the layer structure emphasizing filter is searched for further in the depth direction of the fundus, and the last peak position equal to or larger than the threshold is detected as an initial value of the Bruch's membrane line. A gradient feature was searched for from that initial value in the depth direction of the fundus, and a gradient peak position was detected as the Bruch's membrane line.

By applying Snakes [22] using the detected boundary as the initial position, the boundary shape became smooth.

Data analysis

We evaluated the curvature maps for eyes with foveal retinal detachments (RDs), retinoschisis, mCNV, and severe CRA. In addition, differences in the curvature maps were compared between eyes with staphyloma and eyes without staphyloma. The presence of retinoschisis, RD, CRA, and staphyloma was determined using color fundus photographs and OCT images. FA images were used to identify mCNV. The images of each eye were examined by 2 retina specialists (K.Y and A.T), and any discrepancies were settled by a third specialist (N.Y). Cases showing patchy CRA >3 disc diameters in area were diagnosed as having severe CRA. The eyes with both retinoschisis and RD were classified as RD. Multiple comparisons of numerical values such as patient age and axial length were performed with analysis of variance (ANOVA) and Tukey–Kramer's tests. Single comparisons were performed using an unpaired t-test. The male:female ratio and other 2×2 or 2×3 tables were compared using Fisher's exact test and Tukey's test for post-hoc analysis. A p-value of ≤5% was considered statistically significant.

Results

Among these 113 patients, 37 were men and 76 were women, with a mean age of 61.9±14.1 years. The mean axial length was 28.68±1.74 mm. RD with or without retinoschisis was seen in 13 eyes (7.1%), retinoschisis without RD in 34 eyes (18.7%), mCNV in 33 eyes (18.1%), and severe CRA in 20 eyes (11.0%). The highly myopic patients with retinoschisis, RD, and severe CRA were significantly older than the highly myopic patients without these 3 complications ($P = 1.6 \times 10^{-4}$, 0.0017, 0.0012, respectively). There were more women than men with mCNV, retinoschisis, and CRA (Table 1). Axial length was significantly longer in eyes with retinoschisis, RD, and CRA as compared to eyes without

Table 1. Characteristics of the included eyes according to complications.

Variable		No complications	mCNV	Retinoschisis	RD	CRA	P-value[†]
n		88	33	34	13	20	
Age (years ± SD)		56.2±13.9	60.3±16.1	67.9±11.9	71.0±8.56	68.9±6.51	1.16×10^{-6}
p-value*	No complications	-	0.54	<0.001	0.002	0.001	
	mCNV	-	-	0.13	0.10	0.14	
	Retinoschisis	-	-	-	0.95	1.00	
	RD	-	-	-	-	0.99	
Sex (male:female)		44:44	5:28	6:28	4:9	3:17	2.03×10^{-4}
p-value*	No complications	-	0.002	0.004	0.60	0.02	
	mCNV	-	-	1.00	0.82	1.00	
	Retinoschisis	-	-	-	0.90	1.00	
	RD	-	-	-	-	0.86	
Axial length (mm ± SD)		28.02±1.49	28.35±1.20	29.46±1.54	29.31±1.38	30.96±1.11	5.47×10^{-11}
p-value*	No complications	-	0.82	<0.001	0.04	<0.001	
	mCNV	-	-	0.03	0.31	<0.001	
	Retinoschisis	-	-	-	1.00	0.05	
	RD	-	-	-	-	0.11	

*Tukey-Kramer's multiple comparison.
[†]Analysis of variance.
CNV: choroidal neovascularization, RD: retinal detachment, CRA: chorioretinal atrophy.

complications, while the axial length of eyes with mCNV was not significantly different from eyes without these 4 complications.

Constructing fundus curvature maps

Fundus curvature maps were successfully obtained and super-imposed on color fundus photographs in all 182 cases. In 4 eyes with staphylomas, the entire staphyloma edge could be visualized clearly using this method (Figure 3A and 3B). Because the staphyloma edge must have an inflection point, the edge curvature theoretically ranges from zero to plus, which would be represented on the curvature map as yellow to green shading along the staphyloma edge. The area inside the staphyloma is depicted as red to orange, which represents a relatively high degree of concave curvature. This image can be contrasted with that of a representative normal eye, which yielded a topographical map that was yellow in overall appearance (Figure 1).

In this analysis, however, manual correction was needed in all cases more or less. While we required re-plot of less than 10 points per slice in eyes without staphyloma, re-plot of more than or equal to 10 points per slice was needed in most eyes with staphyloma to

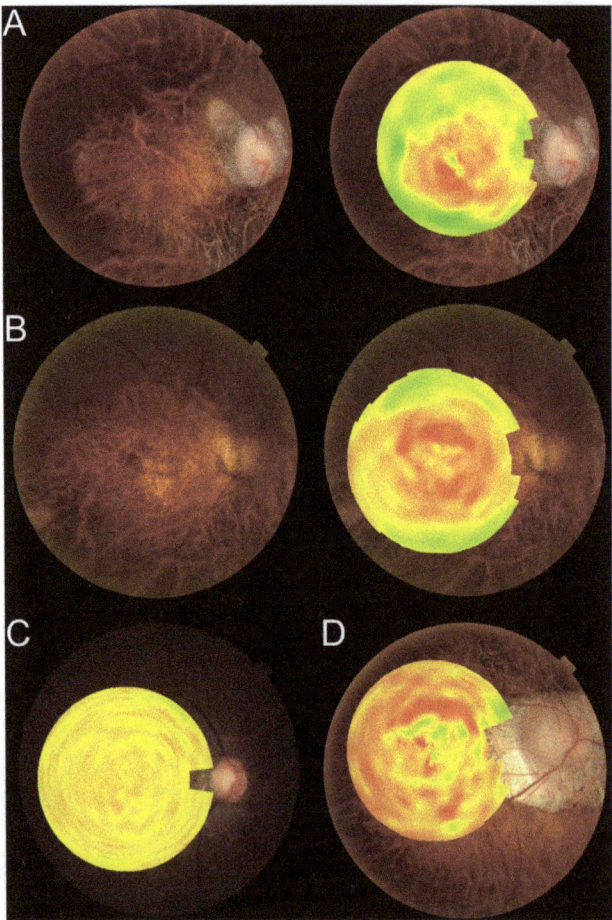

Figure 3. Representative color maps of highly myopic eyes. A, Right eye from a 58-year-old woman with axial length of 29.01 mm. The staphyloma edge is depicted in green-yellow. **B,** Right eye of a 72-year-old woman with axial length of 28.37 mm. Upper and lower edges of the staphyloma can be visualized clearly. **C,** Right eye of a 38-year-old woman, with axial length of 26.38 mm. The yellow-dominant color map represents a relatively flat fundus. **D,** Right eye from a 65-year-old woman with axial length of 34.64 mm. The mosaic color pattern indicates an undulated fundus.

obtain correct curvature of Bruch's membrane. When image inversion towards the edges of the OCT scan existed, we could not construct curvature map at the corresponding area. In the studied eyes, however, mean coverage area was $86.4 \pm 10.2\%$, which corresponds to 87.3%–98.3% coverage of diameter.

Some of the participants underwent several OCT examinations within 3 months. In these eyes, the color map did not show notable change within 3 months, suggesting our method has acceptable repeatability.

Quantitative evaluation of the curvature maps

When we evaluated the color maps for 182 eyes, we found roughly 3 patterns of curvature maps: a yellow dominant curvature map (Figure 3C), a map with an orange-red color at the center (Figure 3A and 3B), and one with a mosaic pattern of red and green (Figure 3D). The comparison between eyes with yellow-dominant curvature maps and eyes that yielded maps with an orange-red color at the center suggested that the degree of staphyloma could be represented by the mean curvature value. In addition, the mosaic patterns of red and green suggested that the smoothness of the staphyloma surface could be represented by the variance in curvature. Hence, we calculated the mean absolute curvature and variance of curvature for each eye as an index for fundus shape. This approach allowed for a quantitative evaluation of the characteristics of fundus shape. With mean curvature values assigned to the horizontal axis and the variance values assigned to the vertical axis, a scatter plot was used to illustrate the consecutive distribution of all eyes evaluated (Figure 4A).

Characteristics of fundus curvature in eyes with myopic complications

Scatter plots showed that each myopic complication evaluated had a specific profile, as represented by mean curvature and variance. Eyes with mCNV exhibited low-to-moderate levels of curvature and minimal variance (Figure 4B). In contrast, eyes with severe CRA exhibited higher levels of both curvature and variance (Figure 4C). When we drew a splitting line at 1.5×10^{-4} for mean curvature and 1×10^{-8} for the variance of curvature, most eyes with mCNV were distributed throughout the left-lower area, while most eyes with CRA were distributed throughout the right-upper area. Eyes with RD and retinoschisis were similar in exhibiting moderate levels of both curvature and variance (Figure 4D).

The quantitative evaluation of mean curvature and variance of curvature revealed additional differences in fundus shape that distinguished each of the complications studied from the others. Mean curvature was significantly larger in eyes with complications than in eyes without any of the complications studied (Table 2). When the values of eyes with RD and eyes with retinoschisis were combined for further analysis, mean curvature values were significantly smaller in eyes with mCNV as compared to eyes with RD or retinoschisis, and significantly smaller in eyes with RD or retinoschisis as compared to eyes with CRA. Similar to the mean curvature results, variance of curvature was significantly larger in eyes with retinoschisis, RD, and CRA than in eyes without complications (Table 3). However, there was no significant difference in the variance of curvature between eyes with mCNV and eyes without complications. Among the eyes with complications, the variance of curvature also showed significant trends: smaller in eyes with mCNV, intermediate in eyes with RD or retinoschisis, and larger in eyes with CRA.

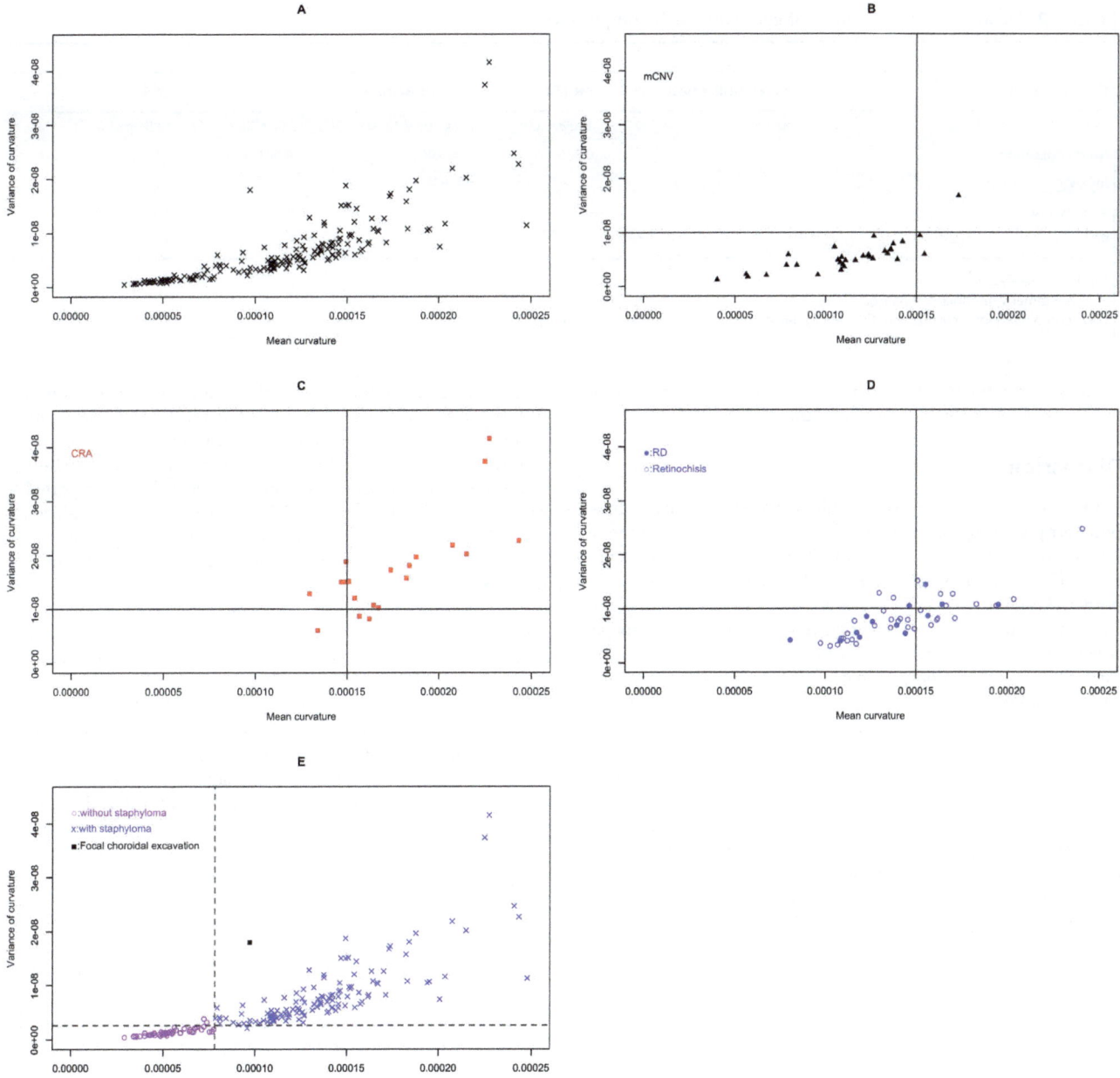

Figure 4. Scatter plot assigning mean curvature to the horizontal axis and variance of curvature to the vertical axis. A, All 182 highly myopic eyes are plotted. **B,** 33 eyes with myopic choroidal neovascularization (mCNV) are highlighted. Most values localize to the lower segment of the splitting line at 0.00015 for mean curvature and 1×10^{-8} for variance of curvature. **C,** 17 eyes with severe chorioretinal atrophy (CRA) are highlighted. Most of these values localize to the higher segment of the splitting line. **D,** 33 eyes with retinoschisis (open circles) and 11 eyes with foveal retinal detachments (filled circles) are plotted. **E,** Eyes with and without staphylomas. The groups are easily separated into 2 groups by broken lines that indicate 0.000078 in mean curvature and 0.26×10^{-8} in curvature variance. One eye without a staphyloma had focal choroidal excavation (square).

Characteristics of fundus curvature in eyes with staphylomas

Of the 182 eyes evaluated, 129 eyes were judged to have staphylomas, while 52 eyes were not. One eye without staphyloma had focal choroidal excavation, which was visualized clearly as a red spot on the color map. When the eye with focal choroidal excavation was excluded from the analysis, the highly myopic patients with staphylomas were found to be older than those without. There were also more women than men with staphylo-

mas (Table 4). Furthermore, eyes with staphylomas had significantly greater axial length, mean curvature, and variance of curvature. Figure 4E shows the distribution of eyes with staphylomas vs. those without in the scatter plot of mean curvature and variance of curvature. When we drew a watershed line at 7.8×10^{-5} for mean curvature and 0.26×10^{-8} for variance of curvature, 98.4% of eyes with staphyloma were distributed in areas of the plot corresponding to greater curvature and greater

Table 2. Mean absolute curvature of eyes with each complication.

Complication	No complications	mCNV	Retinoschisis	RD	CRA
value (x10^5: mean ± SD)	8.61±4.27	11.27±3.01	14.39±3.17	13.64±2.89	17.54±3.28
No complications	-	0.005	<0.001	<0.001	<0.001
mCNV	-	-	0.006	0.29	<0.001
Retinoschisis	-	-	-	0.97	0.02
RD	-	-	-	-	0.03

P-values* are shown.
*Tukey-Kramer's multiple comparison.
CNV: choroidal neovascularization, RD: retinal detachment, CRA: chorioretinal atrophy.

variance, while 96.2% of eyes without staphylomas aggregated to the zones of low curvature and low variance.

Discussion

In the current study, we successfully visualized the shape of the posterior pole by using a novel method to analyze the curvature of 12 lines of 9-mm radial OCT scans. The color map of curvature effectively localized the staphyloma itself as well as the surrounding border. Furthermore, mean curvature and variance of curvature calculations were used to quantitatively evaluate fundus shape, which revealed associations between myopic complications and fundus shape. Our findings suggest that mean curvature and variance of curvature values could be used to define staphylomas and quantitatively evaluate staphylomas.

At present, the process of mCNV development has not been fully elucidated. Lacquer cracks and CRA often lead to mCNV in highly myopic eyes. [23] Curtin and Karlin showed that axial length was associated with the development of lacquer cracks and CRA in high myopia. [24] They also showed that the development of mCNV was not dependent on increases in axial length. Our study also showed that axial length did not differ significantly between highly myopic eyes with mCNV and highly myopic eyes without myopic complications.

The analysis of posterior fundus shape could provide valuable insights for mCNV development. Our findings suggest that mCNV develops in eyes with moderate curvature without undulation. Considering that mCNV was observed in eyes with staphyloma as well as in eyes without staphyloma, the presence of a staphyloma itself was not able to predict the development of mCNV in this study. Previous reports on the relationship between staphyloma and the development of mCNV were inconsistent. Although 2 reports graded staphyloma using B-scan ultrasono-

graphic images, one study reported that the prevalence of mCNV was not associated with staphyloma grade, [13] while another reported that mCNV development was inversely correlated with staphyloma severity. [25] In contrast to these reports using B-scan ultrasonographic images, a study using OCT images reported a direct correlation between mCNV development and staphyloma severity. [18] Quantitative evaluations of the entire posterior pole should elucidate the relationship between eye shape and mCNV development.

In contrast to eyes with mCNV, eyes with severe CRA tended to have severe staphylomas with undulated surfaces. Considering that patchy and diffuse CRA are reported to predispose the patient to the development of mCNV [23,26] while CRA also develops in the area proximal to regressed mCNV, [27,28] it might be expected that eyes with mCNV and eyes with CRA would exhibit similar shape. The observed differences in mean curvature and variance of curvature could be explained by the fact that severe CRA can develop after the inactivation of mCNV, causing concave deformation in the posterior pole [29]. The imaging strategy outlined in this study could be used to capture such temporal changes in fundus shape. The evaluation of time-course changes in fundus shape and the association with mCNV and CRA development might elucidate a causal relationship between mCNV and CRA. Such analysis might also identify factors that can be used to predict progression from mCNV to CRA, or vice versa.

The present study could not detect significant differences in fundus shape between eyes with retinoschisis and eyes with RD. The number of eyes with retinoschisis or RD may not have been sufficient for statistical evaluation. Since RD in highly myopic eyes are reported to originate from retinoschisis [30] while retinoschisis does not always lead to RD, the ability to predict RD development from retinoschisis could prevent severe visual loss in highly myopic

Table 3. Mean variance of curvature for eyes with each complication.

Complication	No complications	mCNV	Retinoschisis	RD	CRA
value (x10^9: mean ± SD)	3.37±3.08	5.53±2.87	8.42±4.29	7.87±3.15	17.40±8.88
No complications	-	0.10	<0.001	0.004	<0.001
mCNV	-	-	0.047	0.45	<0.001
Retinoschisis	-	-	-	0.99	<0.001
RD	-	-	-	-	<0.001

P-values* are shown.
*Tukey-Kramer's multiple comparison.
CNV: choroidal neovascularization, RD: retinal detachment, CRA: chorioretinal atrophy.

Table 4. Characteristics of the included eyes according to the presence of staphylomas.

Variable	without staphyloma	with staphyloma	P-value*
n	52	129	
Age (years ± SD)	49.4±12.5	65.7±12.1	<0.01
Sex (male:female)	29:23	33:96	<0.01[†]
Axial length (mm ± SD)	27.34±1.08	29.24±1.66	<0.01
Mean absolute curvature (x10^5: mean ± SD)	5.36±1.24	13.71±3.50	<0.01
Variance of curvature (x10^9: mean ± SD)	1.35±0.65	8.26±6.03	<0.01

*unpaired t-test.
[†]Fisher's exact test.

eyes. Currently, factors such as age, refractive error, axial length, staphyloma, CRA, and vitreoretinal interface quality are hypothesized to play a role in progression from retinoschisis to RD, [31,32] but the mechanisms involved have not been thoroughly elucidated. Further quantitative study of fundus shape might elucidate mechanisms of the progression form retinoschisis to RD.

Our methodology also allows for the quantification of staphyloma severity. Using the technology described here, staphylomas could be graded objectively on the basis of mean curvature and variance of curvature. Furthermore, our method might be able to distinguish eyes with staphyloma and eyes without staphyloma by the numerical values of mean curvature and variance of curvature. We may be able to define staphyloma by cut-off value of such parameters as well as high myopia by spherical equivalents of ≤ − 5D, ≤ −6D, or ≤ −8D, or axial length of ≥26.0 mm, ≥26.5 mm, or ≥28.0 mm. Similarly, mean curvature and variance of curvature could objectively define staphyloma, and further study should verify the value of mean curvature as $>7.8 \times 10^{-5}$ and the mean variance of curvature as $>0.26 \times 10^{-8}$ used in this study. Currently, staphylomas are usually graded in a subjective manner based on slit-lamp biomicroscopy. [12] Our method with wider OCT could be used to elaborate a standardized system for objective staphyloma classification.

This study has certain limitations. One is a segmentation problem. The auto-segmentation used for this research is accurate when studying the normal eye but not as well when studying highly myopic eyes, because the OCT images obtained in the latter case are often of poor quality. Manual segmentation support was therefore used in such cases presented here. The second issue involves scan width. The 9-mm scan width employed for this study is actually wider than that used in previous studies. However, it was not sufficiently wide to include the entire staphyloma border in all cases. We could detect the entire staphyloma edge only in 4 eyes out of 129 eyes with staphyloma. Third, this study utilized a cross-sectional study design using case series, which precluded causational analysis. Future studies should measure changes in curvature and variance over time. Associations between myopic complications and posterior fundus curvature should be further

examined in high myopic patients without subjective complaint or myopic but not highly myopic eyes. Fourth, in a strict sense, the lines we plotted may not simply be attributed to Bruch's membrane line. Although fourth hyperreflective line in OCT is generally recognized as retinal pigment epithelium and the line we plotted as Bruch's membrane, [33,34] Spaide and Curcio discussed that the origin of the fourth hyperreflective line in OCT remained to be determined. [35] Lastly, the current study is evaluating the curvature of OCT images, not the true curvature of the eyeball. As being reported by Kuo et al., [36] the OCT images were more flattened than MRI images. Indeed, as shown in the Supplemental Note, Bruch's membrane line in OCT becomes considerably steeper after correction. However, since we evaluated the local curvature by every 1,000-μm distance rather than by eye shape as a whole, the curvature map did not notably change after correction (Details are shown in Supplemental Note). For the clinical setting, evaluating OCT images is more practical than evaluating true eye shape, from the viewpoint of accessibility. Considering the minor effect of correction to the local curvature evaluation, it would be more helpful for ophthalmologist to use the OCT image without correction.

Despite these limitations, this novel quantitative approach allowed us to correlate fundus shape and myopic complications. Furthermore, we demonstrated how these maps could be used to evaluate fundus shape. The ability to evaluate staphylomas quantitatively will facilitate investigations into the associations between myopic complications and staphylomas.

Acknowledgments

I am very grateful to Yoshihiko Iwase for his valuable cooperation in developing software.

Author Contributions

Conceived and designed the experiments: MM KY. Performed the experiments: MM. Analyzed the data: MM. Contributed reagents/materials/analysis tools: KY YAK AO AT MH NY. Wrote the paper: MM KY.

References

1. Kempen JH, Mitchell P, Lee KE, Tielsch JM, Broman AT, et al. (2004) The prevalence of refractive errors among adults in the United States, Western Europe, and Australia. Arch Ophthalmol 122: 495–505.
2. Saw SM (2003) A synopsis of the prevalence rates and environmental risk factors for myopia. Clin Exp Optom 86: 289–294.
3. Sawada A, Tomidokoro A, Araie M, Iwase A, Yamamoto T (2008) Refractive errors in an elderly Japanese population: the Tajimi study. Ophthalmology 115: 363–370 e363.
4. Wong TY, Foster PJ, Johnson GJ, Seah SK (2002) Education, socioeconomic status, and ocular dimensions in Chinese adults: the Tanjong Pagar Survey. Br J Ophthalmol 86: 963–968.
5. Jacobi FK, Zrenner E, Broghammer M, Pusch CM (2005) A genetic perspective on myopia. Cellular and molecular life sciences: CMLS 62: 800–808.
6. Chang L, Pan CW, Ohno-Matsui K, Lin X, Cheung GC, et al. (2013) Myopia-related fundus changes in Singapore adults with high myopia. Am J Ophthalmol 155: 991–999 e991.

7. Pan CW, Zheng YF, Anuar AR, Chew M, Gazzard G, et al. (2013) Prevalence of refractive errors in a multiethnic Asian population: the Singapore epidemiology of eye disease study. Invest Ophthalmol Vis Sci 54: 2590–2598.

8. Ohno-Matsui K, Akiba M, Modegi T, Tomita M, Ishibashi T, et al. (2012) Association between shape of sclera and myopic retinochoroidal lesions in patients with pathologic myopia. Invest Ophthalmol Vis Sci 53: 6046–6061.

9. Miyake M, Yamashiro K, Akagi-Kurashige Y, Kumagai K, Nakata I, et al. (2013) Vascular Endothelial Growth Factor Gene and the Response to Anti-Vascular Endothelial Growth Factor Treatment for Choroidal Neovascularization in High Myopia. Ophthalmology.

10. Khor CC, Miyake M, Chen LJ, Shi Y, Barathi VA, et al. (2013) Genome-wide association study identifies ZFHX1B as a susceptibility locus for severe myopia. Hum Mol Genet 22: 5288–5294.

11. Miyake M, Yamashiro K, Nakanishi H, Nakata I, Akagi-Kurashige Y, et al. (2013) Evaluation of pigment epithelium-derived factor and complement factor I polymorphisms as a cause of choroidal neovascularization in highly myopic eyes. Invest Ophthalmol Vis Sci 54: 4208–4212.

12. Curtin BJ (1977) The posterior staphyloma of pathologic myopia. Trans Am Ophthalmol Soc 75: 67–86.

13. Hsiang HW, Ohno-Matsui K, Shimada N, Hayashi K, Moriyama M, et al. (2008) Clinical characteristics of posterior staphyloma in eyes with pathologic myopia. Am J Ophthalmol 146: 102–110.

14. Moriyama M, Ohno-Matsui K, Hayashi K, Shimada N, Yoshida T, et al. (2011) Topographic analyses of shape of eyes with pathologic myopia by high-resolution three-dimensional magnetic resonance imaging. Ophthalmology 118: 1626–1637.

15. Cheng HM, Singh OS, Kwong KK, Xiong J, Woods BT, et al. (1992) Shape of the myopic eye as seen with high-resolution magnetic resonance imaging. Optom Vis Sci 69: 698–701.

16. Atchison DA, Pritchard N, Schmid KL, Scott DH, Jones CE, et al. (2005) Shape of the retinal surface in emmetropia and myopia. Invest Ophthalmol Vis Sci 46: 2698–2707.

17. van Velthoven ME, Faber DJ, Verbraak FD, van Leeuwen TG, de Smet MD (2007) Recent developments in optical coherence tomography for imaging the retina. Prog Retin Eye Res 26: 57–77.

18. Ikuno Y, Jo Y, Hamasaki T, Tano Y (2010) Ocular risk factors for choroidal neovascularization in pathologic myopia. Invest Ophthalmol Vis Sci 51: 3721–3725.

19. Chae JB, Moon BG, Yang SJ, Lee JY, Yoon YH, et al. (2011) Macular gradient measurement in myopic posterior staphyloma using optical coherence tomography. Korean journal of ophthalmology: KJO 25: 243–247.

20. Szkulmowski M, Wojtkowski M, Sikorski B, Bajraszewski T, Srinivasan VJ, et al. (2007) Analysis of posterior retinal layers in spectral optical coherence tomography images of the normal retina and retinal pathologies. J Biomed Opt 12: 041207.

21. Kaluzny JJ, Wojtkowski M, Sikorski BL, Szkulmowski M, Szkulmowska A, et al. (2009) Analysis of the outer retina reconstructed by high-resolution, three-dimensional spectral domain optical coherence tomography. Ophthalmic Surg Lasers Imaging 40: 102–108.

22. Kass M, Witkin A, Terzopoulos D (1988) Snakes: Active contour models. Int J Comput Vision 1: 321–331.

23. Hayashi K, Ohno-Matsui K, Shimada N, Moriyama M, Kojima A, et al. (2010) Long-term pattern of progression of myopic maculopathy: a natural history study. Ophthalmology 117: 1595–1611, 1611 e1591–1594.

24. Curtin BJ, Karlin DB (1971) Axial length measurements and fundus changes of the myopic eye. Am J Ophthalmol 71: 42–53.

25. Steidl SM, Pruett RC (1997) Macular complications associated with posterior staphyloma. Am J Ophthalmol 123: 181–187.

26. Ohno-Matsui K, Yoshida T, Futagami S, Yasuzumi K, Shimada N, et al. (2003) Patchy atrophy and lacquer cracks predispose to the development of choroidal neovascularisation in pathological myopia. Br J Ophthalmol 87: 570–573.

27. Yoshida T, Ohno-Matsui K, Yasuzumi K, Kojima A, Shimada N, et al. (2003) Myopic choroidal neovascularization: a 10-year follow-up. Ophthalmology 110: 1297–1305.

28. Kojima A, Ohno-Matsui K, Teramukai S, Yoshida T, Ishihara Y, et al. (2004) Factors associated with the development of chorioretinal atrophy around choroidal neovascularization in pathologic myopia. Graefe's archive for clinical and experimental ophthalmology = Albrecht von Graefes Archiv fur klinische und experimentelle Ophthalmologie 242: 114–119.

29. Teramura T (1993) [The shape of posterior staphyloma in high myopia]. Nippon Ganka Gakkai Zasshi 97: 873–880.

30. Shimada N, Ohno-Matsui K, Yoshida T, Sugamoto Y, Tokoro T, et al. (2008) Progression from macular retinoschisis to retinal detachment in highly myopic eyes is associated with outer lamellar hole formation. Br J Ophthalmol 92: 762–764.

31. Morita H, Ideta H, Ito K, Yonemoto J, Sasaki K, et al. (1991) Causative factors of retinal detachment in macular holes. Retina 11: 281–284.

32. Wu PC, Chen YJ, Chen YH, Chen CH, Shin SJ, et al. (2009) Factors associated with foveoschisis and foveal detachment without macular hole in high myopia. Eye 23: 356–361.

33. Farsiu S, Chiu SJ, O'Connell RV, Folgar FA, Yuan E, et al. (2013) Quantitative Classification of Eyes with and without Intermediate Age-related Macular Degeneration Using Optical Coherence Tomography. Ophthalmology.

34. Chiu SJ, Izatt JA, O'Connell RV, Winter KP, Toth CA, et al. (2012) Validated automatic segmentation of AMD pathology including drusen and geographic atrophy in SD-OCT images. Invest Ophthalmol Vis Sci 53: 53–61.

35. Spaide RF, Curcio CA (2011) Anatomical correlates to the bands seen in the outer retina by optical coherence tomography: literature review and model. Retina 31: 1609–1619.

36. Kuo AN, McNabb RP, Chiu SJ, El-Dairi MA, Farsiu S, et al. (2013) Correction of ocular shape in retinal optical coherence tomography and effect on current clinical measures. Am J Ophthalmol 156: 304–311.

13

Dual-Phase CT Collateral Score: A Predictor of Clinical Outcome in Patients with Acute Ischemic Stroke

Na-Young Shin[1], Kyung-eun Kim[1], Mina Park[1], Young Dae Kim[2], Dong Joon Kim[1], Sung Jun Ahn[1], Ji Hoe Heo[2], Seung-Koo Lee[1]*

1 Department of Radiology, Severance Hospital, Yonsei University College of Medicine, Seoul, Korea, **2** Department of Neurology, Severance Hospital, Yonsei University College of Medicine, Seoul, Korea

Abstract

Background and Purpose: The presence of good collaterals on CT angiography (CTA) is a well-known predictor for favorable outcome in acute ischemic stroke. Recently, multiphase CT has been introduced as a more accurate method in assessing collaterals. The aim of this study was to assess the ability of dual-phase CT to evaluate collateral status and predict clinical outcome.

Methods: Forty-three patients who underwent both dual-phase CT and transfemoral cerebral angiography (TFCA) for occluded intracranial internal carotid artery (ICA) and/or middle cerebral artery (M1 segment) were recruited from a prospectively collected database. The collateral status on dual-phase CT was graded by using a 4-point scale: grade 0 = no collaterals; 1 = some collaterals with persistence of some defects; 2 = slow but complete collaterals; and 3 = fast and complete collaterals. Univariate and multivariate analysis were performed to define the independent predictors for favorable outcome at 3 months.

Results: Dual-phase CT collateral status ($\rho = 0.744$) showed higher correlation with TFCA collateral status than CTA collateral status ($\rho = 0.596$) and substantial interobserver agreement (weighted $\kappa = 0.776$). In the univariate analysis, age, history of hypertension, collateral scores on CTA, dual-phase CT, and TFCA, occlusion in intracranial ICA, final infarct volume, and symptomatic hemorrhage were significantly associated with outcome. Among them, only the dual-phase CT collateral score was an independent predictor for favorable outcome (OR = 26.342 (2.788–248.864); $P = 0.004$) in the multivariate analysis.

Conclusions: The collateral status on dual-phase CT can be a useful predictor for clinical outcome in acute stroke patients, especially when advanced CT techniques are not available in emergent situations.

Editor: Jean-Claude Baron, INSERM U894, Centre de Psychiatrie et Neurosciences, Hopital Sainte-Anne and Université Paris 5, France

Funding: These authors have no support or funding to report.

Competing Interests: The authors have declared that no competing interests exist.

* Email: slee@yuhs.ac

Introduction

The presence of good collateral circulation to the ischemic territory is a notable predictor for favorable long term clinical outcome as well as small infarct size and good response to treatment in patients with proximal intracranial arterial occlusion [1–6]. These beneficial roles may be attributable to preserve downstream perfusion distal to occluded vessels, to permit access of thrombolytic materials to the distal end of the clot by retrograde flow, and to augment washout of emboli in distal arteries [7–9].

Transfemoral cerebral angiography (TFCA) has been considered as a gold standard to assess collateral status owing to its temporal and spatial resolution. However, global evaluation of pial collateral flow requires catheterization of multiple vessels and, as an invasive investigation with recognized complication rate, is usually only performed when IA treatment is indicated. To aid selection of treatment strategy or to prognosticate, a method of collateral assessment for all stroke patients, not just for those undergoing intra-arterial therapy is warranted. Furthermore, accurate non-invasive assessment of collateral status prior to endovascular therapy would also be advantageous. Therefore, noninvasive assessment of collateral status before IA treatment or in patients who are not candidates for IA treatment may be helpful to select the treatment strategy and predict long term outcome.

Because of short scan times and easy accessibility, computed tomography (CT) is used as the first imaging modality in most patients with acute ischemic stroke. Diverse collateral scoring methods have been suggested in the last decades using CT angiography source images (CTA-SI) [4,5,7,10–14] and CTA maximum intensity projection (MIP) images [6,12,15,16]. Although there is no standard scoring system, CTA allows prediction of clinical outcome with moderate to excellent interobserver agreement [11–13,16,17]. To overcome limitations of CTA such

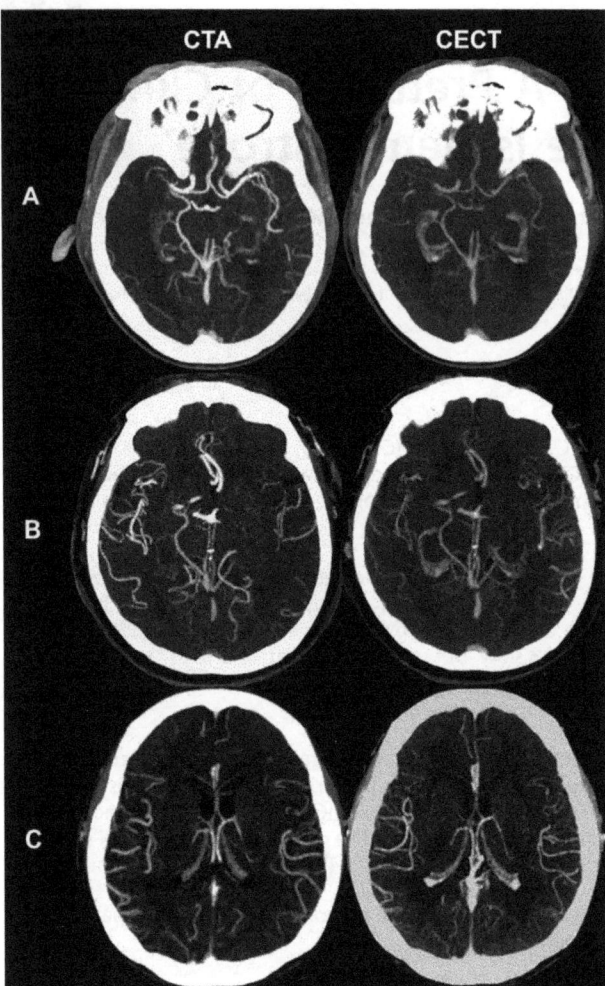

Figure 1. Representative images of collateral status on dual-phase CT. A, Some collaterals to the right MCA territory on CTA with persistence of some defects on CECT (Grade 1). B, Collaterals in part of the left MCA territory on CTA with complete filling on CECT (Grade 2). The collaterals show lower attenuation on CTA with equal to higher attenuation on CECT than unaffected vessels, suggesting slow inflow and washout of collaterals. C, Collaterals in the entire right MCA territory on both CTA and delayed CECT (Grade 3). The collateral vessels show attenuation similar to unaffected vessels on both phase images, suggesting fast velocity of collaterals.

as absence of temporal information from single phase acquisition and possible underestimation of collateral status from faster image acquisition, multi- [18,19] or tri-phase CT [20] and perfusion CT [3,21] have been proposed for assessing collateral status. At our institution, the routine CT protocol consists of noncontrast CT (NCCT), CTA, and delayed contrast enhanced CT (CECT). We empirically found that dual-phase CT composed of CTA and delayed CECT is helpful for predicting clinical outcome in patients with acute stroke. Therefore, the aim of this study was to assess the ability of dual-phase CT to evaluate collateral status and predict clinical outcome.

Materials and Methods

Patients

The patients were retrospectively selected from a prospectively collected neurointerventional database in a single institution. From

February 2011 to June 2013, we recruited consecutive patients who underwent TFCA for possible thrombolysis/mechanical thrombectomy for acute ischemic stroke and met the following inclusion criteria: (1) occlusion of the intracranial ICA or M1 segment; (2) time from symptom onset to admission <6 hours; and (3) presence of a standard local CT protocol including NCCT, CTA, and delayed CECT. Exclusion criteria included bilateral anterior circulation occlusion, posterior circulation occlusion, significant stenosis in contralateral anterior circulation, and past history of stroke.

Clinical data were collected from a prospectively recorded stroke registry database. Type of stroke etiology was classified using Trial of Org 10172 in Acute Stroke Treatment (TOAST) criteria [22]. Functional outcome was assessed using the modified Rankin Scale score (mRS) at 3 months and classified as favorable (≤2) and unfavorable (>2). This study was approved by Severance hospital Institutional Review Board. The Clinical Research Ethics Committee waived the need for written informed consent from the participants because the data released from the hospital database were analyzed anonymously.

Image Acquisition

CT images were obtained on a 64 multi-detector row CT system (Sensation 64; Siemens, Erlangen, Germany). The sequential axial 3-mm NCCT was performed first with the following parameters from the skull base to the vertex: 120 kVp, 300 mAs, field of view (FOV) of 25 cm, feed/rotation 18 mm, 30×0.6 mm collimation and a H30s medium reconstruction kernel. Each of the conventional axial CT images was subsequently reconstructed into 1.2 mm slices and 1.2 mm increments. A nonionic contrast agent was administered followed by a 40 ml saline chaser at a rate of 4 ml/s by using a power injector. A bolus tracking technique was used with a marker placed at the ascending aorta, triggering at 100 Hounsfield Units (HU) above baseline with a 7 s delay prior to image acquisition. CTA from the aortic arch to the vertex was performed with the following parameters: 120 kVp, 160 mA, FOV of 18–20 cm, 0.33 s per rotation, 0.8 pitch, and a 0.6-mm section thickness. Delayed CECT was performed with the same parameters as NCCT 40 s after contrast injection. The effective dose which was calculated by the CTDI volume x the scan range x the conversion factor was 1.8 mSv for NCCT and CECT, respectively, 0.9 mSv for the cranial portion of CTA, and 3.0 mSv for the cervical portion of CTA. Therefore the total effective dose was 5.7mSv.

TFCA was performed using biplane digital subtraction angiograms (Allura Xper FD20/20; Philips Healthcare, Best, Netherlands) in all patients for the purpose of IA thrombolysis/thrombectomy via bilateral ICAs and the dominant vertebral artery.

Routine follow-up MRI was obtained 1 day after the onset of symptoms with the 3-Tesla MR system (Achieva; Philips Healthcare, Best, Netherlands). DWI was performed with single shot echo planar imaging and parameters were as follows: b-value 1000 s/mm2, TR/TE 6500–7000/65–78 ms, slice thickness 3 mm, FOV 230 mm, matrix 128×128, and NEX 1.

Image Analysis

Imaging studies at admission. *CT:* The extent of ischemic lesions on NCCT scan images at admission was rated according to the Alberta Stroke Programme Early CT Score (ASPECTS) [23].

Collaterals on dual-phase CT were graded on CTA and delayed CECT axial MIP images by using a 4-point scale [19]: Grade 0 = no collaterals to the occluded arterial territory; 1 = some collaterals to the occluded arterial territory with persistence of

Table 1. Demographic characteristics according to dual-phase collateral status.

	Collateral status on dual-phase CT				
	Incomplete (G1) (n = 10)	Slow-complete (G2) (n = 23)	Rapid-complete (G3) (n = 10)	P value	Post-hoc analysis
Age, y, mean ± SD	75.9±6.8	70.1±10.7	61.1±11.4	0.010*	G1>G3 (P = 0.008)
Sex, n, M:F	4:3	13:10	6:4	0.974‡	
Risk factors					
Hypertension, n (%)	9 (90.0)	14 (60.9)	1 (10.0)	0.001‡	G1>G3 (P = 0.002)
Diabetes, n (%)	4 (40.0)	5 (21.7)	0 (0.0)	0.109‡	
Hypercholesterolemia, n (%)	3 (30.0)	2 (8.7)	0 (0.0)	0.147‡	
Smoking, n (%)	6 (60.0)	8 (34.8)	6 (60.0)	0.302‡	
Coronary artery disease, n (%)	3 (30.0)	10 (43.5)	3 (30.0)	0.763‡	
Clinical measures at presentation					
SBP, mmHg, median (IQR)	134.0 (111.0–161.0)	135.0 (120.0–146.5)	138.5 (112.0–149.0)	0.947†	
DBP, mmHg, mean ± SD	78.5 mmHg	76.3 mmHg	74.9 mmHg	0.680*	
Glucose, mmol/L, median (IQR)	7.25 (6.9–8.6)	6.7 (5.7–8.3)	7.1 (5.9–8.9)	0.490†	
NIHSS score, median (IQR)	16.5 (12.0–19.0)	17.0 (14.3–19.0)	14.0 (13.0–19.0)	0.210†	
TOAST classification				0.015‡	
Large artery, n (%)	1 (10.0)	2 (8.7)	6 (60.0)		
Cardioembolic, n (%)	7 (70.0)	14 (60.9)	4 (40.0)		
Undetermined, n (%)	2 (20.0)	7 (30.4)	0 (0.0)		
CT					
Time from symptom onset to CT, min, mean ± SD	170.9±106.6	209.0±91.1	170.0±87.1	0.415*	
ASPECTS, mean ± SD	6.3±1.8	7.6±1.2	8.5±1.0	0.002*	G1<G2 (P = 0.038), G1<G3 (P = 0.002)
Occluded segment					
Intracranial ICA, n (%)	5 (50.0)	4 (17.4)	0 (0.0)	0.018‡	
Proximal M1, n (%)	7 (70.0)	16 (69.6)	7 (70.0)	1.000‡	
Distal M1, n (%)	8 (80.0)	20 (87.0)	8 (80.0)	0.753‡	
Thrombus length, mm, median (IQR)	19.3 (11.9–25.5)	15.8 (8.6–18.5)	11.0 (7.3–18.8)	0.298†	
IV tPA					
IV tPA, n (%)	5 (50.0)	11 (47.8)	8 (80.0)	0.275.	
Time from symptom onset to IV tPA, min, mean ± SD	77.8±20.6	108.6±41.4	91.4±38.2	0.301*	
TFCA					
TICI ≥ 2b, n (%)	5 (50.0)	5 (21.7)	2 (20.0)	0.264	
Time from symptom onset to recanalization	385.3±198.2	375.3±106.3	304.0±103.0	0.447	
Outcome					
Final infarct volume, ml, median (IQR)	91.1 (49.1–183.2)	25.0 (10.3–76.7)	12.3 (7.5–27.8)	0.047	G1>G2 (P = 0.012), G1>G3 (P = 0.021)
Symptomatic hemorrhage	3 (30.0)	3 (13.0)	1 (10.0)	0.537	
parenchymal hematoma	5 (50.0)	4 (17.4)	2 (20.0)	0.199	
3m-mRS ≤ 2	0 (0.0)	14 (60.9)	9 (90.0)	<0.001	G1<G2 (P = 0.003), G1<G3 (P<0.001)

ASPECTS indicates Alberta Stroke Program Early CT Score; DBP, diastolic blood pressure; IQR, Interquatile range; mRS, modified Rankin Score; NIHSS, National Institutes of Health Stroke Scale; SBP indicates systolic blood pressure; TICI, thrombolysis in cerebral infarction; TOAST, Trial of Org 10172 in Acute Stroke Treatment; and tPA, tissue plasminogen activator.
* one-way ANOVA; † Kruskal Wallis test; ‡ Fisher's exact test

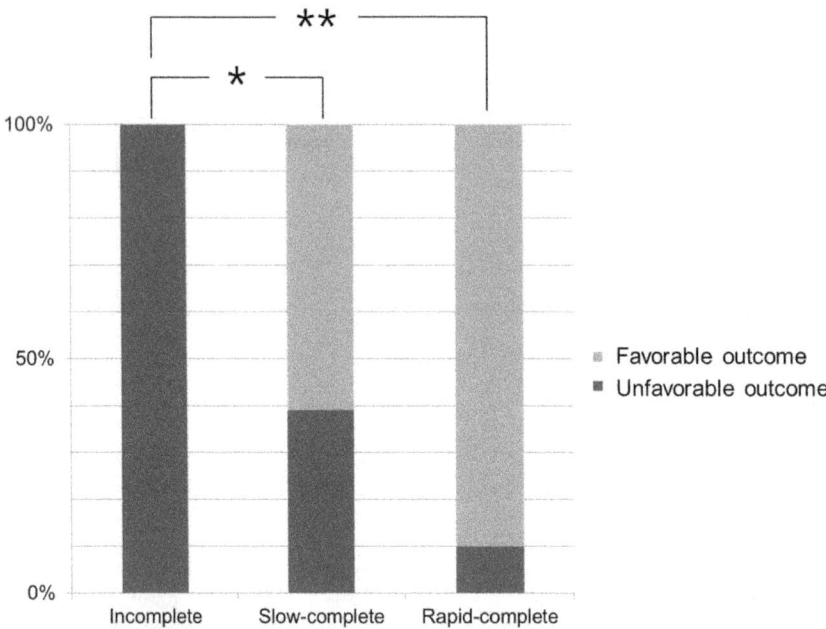

Figure 2. Clinical outcome according to collateral status. All patients with incomplete collaterals showed unfavorable outcome at 3 months. Patients with complete collaterals had favorable clinical outcome more frequently than did patients with incomplete collaterals. * $P = 0.003$; ** $P < 0.001$

some defects; 2 = slow but complete collaterals (detectable only on delayed CECT) without defects; and 3 = fast and complete collaterals (detectable on both CTA and delayed CECT; Figure 1). Collateral vessel scores were assessed on CTA-SI images using a scale of 0–3: 0 = absence of collateral supply to the occluded vascular territory; 1 = collateral supply filling <50% but >0% of the occluded vascular territory; 2 = collateral supply filling >50% but <100% of the occluded vascular territory; and 3 = collateral supply filling 100% of the occluded vascular territory [6]. The collateral scores on both dual-phase CT and CTA were evaluated independently by two neuroradiologist (N.Y.S. with 4 years of experience and M.P. with 1 year of experience) blinded to the clinical data. Disagreements were settled by consensus.

Occluded segments were recorded based on the location of the non-enhanced segment on delayed CECT as follows [24]: intracranial ICA; proximal M1 segment = occlusion at or proximal to the lenticulostriate arteries; and distal M1 segment = occlusion distal to the lenticulostriate arteries before MCA genu. The thrombus length was measured quantitatively on CECT curved multiplanar reformatted (MPR) images by a neuroimaging fellow (K.E.K. with 1 year of experience) blinded to the clinical data.

TFCA: The collateral flow grading system suggested by the Technology Assessment Committees of the American Society of Interventional and Therapeutic Neuroradiology and the Society of Interventional Radiology [24] was used to assess collateral vessels on TFCA: grade 0 = no collaterals to the ischemic region; 1 = slow collaterals to the periphery of the ischemic region with persistence of some defects; 2 = rapid collaterals to the periphery of the ischemic region with persistence of some defects; 3 = slow but complete collaterals to the ischemic bed by the late venous phase; and 4 = complete and rapid collaterals. The assessment of collateral flow was performed through arterial and late venous phases considering all possible collaterals from bilateral carotid and dominant vertebral angiography.

TICI score was recorded to assess recanalization using a 5-point scale [24]: 0 = no perfusion; 1 = penetration of contrast material beyond the occluded segment with minimal perfusion; 2a = partial perfusion (<2/3) of the entire vascular territory; 2b = complete but slow perfusion of the entire vascular territory; and 3 = complete perfusion and rapid clearance comparable to the uninvolved vascular territory. TICI 2b and 3 were considered recanalization.

Imaging outcome. The final infarct volume was measured on diffusion weighted images of 1-day follow-up MRI [25] using semiautomatic segmentation. The hemorrhagic transformation on follow-up CT or MRI was classified into hemorrhagic infarction or parenchymal hematoma and determined if it was symptomatic hemorrhage according to ECASS criteria [26].

Statistics

Nonparametric tests were used for non-normally distributed data. Baseline characteristics were compared according to collateral status on dual-phase CT. Continuous variables are reported as mean ± SD or as the median (interquartile range (IQR)) and were compared using one-way analysis of variance or the Kruskal-Wallis test. Categorical variables are reported as numbers (proportions, %) and were compared using the Fisher's exact test. Post hoc analysis was also performed using the Students' t-test, Mann-Whitney U test, chi-square test, or Fisher's exact test where appropriate with correction for multiple comparisons.

Spearman's rank correlation was used to assess the correlation between collateral status on dual-phase CT or CTA and collateral status on TFCA. Interobserver agreement for assessment of collateral status on CT was determined using weighted Kappa (κ) statistics [27]. The level of agreement was defined as follows: $\kappa \leq$ 0.2, poor; $0.2 < \kappa \leq 0.4$, fair; $0.4 < \kappa \leq 0.6$, moderate; $0.6 < \kappa \leq 0.8$, substantial, and $0.8 < \kappa$, good.

To test the association between various clinical and imaging characteristics including collateral status on dual-phase CT and clinical outcome, univariate logistic regression was performed.

Table 2. Univariate analysis for favorable clinical outcome (mRS ≤2) at 3 months.

	Favorable (n = 23)	Unfavorable (n = 20)	Univariate analysis		
			Odds ratio	95% CI	P value
Age, y, mean ± SD	66.1±10.2	73.4±11.0	0.934	0.874–0.997	0.040
Male, n (%)	16 (69.6)	9 (45.0)	2.794	0.800–9.760	0.107
Risk factors					
Hypertension, n (%)	9 (39.1)	15 (75.0)	0.214	0.058–0.797	0.022
Diabetes, n (%)	4 (17.4)	5 (25.0)	0.632	0.144–2.771	0.542
Hypercholesterolemia, n (%)	1 (4.3)	4 (20.0)	0.182	0.019–1.785	0.143
Smoking, n (%)	12 (52.2)	8 (40.0)	1.636	0.487–5.500	0.426
Coronary artery disease, n (%)	11 (47.8)	5 (25.0)	2.749	0.748–10.102	0.128
Clinical measures at admission					
SBP, mmHg, median (IQR)	135.0 (114.0–144.0)	140.5 (113.5–163.5)	0.980	0.956–1.005	0.114
DBP, mmHg, mean ± SD	73.5±11.0	79.9±17.3	0.967	0.924–1.013	0.157
Glucose, mmol/L, median (IQR)	6.7 (103.0–154.3)	7.25 (121.0–152.5)	1.028	0.793–1.334	0.833
NIHSS score, median (IQR)	15.0 (13.0–16.8)	18.0 (15.5–19.0)	0.873	0.747–1.020	0.088
Delays					
Time from symptom onset to IV tPA, min, mean ± SD	96.8±39.5	96.4±36.7	1.000	0.978–1.023	0.983
Time from symptom onset to CT, min, mean ± SD	198.0±95.7	183.0±93.2	1.002	0.995–1.008	0.596
Time from symptom onset to IA treatment, min, mean ± SD	268.2±107.9	259.2±113.8	1.001	0.995–1.006	0.785
TOAST classification					
Large artery, n (%)	7 (30.4)	2 (10.0)	Reference		0.286
Cardioembolic, n (%)	12 (52.2)	13 (65.0)	0.264	0.046–1.528	0.137
Undetermined, n (%)	4 (17.4)	5 (25.0)	0.229	0.029–1.774	0.158
CT					
ASPECTS, mean ± SD	8.0±0.9	6.9±1.8	1.908	1.135–3.209	0.015
CTA Collateral score	2.0 (2.0–3.0)	1.0 (1.0–2.0)	6.077	1.926–19.167	0.002
0, n (%)	0 (0.0)	0 (0.0)			
1, n (%)	4 (17.4)	14 (70.0)			
2, n (%)	12 (52.2)	5 (25.0)			
3, n (%)	7 (30.4)	1 (5.0)			
Dual-phase CT collateral score	2.4±0.5	1.6±0.6	19.436	2.581–146.371	0.004
0, n (%)	0 (0.0)	0 (0.0)			
1, n (%)	0 (0.0)	10 (50.0)			
2, n (%)	14 (60.9)	9 (45.0)			
3, n (%)	9 (39.1)	1 (5.0)			
Occluded segment					
Intracranial ICA, n (%)	2 (8.7)	7 (35.0)	0.177	0.032–0.985	0.048
Proximal M1, n (%)	14 (60.9)	16 (80.0)	0.389	0.098–1.544	0.179
Distal M1, n (%)	20 (87.0)	16 (80.0)	1.667	0.325–8.549	0.540
Thrombus length, mm, median (IQR)	11.4 (7.4–17.6)	17.9 (10.4–22.8)	0.938	0.871–1.011	0.093
Treatment					
IV tPA only, n (%)	3 (13.0)	0 (0.0)	Reference		0.639
IA only, n (%)	8 (34.8)	11 (55.0)	0.000	0.000	0.999
IV tPA and IA, n (%)	12 (52.2)	9 (45.0)	0.000	0.000	0.999
TFCA					
TFCA collateral score	3.0 (2.3–4.0)	2.0 (1.0–2.0)	3.092	1.537–6.221	0.002
0, n (%)	0 (0.0)	0 (0.0)			
1, n (%)	2 (8.7)	8 (40.0)			

Table 2. Cont.

	Favorable (n = 23)	Unfavorable (n = 20)	Univariate analysis		
			Odds ratio	95% CI	P value
2, n (%)	4 (17.4)	8 (40.0)			
3, n (%)	6 (26.1)	2 (10.0)			
4, n (%)	11 (47.8)	2 (10.0)			
TICI ≥ 2b, n (%)	4 (17.4)	8 (40.0)	0.316	0.078–1.282	0.107
Time from symptom onset to recanalization, min, mean ± SD	352.0±110.6	383.0±152.3	0.998	0.993–1.003	0.998
Imaging outcome					
Final infarct volume, ml, median (IQR)	13.7 (7.2–25.0)	80.7 (34.0–144.8)	0.965	0.943–0.988	0.003
Symptomatic hemorrhage, n (%)	1 (4.3)	6 (30.0)	0.106	0.012–0.977	0.048
Parenchymal hematoma, n (%)	3 (13.0)	8 (40.0)	0.225	0.050–1.016	0.052

ASPECTS indicates Alberta Stroke Program Early CT Score; DBP, diastolic blood pressure; IQR, Interquatile range; mRS, modified Rankin Score; NIHSS, National Institutes of Health Stroke Scale; SBP indicates systolic blood pressure; TFCA, transfemoral cerebral angiography; TICI, thrombolysis in cerebral infarction; TOAST, Trial of Org 10172 in Acute Stroke Treatment; and tPA, tissue plasminogen activator.

Multivariate logistic regression with backward elimination (probability value for elimination of 0.1) was used to identify independent factors for favorable outcome. Variables significantly associated with a favorable outcome in the univariate analysis ($P <$ 0.05) were included in the multivariable model. To assess independent predictors before IA treatment, multivariate analysis with clinical and CT variables was also performed. Receiver operating curve (ROC) comparison was performed to compare the prediction ability of models containing either dual-phase CT collateral (model 1), CTA collateral (model 2), or TFCA collateral (model 3) scores.

All statistical analyses were performed using SAS, version 9.2 (SAS Institute, Cary, NC, USA) and SPSS, version 19 software (IBM Corp., Armonk, NY, USA). ROC curve comparison was performed by using MedCalc, Version 9.3.9.0 software (MedCalc software, Mariakerke, Belgium). P values less than 0.05 were considered statistically significant.

Results

Among 166 patients who underwent TFCA for possible thrombolysis/mechanical thrombectomy for acute ischemic stroke, 123 patients were excluded due to posterior circulation occlusion (n = 34), anterior cerebral arterial occlusion (n = 4), occlusion distal to the M1 segment (n = 41), proximal ICA occlusion only (n = 12), old territorial infarcts (n = 8), multiple territorial infarcts due to cardioembolism (n = 2), significant stenosis in the contralateral M1 segment (n = 1), moyamoya disease (n = 1), and only NCCT acquisition (n = 20). Therefore, a total of 43 patients were recruited for this study. The patients underwent IA treatment with stent-assisted thrombectomy (SAT; n = 29), Penumbra system (n = 1), both SAT and Penumbra system (n = 4), stent placement after mechanical thrombectomy (n = 4), Penumbra system with urokinase infusion (n = 2), and urokinase infusion only (n = 1).

Patient demographic and clinical data according to collateral status on dual-phase CT are summarized in Table 1. Ten (23.3%) patients were grouped as grade 1 (incomplete collaterals); 23 (53.5%) as grade 2 (slow-complete collaterals); and 10 (23.3%) as grade 3 (rapid-complete collaterals). No patients were classified as grade 0 (no collaterals). There was no statistical difference in the time from symptom onset to CT scan between there groups

($P = 0.415$). Patients with incomplete collaterals were older than those with rapid-complete collaterals ($P = 0.008$). Patients with less collaterals had hypertension more often, although other cardiovascular risk factors did not show differences in the prevalence across different collateral patterns. The pattern of leptomeningeal collaterals on dual-phase CT was also associated with the TOAST classification of stroke: cardioembolic infarcts were observed more often in patients with less collaterals than those with large arterial infarcts. Less collaterals were associated with lower ASPECTS on NCCT ($P = 0.002$) and the presence of intracranial ICA occlusion ($P = 0.018$). Final infarct volume was significantly larger in patients with incomplete collaterals (91.1 (IQR, 49.1–183.2) ml) than that in patients with slow-complete (25.0 (IQR, 10.3–76.7) ml) and rapid-complete (12.3 (IQR, 7.5–27.8) ml) collaterals on dual-phase CT ($P = 0.012$ and $P = 0.021$, respectively). Clinical outcome was also more favorable in patients with complete collateral patterns (Figure 2). However, there was no significant difference in recanalization rate or hemorrhagic transformation according to collateral pattern.

The dual-phase collateral scores showed higher correlation with collateral status on TFCA ($\rho = 0.744$; $P<0.001$) than that of the CTA collateral scores ($\rho = 0.596$; $P<0.001$). Interobserver agreement for the collateral scoring on dual-phase CT [weighted $\kappa = 0.776$ (0.619–0.933)] was substantial and better than that on CTA [weighted $\kappa = 0.475$ (0.285–0.665)].

Univariate analysis of patients with good and poor clinical outcome is presented in Table 2. Younger age ($P = 0.040$), absence of history of hypertension ($P = 0.022$), higher collateral scores on CTA ($P = 0.002$), dual-phase CT ($P = 0.004$), and TFCA ($P = 0.002$), absence of occlusion in intracranial ICA ($P = 0.048$), smaller final infarct volume ($P = 0.003$), and absence of symptomatic hemorrhage ($P = 0.048$) were all significantly associated with favorable clinical outcome. Multivariate analysis of all significant variables using backward elimination showed that only the collateral score on dual-phase CT [odds ratio (OR) = 26.342 (2.788–248.864); $P = 0.004$] was an independent predictor for favorable outcome with adjustment for NIHSS scores at admission [OR = 0.834 (0.679–1.025); $P = 0.085$]. Moreover, multivariate analysis with significant clinical and imaging variables before IA treatment also showed the dual-phase CT collateral score [OR = 27.117 (1.519–484.258); $P = 0.025$] as an independent

Table 3. Multivariate analysis for favorable clinical outcome (mRS ≤2) at 3 months.

	Model 1			Model 2			Model 3		
	Odds ratio	95% CI	P value	Odds ratio	95% CI	P value	Odds ratio	95% CI	P value
Age	0.969	0.880–1.067	0.520	0.953	0.877–1.035	0.250	0.958	0.879–1.044	0.332
Hypertension	2.682	0.294–24.508	0.382	1.435	0.187–10.993	0.728	1.164	0.171–7.939	0.877
NIHSS score at admission	0.814	0.648–1.023	0.077	0.868	0.731–1.029	0.103	0.826	0.678–1.006	0.058
ASPECTS	1.504	0.675–3.351	0.318	1.515	0.793–2.893	0.208	1.480	0.734–2.984	0.273
Occlusion of intracranial ICA	0.518	0.057–4.679	0.558	0.273	0.032–2.318	0.234	0.245	0.025–2.371	0.225
Dual-phase CT collateral score	27.117	1.519–484.258	0.025	-	-	-	-	-	-
CTA collateral score	-	-	-	4.456	0.929–21.365	0.062	-	-	-
TFCA collateral score	-	-	-	-	-	-	2.996	1.138–7.890	0.026
AUC	0.922 (0.798–0.981)			0.880 (0.745–0.959)			0.874 (0.737–0.955)		

ASPECTS indicates Alberta Stroke Program Early CT Score; AUC, area under the curve; ICA, internal carotid artery; and NIHSS, National Institutes of Health Stroke Scale.

predictor for clinical outcome even after adjustment of age, presence of hypertension, NIHSS score at admission, ASPECTS, and occlusion of intracranial ICA. Meanwhile, the CTA collateral score in model 2 was not an independent predictor ($P = 0.062$) unlike dual-phase CT collateral score in model 1. Although the TFCA collateral score was also an independent predictor [OR = 2.996 (1.138–7.890); $P = 0.026$], the area under the curve (AUC) of model 3 (0.874) was lower than that of model 1 (0.922). However, it failed to achieve a level of statistical significance ($P = 0.206$; Table 3).

Discussion

The present study suggests collateral status on dual-phase CT may be an independent predictor [OR = 26.342 (2.788–248.864); $P = 0.004$] for clinical outcome in acute ischemic stroke patients who are subjected to IA treatment. Moreover, after adjustment of clinical and CT variables measured before IA treatment, collateral status on dual-phase CT was also an independent predictor for clinical outcome [OR = 25.763 (1.342–494.601); $P = 0.031$]. On the other hand, the CTA collateral score could not independently predict clinical outcome in model 2. Also, although there was no statistical significance, the prediction model with the dual-phase CT collateral score was better than that with TFCA collateral scores.

Leptomeningeal collaterals have been considered as having a beneficial role in patients with acute stroke despite various scoring scales and different imaging modalities [17]. CT, which is noninvasive and widely available in emergency situations, has been used to evaluate collateral status. Above all, CTA-based methods are the most commonly suggested so far [4–6,10–14]. However, the prediction power of these methods can be influenced by small differences in time delay from contrast injection to image acquisition as there is no dynamic information on single phase CTA. Before the era of fast CTA acquisition, CTA images were acquired under an almost steady-state condition with maximal enhancement in arteries and tissues. Therefore, the nonenhanced area on this protocol is associated with decreased cerebral blood volume and can be a predictor for cerebral infarction [11]. After the introduction of multidetector CT that has made fast acquisition of CTA possible, slowly perfused areas via collaterals might not be enhanced on CTA images causing overestimation of infarct core [28] and thrombus length [29] as well as underestimation of collateral status [21,30]. To overcome limitations of single phase CTA, multi- [18,19] and tri-phase [20,31] CT and perfusion CT [3,21] have been suggested as a tool to assess collateral status; but the additional value of these advanced techniques over single phase CTA to predict clinical outcome lacks confirmation. Moreover, lack of ubiquitousness of these advanced sequences and post processing techniques, insufficient scan coverage, and potential radiation hazard caused by additional CT scans might be problems in daily clinical practice.

A previous study using tri-phase CT [31] graded collateral scores on each phase image and focused on identifying the best phase to predict infarct volume. A recent study with time-resolved assessment of collateral status on perfusion CT [21] also scored collateral status on early and peak phases and temporal MIP reconstruction images which were obtained by fusing contrast enhancement across the whole duration of the 4-dimensional CTA. This study classified patients into incomplete, slow-complete, and rapid-complete collateral flow groups by integrating dynamic information from various phase images. In addition, they also showed that complete collateral flow groups achieve favorable clinical outcome more often; however, the effective dose of this CT protocol was 8.5 mSv excluding NCCT. Kim et al. [19] obtained multiphase CT and evaluated collateral status on mid (23 and 32 s after contrast injection) and late (41 and 50 s after contrast injection) phase CECT images by using the same scales that were used in our study. They found high correlation between collateral status on these two phase images and TFCA. However, analysis of the effect of collateral status on multiphase CT on clinical outcome was not conducted. It is worth noting that the time delay between contrast injection and image acquisition of mid and late phases were similar to those of CTA and delayed CECT in the present study. Thus, supporting that only dual-phase CT with optimized time delay from contrast injection may have sufficient dynamic information to show collateral status.

In this study, collateral scores on dual-phase CT showed better correlation with collateral status on TFCA and higher interobserver agreement than did collateral scores on single phase CTA. Also, as mentioned above, collateral status on dual-phase CT was an independent predictor for clinical outcome; however, collateral scores on single phase CTA and even TFCA were not. On dual-phase CT, detection of collateral defects on CTA and delayed CECT was needed. On the other hand, additional detection on the degree (smaller or larger than 50% of the occluded territory) of collateral extent was required on single phase CTA. Therefore, the observers might grade collateral status more consistently on dual-phase CT. Both dual-phase CTA and TFCA provide dynamic information of collaterals; however, it is difficult to evaluate pial collaterals from whole cerebral circulation by TFCA, so the prediction power for clinical outcome might be lower than that of dual-phase CT.

Among the patients with complete collaterals on dual-phase CT, patients with rapid-complete collaterals had higher ASPECT scores at admission (7.6 vs. 8.5), smaller final infarct volume (25.0 ml vs. 12.3 ml), and more frequent favorable clinical outcome (60.9% vs. 90%) than patients with slow-complete collaterals. Although there was no significant differences between the two groups as reported in a previous study [21], the number of patients may have been too small to reach a statistically significant conclusion. Therefore, prospective studies with larger sample size and an optimized CT protocol are warranted to establish the influence of collateral velocity on clinical outcome.

There were several limitations in our study. First, this study was a retrospective study although the patients were recruited from a prospectively collected database. Also a small number of patients

included in the analysis might cause a wide range of 95% CI of OR of dual-phase CT collateral status and its overestimation. Therefore, caution is needed in generalizing the results of this study. Second, more than 50% of patients were treated with IV thrombolysis. As a result of the IV treatment, potential confounding factors may have influenced the assessment of collateral status on TFCA and prediction of clinical outcome. There might be difference in thrombus extent and the collateral status between CT and TFCA. Third, there is the possibility that selection bias may exist. Patients who achieved recanalization only after IV treatment or had substantial ischemic change larger than 1/3 of the middle cerebral artery (MCA) territory were not subjected to IA treatment and excluded from this study. We also excluded considerable number of patients according to the exclusion criteria. However, our results could be applied to a relatively homogenous patient group with occlusion of distal ICA or M1 segments who are indicated for IA treatment. Fourth, we did not perform multiphase CT or perfusion CT, so direct comparison between these advanced techniques and dual-phase CT in predicting clinical outcome was not performed. Finally, our routine CT protocol was not optimized to assess collateral status in patients with acute ischemic stroke. According to a previous study using time-resolved CTA [21], alteration of time delay from contrast injection to image acquisition has the potential to impair outcome prediction. Therefore, efforts to establish an appropriate CT protocol and future studies with this optimized CT protocol in a larger scale are required.

Conclusions

In conclusion, dual-phase CT is feasible for assessing collateral status in patients with acute ischemic stroke, showing substantial interobserver agreement. Collateral status on dual-phase CT can also be a useful predictor for clinical outcome in acute stroke patients subjected to IA treatment, especially when advanced CT techniques are not available in emergency situations.

Author Contributions

Conceived and designed the experiments: NYS SKL. Performed the experiments: NYS KEK MP. Analyzed the data: NYS KEK. Contributed reagents/materials/analysis tools: YDK JHH. Contributed to the writing of the manuscript: NYS. Revising the manuscript: YDK SKL DJK SJA.

References

1. Kucinski T, Koch C, Eckert B, Becker V, Kromer H, et al. (2003) Collateral circulation is an independent radiological predictor of outcome after thrombolysis in acute ischaemic stroke. Neuroradiology 45: 11–18.

2. Bang OY, Saver JL, Kim SJ, Kim GM, Chung CS, et al. (2011) Collateral flow predicts response to endovascular therapy for acute ischemic stroke. Stroke 42: 693–699.

3. Calleja AI, Cortijo E, Garcia-Bermejo P, Gomez RD, Perez-Fernandez S, et al. (2013) Collateral circulation on perfusion-computed tomography-source images predicts the response to stroke intravenous thrombolysis. Eur J Neurol 20: 795–802.

4. Lima FO, Furie KL, Silva GS, Lev MH, Camargo EC, et al. (2010) The pattern of leptomeningeal collaterals on CT angiography is a strong predictor of long-term functional outcome in stroke patients with large vessel intracranial occlusion. Stroke 41: 2316–2322.

5. Maas MB, Lev MH, Ay H, Singhal AB, Greer DM, et al. (2009) Collateral vessels on CT angiography predict outcome in acute ischemic stroke. Stroke 40: 3001–3005.

6. Tan IY, Demchuk AM, Hopyan J, Zhang L, Gladstone D, et al. (2009) CT angiography clot burden score and collateral score: correlation with clinical and radiologic outcomes in acute middle cerebral artery infarct. AJNR Am J Neuroradiol 30: 525–531.

7. Liebeskind DS (2003) Collateral circulation. Stroke 34: 2279–2284.

8. Bang OY, Saver JL, Alger JR, Starkman S, Ovbiagele B, et al. (2008) Determinants of the distribution and severity of hypoperfusion in patients with ischemic stroke. Neurology 71: 1804–1811.

9. Caplan LR, Hennerici M (1998) Impaired clearance of emboli (washout) is an important link between hypoperfusion, embolism, and ischemic stroke. Arch Neurol 55: 1475–1482.

10. Rosenthal ES, Schwamm LH, Roccatagliata L, Coutts SB, Demchuk AM, et al. (2008) Role of recanalization in acute stroke outcome: rationale for a CT angiogram-based "benefit of recanalization" model. AJNR Am J Neuroradiol 29: 1471–1475.

11. Schramm P, Schellinger PD, Fiebach JB, Heiland S, Jansen O, et al. (2002) Comparison of CT and CT angiography source images with diffusion-weighted imaging in patients with acute stroke within 6 hours after onset. Stroke 33: 2426–2432.

12. Tan JC, Dillon WP, Liu S, Adler F, Smith WS, et al. (2007) Systematic comparison of perfusion-CT and CT-angiography in acute stroke patients. Ann Neurol 61: 533–543.

13. Wildermuth S, Knauth M, Brandt T, Winter R, Sartor K, et al. (1998) Role of CT angiography in patient selection for thrombolytic therapy in acute hemispheric stroke. Stroke 29: 935–938.

14. Knauth M, von Kummer R, Jansen O, Hahnel S, Dorfler A, et al. (1997) Potential of CT angiography in acute ischemic stroke. AJNR Am J Neuroradiol 18: 1001–1010.

15. Soares BP, Tong E, Hom J, Cheng SC, Bredno J, et al. (2010) Reperfusion is a more accurate predictor of follow-up infarct volume than recanalization: a proof of concept using CT in acute ischemic stroke patients. Stroke 41: e34–40.

16. Miteff F, Levi CR, Bateman GA, Spratt N, McElduff P, et al. (2009) The independent predictive utility of computed tomography angiographic collateral status in acute ischaemic stroke. Brain 132: 2231–2238.

17. McVerry F, Liebeskind DS, Muir KW (2012) Systematic review of methods for assessing leptomeningeal collateral flow. AJNR Am J Neuroradiol 33: 576–582.

18. Lee SJ, Lee KH, Na DG, Byun HS, Kim YB, et al. (2004) Multiphasic helical computed tomography predicts subsequent development of severe brain edema in acute ischemic stroke. Arch Neurol 61: 505–509.

19. Kim SJ, Noh HJ, Yoon CW, Kim KH, Jeon P, et al. (2012) Multiphasic perfusion computed tomography as a predictor of collateral flow in acute ischemic stroke: comparison with digital subtraction angiography. Eur Neurol 67: 252–255.

20. Lee KH, Cho SJ, Byun HS, Na DG, Choi NC, et al. (2000) Triphasic perfusion computed tomography in acute middle cerebral artery stroke: a correlation with angiographic findings. Arch Neurol 57: 990–999.

21. Frolich AM, Wolff SL, Psychogios MN, Klotz E, Schramm R, et al. (2014) Time-resolved assessment of collateral flow using 4D CT angiography in large-vessel occlusion stroke. Eur Radiol 24: 390–396.

22. Adams HP Jr, Bendixen BH, Kappelle LJ, Biller J, Love BB, et al. (1993) Classification of subtype of acute ischemic stroke. Definitions for use in a multicenter clinical trial. TOAST. Trial of Org 10172 in Acute Stroke Treatment. Stroke 24: 35–41.

23. Barber PA, Demchuk AM, Zhang J, Buchan AM (2000) Validity and reliability of a quantitative computed tomography score in predicting outcome of hyperacute stroke before thrombolytic therapy. ASPECTS Study Group. Alberta Stroke Programme Early CT Score. Lancet 355: 1670–1674.

24. Higashida RT, Furlan AJ, Roberts H, Tomsick T, Connors B, et al. (2003) Trial design and reporting standards for intra-arterial cerebral thrombolysis for acute ischemic stroke. Stroke 34: e109–137.

25. Campbell BC, Tu HT, Christensen S, Desmond PM, Levi CR, et al. (2012) Assessing response to stroke thrombolysis: validation of 24-hour multimodal magnetic resonance imaging. Arch Neurol 69: 46–50.

26. Hacke W, Kaste M, Fieschi C, von Kummer R, Davalos A, et al. (1998) Randomised double-blind placebo-controlled trial of thrombolytic therapy with intravenous alteplase in acute ischaemic stroke (ECASS II). Second European-Australasian Acute Stroke Study Investigators. Lancet 352: 1245–1251.

27. Landis JR, Koch GG (1977) The measurement of observer agreement for categorical data. Biometrics 33: 159–174.

28. Yoo AJ, Hu R, Hakimelahi R, Lev MH, Nogueira RG, et al. (2012) CT angiography source images acquired with a fast-acquisition protocol overestimate infarct core on diffusion weighted images in acute ischemic stroke. J Neuroimaging 22: 329–335.

29. Mortimer AM, Little DH, Minhas KS, Walton ER, Renowden SA, et al. (2013) Thrombus length estimation in acute ischemic stroke: a potential role for delayed contrast enhanced CT. J Neurointerv Surg.

30. Choi JY, Kim EJ, Hong JM, Lee SE, Lee JS, et al. (2011) Conventional enhancement CT: a valuable tool for evaluating pial collateral flow in acute ischemic stroke. Cerebrovasc Dis 31: 346–352.

31. Jung SL, Lee YJ, Ahn KJ, Kim YI, Lee KS, et al. (2011) Assessment of collateral flow with multi-phasic CT: correlation with diffusion weighted MRI in MCA occlusion. J Neuroimaging 21: 225–228.

14

Radioimmunoimaging of Liver Metastases with PET Using a ^{64}Cu-Labeled CEA Antibody in Transgenic Mice

Stefanie Nittka[1]☯, Marcel A. Krueger[5]*☯, John E. Shively[6], Hanne Boll[2], Marc A. Brockmann[2,3], Fabian Doyon[4], Bernd J. Pichler[5], Michael Neumaier[1]

1 Institute for Clinical Chemistry, Medical Faculty Mannheim, University of Heidelberg, Mannheim, Germany, 2 Department of Neuroradiology, Medical Faculty Mannheim, University of Heidelberg, Mannheim, Germany, 3 Department of Diagnostic and Interventional Neuroradiology, University Hospital of the Rheinisch-Westfaehlische Technical University Aachen, Aachen, Germany, 4 Department of Surgery, Medical Faculty Mannheim, University of Heidelberg, Mannheim, Germany, 5 Department of Preclinical Imaging and Radiopharmacy, Werner Siemens Imaging Center, University of Tuebingen, Tuebingen, Germany, 6 Department of Immunology, Beckman Research Institute, City of Hope, Duarte, California, United States of America

Abstract

Purpose: Colorectal cancer is one of the most common forms of cancer, and the development of novel tools for detection and efficient treatment of metastases is needed. One promising approach is the use of radiolabeled antibodies for positron emission tomography (PET) imaging and radioimmunotherapy. Since carcinoembryonic antigen (CEA) is an important target in colorectal cancer, the CEA-specific M5A antibody has been extensively studied in subcutaneous xenograft models; however, the M5A antibody has not yet been tested in advanced models of liver metastases. The aim of this study was to investigate the ^{64}Cu-DOTA-labeled M5A antibody using PET in mice bearing CEA-positive liver metastases.

Procedures: Mice were injected intrasplenically with CEA-positive C15A.3 or CEA-negative MC38 cells and underwent micro-computed tomography (micro-CT) to monitor the development of liver metastases. After metastases were detected, PET/MRI scans were performed with ^{64}Cu-DOTA-labeled M5A antibodies. H&E staining, immunohistology, and autoradiography were performed to confirm the micro-CT and PET/MRI findings.

Results: PET/MRI showed that M5A uptake was highest in CEA-positive metastases. The %ID/cm^3 (16.5%±6.3%) was significantly increased compared to healthy liver tissue (8.6%±0.9%) and to CEA-negative metastases (5.5%±0.6%). The tumor-to-liver ratio of C15A.3 metastases and healthy liver tissue was 1.9±0.7. Autoradiography and immunostaining confirmed the micro-CT and PET/MRI findings.

Conclusion: We show here that the ^{64}Cu-DOTA-labeled M5A antibody imaged by PET can detect CEA positive liver metastases and is therefore a potential tool for staging cancer, stratifying the patients or radioimmunotherapy.

Editor: Christoph E. Hagemeyer, Baker IDI Heart and Diabetes Institute, Australia

Funding: The authors have no funding or support to report.

Competing Interests: The authors have declared that no competing interests exist.

* Email: Marcel.Krueger@med.uni-tuebingen.de

☯ These authors contributed equally to this work.

Introduction

Colorectal cancer is still one of the most common forms of cancer in Germany and the third most common cause of cancer-related deaths worldwide [1,2]. An important target for the detection and monitoring of the recurrence of colon cancer is the human carcinoembryonic antigen (CEA, CEACAM5), a key member of the family of carcinoembryonic antigen-related cell adhesion molecules (CEACAMs) and a GPI-anchored cell surface glycoprotein that has been shown to be useful as a tumor-associated antigen and serum marker [3,4]. The widely demonstrated overexpression of CEA in solid tumors can also be exploited to target tumor lesions by immunological methods [5] or for radioimmunotherapy (RIT) [6].

Radiolabeled antibodies have been frequently used in molecular imaging as PET tracers [7–10]. The fully humanized M5A variant of the murine T84.66 anti-CEA specific antibody can be efficiently labeled with ^{64}Cu-DOTA [11]. Moreover, both M5A and T84.66 possesses a very high affinity for the CEA antigen ($>10^{10}$ M^{-1}) [12] with very low cross reactivity to other members of the CEACAM family and can be used as a whole antibody molecule.

Thus far, the evaluation of the ^{64}Cu-labeled murine antibody T84.66 [13] or the fully humanized form M5A has been restricted to athymic nude mice bearing subcutaneous tumors [11]. In these studies, ^{64}Cu-DOTA-M5A was capable of detecting xenograft tumors in nude mice. Our syngeneic orthotopic tumor model in the transgenic mouse strain C57BL/6 Han TgN (CEA-gen) allows us to study hematogenous liver metastases provoked by the intrasplenic injection of CEA-expressing colon tumor cells [14,15].

These mice express CEA predominantly in the colon and intestine, with a spatial distribution of CEA comparable to that of human tissue [16,17]. One major advantage of this syngeneic orthotopic mouse model is that the metastatic growth in this model, compared to subcutaneous tumor transplantation, is a more accurate model of the anatomic behavior, making this model highly attractive for the evaluation of novel imaging antibodies [18,19].

Our aim was to evaluate the ^{64}Cu-DOTA labeled M5A-antibody as a PET-tracer for imaging of liver metastases. Our approach was to inject C57BL/6-derived colon tumor cells into the spleens of syngeneic mice and then screen for metastases by micro-CT. As soon as lesions were detected, we proceeded with radioimmuno-PET/MRI with ^{64}Cu-DOTA labeled M5A followed by histological confirmation of the imaging findings.

Materials and Methods

Ethical approval

All animal experiments have been conducted according to relevant national and international guidelines and were permitted by the Regierungspraesidium Karlsruhe and Regierungspraesidium Tuebingen and the Institutional Animal Care and Use Committees of the University Hospital Tuebingen and the University of Heidelberg.

Cell lines

The murine cell line MC38, a syngeneic methyl-cholanthrene-induced colon cancer line [20], and the MC38-derivative cell line C15A.3 stably transfected with the CEACAM5 gene coding for human CEA [21], were used to induce a primary tumor in the spleen and hematogenic liver metastases. Both cell lines were grown in DMEM supplemented with 10% FCS, 4 mmol/L glutamine and penicillin/streptomycin (100 units/mL and 10 mg/mL). All media and reagents were bought from PAA (Pasching, Austria).

Animals and tumor cell injections

C57BL/6 Han TgN (CEAgen) HvdP mice were generated as described previously [16]. Briefly, the cosmid clone cosCEA1, encompassing the complete human CEA gene including gene promoter regions sufficient for allowing tissue-specific gene expression [16], was used. Six-week-old female CEA-transgenic mice with a heterozygous CEA genotype were used for our studies. Mice were anesthetized, and $2*10^6$ C57BL/6-derived MC38 or C15A.3 cells in 50 μl PBS were injected into the spleen, giving rise to splenic tumors within 5–10 days post-injection. Prior to injection, CEA surface expression on C15A.3 cells using the murine T84.66 und humanized M5A CEA-specific monoclonal antibodies were tested by flow cytometry. C15A.3 cells were accepted for experiments if >95% were positive for CEA expression compared to MC38 and a mean fluorescence intensity above 80 or below 22, respectively. Mice were kept under standardized conditions and supplied with food and water ad libitum in a 12 h light-dark cycle.

micro-CT Scans

For the time series-studies micro-CT scans were performed from days 9 to 19 and days 18 to 49 post-injection for MC38 or C15A.3 metastases, respectively. For all other experiments micro-CT imaging was performed at day 9 or 18 for the MC38 or C15A.3 cell lines, respectively, to detect liver metastases. If necessary, tumor-growth monitoring was repeated after another 7 days after the first pre-screening micro-CT, depending on the outcome of the first evaluation. Micro-CT was performed as described recently [22,23]. Briefly, micro-CT imaging was performed using an industrial X-ray inspection system (Y.Fox; Yxlon International GmbH, Hamburg, Germany) equipped with a transmission X-ray tube and a 12-bit direct digital flatbed detector (PaxScan 2520; Varian, Palo Alto, CA, USA). A single dose of 100 μl of a liver-specific nanoparticulate contrast agent (VISCOVER ExiTron nano 6000; MiltenyiBiotec, Bergisch-Gladbach, Germany) was injected intravenously 3 hours prior to the first micro-CT scan. Mice were anesthetized, relaxed (Rocuronium, Esmeron, EssexPharma, München), and intubated before liver imaging was performed during a single breath stop within a 40 sec scan time during continuous image acquisition at 30 fps (frames per second) using the following scan parameters: 80 kV; 75 mA; and 180° rotation [22,23]. Relaxation afterwards was reversed by the intra peritoneal (i.p.) injection of 20 mg/kg body weight of sugammadex (BridionH; EssexPharma, Munich, Germany). The acquired projections were reconstructed using a filtered back-projection algorithm with a 512×512×512 matrix using the software Reconstruction Studio (Yxlon International GmbH, Hamburg, Germany). Analysis of reconstructed images was performed using the public domain software OsiriX (v3.5.1; www.osirix-viewer.com).

^{64}Cu Labeling of monoclonal M5A antibody

Humanized hu14.18 monoclonal anti-GD2 antibody as control was conjugated to commercially available NHS-DOTA (Macrocyclics, Dallas, TX, USA) as described previously [10]. The number of chelate molecules per immunoglobulin was not determined. The fully humanized DOTA labeled M5A monoclonal anti-CEA antibody was kindly supplied by John E. Shively (Beckman Research Institute of City of Hope, Duarte, CA) and NHS-DOTA conjugation was performed as described previously. The number of chelate molecules per immunoglobulin was determined to be ~8 as analyzed by MALDI-TOF [11]. The antibody was produced in accordance to GMP-standards through a service available to collaborators with City of Hope (J.E.S.). The purified antibody-DOTA conjugates were labeled with ^{64}Cu as described previously [24]. Briefly, ^{64}Cu was produced in Tuebingen by irradiating ^{64}Ni at a 16 MeV cyclotron (GE Healthcare, Uppsala, Sweden) and isolating it from ^{64}Ni and other metals by using ion exchange chromatography [25]. Radiolabeling of DOTA-M5A and DOTA-hu14.18 was performed by adding ~20 MBq of ^{64}CuCl$_2$ buffered in 10xPBS to ~20 μg of antibody in PBS and incubation for 1 h at 42°C. pH was checked to be at 7.0. Quality control was performed by thin-layer chromatography on Polygram SIL G/UV$_{254\ nm}$ (Machery-Nagel, Dueren, Germany) plates and analyzed on a Cyclone Plus phosphor imager (Perkin Elmer, Waltham, Massachusetts, USA). Only antibody preparations with a labeling efficiency of >90% were used for experiments.

PET- and MR Imaging

Approximately 2–4 days after the first detection of liver metastases by micro-CT imaging, animals were given a tail vein injection of ~13 MBq of ^{64}Cu-labeled anti-CEA mAb M5A-DOTA or anti-GD2 mAb hu14.18-DOTA (~20 μg). For the blocking experiments, 500 μg of unlabeled M5A antibody was injected 3 h prior to the injection of ^{64}Cu-labeled M5A antibody.

Ten-minute static PET scans were obtained at 3, 24 and 48 h after tracer injection on an Inveon dedicated small animal PET scanner (Siemens Preclinical Solutions, Knoxville, Tennessee, USA). Animals were anesthetized with 1.5% isoflurane (Abbott, Wiesbaden, Germany) evaporated in oxygen at a flow of 0.5 L/

min, and body temperature was maintained at 37°C by a heating pad and a rectal temperature sensor. Images were reconstructed with an iterative ordered-subset expectation maximization algorithm. According to our standard protocol for mouse PET imaging, attenuation and scatter correction were not applied. Images were reconstructed in Inveon Acquisition Workplace 1.5.0.28 with OSEM2D with four iterations. The reconstructed voxel size was $0.776 \times 0.776 \times 0.796$ mm. After each PET scan, the animals were transferred to a 7 T ClinScan MR scanner (Bruker, Ettlingen, Germany), and anatomic images were acquired with a 3D turbo-spin-echo (tse) sequence (TE = 205 ms, TR = 3000 ms, voxel size: $0.22 \times 0.22 \times 0.22$ mm^3, matrix size: $160 \times 256 \times 120$).

Analysis of PET and MR images

PET and MR images were overlaid and analyzed in Inveon Research Workplace (Siemens Preclinical Solutions, Erlangen, Germany) by rigid fusion. Images were overlaid by manually overlaying three markers that were filled with ^{64}Cu dissolved in PBS and placed in proximity to the animals during the measurements. Liver lesions, primary tumors and other organs were identified and regions of interest (ROI) were drawn in the MR images. Volumes of interest (VOI) were calculated from these ROI's in Inveon Research Workplace and lesion volumes and %ID/cm^3 were determined over the whole lesion volume.

Determination of ^{64}Cu-DOTA-M5A blood half-life

For determination of blood half-life, ~13 MBq of ^{64}Cu-labeled anti-CEA mAb M5A-DOTA (~20 μg) were injected in mice bearing C15A.3 metastases and PET images were acquired at 3; 24 and 48 h post injection. Volumes of interest were drawn in the right ventricle of the animals and the %ID/cm^3 was determined. A single exponential fit was used to calculate the blood half-life.

Immunohistochemistry for Paraffin sections

Mice were killed immediately after the last 48 h PET/MR imaging and major organs were removed. For some animals organs were fixed in 4% of PBS buffered formalin prior to tissue processing and 3–5 μm thick serial paraffin sections were prepared for immunohistochemistry or routine H&E staining.

For immunohistochemistry, sections were deparaffinized and subjected to antigen retrieval by high temperature technique in 1 mM EDTA-Tris buffer (pH 9.0, 30 minutes at 270 W in a microwave oven). Sections were allowed to cool down to room temperature. After incubation in PBS/0.5% Tween20 for 5 minutes, endogenous peroxidase was blocked by immersion in 3% H$_2$O$_2$/Methanol for 20 minutes. The non-specific binding was blocked by incubation with 5% normal goat serum/2% BSA-PBS for 30 minutes at 37°C. M5A primary antibody was diluted to 2.0 μg/mL in 0.1% BSA-PBS and incubated for 45 minutes at 37°C. Sections were washed with water and incubated in PBS for 5 minutes. This was followed by incubation with the diluted secondary reagent goat anti-human-HRP antibody (1/500; Dianova, Hamburg, Germany) for 45 minutes at 37°C. After an additional washing step, antibody binding was visualized by adding diaminobenzidine and subsequent hematoxylin counterstaining.

Routine H&E staining of at least one section adjacent to slides subjected to immunostaining was performed to assess tissue differentiation as well as position and number of metastases.

All slides were evaluated by microscopy (Diaplan, Leica, Nussloch, Germany) and microphotographs were taken.

Immunochemistry with cryosections and autoradiography

In some cases after the 24 h PET/MRI scan, the liver was immersed in TissueTek (Sakura, Alphen aan den Rijn, Netherlands) and frozen at −20°C and 7 μm or 20 μm thick cryosections were prepared in an alternating fashion to compare adjacent slices in immunohistochemistry, H&E and autoradiography. 20 μm thick frozen sections were subjected to autoradiography and routine H&E staining and 7 μm serial sections were used for immunohistochemistry. A total of 10 sections were prepared for each liver.

For immunohistochemistry with frozen sections, frozen slices were subjected to endogenous peroxidase block using 0.3% H$_2$O$_2$/Methanol for 20 minutes, followed by immunostaining steps as described for paraffin sections.

For autoradiography frozen slices were fixed on SuperFrost microscope slides (R. Langenbrick, Emmendingen, Germany) and placed in a shielded cassette (Amersham, Glattbrugg, Switzerland) where a phosphoscreen (Amersham) was exposed to the samples for 24 h. Subsequently the screens were analyzed on a Storm 840 Phospho Imager (Amersham) with a resolution of 50 μm.

All slides were evaluated by microscopy (Diaplan) and microphotographs were taken.

Statistical Analysis

For statistical analysis an ANOVA with a Fisher LSD test was performed. Values were considered to be statistically significantly different at P values of 0.05 or lower.

Quantitative values are reported as mean $+/-$ one standard deviation.

Results

Tumor cells and development of liver metastases

CEA transgenic mice were injected with either CEA-expressing (C15A.3) or CEA-negative (MC38) cells and subsequently micro-CT scans were performed as a pre-screening method. Typically, 9–16 days post-injection, the first metastases were present in the mice injected with MC38 cells, whereas metastases originating from the C15A.3 cells were usually detectable between days 18–25. Micro-CT imaging with ExiTron nano 6000 allowed observation of the development of metastases as demonstrated in Figure 1 over a time course of 31 days. Lesions as small as 0.9 mm in diameter could easily be identified as dark round structures (Figure 1). For all animals, primary tumors were detected in the spleen, ranging from 0.9 mm to 12.0 mm in diameter. No visual correlation was found between the size of the primary tumor and the size or number of metastases.

Immunohistological characterization of liver metastases

To further characterize our tumor model and to independently confirm the findings in micro-CT, we performed histological staining of the liver and other organs. At least 3 sections of each organ were evaluated by standard H&E staining, but metastases were found exclusively in the liver of the animals. The metastases had substantial size and diameter variability. As already suspected on the basis of the micro-CT scans, metastases originating from MC38 tumor cells were smaller but more frequent than those derived from C15A.3 tumor cells.

Tissue sections from the liver and spleen were immunostained using the M5A monoclonal antibody, and CEA-immunoreactivity could be demonstrated for all C15A.3 metastases but not for the MC38 CEA-negative metastases.

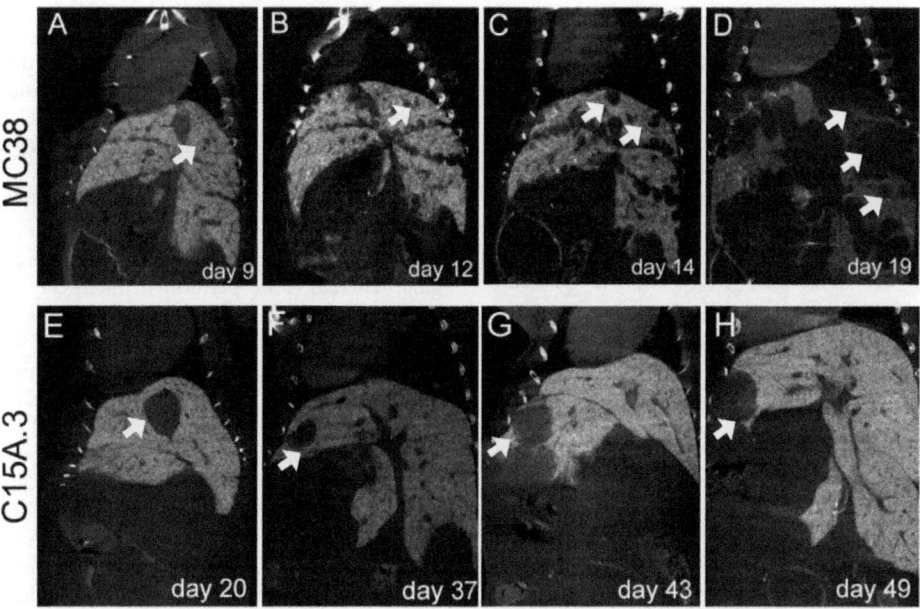

Figure 1. The development of liver metastases in mice monitored by micro-CT. To establish a suitable pre-screening routine, a separate group of animals was subjected to a time-series of micro-CT scans. Images were acquired 3 h post injection of a single dose of hepatocyte-specific contrast agent (ExiTron nano 6000) without the use of additional injections for follow-up. Images were collected at days 9 to 19 and days 20 to 49 for CEA-negative MC38 or CEA-positive C15A.3 metastases, respectively. Arrows indicate the same metastases at different time points for both cell lines. Note the differences in the size and number of metastases originating from MC38 (upper row) compared to C15A.3 (lower row).

The staining patterns for C15A.3 liver metastases appeared to be heterogeneous. The central areas of larger liver metastases were sometimes interspersed with necrotic cells, which are easily recognized by their small condensed or fragmented nuclei (Figure 2).

Detection of liver metastases by ^{64}Cu-labeled M5A-DOTA and *in vivo* biodistribution

Despite the fact that ^{64}Cu-DOTA-labeled antibodies are known to show high nonspecific background in liver tissue [10], the excellent binding properties of the CEA-specific M5A antibody reported in previous studies [11] encouraged us to test this antibody for the detection of CEA-expressing liver lesions.

To test the M5A antibody in our model, we injected ^{64}Cu-DOTA-labeled M5A into mice, which were identified as positive for liver metastases by micro-CT within 3 days. PET/MRI studies were performed at three time-points (3; 24 and 48 h) after antibody injection. Liver lesions were easily detected by MRI at all time points and ranged from 1 mm to 13 mm. Antibody uptake was visible at 3 hours post injection but sufficient uptake in liver metastases was reached after 24 h of tracer uptake. The %ID/cm^3 in CEA-expressing C15A.3 metastases at 24 h post injection was 16.5% ±6.3% and was significantly higher than in healthy liver tissue in the same animals (8.6%±0.9%) and CEA-negative MC38 metastases in control animals (6.0%±0.8%; p≤0.05) (Figure 3). Somewhat unexpectedly, the uptake decreased after the 24 h time point.

The ratio of the %ID/cm^3 between the C15A.3-derived metastases and healthy liver tissue was 1.9±0.7, while the ratio of the MC38 metastases and healthy liver tissue was significantly lower (0.9±0.2; p≤0.05). Thus, we could visually discriminate between healthy liver tissue and CEA-positive lesions (Figure 4).

Additionally in all animals injected with C15A.3 cells and the M5A antibody, several organs were analyzed for M5A uptake in *in*

vivo whole body PET images at the three time-points. We could clearly see that in all organs analyzed, except liver and metastases, the uptake decreased over time. In liver the %ID/cm^3 stayed relatively stable over the time analyzed (Figure 3).

To determine the blood half-life time of the ^{64}Cu-DOTA-labeled M5A antibody, the %ID/cm^3 in the right ventricle was determined 3; 24 and 48 h after antibody injection and a blood half-life of 18.7 h was calculated.

Verification of M5A specificity

To prove the specific binding of the M5A antibody in CEA-expressing metastases and to exclude nonspecific enhanced perfusion and retention (EPR) effects, we repeated these experiments with the fully humanized GD2-specific hu14.18 antibody, which should not bind to C15A.3 tumors and metastases. Thus, the GD2-specific hu14.18 antibody signal represents the level of nonspecific background binding of antibodies in this tissue. We did not observe a significant increase in the %ID/cm^3 over time for the control antibody in C15A.3 lesions, but we did detect a significantly lower uptake of the control antibody in the C15A.3-derived liver metastases after 24 h of tracer injection (5.3%±0.5% ID/cm^3) compared to M5A (Figure 3).

Additionally, we tested M5A specificity with blocking experiments. We injected mice bearing C15A.3 liver metastases with unlabeled M5A antibody 3 h prior to the injection of the ^{64}Cu-DOTA-labeled M5A antibody. The large amount of unlabeled M5A was expected to bind most of the available specific binding sites within the metastases, decreasing the enrichment of the labeled M5A. PET and MRI scans were performed at different time points post injection of the labeled M5A. There was a significant reduction in the uptake of the M5A antibody into the C15A.3 metastases and tumor tissue from 16.5±6.3%ID/cm^3 to 4.3±1.0%ID/cm^3 at 24 h post injection of ^{64}Cu-DOTA-M5A (Figure 3). These results clearly show that the high uptake of M5A

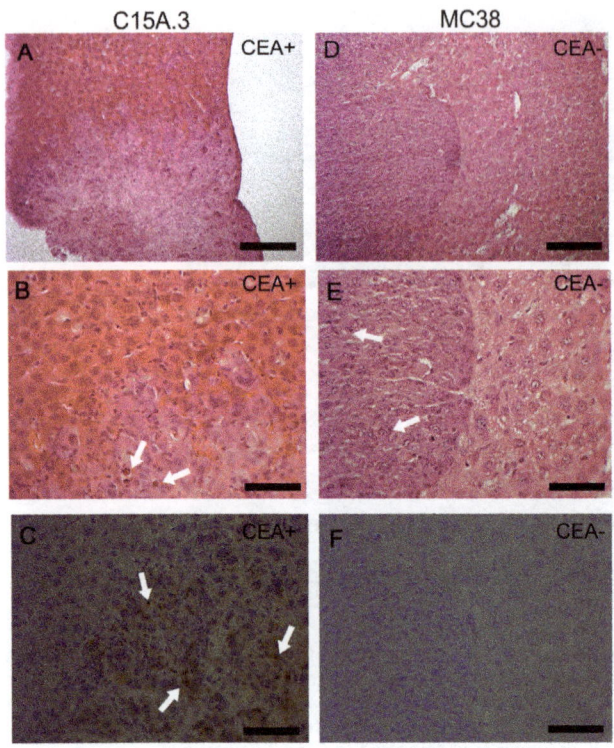

Figure 2. Liver histopathology of metastases derived from CEA-positive C15A.3 murine tumor cells (A–C) or CEA-negative parental MC38 colon tumor cells (D–F). (A, D) H&E staining of liver metastases surrounded by normal tissue. (B, E) Higher magnification, emphasizing the difference in the tumor cell growth patterns with respect to the normal-to-tumor tissue border. (C, F) Immunohisto-chemistry of serial sections stained for CEA with CEA-specific M5A antibody confirming the CEA-expression status of the metastases. Note many central necrotic cells as indicated by arrows in B, C and E in both metastases. Bar size (A, D) 125 µm, all other 50 µm.

after 24 h in the C15A.3 metastases is not due to nonspecific tissue-related effects.

Correlation of the histological findings and PET imaging results

Closer examination of the PET imaging results showed central lesion regions with low tracer-related signals for some of the larger liver metastases (Figure 4). This finding was in agreement with our histological findings described earlier but was still subjected to intensive *ex vivo* examination.

For this purpose, animals were killed immediately after the 24 h PET/MR scan, which showed a peak in M5A uptake. The livers were removed, and autoradiography, H&E staining and immu-nochemistry were performed on cryosections of the liver.

In general, the autoradiography findings confirmed the heterogeneous antibody distribution in the large liver metastases, as seen in *in vivo* PET scans. We also noted a pronounced immunohistochemical signal at the border of the larger metastases, indicating higher antigen expression or antibody binding in these areas. H&E staining revealed necrotic areas in the center of large lesions (Figure 5). In general, areas of high CEA expression as seen by immunochemistry correlated with areas of high signal in autoradiography, whereas areas of necrosis shown by H&E correlated inversely with the autoradiography signal.

Discussion

It has been previously reported that the M5A antibody shows outstanding binding characteristics in subcutaneous CEA tumor models [11]. Therefore, we decided to use this promising antibody in a more challenging and novel model of syngeneic liver metastases.

Obviously, when testing a tumor-specific PET probe for the screening or monitoring of liver lesions *in vivo*, it is necessary to select a suitable time point for the beginning of the immunoima-ging. Therefore, we performed micro-CT scans to confirm the presence of liver lesions in the animals used for further immunoimaging studies. To confirm CEA expression in our model of liver metastases, we performed immunostainings with M5A after the final micro-CT or PET/MRI-scan. These experiments showed CEA expression in all C15A.3-derived liver metastases, supporting the usefulness of our syngeneic tumor model in testing novel CEA-targeting PET tracers.

The ^{64}Cu-DOTA-M5A antibody in our tumor model showed high M5A uptake in CEA-positive C15A.3 lesions 24 h after antibody injection, while uptake in CEA-negative MC38 lesions stayed at a background level. The uptake in C15A.3 lesions was lower than in subcutaneous LS-174T tumors as reported by Li et al. [11]. The differences in the cell type and tumor location could both contribute to a different tumor microenvironment, explaining the discrepancy in the results.

We are aware of the fact that the ^{64}Cu-DOTA complex is unstable *in vivo* and release of ^{64}Cu will lead to enhanced uptake in healthy liver, which is the organ of interest in this study [10,26]. Other chelators like NOTA, crossbridged cyclams, and others [27–30] have been shown to give better tumor to liver ratios *in vivo*, but since the M5A antibody has already been labeled with DOTA under GMP conditions and clinical studies have been performed with ^{64}Cu-DOTA-M5A, we still decided to use DOTA in this work to increase the clinical relevance of this study. Therefore it is especially notable that the lesion-to-liver-ratio of tracer uptake for C15A.3 lesions allowed clear identification of lesions in PET/MR-images. Although for clinical studies a higher lesion-to-liver ratio would be appreciated, we still believe that for diagnostic purposes a lesion-to-liver ratio of ~2 is for most cases sufficient for stratification. Alternatively for future studies other chelators could be used. For RIT it would be important to perform similar biodistribution studies with therapeutic isotopes like ^{177}Lu or ^{90}Y, since the high unspecific background observed here is probably to large parts due to free ^{64}Cu released from the DOTA complex. Therefore a translation of the observed lesion-to-liver ratios to other isotopes is speculative, since the complex stability of these isotopes with DOTA is different from ^{64}Cu.

Interestingly, the lesion-to-liver ratio observed here with the full M5A antibody outcompetes the ratios reached with a ^{64}Cu-DOTA labeled T84.66 derived 80 kDa minibody (T84.66 is the parental antibody of M5A) [31], although smaller antibody formats are commonly expected to have better pharmacokinetic properties when used as imaging probes [32]. One possible explanation for this might be the higher affinity of the M5A antibody compared to the minibody (1.1×10^{10} vs.2–$3\times10^{9}M^{-1}$ respectively) [33,34].

Although both cell lines used were based on the same cellular background (MC38 or MC38 stably expressing human CEA), we could see differences in the size, number and growth rate of liver metastases by micro-CT, histology and PET/MRI. MC38 cells generated smaller but more frequent metastases that appeared more quickly than C15A.3-derived metastases (data not shown). This result is comparable with findings by Hand et al. [35], who

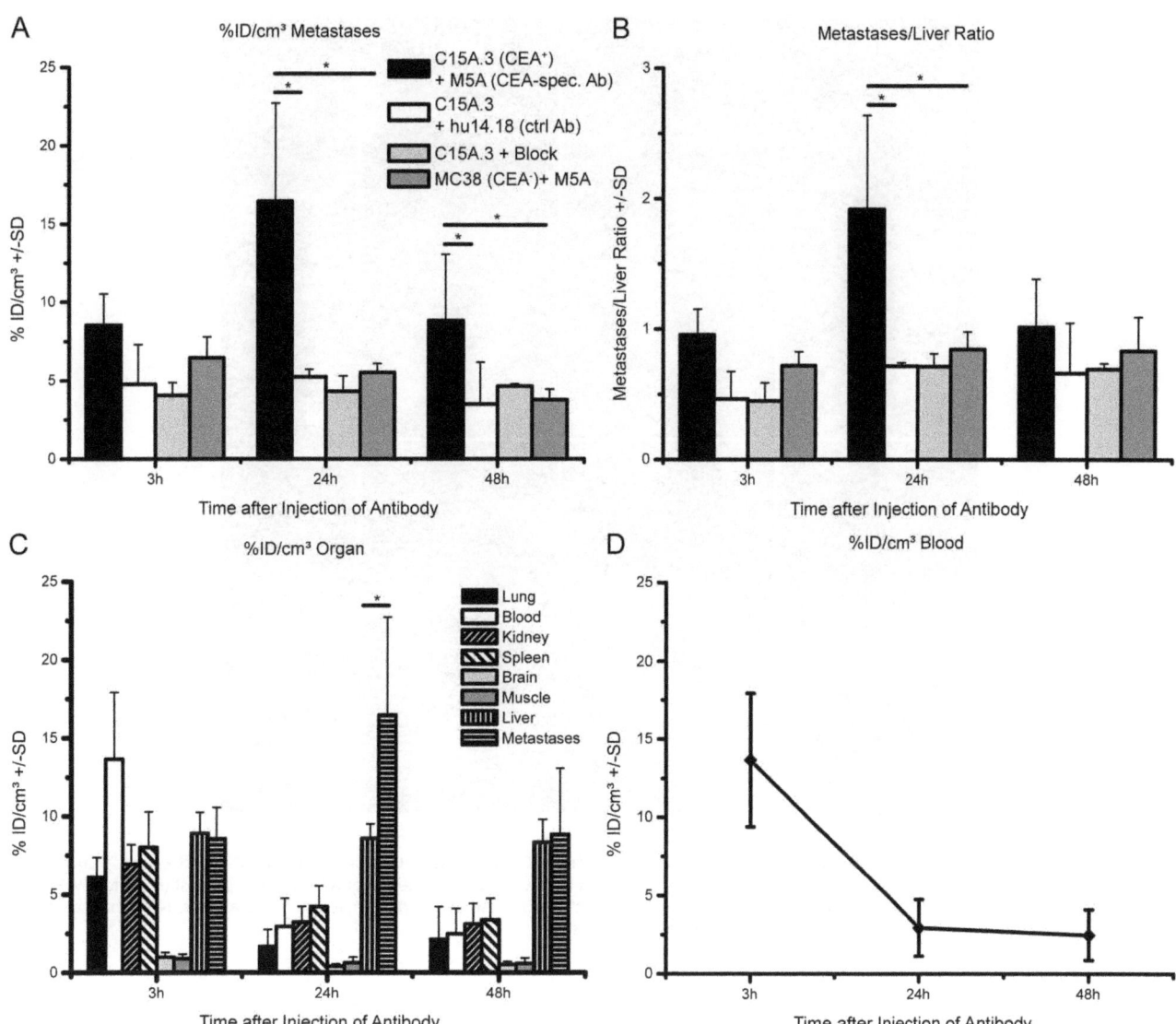

Figure 3. Uptake of the ^{64}Cu-DOTA-labeled M5A antibody in CEA-positive C15A.3- and CEA-negative MC38-derived liver metastases. (A) Depicted are the %ID/cc of the labeled M5A antibody in either C15A.3 or MC38 derived metastases and the uptake of the control antibody hu14.18 at three different time points post injection of antibodies. For blocking experiments, 500 µg of unlabeled M5A was injected 3 h prior to labeled M5A. (B) The ratio of the antibody uptake between metastases and healthy liver. For A+B n = 8 animals for C15A.3+M5A, n = 7 animals for MC38+M5A, n = 2 animals for blocking and n = 4 animals for control antibody (hu14.18). All animals were scanned at every time-point. (C) %ID/cm^3 of ^{64}Cu-DOTA-labeled M5A antibody in several organs at different time points. (D) Focus on the %ID/cm^3 of ^{64}Cu-DOTA-labeled M5A in the right ventricle. For C+D n = 7 at all time points. Statistically significant results are designated with * when p≤0.05.

showed reduced growth rates of subcutaneous tumors positive for human CEA in C57BL/6 mice.

The differences in the size and number of metastases made us question whether MC38-derived tumors or metastases are a suitable control for our purposes because antibody uptake in tumors is well known to be strongly affected by factors such as tumor size, vascularization or interstitial pressure [36]. Since the amount of vascularization, interstitial pressure and other factors were not determined for the liver metastases of either origin and the tumor size can affect the antibody uptake due to partial volume effects, necrotic areas or decreased perfusion in larger tumors, we also injected the GD$_2$-specific hu14.18 antibody into animals bearing C15A.3 lesions, which are GD$_2$-negative. Since the uptake of this control antibody stayed at a background level, we were able to exclude the possibility of high M5A uptake in

C15A.3 lesions due to physiological reasons. Furthermore, blocking experiments were performed, showing that M5A uptake can be decreased by pre-injecting unlabeled M5A, again showing that the high uptake of M5A in C15A.3 lesions does not depend on nonspecific differences in tumor physiology, indicating the specificity of M5A.

In several PET images, we could clearly identify a heterogeneous distribution of ^{64}Cu-DOTA-M5A in C15A.3 lesions, especially within larger liver metastases. When this phenomenon occurred, the rims of the lesions showed high signal, and the cores showed low signal. These findings could be supported by autoradiographies of livers performed after PET/MRI scans. In some cases, the M5A immunostaining of the same livers used for the autoradiographies showed increased CEA expression in the rims, correlating with the findings in PET and autoradiography.

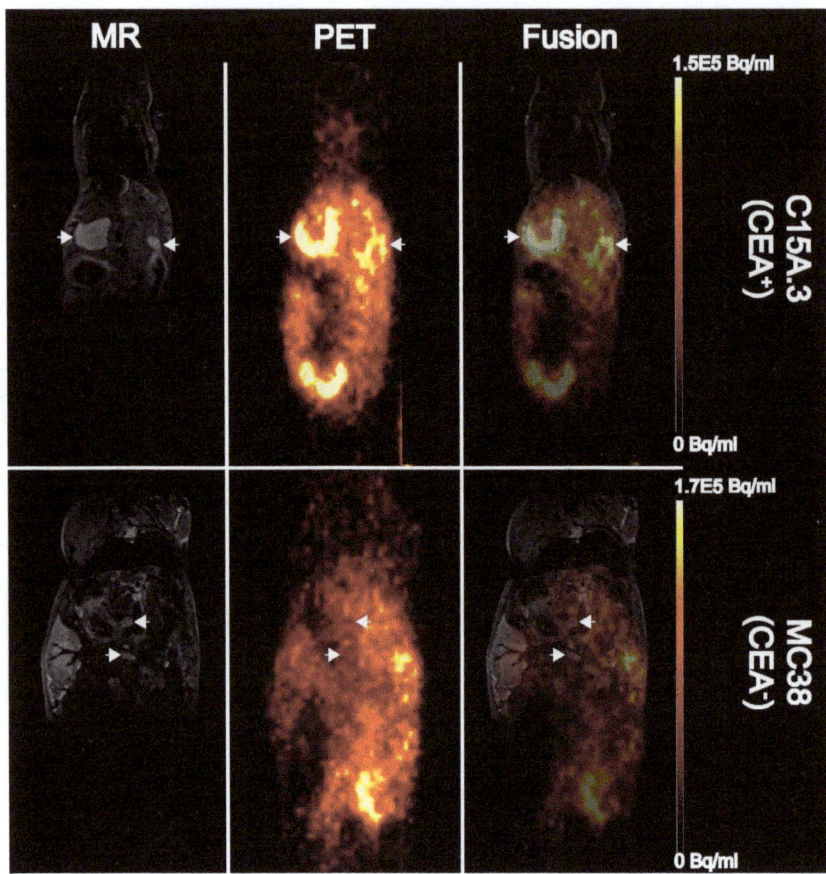

Figure 4. MRI and PET scan results for liver metastases originating from C15A.3 and MC38 cells 24 h post-injection of ^{64}Cu-DOTA-M5A antibody. MRI images clearly show the location of the liver metastases (arrows) and were used to draw regions of interest (ROIs) for evaluating the PET data. Immuno-PET images indicate strong signals in the areas of the CEA-positive C15A.3-derived liver metastases. No enhanced tracer uptake was observed in the areas of CEA-negative MC38 derived metastases.

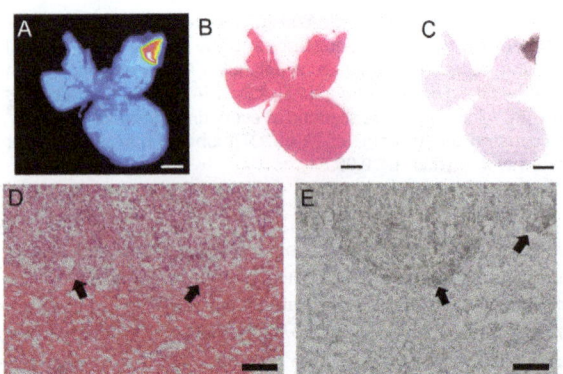

Figure 5. *Ex vivo* autoradiography (A), H&E staining (B, D) and M5A-immunohistochemistry (C, E) of the CEA-positive C15A.3-derived metastases. Evaluation of the cryosections was performed 24 h post-injection of ^{64}Cu-DOTA-M5A antibody. (A) Autoradiography shows the heterogeneous distribution of M5A within metastases. (B, C) The location of metastases in H&E and immunostaining correlates with the location of the metastases shown in (A). Note the intense, dark staining of the C15A.3 tumor cells near the tumor-to-normal border (D, E arrows). Bar size A-C 3 mm and C-D 200 μm respectively.

Furthermore, H&E staining of the autoradiography sections revealed necrotic areas in the centers of the metastases, which might be poorly perfused. Therefore, both effects might account for the heterogeneous tracer distribution within liver metastases. Additionally, these observations could be attributed to the high affinity of M5A [33], which could lead to a rapid sequestration of the antibody to the antigen and interfere with the free diffusion of M5A into the lesions, thus preventing antibody uptake into the tumor core. This effect is known as a 'binding-site barrier' effect, which was first described by Fujimori et al. [37].

Since the ROIs in this study were drawn based on the MR images and no necrosis was visible in the MR images, lesion areas with low PET signal were included in the %ID/cm^3, making the high M5A-uptake for C15A.3 metastases even more impressive.

Finally, we observed a wash-out effect of M5A between the 24 h and 48 h time point. Our results stand in contrast to data generated by Li et al. [11] for subcutaneous LS-174T tumors in which there was an increase in antibody uptake over the first 48 h upon injection. However, this discrepancy might again be due to the differences in the tumor models used.

Conclusions

The binding properties of M5A were analyzed for the first time in a syngeneic orthotopic model of liver metastases that matches the scenario for human patients much more closely than common subcutaneous tumor models. The outstanding binding properties of the M5A antibody enabled us to generate signal-to-noise ratios in the liver that were high enough to clearly identify CEA-expressing liver metastases. This is the first report showing the characterization of liver lesions with a ^{64}Cu-DOTA-labeled antibody despite the high nonspecific background in healthy liver tissue. Therefore, this study proposes that the M5A antibody, which is currently undergoing clinical Phase I/II RIT trials [6],

could be a useful tool to diagnose CEA-positive liver metastases for patient stratification and subsequent RIT.

Author Contributions

Conceived and designed the experiments: MAK SN MN. Performed the experiments: MAK SN HB MAB FD. Analyzed the data: MAK SN HB MAB. Contributed reagents/materials/analysis tools: JES MN BJP. Contributed to the writing of the manuscript: MAK SN.

References

1. Ferlay J, Parkin DM, Steliarova-Foucher E (2010) Estimates of cancer incidence and mortality in Europe in 2008. Eur J Cancer 46: 765–781.
2. Pancione M, Forte N, Fucci A, Sabatino L, Febbraro A, et al. (2010) Prognostic role of beta-catenin and p53 expression in the metastatic progression of sporadic colorectal cancer. Hum Pathol 41: 867–876.
3. Hammarström S (1999) The carcinoembryonic antigen (CEA) family: structures, suggested functions and expression in normal and malignant tissues. Seminars in Cancer Biology 9: 67–81.
4. Blumenthal RD, Leon E, Hansen HJ, Goldenberg DM (2007) Expression patterns of CEACAM5 and CEACAM6 in primary and metastatic cancers. BMC Cancer 7: 218–225.
5. Szalai G, Williams LE, Primus FJ (2000) Tumor targeting with radiolabeled antibodies in a human carcinoembryonic antigen transgenic mouse model. Int J Cancer 85: 751–756.
6. Yazaki PJ, Lee B, Channappa D, Cheung CW, Crow D, et al. (2013) A series of anti-CEA/anti-DOTA bispecific antibody formats evaluated for pre-targeting: comparison of tumor uptake and blood clearance. Protein Eng Des Sel 26: 187–193.
7. Wadas TJ, Wong EH, Weisman GR, Anderson CJ (2007) Copper chelation chemistry and its role in copper radiopharmaceuticals. Current pharmaceutical design 13: 3–16.
8. Li L, Yazaki PJ, Anderson A-l, Crow D, Colcher D, et al. (2006) Improved Biodistribution and Radioimmunoimaging with Poly (ethylene glycol) -DOTA-Conjugated Anti-CEA Diabody Improved Biodistribution and Radioimmunoimaging with Poly (ethylene glycol) -DOTA-Conjugated Anti-CEA Diabody. Bioconjugate Chemistry 17: 68–76.
9. Anderson C, Ferdani R (2009) Copper-64 radiopharmaceuticals for PET imaging of cancer: advances in preclinical and clinical research. Cancer Biother Radiopharm 24: 379–393.
10. Elsasser-Beile U, Reischl G, Wiehr S, Buhler P, Wolf P, et al. (2009) PET imaging of prostate cancer xenografts with a highly specific antibody against the prostate-specific membrane antigen. J Nucl Med 50: 606–611.
11. Li L, Bading J, Yazaki PJ, Ahuja AH, Crow D, et al. (2008) A versatile bifunctional chelate for radiolabeling humanized anti-CEA antibody with In-111 and Cu-64 at either thiol or amino groups: PET imaging of CEA-positive tumors with whole antibody. Bioconjugate Chemistry 19: 89–96.
12. Wong JY, Thomas GE, Yamauchi D, Williams LE, Odom-Maryon TL, et al. (1997) Clinical evaluation of indium-111-labeled chimeric anti-CEA monoclonal antibody. J Nucl Med 38: 1951–1959.
13. Bryan JN, Jia F, Mohsin H, Sivaguru G, Anderson CJ, et al. (2011) Monoclonal antibodies for copper-64 PET dosimetry and radioimmunotherapy. Cancer Biol Ther 11: 1001–1007.
14. Jain RK, Munn LL, Fukumura D (2012) Liver tumor preparation in mice. Cold Spring Harb Protoc 2012.
15. Brand MI, Casillas S, Dietz DW, Milsom JW, Vladisavljevic A (1996) Development of a reliable colorectal cancer liver metastasis model. J Surg Res 63: 425–432.
16. Eades-Perner AM, van der Putten H, Hirth A, Thompson J, Neumaier M, et al. (1994) Mice transgenic for the human carcinoembryonic antigen gene maintain its spatiotemporal expression pattern. Cancer Research 54: 4169–4176.
17. Wilkinson RW, Ross EL, Ellison D, Zimmermann W, Snary D, et al. (2002) Evaluation of a transgenic mouse model for anti-human CEA radioimmunotherapeutics. J Nucl Med 43: 1368–1376.
18. Du X, Jin R, Ning N, Li L, Wang Q, et al. (2012) In vivo distribution and antitumor effect of infused immune cells in a gastric cancer model. Oncol Rep 28: 1743–1749.
19. Salavatifar M, Amin S, Jahromi ZM, Rasgoo N, Rastgoo N, et al. (2011) Green fluorescent-conjugated anti-CEA single chain antibody for the detection of CEA-positive cancer cells. Hybridoma (Larchmt) 30: 229–238.
20. Corbett TH, Griswold DP, Jr., Roberts BJ, Peckham JC, Schabel FM, Jr. (1975) Tumor induction relationships in development of transplantable cancers of the colon in mice for chemotherapy assays, with a note on carcinogen structure. Cancer Res 35: 2434–2439.
21. Clarke P, Mann J, Simpson JF, Rickard-Dickson K, Primus FJ (1998) Mice transgenic for human carcinoembryonic antigen as a model for immunotherapy. Cancer Res 58: 1469–1477.
22. Boll H, Nittka S, Doyon F, Neumaier M, Marx A, et al. (2011) Micro-CT based experimental liver imaging using a nanoparticulate contrast agent: a longitudinal study in mice. PloS one 6: e25692.
23. Boll H, Bag S, Schambach SJ, Doyon F, Nittka S, et al. (2010) High-speed single-breath-hold micro-computed tomography of thoracic and abdominal structures in mice using a simplified method for intubation. Journal of computer assisted tomography 34: 783–790.
24. Lin Yc SD, Juselius J, Cui LF, Li X, Zhai H-J, Wang LS (2006) Experimental and computational studies of alkali-metal coinage-metal clusters. J Phys Chem A 110: 4244–4250.
25. McCarthy DW, Shefer RE, Klinkowstein RE, Bass LA, Margeneau WH, et al. (1997) Efficient production of high specific activity 64Cu using a biomedical cyclotron. Nucl Med Biol 24: 35–43.
26. Vavere AL, Butch ER, Dearling JL, Packard AB, Navid F, et al. (2012) 64Cu-p-NH2-Bn-DOTA-hu14.18K322A, a PET radiotracer targeting neuroblastoma and melanoma. J Nucl Med 53: 1772–1778.
27. Anderson CJ, Wadas TJ, Wong EH, Weisman GR (2008) Cross-bridged macrocyclic chelators for stable complexation of copper radionuclides for PET imaging. Q J Nucl Med Mol Imaging 52: 185–192.
28. Zhang Y, Hong H, Engle JW, Bean J, Yang Y, et al. (2011) Positron emission tomography imaging of CD105 expression with a 64Cu-labeled monoclonal antibody: NOTA is superior to DOTA. PLoS One 6: e28005.
29. Ferdani R, Stigers DJ, Fiamengo AL, Wei L, Li BT, et al. (2012) Synthesis, Cu(II) complexation, 64Cu-labeling and biological evaluation of cross-bridged cyclam chelators with phosphonate pendant arms. Dalton Trans 41: 1938–1950.
30. Zeng D, Ouyang Q, Cai Z, Xie XQ, Anderson CJ (2014) New cross-bridged cyclam derivative CB-TE1K1P, an improved bifunctional chelator for copper radionuclides. Chem Commun (Camb) 50: 43–45.
31. Wu AM, Yazaki PJ, Tsai S, Nguyen K, Anderson AL, et al. (2000) High-resolution microPET imaging of carcinoembryonic antigen-positive xenografts by using a copper-64-labeled engineered antibody fragment. Proc Natl Acad Sci U S A 97: 8495–8500.
32. Chakravarty R, Goel S, Cai W (2014) Nanobody: the "magic bullet" for molecular imaging? Theranostics 4: 386–398.
33. Yazaki PJ, Sherman Ma, Shively JE, Ikle D, Williams LE, et al. (2004) Humanization of the anti-CEA T84.66 antibody based on crystal structure data. Protein engineering, design & selection: PEDS 17: 481–489.
34. Hu S, Shively L, Raubitschek A, Sherman M, Williams LE, et al. (1996) Minibody: A novel engineered anti-carcinoembryonic antigen antibody fragment (single-chain Fv-CH3) which exhibits rapid, high-level targeting of xenografts. Cancer Res 56: 3055–3061.
35. Hand PH, Robbins PF, Salgaller ML, Poole DJ, Schlom J (1993) Evaluation of human carcinoembryonic-antigen (CEA)-transduced and non-transduced murine tumors as potential targets for anti-CEA therapies. Cancer Immunol Immunother 36: 65–75.
36. Heine M, Freund B, Nielsen P, Jung C, Reimer R, et al. (2012) High interstitial fluid pressure is associated with low tumour penetration of diagnostic monoclonal antibodies applied for molecular imaging purposes. PloS one 7: e36258.
37. Fujimori K, Covell DG, Fletcher JE, Weinstein JN (1989) Modeling analysis of the global and microscopic distribution of immunoglobulin G, F(ab')2, and Fab in tumors. Cancer Research 49: 5656–5663.

15

Facilitating Surveillance of Pulmonary Invasive Mold Diseases in Patients with Haematological Malignancies by Screening Computed Tomography Reports Using Natural Language Processing

Michelle R. Ananda-Rajah[1]*, David Martinez[2], Monica A. Slavin[3,4], Lawrence Cavedon[5], Michael Dooley[6,7], Allen Cheng[1,8], Karin A. Thursky[3,4]

1 Infectious Diseases Unit, Alfred Health, Melbourne, Victoria, Australia, 2 Computing and Information Systems, University of Melbourne, Melbourne, Victoria, Australia, 3 Victorian Infectious Diseases Service, Peter Doherty Centre, Melbourne, Victoria, Australia, 4 Infectious diseases department, Peter MacCallum Cancer Institute, Melbourne, Victoria, Australia, 5 School of Computer Science and IT, RMIT University, Melbourne, Victoria, Australia, 6 Pharmacy Department, Alfred Health, Melbourne, Victoria, Australia, 7 Faculty of Pharmacy & Pharmaceutical Science, Monash University, Melbourne, Victoria, Australia, 8 Department of Epidemiology and Preventative Medicine, Monash University, Melbourne, Victoria, Australia

Abstract

Purpose: Prospective surveillance of invasive mold diseases (IMDs) in haematology patients should be standard of care but is hampered by the absence of a reliable laboratory prompt and the difficulty of manual surveillance. We used a high throughput technology, natural language processing (NLP), to develop a classifier based on machine learning techniques to screen computed tomography (CT) reports supportive for IMDs.

Patients and Methods: We conducted a retrospective case-control study of CT reports from the clinical encounter and up to 12-weeks after, from a random subset of 79 of 270 case patients with 33 probable/proven IMDs by international definitions, and 68 of 257 uninfected-control patients identified from 3 tertiary haematology centres. The classifier was trained and tested on a reference standard of 449 physician annotated reports including a development subset (n = 366), from a total of 1880 reports, using 10-fold cross validation, comparing binary and probabilistic predictions to the reference standard to generate sensitivity, specificity and area under the receiver-operating-curve (ROC).

Results: For the development subset, sensitivity/specificity was 91% (95%CI 86% to 94%)/79% (95%CI 71% to 84%) and ROC area was 0.92 (95%CI 89% to 94%). Of 25 (5.6%) missed notifications, only 4 (0.9%) reports were regarded as clinically significant.

Conclusion: CT reports are a readily available and timely resource that may be exploited by NLP to facilitate continuous prospective IMD surveillance with translational benefits beyond surveillance alone.

Editor: Rossella Rota, Ospedale Pediatrico Bambino Gesu', Italy

Funding: This study was supported by the National Health and Medical Research Council (NHMRC) post-graduate medical scholarship to MAR, and AC is funded by a NHMRC Career Development Fellowship. The funders had no role in study design, data collection and analysis, decision to publish, or preparation of the manuscript.

Competing Interests: The authors have declared that no competing interests exist. There is no patent applicable to the classifier.

* Email: m.ananda-rajah@alfred.org.au

Introduction

Despite the high health and economic burden [1] of invasive mold diseases (IMDs) and effort invested in preventing them, prospective continuous epidemiological surveillance as advocated by professional societies and practice guidelines [2–4] is rarely performed. Prospective epidemiological surveillance in routine practice [5] is an onerous and costly task for hospitals principally because IMDs lack an easily identifiable and consistent laboratory prompt such as a positive blood culture. Case finding, like

diagnosis, relies on a constellation of findings from clinical review in conjunction with radiology and microbiology with adjudication by experts using complicated case definitions [6] making it a time-consuming and therefore costly exercise that is not widely performed outside research protocols [7–10].

For surveillance in general, the primary screening method should have a high sensitivity in order to minimise the burden of case finding while maximising case capture. However, for epidemiological surveillance of IMDs the ideal screening method is undefined. Laboratory-based surveillance is subject to significant underreporting because IMDs may be diagnosed with or without microbiological confirmation corresponding to probable/proven and possible categories respectively [6]. Indeed possible infections may predominate in some settings [11–13] due to the difficulties in establishing a microbiological diagnosis given that conventional microbiology for *Aspergillus* and hyaline molds is positive in 50% or fewer of cases [14] and patient acuity often contraindicates invasive diagnostic procedures. Microbiological confirmation is further hampered by the fact that non-culture based tests (NCBTs) such as galactomannan (GM) or polymerase chain reaction (PCR) are not widely available and have a suboptimal sensitivity [15,16] which is further compromised by concomitant antifungal therapy administered for either treatment or prophylaxis [17]. Administrative data such as coding diagnoses is unreliable for IMD surveillance [18] and neither timely nor informative enough for outbreak detection. In practice, no single method will be adequate for epidemiological surveillance of IMDs and complete case capture will require, the pooling of data from multiple sources [7,8,18]. However, the combination of laboratory based data with clinical or bed-side surveillance to best characterize total disease burden is not feasible for many centers to perform in real-time as it is a labour and time intensive task.

Although the optimal screening method for epidemiological surveillance of IMDs is undefined, the high frequency of pulmonary involvement makes chest computed tomography (CT) imaging an attractive target for screening. Chest CT is routinely performed when IMD is suspected as it is a non-invasive test that is widely available with results reported within hours rather than days and pulmonary involvement is present in 90% to 100% of patients with IA [7,8,10]. Although lung sampling and other laboratory indicators could be used for epidemiological surveillance and may upgrade possible cases to probable/proven categories they are not performed with the same frequency of CT. The major shortcomings of CT, however, are its poor specificity for IMDs [19] and extracting meaning from free-text reports.

We hypothesized that epidemiological surveillance of IMDs that is cost-effective and sustainable could be facilitated by technology. Natural language processing (NLP) is a computational method of analyzing human language that has detected several medical conditions [20–24] from the wealth of unstructured data in hospitals, with an accuracy comparable to human interpretation [24–26]. We developed a classifier that uses NLP based on machine learning techniques, to flag suspicious CT reports performed during routine clinical practice as a means of facilitating prospective IMD epidemiological surveillance in hospitals.

Methods

Study Design and Setting

This was a retrospective case-control cohort study of patients from three tertiary adult university-affiliated hospitals (Alfred Health, AH; Peter MacCallum Cancer Institute, PM; Royal Melbourne Hospital, RMH). AH and RMH operate statewide haematopoietic stem cell transplant (HSCT) services which collectively perform approximately100 allogeneic transplants/ year. De-identified patient records were used and the human research ethics committees at each site who granted permission for the study, waived patient consent.

Inclusion and Exclusion Criteria

Case and uninfected control patients from 2003 to 2011 inclusive were identified from previously completed clinical mycology studies [1,12,27,28] (Ananda-Rajah et. al. Unpublished

work: Prophylactic Effectiveness & Safety Of Intermittent Liposomal Amphotericin In High Risk Haematological Patients Abstract no M-280 51st Interscience Conference on Antimicrobial Agents and Chemotherapy ASM, Chicago 2011) pharmacy dispensing records, antimicrobial stewardship, HSCT, infectious diseases databases and microbiology records. Patients lacking CT scan reports were excluded, as were exclusively brain scans in order to focus detection of sino-pulmonary disease. Because detection of IMDs was the intent, patients with isolated candidaemia were excluded as laboratory-based surveillance is suitable for this infection.

Clinical Data and Definitions

CT reports from haematology/HSCT patients with (i.e. cases) and without IMDs (i.e. controls) were manually downloaded from each hospital as de-identified text files. CT reports, from performance of the diagnostic scan and for 12 weeks thereafter (in order to evaluate radiological progression) performed during the clinical encounter were included. The clinical encounter was defined from admission to either discharge, death or transfer. Clinical information was extracted from aforementioned study datasets and hospital records. IMDs were classified according to consensus definitions by expert reviewers [6]. Date of diagnosis was defined as the first day of suspicious radiological abnormality for possible cases or for probable/proven cases, a positive microbiological or histopathological test.

Development of the Reference Standard

A randomly selected convenience subset of reports from case and control patients were annotated at sentence and scan level by three infectious diseases physicians (MAR, KT, MS). The primary reviewer (MAR) annotated all case and control reports. Secondary review of case reports was undertaken by two physicians (KT, MS). The secondary reviewers served to validate the primary reviewer's analysis through measures of agreement. Pre-specified annotation guidelines were refined with differences in opinion resolved by discussion at face-to-face meetings. An iterative process of annotation ensued with reports from case patients annotated twice or three times over, while those from control patients (from the outset regarded as less challenging to interpret) were annotated once by the primary reviewer (MAR).

For annotation, each sentence within a report and each report was treated as an independent observation, meaning that for sentence level annotation, sentences rather than specific words were coded according to the following contextual features: specificity for IMD (specific vs non-specific features e.g. macro-nodules, halo vs. infiltrates, ground-glass, consolidation); certainty (suggestive, equivocal or not supportive of IMD); directionality/ change (negation, stable, resolution, progression); temporality (recent, past); alternative processes (e.g. pulmonary emboli, edema) and clinical alerts (i.e. urgent follow-up required). Scan level annotation referred to classification of the entire report as being either supportive or not for IMD with equivocal scans subsequently merged with supportive reports. Supportive reports had specific features of IMD including halo, nodule, cavity, focal mass, wedge-shaped lesions, bony sinus erosions. Negative reports had none of the above features while equivocal reports included infiltrate, consolidation, ground glass change, effusions or uncertainty by the reporting radiologist.

Importantly, the reference standard was informed by the opinion of clinician experts rather than radiologists given that the guiding principle was to flag reports of concern to end-users irrespective of the final diagnostic outcome.

Table 1. Characteristics of patients with and without invasive mold diseases (IMDs).

Characteristic	IMD group n (%)	Control group n (%)
No. of patients	79	68
No. of clinical encounters[1]	79 (51)	75 (49)
Male gender	48 (61)	35 (51)
Age, mean (range) years	53 (20–89)	51 (18–89)
Underlying disease		
AML	32 (41)	35 (51)
ALL	14 (18)	14 (19)
Lymphoma	15 (19)	12 (16)
Chronic leukaemia	7 (8.9)	1 (1.3)
MDS/transformed MDS	6 (7.6)	2 (2.7)
Multiple myeloma	3 (3.8)	3 (4)
Other	2 (2.5)	5 (6.7)
Neutropenia (≤0.5 cells/L) present	65 (82)	56 (75)
Median duration of neutropenia (IQR), days	18 (8–45)	19 (5–39)
HSCT	36 (46)	39 (52)
Allogeneic	31/36 (86)	30/39 (77)
Autologous	5/36 (14)	9/39 (23)
Characteristics of IMDs, n = 79		NA
Probable/proven IMDs	33 (42)	
Possible IMDs	46 (58)	
Site of infection		
Lung	67 (85)	
Sino-pulmonary	3 (3.8)	
Sinus	2 (2.5)	
Hepatosplenic	2 (2.5)	
Disseminated	4 (5.1)	
Organism		
Aspergillus fumigatus	13	
Non-fumigatus *Aspergillus* species (*A. niger, A. flavus*)	4	
Fungal hyphae resembling *Aspergillus* species	3	
Scedosporium species	4	
Any positive PCR	2	
Rhizopus species	4	
Other molds (*Acrophialophora fusispora, Paecilomyces lilacinus*)	2	
Candida glabrata (co-infection with *S. Prolificans* fungaemia)	1	

Abbreviations: AML, acute myeloid leukemia; ALL, acute lymphoblastic leukemia; MDS, myelodysplastic syndrome; IQR, inter-quartile range; HSCT, haematopoietic stem cell transplant.
[1]Clinical encounter defined from admission to either discharge, death or transfer and for up to 12-weeks after where applicable.

Development of the Classifier

Reports were classified in a binary fashion as being supportive or not supportive of IMD (i.e. positive/negative). A multi-class classification approach at sentence level was used: each sentence allocated one of a number of classes, with all sentence-level classifications subsequently informing the report level decision.

Text was analyzed as groups of words ("bag-of-words"), phrases ("bag-of-phrases") and concepts ("bag-of-concepts") [29] which were extracted from the annotated reports. The bag-of-words framework collates unordered sets of words, mapping dates and numbers to date and number features respectively. The bag-of-phrases framework uses phrases identified by MetaMap [29]

corresponding to concepts from the Unified Medical Language System (UMLS) Metathesaurus. The version of MetaMap employed leverages the Negex tool [30] to determine negation of a concept (e.g., "… is not consistent with …"). The bag-of-concepts framework used Metathesaurus concepts mapped by MetaMap, noting that multiple phrases may map to the same concept.

We adopted a supervised machine learning approach experimenting with several machine learning algorithms including Support Vector Machines (SVM), Naïve Bayes, Random Forests, and Bayesian Nets, as implemented in the Weka 3.6.0 [31] and LibSVM 3.11 [32] toolkits. Briefly, supervised machine learning is a group of computational methods which use algorithms to

Table 2. Characteristics of the physician expert annotated and unannotated reports.

Characteristic	Annotated reports n (%)	Unannotated reports n (%)
No. of reports	449	1431
Held-out reports[1]	83 (18)	NA
No. of patients total	147	380
No. of IMD patients	79	191
No. reports from IMD patients	294 (65)	905 (63)
No. reports from control patients	155 (35)	526
Chest (alone or in combination with sinus, abdo/pelvis, brain etc)	375 (84)	865 (60)
Sinus (alone or brain-sinus, orbits, abdo/pelvis)	38 (8.5)	44
Other (abdo, abdo pelvis, liver, aorta, neck)	36 (8.0)	408
No. of reports according to study site		
Hospital A	226 (50)	713
Hospital B	131 (29)	422
Hospital C	92 (20)	296
No. of words per report according to study site		
Hospital A	211	229
Hospital B	126	128
Hospital C	314	348

Abbreviation: IMD, invasive mold disease.
[1]Held out reports were annotated at scan level only as being supportive, unequivocal or negative for IMD.

automatically construct a model from labeled/annotated training data that is then used to predict classification in unseen/unlabeled examples [33]. Of the algorithms tested, SVM performed best and was selected for the final classifier.

Physician annotated reports were divided into development (n = 366) and held-out sets (n = 83), the latter annotated at scan level only. We used 10-fold cross validation on the development set with the optimal classifier identified from experiments, tested against the held-out set which served as an additional validation step. Cross-validation is an accepted method within the machine learning domain that maximizes limited gold standard data while minimizing the risk of overfitting associated with training on the test set [34].

Statistical Analysis

The results of each manually annotated report was compared to the binary and probabilistic predictions of the classifier allowing calculation of sensitivity, specificity and receiver operating curve (ROC).

Hypothetical IMD prevalence rates of 5%, 10% and 20% were used to estimate positive and negative predictive values (PPV, NPV). Inter-annotator agreement was assessed using Cohen's

kappa coefficient, a chance corrected index of agreement [35]. All analyses used Stata 11.0 software (Stata Corp, College Station, Texas, USA).

Results

Patient Characteristics

A total of 147 patients were included in the annotated subset of 449 reports; 79 (54%) had IMDs and 68 (46%) were control patients (Table 1). Neutropenia ($\leq 0.5 \times 10^9$ cells/L) was present in 82% and 75% of clinical encounters among case and control patients respectively and was prolonged (median 18 and 19 days respectively). A history of HSCT was present in 46% and 52% of case and control patients, being allogeneic in 86% and 77% of patients respectively.

IMDs were probable/proven in 33/79 (42%) and possible infections in 46/79 (58%). Sinus and/or pulmonary disease occurred in 91% of case-patients. IA comprised 20/33 (61%) of microbiologically confirmed cases with rare molds including *Scedosporium* and *Rhizopus* species identified in 10/33 (30%).

Table 3. Performance characteristics of the classifier.

Characteristic	TP	FP	TN	FN	Sn, % (95%CI)	Sp, % (95%CI)
Development dataset, reports n = 366	197	32	117	20	91 (86 to 94)	79 (71 to 84)
[1]Held-out dataset, reports n = 83	35	13	30	5	88 (74 to 95)	70 (55 to 81)
All reports, n = 449	232	45	147	25	90 (86 to 93)	77 (70 to 82)

[1]Held out dataset were annotated at report level only as being positive, negative or equivocal for IMD.
Abbreviations: TN, true positives; FP, false positives; TN, true negatives; FN, false negatives; Sn, sensitivity; Sp, specificity; CI, confidence interval.

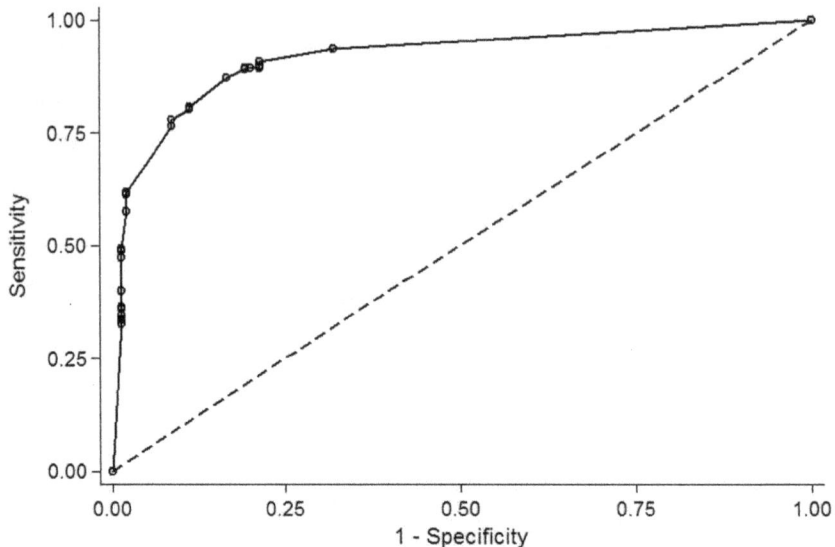

Figure 1. Receiver operating characteristic (ROC) curve for 321 inpatient reports comparing the probabilistic output of the classifier to expert opinion. Area under the ROC curve = 0.90 (95%CI 0.86 to 0.93). Abbreviation: CI, confidence interval.

Characteristics of the Dataset of CT Reports

Overall, 1880 reports were retrieved from 527 patients (51% with IMDs) (Table 2). A total of 7083 sentences were annotated at sentence level according to pre-defined contextual features. Mean report length per hospital was 314, 211 and 126 words reflecting inter-institutional variations in reporting styles. Hospital A supplied 50% of annotated reports. The annotated dataset predominantly comprised chest 375/449 (84%) and sinus scans (alone or in combination with other sites) 28/449 (8.5%). In the annotated subset, there were 10 reports from 5 outpatients, all of who were control patients not subsequently diagnosed with IMD.

Inter-annotator agreement between primary reviewer and the two secondary reviewers combined, was fair at sentence level for distinguishing certainty from equivocal/negative labels (K = 0.64) but improved at report level for the same classification (0.83) given that K levels ≥0.75 represent excellent agreement [35].

Performance of the Classifier

Classifier performance among development and held-out sets respectively, was as follows (Table 3): sensitivity (i.e. concordance between classifier and physician annotation for reports supportive of IMD) was 91% (95%CI 86% to 94%)/88% (95%CI 74% to 95%); specificity was 79% (95%CI 71% to 84%)/70% (95%CI 55% to 81%); false negative rates were 20/366 (9.2%) and 5/83 (12.5%). The area under the ROC for the development set was 0.92 (95%CI 0.89 to 0.94) and 0.90 (95%CI 0.86 to 0.93) for the inpatient subset (n = 321) only (Figure 1). For the inpatient subset, sensitivity was 85% (95% CI 79% to 90%) and specificity was 86% (95% CI 81% to 93%). Using a sensitivity of 90% and specificity of 77% from the entire dataset of 449 reports at IMD prevalence's of 5%, 10%, 20%, estimated PPVs were 17%, 30%, 49% and NPVs were 99%, 99%, 97%.

Error Analysis

Of the 25 missed cases (false negatives), 4 (4/449, 0.9%) were significant as shown in Figure 2. Reports from patients subsequently not diagnosed with IMD were disregarded (n = 10). The remaining 15 reports from case-patients comprised 10 inpatient reports including 6 progress reports whose antecedents were

appropriately flagged. Five scans from case patients performed outside admission were follow up scans that provided information on clinical progress. Among the 4 significant missed notifications, one was a sinus scan in combination with a chest scan, the latter being flagged appropriately.

Review of 45 false positive reports revealed several sources of systematic error described in Table 4. Unsystematic errors were the result of three reports inappropriately annotated negative, two with sinus mucosal thickening and one describing ground glass pulmonary changes with a fungal aetiology entertained by the radiologist.

Discussion

Mold infections are not well suited to prospective detection using manual methods of epidemiological surveillance due to the absence of an easily identifiable electronic prompt but may be rendered amenable to real-time detection using NLP of CT reports. Our classifier flagged reports suggestive of IMD from a variety of anatomic sites but overwhelmingly the sino-pulmonary tract (92%), the site most commonly involved by IA [8,10,36], achieving a sensitivity in the development subset, of 91% (95%CI 86% to 94%), specificity of 79% (95%CI 71% to 84%) and good overall accuracy with an area under the ROC of 0.92 [37]. Performance of the classifier was validated two ways, by cross-validation of development data in addition to held-out data, importantly with both methods using unseen data and producing similar findings (Table 3), lending robustness to the results.

For screening purposes, sensitivity is favoured over specificity especially for uncommon events like IMDs because missed cases are less tolerable than the resources spent following up false notifications [23]. The 25/449 (5.6%) missed notifications occurred at the expense of a modest number of false positive reports (45/449, 10%). Inpatient reports took precedence over the few outpatient reports given the higher clinical acuity of inpatients and the remote but real risk of nosocomial acquisition, resulting in a few missed notifications from case patients regarded as clinically significant (0.9%). False notifications were expected as the classifier was tuned for sensitivity, with inclusion of reports annotated

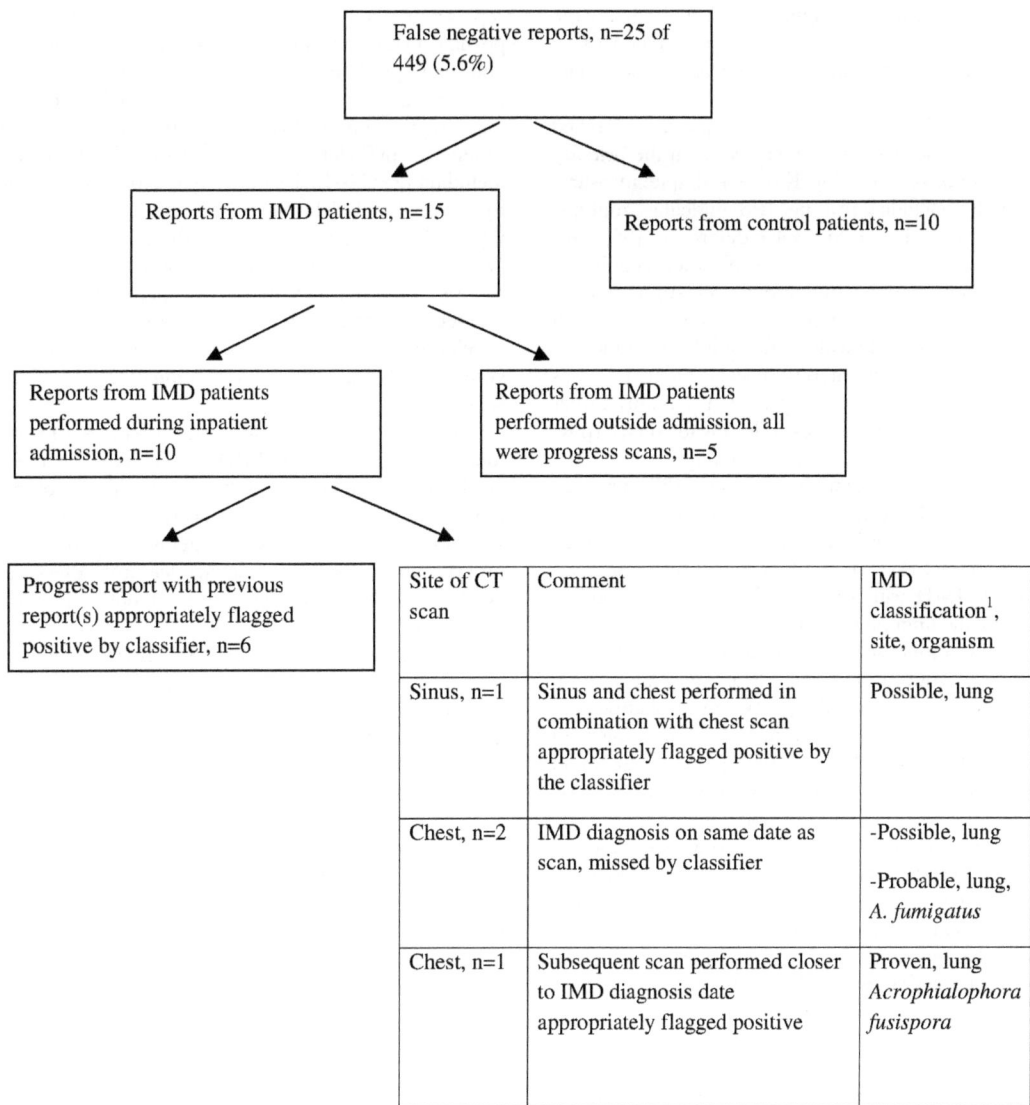

Figure 2. Error analysis of reports annotated supportive for invasive mold disease (IMD) but missed by the classifier. Abbreviations: CT, computed tomography.

Table 4. Major systematic errors in the false notifications (false positives) for invasive mold diseases among computed tomography reports by the classifier.

Reason for misinterpretation	No. of reports	Characteristics
Inconsequential nodules	10	<1 cm nodules, granulomas
Abdominal scans	9	Non-specific hepatic or splenic lesions
Progress scans	9	Change in lesions rather than diagnosis the focus, therefore reports annotated negative by experts
Non-specific pulmonary/thoracic lesion	8	Atelectasis, scarring, mediastinal neoplastic mass
Misclassification	3	Pulmonary oedema, septic emboli, pulmonary lesions consistent with graft versus host disease

equivocal included in the positive training bucket. Accordingly the classifier, like the physician annotators, was not designed to be conservative, assigning a positive label if there was any possibility of IMD.

In the absence of a gold standard for IMD reporting we relied upon peer review. Sentence level agreement between the primary and secondary annotator pair was fair (K = 0.64) despite measures mitigating unreliability including pre-specified guidelines, multiple experts and repeated consultation to resolve differences [35]. Our inter-annotator agreement is consistent with other cognitively challenging tasks such as ascribing pneumonia [38–40] or central-line associated blood stream infection [21] because deciding if clinical narratives are compatible with these complex conditions is sometimes difficult. Importantly, at report level, agreement was excellent (K = 0.83), noting that this endpoint (i.e. report rather than sentence level classification) is most relevant for the purpose of real-time surveillance or clinical decision support.

Our classifier has several limitations. Its poor PPV was not unexpected as PPV is highly conditional upon disease prevalence and, for uncommon events like IMDs, will be low despite a high sensitivity, as we observed [41]. High NPVs meant that a negative result could exclude IMD with some confidence. False notifications could potentially undermine confidence in a surveillance system and may be minimised (i.e. improving specificity) by including adjunctive sources of data (e.g. antifungal drug dispensing, microbiology) or by raising pre-test probability by filtering reports [41] based on clinical context (a clinical query of fever for example). It is possible but unlikely that changes in clinical practice over the long observational period of the study may have affected the radiological manifestations of IMD. The opinion of expert physicians rather than radiologists informed development of the classifier. However, these are the end users whose clinical acumen we sought to emulate and for similar syndromes such as pneumonia, albeit in chest radiograph reports, clinicians have demonstrated comparable performance to radiologists [25]. Annotation was unblinded, but informed by annotation guidelines that were developed in an iterative process. No conclusions can be drawn regarding classifier performance for subgroups with small numbers of reports such as sinus disease or hepatosplenic candidiasis. We confined ourselves to haematology-oncology population as this group is at highest risk for IMD [8,42] and thus our findings may not be generalizable to other risk groups.

Further improvements in specificity may be achieved by omitting progress reports given their overrepresentation among false notifications. Experts often annotated progress reports negative because diagnostic radiological features may not always be re-iterated in a progress report. Non-specific pulmonary lesions such as atelectasis or scarring could be disregarded with the creation of handcrafted rules. Pulmonary nodules of questionable significance are more challenging to address, as size of lesions was not taken into account by the classifier. The development dataset did not exclusively comprise proven/probable-IMDs (despite these

representing a higher degree of certainty) for several reasons: possible IMDs constitute a substantial burden in clinical practice and may predominate (up to 90%) in some centres [11,12]; possible IMDs consume similar health-care resources (e.g. diagnostics, antifungal drugs) and their exclusion would underestimate true prevalence. Notably, all cases in our reference standard including possible-IMDs underwent expert adjudication according to international definitions [6]. Although we used a sample of reports from the entire dataset, the narrow confidence intervals around overall performance measures suggests that additional reports would not have made an appreciable difference. Finally, a dataset enriched with positive cases was used for classifier development yielding results acceptable for subsequent human verification but prospective validation of the classifier in the field is required.

The classifier is not a diagnostic adjunct but rather a screening tool designed to facilitate IMD case finding by exploiting routinely available clinical data [5,7,10]. The classifier's strengths include its multi-site derivation; machine learning algorithms which unlike rule or knowledge based systems do not require manual programming of specific language features [43,44] and consistency, by avoiding subjective interpretations of complicated case definitions [6].

Epidemiological surveillance for IMDs is needed for many reasons, including antifungal stewardship [45], clinical trial design, clinical audit, clinical registry development, intra and inter-facility comparisons. However, it is rarely performed in routine clinical practice, partly due to a lack of validated tools. Traditionally most IMD surveillance has relied on microbiological/histological diagnoses (which are not sensitive) with or without the addition of clinical diagnoses (which lack specificity). The intention of the classifier is to improve sensitivity i.e. case finding, with the advantage of early detection. This classifier is an additional tool to be used in combination with other methods to enable comprehensive surveillance of IMDs to be performed with minimal additional effort.

Acknowledgments

The authors thank Dr Orla Morrissey for her assistance in identifying study participants and Dr Tim Spelman for his statistical contribution.

Contributions by DM and LC were while employed at National Information and Communication Technology Australia (NICTA). NICTA is funded by the Australian Government as represented by the Department of Broadband, Communications and the Digital Economy and the Australian Research Council through the ICT Centre of Excellence program.

Author Contributions

Conceived and designed the experiments: MAR DM LC AC MS KT. Performed the experiments: MAR DM LC KT MS. Analyzed the data: MAR DM LC AC KT MS MD. Contributed reagents/materials/analysis tools: MD AC MAR MS KT LC. Wrote the paper: MAR DM AC LC KT MS MD.

References

1. Ananda-Rajah MR, Cheng A, Morrissey CO, Spelman T, Dooley M, et al. (2011) Attributable hospital cost and antifungal treatment of invasive fungal diseases in high-risk hematology patients: an economic modeling approach. Antimicrob Agents Chemother 55: 1953–1960.

2. Guidelines on the management of invasive fungal infection during therapy for haematological malignancy. Writing Group of the British Committee on Standards in Haematology (2008) Available at: www.bcshguidelines.com/. Accessed 2013 January 16.

3. Tomblyn M, Chiller T, Einsele H, Gress R, Sepkowitz K, et al. (2009) Guidelines for preventing infectious complications among hematopoietic cell

transplantation recipients: a global perspective. Biol Blood Marrow Transplant 15: 1143–1238.

4. Yokoe D, Casper C, Dubberke E, Lee G, Munoz P, et al. (2009) Infection prevention and control in health-care facilities in which hematopoietic cell transplant recipients are treated. Bone Marrow Transplant 44: 495–507.

5. Fourneret-Vivier A, Lebeau B, Mallaret MR, Brenier-Pinchart MP, Brion JP, et al. (2006) Hospital-wide prospective mandatory surveillance of invasive aspergillosis in a French teaching hospital (2000–2002). J Hosp Infect 62: 22–28.

6. De Pauw B, Walsh TJ, Donnelly JP, Stevens DA, Edwards JE, et al. (2008) Revised definitions of invasive fungal disease from the European Organization for Research and Treatment of Cancer/Invasive Fungal Infections Cooperative

Group and the National Institute of Allergy and Infectious Diseases Mycoses Study Group (EORTC/MSG) Consensus Group. Clin Infect Dis 46: 1813–1821.

7. Kontoyiannis DP, Marr KA, Park BJ, Alexander BD, Anaissie EJ, et al. (2010) Prospective surveillance for invasive fungal infections in hematopoietic stem cell transplant recipients, 2001–2006: overview of the Transplant-Associated Infection Surveillance Network (TRANSNET) Database. Clin Infect Dis 50: 1091–1100.

8. Lortholary O, Gangneux JP, Sitbon K, Lebeau B, de Monbrison F, et al. (2011) Epidemiological trends in invasive aspergillosis in France: the SAIF network (2005–2007). Clin Microbiol Infect 17: 1882–1889.

9. Steinbach WJ, Marr KA, Anaissie EJ, Azie N, Quan SP, et al. (2012) Clinical epidemiology of 960 patients with invasive aspergillosis from the PATH Alliance registry. J Infect 65: 453–464.

10. Nicolle MC, Benet T, Thiebaut A, Bienvenu AL, Voirin N, et al. (2011) Invasive aspergillosis in patients with hematologic malignancies: incidence and description of 127 cases enrolled in a single institution prospective survey from 2004 to 2009. Haematologica 96: 1685–1691.

11. Neofytos D, Treadway S, Ostrander D, Alonso CD, Dierberg KL, et al. (2013) Epidemiology, outcomes, and mortality predictors of invasive mold infections among transplant recipients: a 10-year, single-center experience. Transpl Infect Dis 15: 233–242.

12. Ananda-Rajah MR, Grigg A, Downey MT, Bajel A, Spelman T, et al. (2012) Comparative clinical effectiveness of prophylactic voriconazole/posaconazole to fluconazole/itraconazole in patients with acute myeloid leukemia/myelodysplastic syndrome undergoing cytotoxic chemotherapy over a 12-year period. Haematologica 97: 459–463.

13. Pagano L, Caira M, Candoni A, Aversa F, Castagnola C, et al. (2012) Evaluation of the practice of antifungal prophylaxis use in patients with newly diagnosed acute myeloid leukemia: results from the SEIFEM 2010-B registry. Clin Infect Dis 55: 1515–1521.

14. Denning DW (2000) Early diagnosis of invasive aspergillosis. Lancet 355: 423–424.

15. Mengoli C, Cruciani M, Barnes RA, Loeffler J, Donnelly JP (2009) Use of PCR for diagnosis of invasive aspergillosis: systematic review and meta-analysis. Lancet Infect Dis 9: 89–96.

16. Pfeiffer CD, Fine JP, Safdar N (2006) Diagnosis of invasive aspergillosis using a galactomannan assay: a meta-analysis. Clin Infect Dis 42: 1417–1427.

17. Maertens J, Groll AH, Cordonnier C, de la Cámara R, Roilides E, et al. (2011) Treatment and timing in invasive mould disease. Journal of Antimicrobial Chemotherapy 66: i37–i43.

18. Chang DC, Burwell LA, Lyon GM, Pappas PG, Chiller TM, et al. (2008) Comparison of the use of administrative data and an active system for surveillance of invasive aspergillosis. Infect Control Hosp Epidemiol 29: 25–30.

19. Marom EM, Kontoyiannis DP (2011) Imaging studies for diagnosing invasive fungal pneumonia in immunocompromised patients. Curr Opin Infect Dis 24: 309–314.

20. Elkin PL, Froehling D, Wahner-Roedler D, Trusko B, Welsh G, et al. (2008) NLP-based identification of pneumonia cases from free-text radiological reports. AMIA Annu Symp Proc: 172–176.

21. Hota B, Lin M, Doherty JA, Borlawsky T, Woeltje K, et al. (2009) Formulation of a model for automating infection surveillance: algorithmic detection of central-line associated bloodstream infection. J Am Med Inform Assoc 17: 42–48.

22. Hazlehurst B, Naleway A, Mullooly J (2009) Detecting possible vaccine adverse events in clinical notes of the electronic medical record. Vaccine 27: 2077–2083.

23. Elkin PL, Froehling DA, Wahner-Roedler DL, Brown SH, Bailey KR (2012) Comparison of natural language processing biosurveillance methods for identifying influenza from encounter notes. Ann Intern Med 156: 11–18.

24. Murff HJ, FitzHenry F, Matheny ME, Gentry N, Kotter KL, et al. (2011) Automated identification of postoperative complications within an electronic medical record using natural language processing. JAMA 306: 848–855.

25. Hripcsak G, Friedman C, Alderson PO, DuMouchel W, Johnson SB, et al. (1995) Unlocking clinical data from narrative reports: a study of natural language processing. Ann Intern Med 122: 681–688.

26. Elkins JS, Friedman C, Boden-Albala B, Sacco RL, Hripcsak G (2000) Coding neuroradiology reports for the Northern Manhattan Stroke Study: a comparison of natural language processing and manual review. Comput Biomed Res 33: 1–10.

27. Cooley L, Spelman D, Thursky K, Slavin M (2007) Infection with Scedosporium apiospermum and S. prolificans, Australia. Emerg Infect Dis 13: 1170–1177.

28. Morrissey CO, Chen SC, Sorrell TC, Milliken S, Bardy PG, et al. (2013) Galactomannan and PCR versus culture and histology for directing use of antifungal treatment for invasive aspergillosis in high-risk haematology patients: a randomised controlled trial. Lancet Infect Dis 13: 519–528.

29. Aronson AR (2001) Effective mapping of biomedical text to the UMLS Metathesaurus: the MetaMap program. Proc AMIA Symp: 17–21.

30. Chapman WW, Bridewell W, Hanbury P, Cooper GF, Buchanan BG (2001) Evaluation of negation phrases in narrative clinical reports. Proc AMIA Symp: 105–109.

31. Frank E, Hall M, Trigg L, Holmes G, Witten IH (2004) Data mining in bioinformatics using Weka. Bioinformatics 20: 2479–2481.

32. LIBSVM A library for support vector machines at http://ntu.csie.org/~cjlin/papers/libsvm.pdf. Accessed 2012 January 6.

33. Cohen KB, Hunter L (2008) Getting started in text mining. PLoS Comput Biol 4: e20.

34. Stone M (1974) Cross-validation choice and assessment of statistical predictions (with Discussion). Journal of the Royal Statistical Society 36: 111–147.

35. Goldman RL (1992) The reliability of peer assessments of quality of care. JAMA 267: 958–960.

36. Pagano L, Caira M, Candoni A, Offidani M, Martino B, et al. (2010) Invasive aspergillosis in patients with acute myeloid leukemia: a SEIFEM-2008 registry study. Haematologica 95: 644–650.

37. Altman DG, Bland JM (1994) Diagnostic tests 3: receiver operating characteristic plots. BMJ 309: 188.

38. Hripcsak G, Kuperman GJ, Friedman C, Heitjan DF (1999) A reliability study for evaluating information extraction from radiology reports. J Am Med Inform Assoc 6: 143–150.

39. Fiszman M, Chapman WW, Aronsky D, Evans RS, Haug PJ (2000) Automatic detection of acute bacterial pneumonia from chest X-ray reports. J Am Med Inform Assoc 7: 593–604.

40. Haas JP, Mendonca EA, Ross B, Friedman C, Larson E (2005) Use of computerized surveillance to detect nosocomial pneumonia in neonatal intensive care unit patients. Am J Infect Control 33: 439–443.

41. McKnight LK, Wilcox A, Hripcsak G (2002) The effect of sample size and disease prevalence on supervised machine learning of narrative data. Proc AMIA Symp: 519–522.

42. Azie N, Neofytos D, Pfaller M, Meier-Kriesche HU, Quan SP, et al. (2012) The PATH (Prospective Antifungal Therapy) Alliance(R) registry and invasive fungal infections: update 2012. Diagn Microbiol Infect Dis 73: 293–300.

43. D'Avolio LW, Nguyen TM, Farwell WR, Chen Y, Fitzmeyer F, et al. (2009) Evaluation of a generalizable approach to clinical information retrieval using the automated retrieval console (ARC). J Am Med Inform Assoc 17: 375–382.

44. Wang Z, Shah AD, Tate AR, Denaxas S, Shawe-Taylor J, et al. (2012) Extracting diagnoses and investigation results from unstructured text in electronic health records by semi-supervised machine learning. PLoS One 7: e30412.

45. Ananda-Rajah MR, Slavin MA, Thursky KT (2012) The case for antifungal stewardship. Curr Opin Infect Dis 25: 107–115.

16

Nonlinear Dual Reconstruction of SPECT Activity and Attenuation Images

Huafeng Liu[1], Min Guo[1], Zhenghui Hu[1], Pengcheng Shi[2], Hongjie Hu[3]*

1 State Key Laboratory of Modern Optical Instrumentation, Department of Optical Engineering, Zhejiang University, Hangzhou, China, **2** B. Thomas Golisano College of Computing and Information Sciences, Rochester Institute of Technology, Rochester, New York, United States of America, **3** Department of Radiology, Sir Run Run Shaw Hospital, College of Medicine, Zhejiang University, Hangzhou, China

Abstract

In single photon emission computed tomography (SPECT), accurate attenuation maps are needed to perform essential attenuation compensation for high quality radioactivity estimation. Formulating the SPECT activity and attenuation reconstruction tasks as coupled signal estimation and system parameter identification problems, where the activity distribution and the attenuation parameter are treated as random variables with known prior statistics, we present a nonlinear dual reconstruction scheme based on the unscented Kalman filtering (UKF) principles. In this effort, the dynamic changes of the organ radioactivity distribution are described through state space evolution equations, while the photon-counting SPECT projection data are measured through the observation equations. Activity distribution is then estimated with sub-optimal fixed attenuation parameters, followed by attenuation map reconstruction given these activity estimates. Such coupled estimation processes are iteratively repeated as necessary until convergence. The results obtained from Monte Carlo simulated data, physical phantom, and real SPECT scans demonstrate the improved performance of the proposed method both from visual inspection of the images and a quantitative evaluation, compared to the widely used EM-ML algorithms. The dual estimation framework has the potential to be useful for estimating the attenuation map from emission data only and thus benefit the radioactivity reconstruction.

Editor: Mark G. Kuzyk, Washington State University, United States of America

Funding: This work was supported in part by the National Basic Research Program (2010CB732500, 2010CB732504), the National Natural Science Foundation of China (61271083), and the Natural Science Foundation of Zhejiang (R12F030004). The funders had no role in study design, data collection and analysis, decision to publish, or preparation of the manuscript.

Competing Interests: The authors have declared that no competing interests exist.

* Email: hongjiehu@zju.edu.cn

Introduction

Single photon emission computed tomography (SPECT) has become an indispensable tool in clinical trials and medical practice. Attenuation correction in SPECT has significant values to better understand the physiological processes associated with the disease (i.e. cancers, heart diseases) and to provide improvement in patient diagnosis and treatment. However, even with ample efforts devoted to the development of various attenuation estimation and compensation techniques, it remains one of the key open issues in SPECT imaging [1–11].

Tissue attenuation map is usually estimated based on transmission data by scanning the patient with a rotating external radionuclide source [3,5,6,12], or obtained from X-ray computed tomography (CT) system [10,11,13–16]. However, transmission based attenuation correction clearly increases the patient's dose, and requires maintaining additional radioactive sources. Further, if multiple imaging sessions are needed, it may be difficult for some patients to tolerate for a longer scan at one time, and leads to co-registration problem in emission image reconstruction, especially for deformed tissues and organs. In addition to the added

equipment cost and the well-known beam hardening problem, similar registration issue exists for CT attenuation data.

It has been the goal of many recent research efforts to simultaneously estimate the activity and attenuation distributions from emission data. Iterative statistical methods have been extensively studied, with the main incentive being that they explicitly take into account the specific SPECT data statistics. Some of the most notable works include the use of differential attenuation method [17], gradient ascent [18], Tikhonov regularization [19], and expectation maximization (EM) [20–23]. With the SPECT imaging and measurement processes in state space representation, a recent work has adopted the extended Kalman filtering (EKF) procedures to linearize the augmented state representation to provide the joint estimates in the minimum-mean-square-error sense [24]. Such EKF based framework, however, has several potential drawbacks. First, the derivation of the Jacobian matrices, the linear approximations to the nonlinear functions, often leads to filter instability. Furthermore, it has been shown that estimation bias may originate from a coupling between the state variables and the model parameters, which suggests that if the system parameters can be separated from the system state variables, the precision of the estimation could be improved.

Following the same spirit while addressing the limitations, we present a robust unscented Kalman filter framework for the joint estimation of SPECT activity and attenuation parameters. Instead of linearizing using the Jacobian matrices and thus overcoming the associated shortcomings, our effort deals with the nonlinear estimation process by using a deterministic sampling approach to capture the mean and covariance estimates [25]. In addition, two iteratively coupled filters are used to sequentially estimate the activity variables (with fixed attenuation estimates from the last iteration) and the attenuation map (with fixed activity values from the previous estimation). Furthermore, such framework can explicitly recognize the uncertainties in the measurement data and the model structure, thus has the potential to produce more robust reconstructions.

Materials and Methods

SPECT Emission Scan Model

In SPECT imaging, once radio-tracers are injected into the subjects, they are delivered to the tissues/organs by the blood flow and participate in the related physiologic/metabolic processes. The general mathematical model for the emission scan can be stated as

$$y(t) = Gx(t) + e_o \tag{1}$$

where column vector $x(t) = \{x_j | j = 1,...,N\}$ is the radiopharmaceutical concentration of the object, e_o is the background noises (e.g. scatter events), and y is the emission measurement data that is acquired by a rotating detector head around the patient at each angle and represented lexicographically as a column vector $y(t) = \{y_i | i = 1,...,M\}$. Here, i indicates different projection defined by rotating angle and different detector bin, and M is the total number of projections. G represents the emission system matrix including attenuation effects, and its element indicates the probability that a photon emitted from pixel gets detected in a specific detector bin.

Let the attenuation map be given by column vector $\mu = \{\mu_k | k = 1,...,N\}$, we may explicitly account for the attenuation effects in the system matrix G by factoring it as

$$G = (A \cdot D) = \left(e^{-[L\mu]} \cdot D \right) \tag{2}$$

Here, The symbol '·' means the dot product of two matrices. $[L]_{ijk} = l_{ijk}$ represents the length of the ray through voxel k with respect to a photon emitted from voxel i being detected in projection bin j. The photon survival probability considering attenuation can now be represented by a matrix A with elements $[A]_{ij} = a_{ij}$ as

$$a_{ij} = \exp\left(-\sum_k l_{ijk} \mu_k \right) \tag{3}$$

The term D, with elements $[D]_{ij} = d_{ij}$, is the photon-detection probability without taking into account the attenuation effects.

The mathematical model of the SPECT emission measurement (Eqn. (1)) can now be rewritten as

$$y = Gx + e_o = \left(e^{-[L\mu]} \cdot D \right) x + e_o \tag{4}$$

or in discrete form

$$y_i = \sum_j \left[\exp\left(-\sum_k l_{ijk} \mu_k \right) d_{ij} x_j \right] + e_o \tag{5}$$

In the following sections, we will present the dual estimation method which works by alternating between using the UKF state-filter to estimate the radioactivity based on fixed attenuation parameters, and the UKF parameter-filter to estimate the attenuation coefficients given previously estimated activity states. Although two separate state-space representations are constructed for the activity and attenuation estimation problems, both of them use the same emission scan model (Eqn. (4) or (5)) as the measurement equation.

Activity Estimation: UKF State Filter

State Space Representation for Radioactivity. In emission tomography, the goal is to reconstruct the radioactivity distribution $x(t)$ from the measurement data $y(t)$. The system equation of the SPECT imaging system, which describes the radioactivity evolution of the pixels, can be written in the form of

$$x(t+1) = Sx(t) + v_s \tag{6}$$

with initial activity x_0 and system noise v_s that accounts for the statistical uncertainty of the imaging model. In general, Eqn. (6) represents the dynamic changes of the state variable $x(t)$, and it reduces to the conventional static reconstruction problem when the transition matrix S is an identity. The associated measurement equation, which describes the observations provided by the imaging data $y(t)$, is given by Eqn. (4). And now we have the following state space representation for radioactivity distribution:

$$x(t+1) = x(t) + v_s \tag{7}$$

$$y(t) = G(\mu(t))x(t) + e_o = h(x(t), \mu(t)) + e_o \tag{8}$$

where v_s and e_o, with covariance matrices Q_s and R_o, model the uncertainties of the imaging system and the measurement data respectively.

Two important observations on the nonlinear SPECT imaging system represented by Eqns. (7) and (8). First, since the noises in emission sinogram are typically Poisson distributed, it is difficult to perform standard estimation on such non-Gaussian system. By applying the Anscombe transformation [26], however, the Poisson noise could be converted into a Gaussian one, and various Kalman filtering techniques become viable options. Secondly, the EKF, probably the most widely used estimation algorithm for nonlinear systems, has several drawbacks. EKF requires the system is almost linear on the time scale of the updates, and is difficult to implement and to set proper parameters due to the cross-talk between state and parameter. To overcome such limitations, we have adopted the unscented transformation (UT) to accurately propagate mean and covariance information through nonlinear transformations [25], with little additional computational cost.

UKF State-Filter. For the SPECT imaging system given by Eqns. (7) and (8), the purpose of the UKF state-filtering is to search for the optimal estimates of radio-tracer variable $x(t)$, given fixed attenuation values $\mu(t)$. Since detailed discussion of the unscented Kalman filtering is certainly beyond the scope of this paper [25], we present here a more algorithmic description while ignoring some theoretical considerations.

The unscented transformation is a method for calculating the statistics of a random variable. Given a random variable $\mathbf{x}$ (dimension L) with mean $\bar{\mathbf{x}}$ and covariance $\mathbf{P_x}$ through a nonlinear function $\mathbf{y} = \mathbf{f(x)}$. To compute the statistics of $\mathbf{y}$, we form a sigma point matrix $\mathcal{X}$ and their weights according to the following:

$$\mathcal{X}_0 = \mathbf{x}$$

$$\mathcal{X}_i = \mathbf{x} + \left(\sqrt{(L+\lambda)\mathbf{P_x}}\right)_i, i = 1,...,L$$

$$\mathcal{X}_i = \mathbf{x} - \left(\sqrt{(L+\lambda)\mathbf{P_x}}\right)_{i-L}, i = L+1,...,2L$$

$$w_0^{(m)} = \frac{\lambda}{L+\lambda}, i = 0 \qquad (9)$$

$$w_0^{(c)} = \frac{\lambda}{L+\lambda} + (1-\alpha^2+\beta), i = 0$$

$$w_i^{(m)} = w_i^{(c)} = \frac{1}{2(L+\lambda)}, i = 1,...,2L$$

where $\lambda = \alpha^2(L+\kappa)-L$. The parameter $\alpha \in [0,1]$ determines the spread of the sigma points, $\beta \geq 0$ is used to incorporate any prior knowledge about the distribution of $\mathbf{x}$, and κ is a scaling parameter and is often set to be zero. Once having the above definitions, the UKF state-filter is initialized with $\hat{x}(0) = \hat{x}_0$ and covariance matrix $P_{x(0)}$, the state estimates and their error covariance matrices are computed sequentially until convergence:

1. Calculate the sigma point weights as in (9);
2. Project the state variable $x(t)$ ahead:

$$\hat{x}(t|t-1) = \hat{x}(t-1) \qquad (10)$$

3. Project the error covariance $P_{x(t)}$ ahead:

$$P_{x(t|t-1)} = P_{x(t-1)} + Q_s \qquad (11)$$

4. Calculate the sigma points as defined in Eqn. (9):

$$\mathcal{X}(t|t-1) = [\hat{x}(t|t-1), \hat{x}(t|t-1) +$$

$$\sqrt{(L+\lambda)P_{x(t|t-1)}}, \hat{x}(t|t-1) -$$

$$\sqrt{(L+\lambda)P_{x(t|t-1)}}] \qquad (12)$$

5. Filtering of the measurement equations:

$$\mathcal{Y}(t|t-1) = h(\mathcal{X}(t|t-1), \hat{\mu}(t-1)) \qquad (13)$$

$$\hat{y}(t|t-1) = \sum_{i=0}^{2L} w_i^{(m)} \mathcal{Y}(i,t|t-1) \qquad (14)$$

$$P_{yx(t)} = \sum_{i=0}^{2L} w_i^{(c)}(\mathcal{Y}(i,t|t-1)$$
$$-\hat{y}(t|t-1))(\mathcal{Y}(i,t|t-1)$$
$$-\hat{y}(t|t-1))^T + R_o \qquad (15)$$

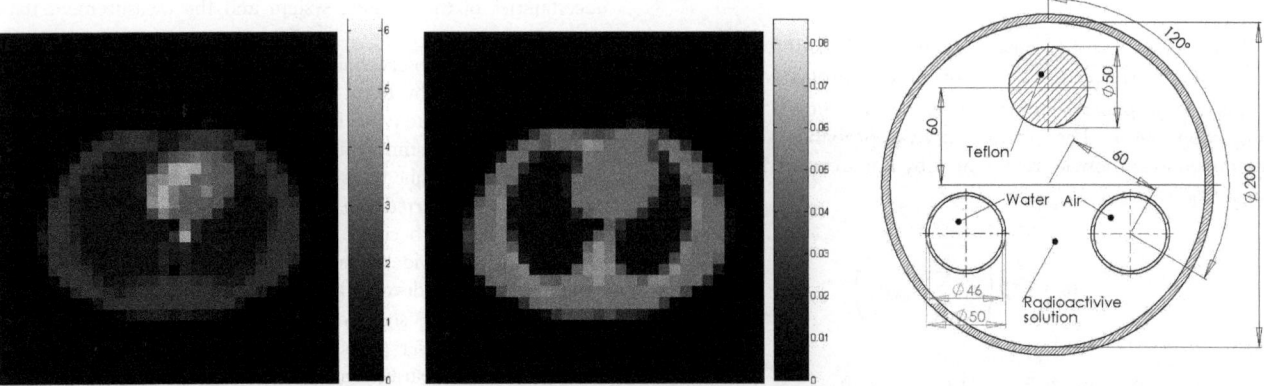

Figure 1. Simulated and physical phantom used in the experiments. From left to right: activity (*left*) and attenuation (*middle*) distributions of simulated Zubal phantom, physical imaging phantom with three different material rods inside. (*right*)

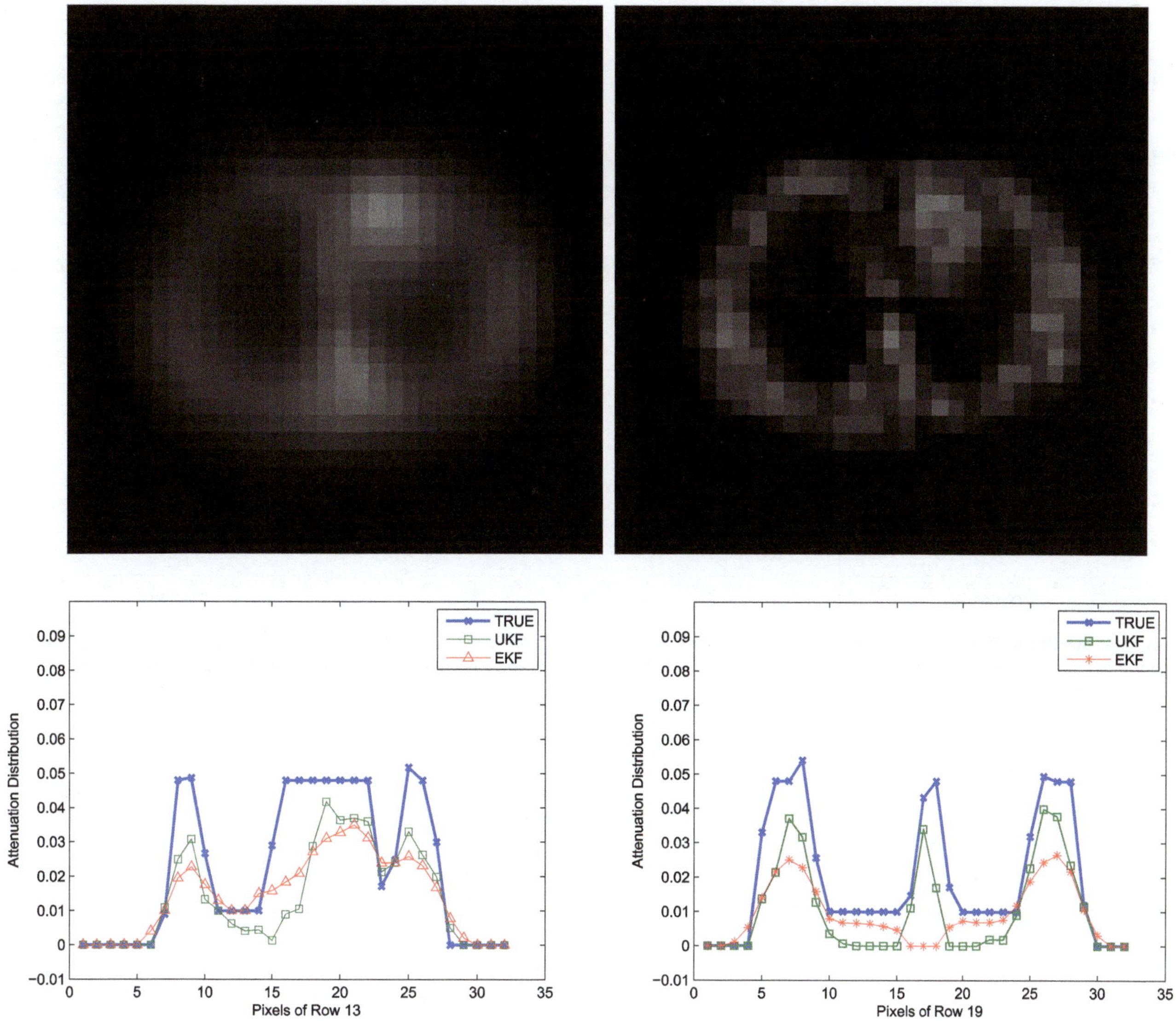

Figure 2. Synthetic Data. Top: Attenuation maps recovered by the EKF (*left*) and dual UKF (*right*) frameworks for low count measurements. Bottom: Horizontal profiles along the 13th (*left*) and 19th (*right*) rows of the recovered attenuation maps.

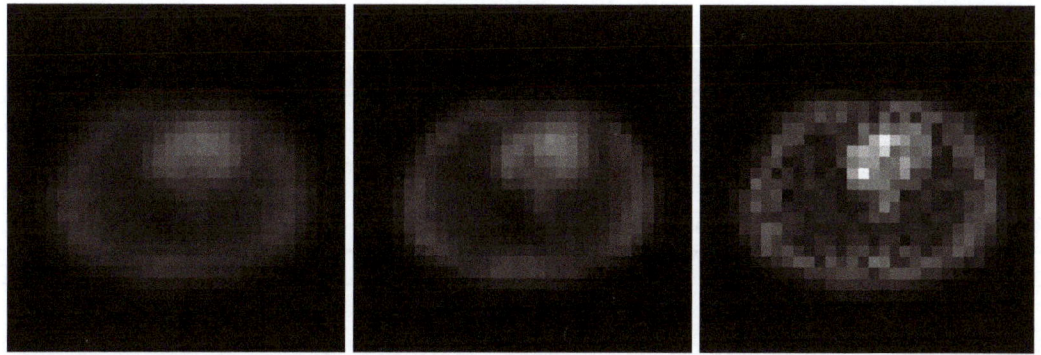

Figure 3. Synthetic Data. From left to right: activity maps recovered by FBP, EM-ML, and UKF methods for high count measurements.

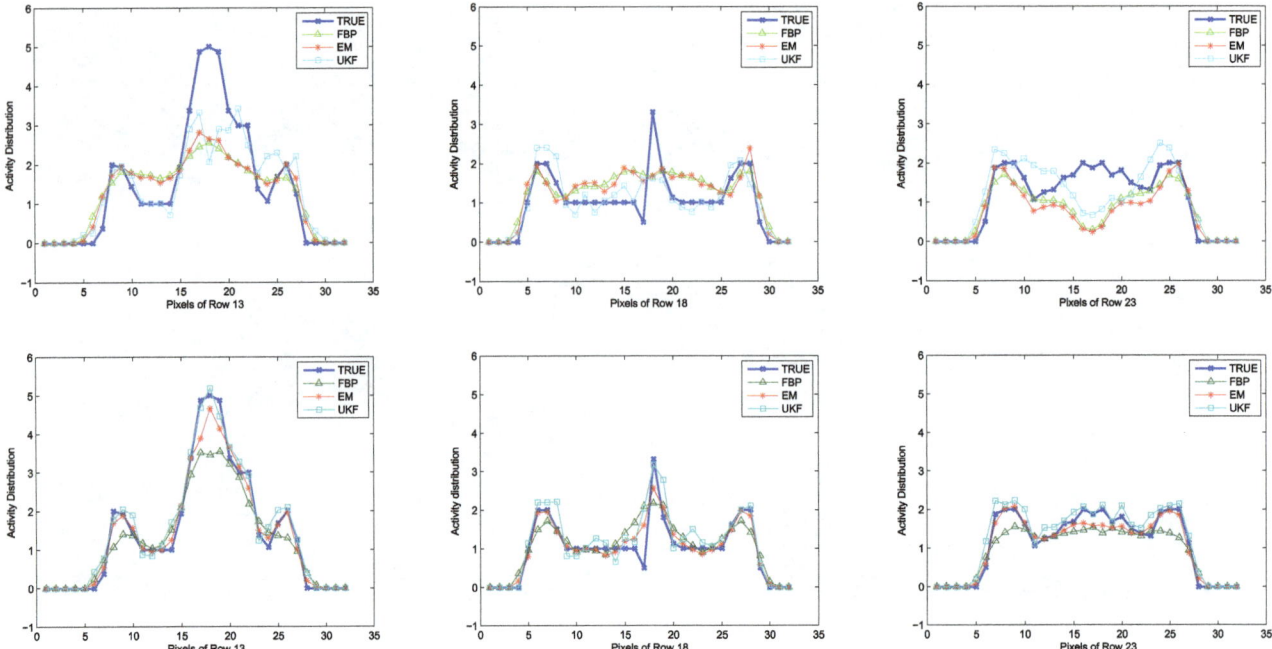

Figure 4. Synthetic Data. Top: Horizontal profiles along the 13th (*left*), 18th (*middle*), and 23rd (*right*) rows of the recovered activity maps for low count measurements. Bottom: Horizontal profiles along the 13th (*left*), 18th (*middle*), and 23rd (*right*) rows of the recovered activity maps for high count measurements.

6. Compute the Kalman Gain:

$$P_{x(t)y(t)} = \sum_{i=0}^{2L} w_i^{(c)} (\mathcal{X}(i,t|t-1)$$
$$- \hat{x}(t|t-1))(\mathcal{Y}(i,t|t-1)$$
$$- \hat{y}(t|t-1))^T \tag{16}$$

$$K_x(t) = P_{x(t)y(t)} P_{yx(t)}^{-1} \tag{17}$$

7. Update the estimate with the measurement:

$$\hat{x}(t) = \hat{x}(t|t-1) + K_x(t)(y(t) - \hat{y}(t|t-1)) \tag{18}$$

8. Update the error covariance:

$$P_{x(t)} = P_{x(t|t-1)} - K_x(t) P_{yx(t)} K_x(t)^T \tag{19}$$

Here, the previously stored information in the prediction step is combined with the new information coming from the next measurement $y(t)$ and the Kalman gain matrix to refine $\hat{x}(t)$ and $P_{x(t)}$ in the correction step. The covariance of the measurement error R_o and system error Q_s is assumed to be known and set to time-invariant.

Attenuation Estimation: UKF Parameter Filter

Once the UKF state-filter converges, it is followed by the estimation of a coupled UKF parameter-filter aiming to recover the attenuation map of the object being imaged, given the estimated radioactivity map. The system equations for the parameter-filter are

$$\mu(t+1) = \mu(t) + \upsilon_p \tag{20}$$

$$y(t) = h(x(t), \mu(t)) + e_o \tag{21}$$

Here, υ_p is the process noise with covariance matrix Q_p, and we assume that the attenuation parameter vector μ is temporally

Table 1. RMSE values of estimated activity maps for the synthetic data.

	FBP	EM	EKF	UKF
low count measurement	0.6724	0.5469	0.4152	0.3660
high count measurement	0.5252	0.3933	0.3710	0.3575

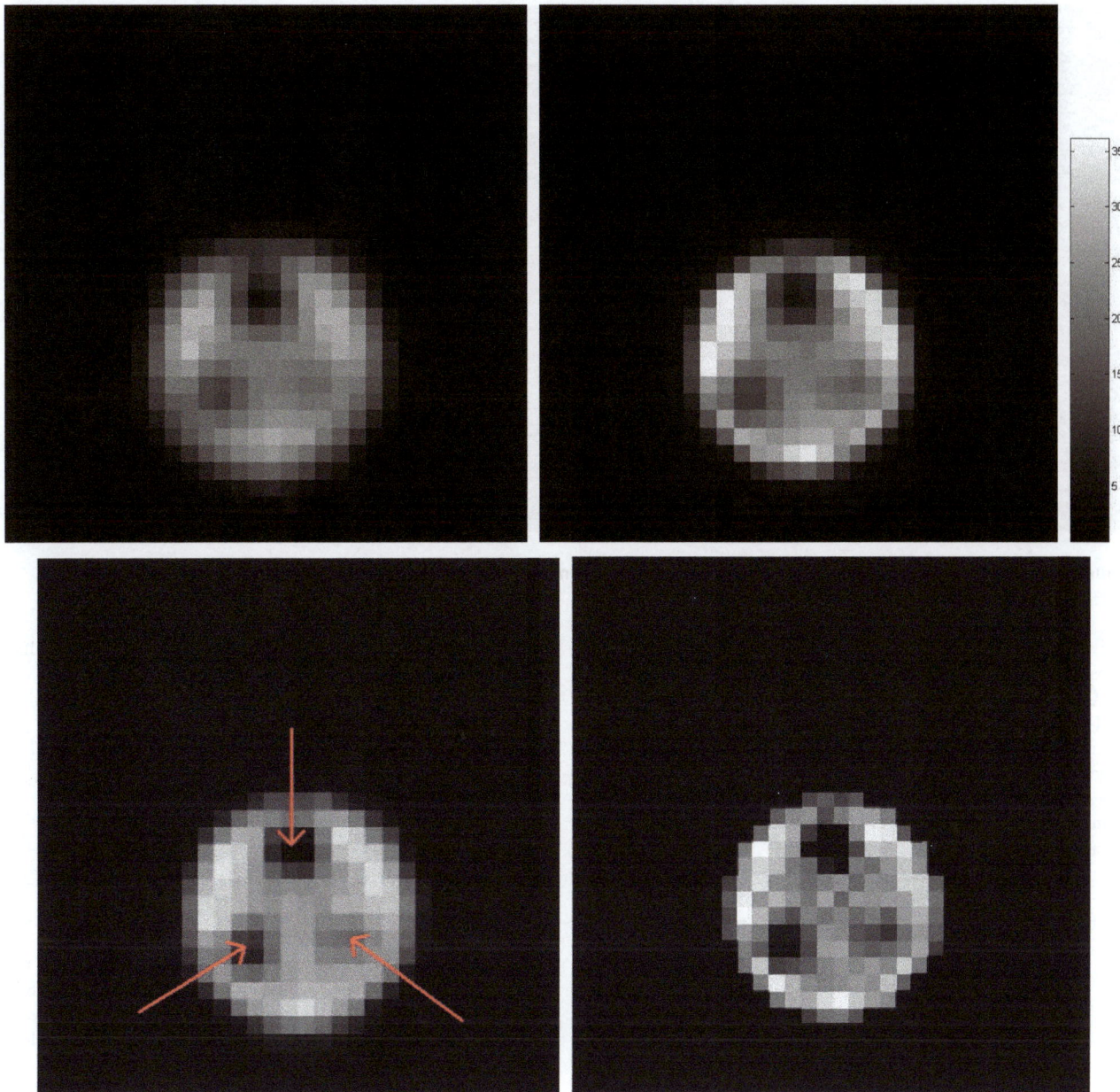

Figure 5. Reconstructed activity map of the physical phantom by FBP (*top left*), EM-ML (*top right*), EKF (*bottom left*) and UKF(*bottom right*) (arrows indicate cold areas), and the associated color scale.

constant. Initializing the unscented parameter filter with $\hat{\mu}(0) = \hat{\mu}_0$ and covariance matrix $P_{\mu(0)}$, the parameter-filter follows similar recursion steps as the state-filter (Eqns. (9)–(17)) until convergence, given the sigma point calculation scheme of Eqn. 9.

The coupled radioactivity state and attenuation parameter estimation processes are iteratively repeated as necessary, until stable results are achieved. The final optimal estimates then become the reconstructed SPECT activity and attenuation maps.

Results

Validation with Synthetic Data

Synthetic Zubal phantom is used to quantitatively evaluate the accuracy and robustness of the framework, where a simplified

human thorax with two lungs is represented by 32×32 attenuation and activity (Fig. 1). Specifically, while both lungs have average attenuation coefficient of 0.04/cm, attenuation of the left lung is nonuniform but that of the right lung is uniform. SPECT projection data have been generated for a parallel beam geometry and 90 views uniformly spaced over 360 degrees. To generate realistic data, simulations in our study are performed using toolbox GATE [27], which can provide a relatively accurate reference for the assessment of new image reconstruction algorithms. And we have performed two studies, one with mean activities of 50 counts/pixel (low count), and the other with 200 counts/pixel (high count).

For these two sets of synthetic projection data, the radioactivity maps are reconstructed using four reconstruction methods: FBP

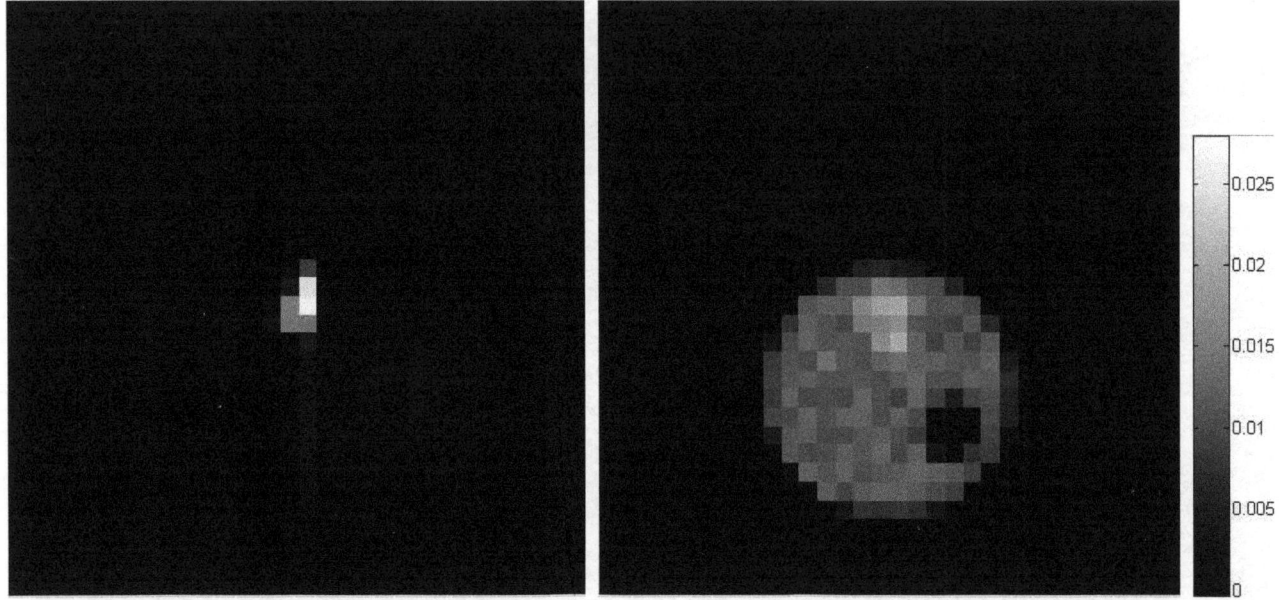

Figure 6. Reconstructed attenuation map of the physical phantom by EKF (*left*) and UKF (*right*), and the associate color scale.

[28], EM-ML [29], EKF [24], and dual UKF (The attenuation maps are also reconstructed for the EKF and UKF methods). For the UKF framework, the state (activity map) is estimated by the UKF state-filter, where, for the first iteration, the attenuation parameters come from the initial guess. Otherwise, we use the values estimated in the last iteration from the UKF parameter-filter. Consequently, these state estimates are used by the UKF parameter-filter to recover the attenuation coefficients. This process is executed iteratively until it meets the convergence criterion, which is defined using two consecutive normalized errors $\chi(t+1)$ and $\chi(t)$ through $\|\chi(t+1) - \chi(t)\| < \varsigma$ with ς being a small constant, and χ defines the normalized error between the estimated and the exact value ($\Xi = x$ for the state-filter process, $\Xi = \mu$ for the parameter-filter process) with

$$\chi = \left(\frac{1}{N} \frac{\sum_{i=1}^{N} |\Xi_i^t - \Xi_i^r|^2}{\sum_{i=1}^{N} |\Xi_i^t|^2} \right)^{0.5} \tag{22}$$

where Ξ_i^t is the estimated value, Ξ_i^r is the corresponding true value, and i indicates the pixel.

A detailed statistical analysis on the estimation results against the ground truth phantom map is performed. Let N_p and $\hat{x}$ be the total number of pixels in the region of interest(ROI), e.g. body anatomy, and the final reconstruction results respectively, and x_{tr} be the ground truth, we have the following error definitions:

$$RMSE = \left(\frac{1}{N_p} \sum (\hat{x} - x_{tr})^2 \right)^{0.5} \tag{23}$$

The results for the reconstruction of the attenuation maps are shown in Fig. 2 for the low count case. Visually, the UKF-reconstructed attenuation image clearly shows all relevant anatomical structures, where the lungs are easily seen with clear shape and size. The RMSE values in ROI of body anatomy using the UKF method are 0.0190 (low counts) and 0.0187 (high

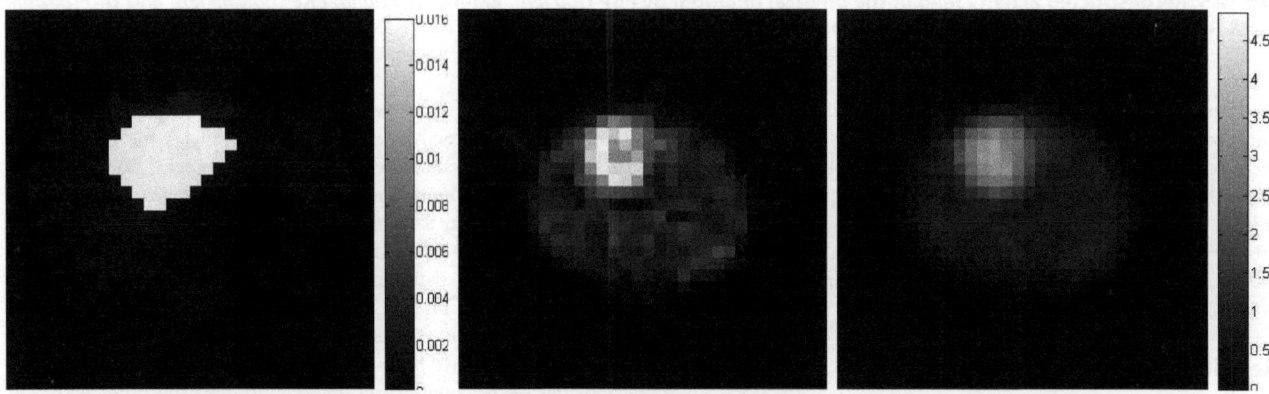

Figure 7. Reconstructed attenuation (*left*, by UKF) and activity maps of the patient by UKF (*middle*) and FBP (*right*), and the associated color scales.

counts), which, though not as impressive, are still somewhat smaller than the corresponding values of 0.0204 (low counts) and 0.0199 (high counts) obtained by the EKF method (note that the true average attenuation coefficient is 0.04). The worse performance of the EKF strategy could be caused by the first-order Taylor approximations of state transition that provided insufficiently accurate representations.

The results for the reconstruction of the activity maps are presented in Fig. 3, and the quantitative tabulation of the reconstruction accuracy is in Table 1. These figures and results illustrate that traditional EM-ML and FBP methods, with unknown attenuation map settings, produce some noticeable errors. The dual UKF estimation framework, on the other hand, consistently yields the best quality radioactivity estimates for both high and low count data. Same conclusion can be drawn from the visual examples of the selected horizontal profiles, as shown in Fig. 4.

Reconstruction from Physical Phantom Scanning Data

The second data set used for validation has been on a real cylinder phantom. The dimension of the phantom is 200 mm (diameter) × 290 mm (depth). A Teflon rod and two hollow PMMA cylinders with diameters of $50mm$ are inserted in the phantom's volume, as shown in Fig. 1. The phantom is filled with ^{99m}Tc concentration with a total radioactivity of 20mCi (100kBq/cc) and the two hollow cylinder rods are filled with air and pure water respectively. The phantom was scanned with a Siemens ECam^{duet} ECT scanner by two detector head rotating at total 64 angle position around 180 degree and the acquiring time at each position is 30 seconds. The final sinogram data has 64×128 projections for each slice. Once again, FBP, EM-ML, EKF and dual UKF strategies have been used to reconstruct activity maps from the measurement data, as shown in Fig. 5. Visually, it is evident that the UKF method produces the best reconstruction results, especially for the three cold areas. The results of EKF and UKF reconstructed attenuation map are shown in Fig. 6, with RMSE values of 0.0007 for UKF and 0.0044 for EKF.

Reconstruction from Real Patient Scanning Data

The dual reconstruction strategy has also been evaluated on clinical studies, where the patients are undergoing ^{99m}Tc sestamibi stress tests. Using a Siemens ECam^{duet} scanner, all projections are acquired over 120 angles covering a circular 360 degrees acquisition orbit in a continuous step-and-shoot mode. With an acquisition time of 16s/frame, the total photon counts for each slice are 148761. The dual reconstruction of activity and attenuation maps are shown in Fig. 7, and the clinically standard FBP reconstruction (without attenuation correction) is also shown for comparison. Since the transmission data is not available from this imaging site, we can only make qualitative visual inspection of the images. It is quite clear, however, that the estimated attenuation map agrees with general knowledge of the imaged area, and the UKF estimated activity map exhibits improved contrast between heart and soft tissue.

There is usually a considerable increase in computation for improved performance. The computational load increases when moving from the EM to the UKF. However, as the UKF gives a better approximation in time update step, the UKF estimate is able to converge quite faster comparing to the EM. Furthermore, this proposed approach runs efficiently on graphics processing units(GPUs) since large amounts of computations are done in matrix forms. Further investigations on the implementation with GPUs are underway.

Conclusions

A dual UKF strategy has been derived for joint reconstruction of the attenuation map and activity distribution solely from SPECT emission sinograms. Constructing the state transition of the activity distribution through state space evolution equations and the photon-counting measurements through observation equations, we rely on the unscented Kalman filter principles to first generate estimates of activity maps with sub-optimal attenuation parameter estimates, and then recover the attenuation maps given these activity estimates. These coupled iterative steps are repeated as necessary until convergence. Simulated and physical phantoms, as well as real patient data, are used to evaluate the proposed strategy.

Author Contributions

Conceived and designed the experiments: HL PS. Performed the experiments: HL ZH MG. Analyzed the data: ZH MG HH. Contributed reagents/materials/analysis tools: HH HL. Contributed to the writing of the manuscript: HL MG.

References

1. King MA, Tsui BM, Pan T (1995) Attenuation compensation for cardiac single-photon emission computed tomography imaging: Part 1. Impact of attenuation and methods of estimating attenuation maps. J Nucl Cardiol 2: 513–524.
2. Welch A, Clack R, Natterer F, Gullberg G (1997) Toward accurate attenuation correction in SPECT without transmission measurements. IEEE Trans Med Imag 16: 532–541.
3. Zaidi H, Hasegawa B (2003) Determination of the attenuation map in emission tomography. J Nucl Med 44: 291–315.
4. Ficaro E, Corbett J (2004) Advances in quantitative perfusion SPECT imaging. J Nucl Cardiol 11: 62–70.
5. Celler A, Dixon KL, Chang Z, Blinder S, Powe J, et al. (2005) Problems created in attenuation-corrected SPECT images by artifacts in attenuation maps: A simulation study. J Nucl Med 46: 335–343.
6. Feng B, Fessler JA, King MA (2006) Incorporation of system resolution compensation (RC) in the ordered-subset transmission (OSTR) algorithm for transmission imaging in SPECT. IEEE Trans Med Imag 25: 941–949.
7. Nunez M, Prakash V, Vila R, Mut F, Alonso O, et al. (2009) Aattenuation correction for lung SPECT: evidence of need and validation of an attenuation map derived from the emission data. European Journal of Nuclear Medicine and Molecular Imaging 36: 1076–1089.
8. Cuocolo A (2011) Attenuation correction for myocardial perfusion spect imaging: still a controversial issue. European journal of nuclear medicine and molecular imaging 38: 1887–1889.
9. Garcia EV (2007) Spect attenuation correction: an essential tool to realize nuclear cardiologys manifest destiny. Journal of nuclear cardiology 14: 16–24.
10. Wu C, van Andel HAG, Laverman P, Boerman OC, Beekman FJ (2013) Effects of attenuation map accuracy on attenuation-corrected micro-spect images. EJNMMI research 3: 1–11.
11. Ishii K, Hanaoka K, Okada M, Kumano S, Komeya Y, et al. (2012) Impact of ct attenuation correction by spect/ct in brain perfusion images. Annals of nuclear medicine 26: 241–247.
12. McGowan SE, Greaves CD, Evans S (2012) An investigation into truncation artefacts experienced in cardiac imaging using a dedicated cardiac spect gamma camera with transmission attenuation correction. Nuclear medicine communications 33: 1287–1291.
13. Fleming JS (1989) A technique for using CT images in attenuation correction and quantification in SPECT. Nucl Med Commun 10: 83–97.
14. Kalki K, Blankespoor SC, Brown JK, Hasegawa BH, et al. (1997) Myocardial perfusion imaging with a combined x-ray CT and SPECT system. J Nucl Med 38: 1535–1540.
15. Kinahan PE, Townsend DW, Beyer T, Sashin D (1998) Attenuation correction for a combined 3D PET/CT scanner. Med Phys 25: 2046–2053.
16. Willowson K, Bailey D, Baldock C (2008) Quantitative SPECT reconstruction using CT-derived corrections. Phys Med Biol 53: 3099–3112.
17. Kaplan MS, Haynor RS, Vija H (1999) A differential attenuation method for simultaneous estimation of SPECT activity and attenuation distributions. IEEE Nucl Sci 46: 535–541.
18. Nuyts J, Dupont P, Stroobants S, Benninck R, Mortelmans L, et al. (1999) Simultaneous maximum a posteriori reconstruction of attenuation and activity distributions from emission sinograms. IEEE Trans Med Image 18: 393–403.

19. Dicken V (1999) A new approach towards simultaneous activity and attenuation reconstruction in emission tomography. Inverse Problem 15: 931–960.
20. Krol A, Bowsher JE, Manglos SH, Feiglin DH, Tomai MP, et al. (2001) An EM algorithm for estimating SPECT emission and transmission parameters from emissions data only. IEEE Trans Med Imag 20: 218–232.
21. Gourion D, Noll D, Gantet P, Celler A, Esquerre J (2002) Attenuation correction using SPECT emission data only. IEEE Trans on Nuclear Science 49: 2172–2179.
22. Jha AK, Clarkson E, Kupinski MA, Barrett HH (2013) Joint reconstruction of activity and attenuation map using lm spect emission data. In: SPIE Medical Imaging. International Society for Optics and Photonics, pp. 86681W–86681W.
23. Salomon A, Goedicke A, Aach T (2011) Attenuation corrected cardiac spect imaging using simultaneous reconstruction and a priori information. IEEE Transactions on Nuclear Science 58: 527–536.
24. Tian Y, Liu HF, Shi P (2006) Simultaneous reconstruction of tissue attenuation and radioactivity maps in SPECT. MICCAI I: 397–404.
25. Julier SJ, Uhlmann JK (2004) Unscented filtering and nonlinear estimation. Proceedings of the IEEE Aerospace and Electronic Systems 92: 401–422.
26. Anscombe FJ (1948) The transformation of poisson, binomial and negative-binomial data. Biometrika 35: 246–254.
27. Jan S, Santin G, Strul D, Staelens S, Assie K, et al. (2004) GATE: a simulation toolkit for PET and SPECT. Physics in Medicine and Biology : 4543–4561.
28. Kak AC, Slaney M (2001) Principles of computerized tomographic imaging. Society for Industrial and Applied Mathematics.
29. Shepp LA, Vardi Y (1982) Maximum likelihood reconstruction for emission tomography. IEEE Transactions on Medical Imaging 1: 113–122.

17

Neutrophil/Lymphocyte Ratio Is Associated with Non-Calcified Plaque Burden in Patients with Coronary Artery Disease

Lennart Nilsson[1,2]*, **Wouter G. Wieringa[4]**, **Gabija Pundziute[4]**, **Marcus Gjerde[1,2]**, **Jan Engvall[1,3]**, **Eva Swahn[1,2]**, **Lena Jonasson[1,2]**

1 Department of Medical and Health Sciences, Linköping University, Linköping, Sweden, **2** Department of Cardiology, Linköping University, Linköping, Sweden, **3** Department of Clinical Physiology, Linköping University, Linköping, Sweden, **4** University of Groningen, University Medical Center Groningen, Department of Cardiology, Groningen, The Netherlands

Abstract

Background: Elevations in soluble markers of inflammation and changes in leukocyte subset distribution are frequently reported in patients with coronary artery disease (CAD). Lately, the neutrophil/lymphocyte ratio has emerged as a potential marker of both CAD severity and cardiovascular prognosis.

Objectives: The aim of the study was to investigate whether neutrophil/lymphocyte ratio and other immune-inflammatory markers were related to plaque burden, as assessed by coronary computed tomography angiography (CCTA), in patients with CAD.

Methods: Twenty patients with non-ST-elevation acute coronary syndrome (NSTE-ACS) and 30 patients with stable angina (SA) underwent CCTA at two occasions, immediately prior to coronary angiography and after three months. Atherosclerotic plaques were classified as calcified, mixed and non-calcified. Blood samples were drawn at both occasions. Leukocyte subsets were analyzed by white blood cell differential counts and flow cytometry. Levels of C-reactive protein (CRP) and interleukin(IL)-6 were measured in plasma. Blood analyses were also performed in 37 healthy controls.

Results: Plaque variables did not change over 3 months, total plaque burden being similar in NSTE-ACS and SA. However, non-calcified/total plaque ratio was higher in NSTE-ACS, 0.25(0.09–0.44) vs 0.11(0.00–0.25), p<0.05. At admission, levels of monocytes, neutrophils, neutrophil/lymphocyte ratios, CD4+ T cells, CRP and IL-6 were significantly elevated, while levels of NK cells were reduced, in both patient groups as compared to controls. After 3 months, levels of monocytes, neutrophils, neutrophil/lymphocyte ratios and CD4+ T cells remained elevated in patients. Neutrophil/lymphocyte ratios and neutrophil counts correlated significantly with numbers of non-calcified plaques and also with non-calcified/total plaque ratio (r=0.403, p=0.010 and r=0.382, p=0.024, respectively), but not with total plaque burden.

Conclusions: Among immune-inflammatory markers in NSTE-ACS and SA patients, neutrophil counts and neutrophil/lymphocyte ratios were significantly correlated with non-calcified plaques. Data suggest that these easily measured biomarkers reflect the burden of vulnerable plaques in CAD.

Editor: Carmine Pizzi, University of Bologna, Italy

Funding: The authors have no support or funding to report.

Competing Interests: The authors have declared that no competing interests exist.

* Email: lennart.nilsson@liu.se

Introduction

Coronary artery disease (CAD) is the leading cause of death in the western world. Although multifactorial in its origin, inflammatory and immunological events are considered to play central roles in initiation and progression of atherosclerotic plaques [1]. Indeed, elevations in soluble markers of inflammation as well as changes in leukocyte subset distribution are frequently reported in patients with CAD [2–5]. However, studies on relationships between markers of inflammation and severity of CAD have yielded disparate results [6–9].

In recent years, several studies have demonstrated the important role of neutrophils in all stages of atherosclerosis and plaque destabilization leading to acute coronary syndromes (ACS) [10]. Accordingly, neutrophil infiltration has been detected in very early stages of atherosclerosis as well as in shoulder regions of plaques prone to rupture [11,12]. Circulating neutrophil counts and neutrophil/lymphocyte ratios are emerging markers of the presence and severity of CAD [13–15]. Furthermore, they are independent predictors of mortality and cardiovascular events in high-risk groups and a broad range of CAD patients [14,16–19].

CAD severity is not only a question about the extent of obstructive stenosis, but the risk of plaque rupture and ACS largely depends on plaque composition [20]. Coronary computed tomography angiography (CCTA) is a non-invasive method allowing accurate assessment of CAD [21]. In contrast to invasive coronary angiography (ICA), CCTA provides information about the vessel wall and composition of plaques in addition to degree of stenosis. CCTA may therefore provide valuable information about the burden of CAD with prognostic implications as well as assessing the morphological aspects of the disease process [22–24]. The identification of circulating immune-inflammatory markers that are associated with the atherosclerotic disease process in coronary arteries may provide additive information. The aim of the study was to investigate if neutrophil counts, neutrophil/lymphocyte ratio or other immune-inflammatory markers were related to plaque burden, as assessed by CCTA in patients with stable angina (SA) and ACS.

Methods

Study design and population

This study is a single-center, prospective, pilot study. The study population consisted of 30 patients with SA, 20 patients with non-ST-elevation acute coronary syndrome (NSTE-ACS), and 37 healthy control subjects. In order to assess coronary atherosclerosis the patients underwent CCTA prior to ICA and revascularization (percutaneous coronary intervention (PCI) or coronary artery bypass grafting). A follow-up CCTA was performed at three months following revascularization in order to reevaluate the plaque burden and plaque composition. Blood samples were collected at baseline (prior to CCTA and ICA), and at three months follow-up. Inclusion criteria were as follows: 1) patients with planned ICA due to SA, defined as clinically probable angina pectoris and positive exercise test or myocardial perfusion imaging; 2) NSTE-ACS, defined as unstable angina or non-ST-elevation myocardial infarction, according to universally accepted definitions [25,26]. The exclusion criteria were: 1) inability to perform CCTA (contraindications to betablockers or nitroglycerine, allergy to contrast medium, pregnancy, permanent atrial fibrillation); 2) renal dysfunction (creatinine >150 μmol/L) or risk factors for contrast induced acute kidney injury (treatment with metformin, high dose diuretics); 3) known factors influencing immunological and inflammatory markers (active immunologic or inflammatory disease, infection with fever or use of antibiotics during the last 30 days, immunosuppressive treatment); and 4) major trauma, surgery or PCI in the last 30 days. The control subjects, randomly invited from the Swedish Population Register and representative for hospital recruitment area, were clinically healthy and received no medication.

Ethical Considerations

The study protocol was approved by the Regional Ethical Review Board in Linköping and written informed consent was obtained from all study participants. The study was conducted in accordance with the ethical guidelines set forth in the Declaration of Helsinki.

Coronary computed tomography angiography: image acquisition

Patients underwent CCTA within twenty-four hours after inclusion using a 16-slice multi-slice CT scanner or a 64-slice dual-source CT scanner (Sensation or Somatom Definition, Siemens Healthcare, Forchheim, Germany). During CTA acquisition non-ionic contrast medium was administered (Iomeron 400,

Bracco, Altana, Pharma, Konstanz, Germany). Beta-blocker treatment (orally or intravenously) and nitroglycerine was administered to achieve optimal image quality. In order to reduce radiation exposure, electrocardiogram-gated current modulation was used in all patients. The following scan parameters were used: 1. For the 16-slice multi-slice scanner: 16×0.75 mm collimation, gantry rotation time of 375 ms, temporal resolution of 188 ms, tube voltage 100 or 120 kV, and maximal tube current of 650 mAs; 2. For the 64-slice dual-source CT scanner: $64 \times 2 \times 0.6$ mm collimation, gantry rotation time of 330 ms, temporal resolution of 83 ms, tube voltage 100 or 120 kV, and maximal tube current of 560 mAs. Upon completion of the scan, images were reconstructed, if possible in several phases of the R-R interval, to obtain motion-free images of the coronary arteries.

Coronary computed tomography angiography: image analysis

Evaluation of CCTA images was performed on a remote workstation with dedicated software (QAngio CT, Medis Medical Imaging Systems, Leiden, the Netherlands) [27], side by side in consensus by two experienced observers blinded to baseline patient characteristics and ICA results. A predefined window and level setting (window 900 HU, level 250 HU) was used for analysis of lumen and plaque [28]. Coronary segments were differentiated into seventeen segments, according to a modified American Heart Association classification [29]. Segments of insufficient quality for evaluation were scored as non-evaluable and excluded from analysis. The CT scan was considered unevaluable if 2 vessels had 3 or more segments that were non-evaluable. Presence of plaques was visually assessed. Coronary atherosclerosis was defined as tissue structures >1 mm2 within or adjacent to the coronary artery lumen but distinctive from surrounding pericardial or epicardial tissue. Per segment, one coronary plaque was selected. The degree of luminal narrowing of the coronary artery was quantified visually, based on comparison of the luminal diameter of the plaque containing segment to the luminal diameter of the most normal-appearing site immediately proximal to the plaque. Plaques with ≥50% luminal narrowing were classified as obstructive. In addition, plaque composition was assessed. Three types of plaques were classified: 1) Non-calcified plaque (plaques with lower density compared to contrast-enhanced lumen), 2) calcified plaque (plaques with high density structures compared to contrast-enhanced lumen), or 3) mixed plaque (non-calcified and calcified constituents in single plaque) [30]. The number of any plaques (total plaque burden), as well as plaques with different features was calculated per patient.

Invasive coronary angiography: image acquisition and analysis

Since the assessment of degree of stenosis with 16-slice CCTA is only moderately accurate, ICA was used to assess the obstructive plaque burden. ICA of left and right coronary arteries was performed in multiple views by using the transfemoral approach. Coronary segments were scored in the same manner as on CCTA images, and a diameter stenosis of ≥50% was classified as obstructive. Digital angiograms were analyzed off-line with dedicated software (Coronary Artery Analysis System 9, Pie Medical Imaging, Maastricht, The Netherlands). All segments > 1.5 mm in diameter with a <100% diameter stenosis were measured on the angiograms. The contrast-filled non-tapered catheter tip was used for calibration. The proximal and distal reference vessel diameters and minimal lumen diameter of the

Table 1. Baseline clinical and biochemical characteristics of patients and controls.

	SA	NSTE-ACS	Controls	P-value
	N = 30	N = 20	N = 37	
Age (years)	64±9	67±10	64±8	NS
Female	4 (13)	5 (25)	9 (24)	NS
Waist circumference (cm)	102±11	99±13	95±9	0.003[ψ]
Current or previous smoker	22 (73)	15 (75)	1 (3)	<0.001[ψγ]
Hypertension	21 (70)	7 (35)	0	<0.001[ψγ], 0.015[Φ]
Diabetes mellitus	4 (13)	1 (5)	0	0.022[ψ]
History of MI	6 (20)	2 (10)	0	0.004[ψ]
Statin treatment	24 (80)	6 (30)	0	<0.001[ψ,Φ]
Plasma cholesterol (mmol/L)	5.1±1.0	5.4±1.3	5.5±1.1	NS
Plasma LDL-cholesterol (mmol/L)	2.9±0.8	3.2±1.2	3.4±0.9	0.013[ψ]
Plasma HDL-cholesterol (mmol/L)	1.2±0.2	1.3±0.4	1.4±0.4	0.010[ψ]
Triglycerides (mmol/L)	1.4 (1.1,2.1)	1.4 (1.2,1.7)	1.1 (0.9,1.6)	0.018[ψ], 0.038[γ]

The data are presented as mean ±SD, median (25th, 75th percentile), or numbers (%). SA = stable angina; ACS = acute coronary syndrome; MI = myocardial infarction; LDL = low density lipoprotein, HDL = high density lipoprotein. NS = non-significant ($p \geq 0.05$). For comparisons between groups, p-values indicating significant differences are denoted by ψ (controls vs SA), γ (controls vs NSTE-ACS) and Φ (SA vs NSTE-ACS), respectively.

suspected lesion were recorded. The percentage of diameter stenosis was calculated.

Blood sampling, biochemical analysis and flow cytometry

Venous blood samples were collected in vacutainer tubes (using sodium heparin as anticoagulant). Baseline blood samples of NSTE-ACS patients were received within 24 hours of hospital admission. For all CAD patients, the samples at baseline and at three months were collected prior to CCTA and ICA. Samples were centrifuged within 30 minutes to separate plasma, which then was stored immediately at −70°C until analyzed. White blood cell differential counts were determined in whole blood by Cell-Dyn Sapphire™ (Abbot Diagnostics). Leukocyte subset distributions were analyzed in whole blood by flow cytometry as previously described [31,32]. Briefly, monoclonal antibodies against CD3, CD4, CD8, CD19, CD16 and CD56 were purchased from BD Biosciences, San José, CA, US. The antibodies were marked with one of 3 fluorochromes: fluorescein isothiocyanate, phycoerythrin and peridinin chlorophyll protein. The cells were identified by combinations as follows: CD3/CD4/CD8 (T helper cells and cytotoxic T cells), CD19 (B cells) and CD3/CD16/CD56 (NK cells). Whole blood and antibodies were incubated for 15 minutes at room temperature, thereafter erythrocytes were lysed with FACS™ Lysing Solution (BD Biosciences) for 15 minutes at room temperature. Samples were analyzed on a FACSCanto II (BD Biosciences) equipped with 3 lasers, a blue 488 nm, a red 633 nm and a violet 405 nm. Analysis of samples was stopped when 10 000 cells were collected in the lymphocyte gate. Data were analyzed and subpopulations gated with FACSDiva™ 6.1.2 software (BD Biosciences). C-reactive protein (CRP) was measured in serum using a highly sensitive latex-enhanced turbidimetric immunoassay (Roche Diagnostics GmbH, Vienna, Austria) with a lower limit of detection of 0.03 mg/L. IL-6 levels in plasma were measured using an ELISA (R&D Systems Europe, Abingdon, United Kingdom) with a lower limit of detection of 0.48 pg/mL.

Statistical analysis

Categorical variables are presented as numbers (percentages) and were compared between groups using chi-square or Fisher's exact tests. When normally distributed, continuous variables are expressed as mean ±SD and were compared using one-way ANOVA and Students t-test for independent samples. When non-Gaussian distributed, continuous variables are presented as medians with 25th and 75th percentiles and were compared using the nonparametric Kruskal-Wallis test and Mann-Whitney-U test. Wilcoxon signed-rank test was used for paired comparisons. Bivariate correlations were performed to assess the associations between continuous variables using Spearman's correlation coefficient. A p-value of <0.05 was considered statistically significant. Statistical analyses were performed using SPSS version 20 (Chicago, IL, USA) and STATA version 11.0 (College Station, TX, USA).

Results

Study population

During the study period from March 2006 till January 2009 a total of 64 patients were initially included in the study. Fourteen patients were excluded from analysis: 11 patients did not complete any CCTA examination and in 3 patients the CCTA was of non-diagnostic quality. Baseline clinical characteristics of all patients are listed in Table 1. Revascularization was performed in 22 of 30 SA patients (8 PCI and 14 CABG) and in 13 of 20 NSTE-ACS patients (9 PCI and 4 CABG) within the first two months after study inclusion. All CAD patients were treated with statin therapy after admission.

Coronary computed tomography angiography

Data of the baseline CCTAs are summarized in Table 2. A 16-slice CCTA was used in 10 and a 64-slice CCTA in 40 of the 50 patients. Typical CCTA images of coronary plaques are shown in Figure 1. The total plaque burden (i.e. the total number of any plaque) did not differ between SA and NSTE-ACS patients neither did plaque characteristics differ significantly between the patient groups. However, there was a trend towards more calcified plaques in SA patients, whereas NSTE-ACS patients tended to have more non-calcified plaques. As a measure of vulnerable plaques, the ratio between non-calcified plaques and total plaques was calculated. This ratio was significantly higher in ACS patients as compared to SA patients.

Follow-up CCTA at 3 months was available in 41 patients (26 SA and 15 NSTE-ACS patients), 9 performed by a 16-slice CCTA and 32 by a 64-slice CCTA. There were no differences in total plaque burden or plaque characteristics between baseline and 3 months. Total plaque burden and non-calcified plaque/total plaque ratio were 9 (5, 11) and 0.16 (0.00, 0.26), respectively, in SA patients, and 8 (3, 10) and 0.25 (0.09, 0.44), respectively, in NSTE-ACS patients, at 3 months.

Invasive coronary angiography

The findings on ICA are presented in Table 2. There was no difference in the number of coronary artery segments with obstructive lesions in SA patients as compared to NSTE-ACS patients. Strong positive correlations were found between the number of obstructive stenosis on ICA and total plaque burden as well as number of non-calcified plaques on CCTA ($r = 0.694$, $p < 0.001$, and $r = 0.398$, $p = 0.004$, respectively). On the other hand, the non-calcified plaque/total plaque ratio was not associated with the number of obstructive lesions on ICA ($r = 0.163$, NS).

Immune-inflammatory markers

At admission, levels of leukocytes, neutrophils, monocytes, neutrophil/lymphocyte ratios, CD4+ T cells, and plasma levels of CRP and IL-6 were significantly elevated, while levels of NK cells were reduced, in SA and NSTE-ACS patients as compared to controls (Table 3). Plasma CRP in SA and NSTE-ACS patients declined over time reaching similar levels as control subjects at 3 months (0.9 (0.3, 2.8), 0.7 (0.3, 1.9) and 0.7 (0.4, 1.2) ng/mL, respectively, NS). Similarly, plasma IL-6 in SA and NSTE-ACS patients did not differ significantly from controls at follow-up (2.4 (1.1, 2.9), 1.7 (1.2, 3.1) and 1.4 (1.0, 2.2) ng/mL, respectively, NS).

At 3 months, neutrophil counts were still significantly higher in SA and NSTE-ACS patients as compared to control subjects (4.0 ± 1.6, 4.0 ± 1.4 and $3.0 \pm 1.0 \times 10^9$/L, respectively, $p = 0.006$), as were the neutrophil/lymphocyte ratios (2.0 ± 0.8, 2.2 ± 0.7 and

1.5 ± 0.7, respectively, $p = 0.030$). Also, levels of monocytes and CD4+ T cells remained unchanged at 3 months whereas NK cell levels increased (data not shown). Of note, SA and NSTE-ACS patients did not differ significantly in any immune-inflammatory markers at 3 months.

Correlations of coronary computed tomography angiography and invasive coronary angiography with immune-inflammatory markers

Neutrophil/lymphocyte ratios and neutrophil counts correlated with numbers of non-calcified plaques ($r = 0.302$, $p = 0.028$ and $r = 0.327$, $p = 0.017$) and also with non-calcified plaque/total plaque ratio ($r = 0.403$, $p = 0.010$ and $r = 0.382$, $p = 0.024$, respectively), but not with total plaque burden on CCTA (Figure 2). Furthermore, neutrophil/lymphocyte ratios and neutrophil counts did not correlate with number of obstructive lesions on ICA. Other leukocyte subsets did not show any correlations with any of the plaque variables, neither did CRP or IL-6 (data not shown).

Discussion

This study investigated associations between immune-inflammatory markers and plaque burden, as assessed by CCTA in patients with stable and unstable conditions of CAD. The main finding of this study was the consistent and significant correlation of neutrophil counts and neutrophil/lymphocyte ratios with numbers of non-calcified plaques and non-calcified plaque/total plaque ratio, but not with total plaque burden.

Neutrophils and neutrophil/lymphocyte ratios were significantly higher in both SA and NSTE-ACS patients as compared to controls, not only at admission but also at 3 months. The contribution of immune cells such as monocytes/macrophages and T cells to atherosclerosis and plaque progression has been firmly established over the years [33]. Howere, while being the most abundant white blood cell in the circulation, circulation, neutrophils are rarely detected in atherosclerotic plaques and therefore have attracted less attention. Nevertheless, over the past couple of years numerous studies have lent support to an important role of neutrophils in all stages of atherosclerosis [10]. Neutrophil count and neutrophil/lymphocyte ratio are

Table 2. Baseline coronary computed tomography angiography and invasive coronary angiography.

	SA; N = 30	NSTE-ACS; N = 20	P-value
CCTA characteristics at admission			
Number of segments	15 (15,16)	16 (15,16)	NS
Total plaque burden	9 (6,11)	8 (6,10)	NS
Non-calcified plaque	1 (0,2)	2 (1,4)	NS
Mixed plaque	3 (1,5)	4 (1,6)	NS
Calcified plaque	3 (2,5)	2 (0,3)	NS
Non-calcified & mixed plaque	4 (3,7)	6 (2,8)	NS
Ratio non-calcified plaque/plaque burden	0.13 (0.00,0.25)	0.25 (0.10,0.44)	0.049
ICA characteristics at admission			
Number of segments	15 (15,16)	16 (15,16)	NS
Segments with significant stenosis (>50%)	3 (2,6)	2 (1,4)	NS
Segments without significant stenosis	12 (9,14)	14 (11,15)	NS

The data are presented as median (25th, 75th percentile). CCTA = coronary computed tomography angiography; ICA = invasive coronary angiography; SA = stable angina; ACS = acute coronary syndrome. NS = non-significant ($p \geq 0.05$).

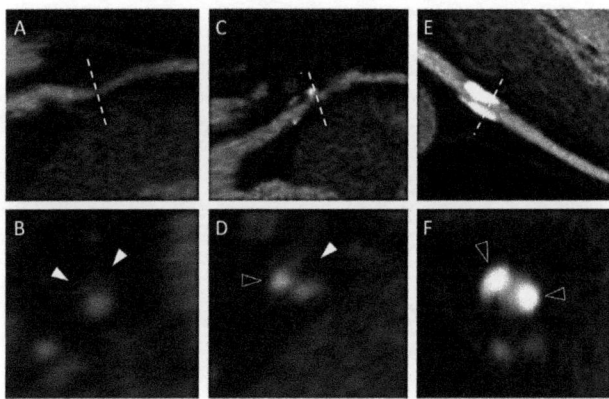

Figure 1. Different plaque compositions as seen by CCTA. The different types of coronary plaque are shown in longitudinal views, with cross-sectional views at the level of the dotted line. A non-calcified plaque is shown on the left (A and B), with white arrowheads pointing at the non-calcified plaque component. A mixed plaque is shown in the middle (C and D), with a white arrowhead indicating the non-calcified plaque component and a black arrowhead indicating the calcified component. A large calcified plaque is shown on the right side (E and F), with black arrowhead indicating the calcifications.

emerging markers of presence and severity of CAD [13–15,34]. They are both independent predictors of mortality and future cardiovascular events in healthy populations, high-risk groups and a broad range of CAD patients [14,16–19,35,36].

Neutrophil counts and neutrophil/lymphocyte ratios have been associated with the presence, severity and progression of coronary atherosclerosis as assessed by various modes of coronary imaging [14,15,37]. In a large cohort study of 3005 consecutive patients undergoing ICA for various indications, neutrophil count and neutrophil/lymphocyte ratio correlated significantly with the number of diseased vessels [14]. Moreover, a higher neutrophil/lymphocyte ratio was associated with higher coronary calcium scores measured by multidetector CT in 849 clinically healthy individuals participating in a health promotion program [37].

However, neither ICA nor coronary calcium score, provide any information about the plaque composition. Correlations of neutrophil counts and neutrophil/lymphocyte ratios with plaque composition on CCTA have not previously been performed.

By using CCTA it has been possible to show that plaque morphology is an independent predictor of prognosis [22,24,38]. Several studies have found that non-calcified plaques are associated with worse outcomes [23,39–40]. Among 3,499 consecutive symptomatic SA patients who underwent CCTA, 1,102 subjects with non-obstructive CAD were prospectively followed for a mean of 78 months. The death rate of these patients was 3.1%, increasing incrementally from calcified plaque (1.4%) to mixed plaque (3.3%) to non-calcified plaque (9.6%) [23]. Our present data indicate that the absolute neutrophil count as well as the neutrophil/lymphocyte ratio, obtained by a white blood cell differential test, reflects the burden of high-risk plaques, rather than the crude number of plaques. Combining these easily available biomarkers and CCTA may be of supplemental value in the identification of patients with vulnerable atherosclerotic plaques. It opens up the potential for early selective treatment and prevention of future myocardial damage.

The increased levels of CD4+ T cells and dynamic changes of NK cells in the patient population of the present study have been described recently [32,41]. However, we did not find any association between these cell subsets and CCTA plaque characteristics. Neither were there any relationships between the well-established inflammatory markers, CRP and IL-6, and the CCTA findings. Only one previous CCTA study has investigated immune cells in relation to plaque burden and plaque composition. Kashiwagi et al found that an increased level of the proinflammatory CD14+ CD16+ monocyte subset, but not the total number of monocytes or CRP, is related to the presence of vulnerable plaques in patients with stable angina pectoris [42]. Unfortunately, we did not measure monocyte subsets, but the lack of association between total number of monocytes, CRP and the presence of vulnerable plaques on CCTA was also found in our study.

A few studies have been performed in search of associations between other inflammatory markers and CCTA characteristics [43,44]. Bamberg et al determined the association between several

Table 3. Baseline leukocyte subsets and plasma cytokines of patients and controls.

	SA	NSTE-ACS	Controls	P-value
	N = 30	N = 20	N = 37	
Leukocytes (x10⁹/L)	7.1±2.2	7.7±2.3	5.5±1.4	<0.001$^{\psi\gamma}$
Neutrophils (x10⁹/L)	4.1±1.5	4.5±1.7	3.0±1.0	<0.001$^{\psi\gamma}$
Monocytes (x10⁹/L)	0.6±0.2	0.6±0.3	0.4±0.1	<0.001$^{\psi\gamma}$
Lymphocytes (x10⁹/L)	2.2±1.0	2.4±0.9	2.0±0.6	NS
CD19+ cells, % of lymphocytes	10 (7,12)	10 (8,15)	10 (7,14)	NS
CD4+ cells, % of lymphocytes	49 (42,54)	50 (44,54)	39 (33,48)	0.005$^{\psi}$, 0.001$^{\gamma}$
CD8+ cells, % of lymphocytes	25 (20,31)	25 (17,31)	23 (19,29)	NS
NK cells, % of lymphocytes	12 (9,18)	12 (7,15)	18 (11,28)	0.023$^{\psi\gamma}$
Neutrophil/lymphocyte ratio	2.1 (1.4,2.4)	2.0 (1.5,2.5)	1.5 (1.2,1.9)	0.012$^{\psi}$, 0.027$^{\gamma}$
Plasma IL-6, pg/mL	3.1 (2.0,5.7)	4.9 (2.9,8.0)	1.4 (1.0,2.2)	<0.001$^{\psi\gamma}$
Plasma CRP, mg/L	1.2 (0.3,3.2)	3.2 (2.2,5.0)	0.7 (0.4,1.2)	0.023$^{\Phi}$, <0.001$^{\gamma}$

The data are presented as mean ±SD or median (25th, 75th percentile). SA = stable angina; NSTE-ACS = non-ST-elevation acute coronary syndrome; CD19+ cells, B cells; CD4+ cells, T helper cells; CD8+ cell, cytotoxic T cell; NK = Natural killer; IL = interleukin; CRP = C-reactive protein. NS = non-significant (p≥0.05). For comparisons between groups, p-values indicating significant differences are denoted by ψ (controls vs SA), γ (controls vs NSTE-ACS) and Φ (SA vs NSTE-ACS), respectively.

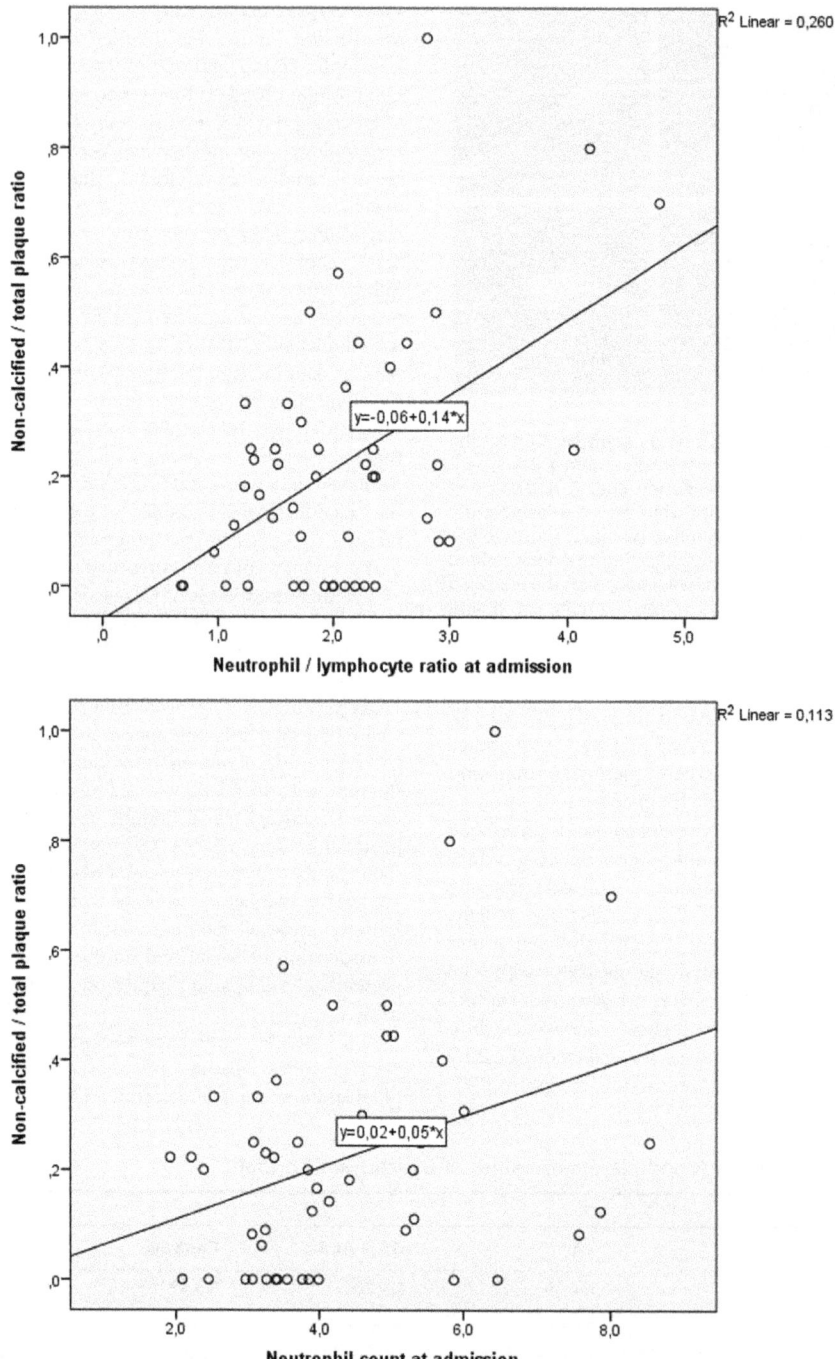

Figure 2. Neutrophils and coronary plaques on CCTA. Scatterplots demonstrating the associations between non-calcified/total plaque ratio on baseline CCTA and neutrophil/lymphocyte ratio and neutrophil counts at admission. Neutrophil counts are given as $\times 10^9$/L.

plasma biomarkers and coronary plaque burden assessed by CCTA in 313 patients with acute chest pain who ultimately had no evidence of ACS [43]. Only 25% of study individuals were on statins and those with prior CAD were excluded. Interestingly, they found higher levels of CRP and oxidized LDL cholesterol and lower levels of adiponectin in patients with exclusively non-calcified plaques as compared to those with any calcified plaque or no plaque at all. In our study, 60% of all patients were on statin treatment at the time of inclusion. This may explain the absence of

correlations between CRP and plaque characteristics, since statins are known to markedly reduce CRP levels [45]. Another study by Harada et al included 178 non-ACS acute chest pain patients, who underwent CCTA examination [44]. In contrast to the study by Bamberg et al, they found an association between CRP and the presence of calcified rather than non-calcified plaques.

This study has some major limitations. First, the size of the study population was small. On the other hand, we included both SA and ACS patients, who were examined by CCTA and blood sample analysis prior to ICA and revascularization as well as in the stabilized phase at 3 months. Secondly, this study was performed between 2006 and 2009, first using a 16-slice and later a 64-slice CCTA. The 16-slice CCTA is less accurate than the 64-slice CCTA in measuring degree of stenosis and plaque composition. However, we did use ICA as well to assess obstructive and non-obstructive plaque burden and CCTA was performed twice in a majority of patients yielding identical results. Thus, in order not to reduce the size of the study population, all study patients irrespective of CT-scanner used were included in the data analysis.

To conclude, both neutrophil counts and neutrophil/lymphocyte ratio were significantly correlated with non-calcified plaque burden and non-calcified plaque/total plaque ratio. The results highlight the potential utility of these easily measured cellular markers in the risk assessment and monitoring of CAD patients.

Acknowledgments

The authors thank Elisabeth Logander, RN, for coordinating patient logistics, Petter Quick, RN, and the radiology technicians at CMIV for performing CCTA, and Karin Backteman, PhD, for performing flow cytometri.

Author Contributions

Conceived and designed the experiments: LN MG JE ES LJ. Performed the experiments: LN WW GP MG LJ. Analyzed the data: LN WW GP MG JE ES LJ. Contributed reagents/materials/analysis tools: LN GP JE LJ. Wrote the paper: LN WW GP JE ES LJ.

References

1. Hansson GK (2005) Inflammation, atherosclerosis, and coronary artery disease. N Engl J Med 352: 1685–95.
2. Pai JK, Pischon T, Ma J, Manson JE, Hankinson SE, et al. (2004) Inflammatory markers and the risk of coronary heart disease in men and women. N Engl J Med 351: 2599–610.
3. Nijm J, Wikby A, Tompa A, Olsson AG, Jonasson L (2005) Circulating levels of proinflammatory cytokines and neutrophil-platelet aggregates in patients with coronary artery disease. Am J Cardiol 95(4): 452–6.
4. Jonasson L, Backteman K, Ernerudh J (2005) Loss of natural killer cell activity in patients with coronary artery disease. Atherosclerosis 183(2): 316–21.
5. Packard RR, Libby P (2008) Inflammation in atherosclerosis: from vascular biology to biomarker discovery and risk prediction. Clin Chem 54(1): 24–38.
6. Abdelmouttaleb I, Danchin N, Ilardo C, Aimone-Gastin I, Angioï M, et al. (1999) C-Reactive protein and coronary artery disease: additional evidence of the implication of an inflammatoryprocess in acute coronary syndromes. Am Heart J 137(2): 346–51.
7. Rifai N, Joubran R, Yu H, Asmi M, Jouma M (1999) Inflammatory markers in men with angiographically documented coronary heart disease. Clin Chem 45(11): 1967–73.
8. Bamberg F, Truong QA, Koenig W, Schlett CL, Nasir K, et al. (2012) Differential associations between blood biomarkers of inflammation, oxidation, and lipid metabolism with varying forms of coronary atherosclerotic plaque as quantified by coronary CT angiography. Int J Cardiovasc Imaging 28: 183–92.
9. Harada K, Amano T, Uetani T, Yoshida T, Kato B, et al. (2013) Association of inflammatory markers with the morphology and extent of coronary plaque as evaluated by 64-slice multidetector computed tomography in patients with stable coronary artery disease. Int J Cardiovasc Imaging 29: 1149–58.
10. Soehnlein O (2012) Multiple roles for neutrophils in atherosclerosis. Circ Res 110(6): 875–88.
11. Drechsler M, Megens RT, van Zandvoort M, Weber C, Soehnlein O (2010) Hyperlipidemia-triggered neutrophilia promotes early atherosclerosis. Circulation 122(18): 1837–45.
12. Rotzius P, Thams S, Soehnlein O, Kenne E, Tseng CN, et al. (2010) Distinct infiltration of neutrophils in lesion shoulders in ApoE-/- mice. Am J Pathol 177(1): 493–500.
13. Kawaguchi H, Mori T, Kawano T, Kono S, Sasaki J, et al. (1996) Band neutrophil count and the presence and severity of coronary atherosclerosis. Am Heart J 132(1 Pt 1): 9–12.
14. Arbel Y, Finkelstein A, Halkin A, Birati EY, Revivo M, et al. (2012) Neutrophil/lymphocyte ratio is related to the severity of coronary artery disease and clinical outcome in patients undergoing angiography. Atherosclerosis 225: 456–60.
15. Kalay N, Dogdu O, Koc F, Yarlioglues M, Ardic I, et al. (2012) Hematologic parameters and angiographic progression of coronary atherosclerosis. Angiology 63: 213–7.
16. Duffy BK, Gurm HS, Rajagopal V, Gupta R, Ellis SG, et al. (2006) Usefulness of an elevated neutrophil to lymphocyte ratio in predicting long-term mortality after percutaneous coronary intervention. Am J Cardiol 97(7): 993–6.
17. Papa A, Emdin M, Passino C, Michelassi C, Battaglia D, et al. (2008) Predictive value of elevated neutrophil-lymphocyte ratio on cardiac mortality in patients with stable coronary artery disease. Clin Chim Acta 395: 27–31.
18. Guasti L, Dentali F, Castiglioni L, Maroni L, Marino F, et al. (2011) Neutrophils and clinical outcomes in patients with acute coronary syndromes and/or cardiac revascularisation. A systematic review on more than 34,000 subjects. Thromb Haemost 106(4): 591–9.
19. Azab B, Chainani V, Shah N, McGinn JT (2013) Neutrophil-lymphocyte ratio as a predictor of major adverse cardiac events among diabetic population: a 4-year follow-up study. Angiology 64(6): 456–65.
20. Kolodgie FD, Burke AP, Farb A, Gold HK, Yuan J, et al. (2001) The thin-cap fibroatheroma: A type of vulnerable plaque: The major precursor lesion to acute coronary syndromes. Curr Opin Cardiol 16: 285–92.
21. Voros S, Rinehart S, Qian Z, Joshi P, Vazquez G, et al. (2011) Coronary atherosclerosis imaging by coronary CT angiography: Current status, correlation with intravascular interrogation and meta-analysis. JACC Cardiovasc Imaging 4: 537–48.
22. Russo V, Zavalloni A, Bacchi Reggiani ML, Buttazzi K, Gostoli V, et al. (2010) Incremental prognostic value of coronary CT angiography in patients with suspected coronary artery disease. Circ Cardiovasc Imaging 3: 351–9.
23. Ahmadi N, Nabavi V, Hajsadeghi F, Flores F, French WJ, et al. (2011) Mortality incidence of patients with non-obstructive coronary artery disease diagnosed by computed tomography angiography. Am J Cardiol 107: 10–16.
24. Pundziute G, Schuijf JD, Jukema JW, Boersma E, de Roos A, et al. (2007) Prognostic value of multislice computed tomography coronary angiography in patients with known or suspected coronary artery disease. J Am Coll Cardiol 49: 62–70.
25. The Joint European Society of Cardiology/American College of Cardiology Committee for the redefinition of myocardial infarction (2000) Myocardial infarction redefined - a consensus document of The Joint European Society of Cardiology/American College of Cardiology Committee for the redefinition of myocardial infarction. Eur Heart J 21(18): 1502–13.
26. Luepker RV, Apple FS, Christenson RH, Crow RS, Fortmann SP, et al. (2003) Case definitions for acute coronary heart disease in epidemiology and clinical research studies. Circulation 108(20): 2543–9.
27. Boogers MJ, Schuijf JD, Kitslaar PH, van Werkhoven JM, de Graaf FR, et al. (2010) Automated quantification of stenosis severity on 64-slice CT: A comparison with quantitative coronary angiography. JACC Cardiovasc Imaging 3: 699–709.
28. Leber AW, Knez A, Becker A, Becker C, von Ziegler F, et al. (2004) Accuracy of multidetector spiral computed tomography in identifying and differentiating the composition of coronary atherosclerotic plaques: A comparative study with intracoronary ultrasound. J Am Coll Cardiol 43: 1241–7.
29. Austen WG, Edwards JE, Frye RL, Gensini GG, Gott VL, et al. (1975) A reporting system on patients evaluated for coronary artery disease. report of the ad hoc committee for grading of coronary artery disease, council on cardiovascular surgery, american heart association. Circulation 51: 5–40.
30. Kitagawa T, Yamamoto H, Horiguchi J, Ohhashi N, Tadehara F, et al. (2009) Characterization of noncalcified coronary plaques and identification of culprit lesions in patients with acute coronary syndrome by 64-slice computed tomography. JACC Cardiovasc Imaging 2: 153–60.
31. Backteman K, Ernerudh J (2007) Biological and methodological variation of lymphocyte subsets in blood of human adults. J Immunol Methods 322: 20–7.
32. Bergstrom I, Backteman K, Lundberg A, Ernerudh J, Jonasson L (2012) Persistent accumulation of interferon-gamma-producing CD8+CD56+ T cells in blood from patients with coronary artery disease. Atherosclerosis 224: 515–20.
33. Galkina E, Ley K (2009) Immune and inflammatory mechanisms of atherosclerosis. Annu Rev Immunol 27: 165–97.
34. Wheeler JG, Mussolino ME, Gillum RF, Danesh J (2004) Associations between differential leucocyte count and incident coronary heart disease: 1764 incident cases from seven prospective studies of 30,374 individuals. Eur Heart J 25(15): 1287–92.
35. Rana JS, Boekholdt SM, Ridker PM, Jukema JW, Luben R, et al. (2007) Differential leucocyte count and the risk of future coronary artery disease in healthy men and women: the EPIC-Norfolk Prospective Population Study. J Intern Med 262(6): 678–89.
36. Madjid M, Awan I, Willerson JT, Casscells SW (2004) Leukocyte count and coronary heart disease: implications for risk assessment. J Am Coll Cardiol 44(10): 1945–56.
37. Park BJ, Shim JY, Lee HR, Lee JH, Jung DH, et al. (2011) Relationship of neutrophil-lymphocyte ratio with arterial stiffness and coronary calcium score. Clin Chim Acta 412: 925–9.
38. Hadamitzky M, Freissmuth B, Meyer T, Hein F, Kastrati A, et al. (2009) Prognostic value of coronary computed tomographic angiography for prediction

of cardiac events in patients with suspected coronary artery disease. JACC Cardiovasc Imaging 2: 404–11.

39. van Werkhoven JM, Schuijf JD, Gaemperli O, Jukema JW, Kroft IJ, et al. (2009) Incremental prognostic value of multi-slice computed tomography coronary angiography over coronary artery calcium scoring in patients with suspected coronary artery disease. Eur Heart J 30: 2622–9.

40. Gaemperli O, Valenta I, Schepis T, Husmann L, Scheffel H, et al. (2008) Coronary 64-slice CT angiography predicts outcome in patients with known or suspected coronary artery disease. Eur Radiol 18: 1162–73.

41. Backteman K, Ernerudh J, Jonasson L (2014) Natural killer (NK) cell deficit in coronary artery disease: no aberrations in phenotype but sustained reduction of NK cells is associated with low-grade inflammation. Clin Exp Immunol 175(1): 104–12.

42. Kashiwagi M, Imanishi T, Tsujioka H, Ikejima H, Kuroi A, et al. (2010) Association of monocyte subsets with vulnerability characteristics of coronary plaques as assessed by 64-slice multidetector computed tomography in patients with stable angina pectoris. Atherosclerosis 212(1): 171–6.

43. Bamberg F, Truong QA, Koenig W, Schlett CL, Nasir K, et al. (2012) Differential associations between blood biomarkers of inflammation, oxidation, and lipid metabolism with varying forms of coronary atherosclerotic plaque as quantified by coronary CT angiography. Int J Cardiovasc Imaging 28: 183–92.

44. Harada K, Amano T, Uetani T, Yoshida T, Kato B, et al. (2013) Association of inflammatory markers with the morphology and extent of coronary plaque as evaluated by 64-slice multidetector computed tomography in patients with stable coronary artery disease. Int J Cardiovasc Imaging 29: 1149–58.

45. Jialal I, Stein D, Balis D, Grundy SM, Adams-Huet B, et al. (2001) Effect of hydroxymethyl glutaryl coenzyme a reductase inhibitor therapy on high sensitive C-reactive protein levels. Circulation 103(15): 1933–5.

18

Interactive Local Super-Resolution Reconstruction of Whole-Body MRI Mouse Data: A Pilot Study with Applications to Bone and Kidney Metastases

Oleh Dzyubachyk[1][9][¶], Artem Khmelinskii[1,2][9][¶], Esben Plenge[3][9][¶], Peter Kok[1,4][9][¶], Thomas J. A. Snoeks[1], Dirk H. J. Poot[3,5], Clemens W. G. M. Löwik[1], Charl P. Botha[1,4], Wiro J. Niessen[3,5], Louise van der Weerd[1,6], Erik Meijering[3], Boudewijn P. F. Lelieveldt[1,4]*

1 Department of Radiology, Leiden University Medical Center, Leiden, the Netherlands, 2 Percuros B.V., Enschede, the Netherlands, 3 Departments of Radiology and Medical Informatics, Erasmus MC — University Medical Center Rotterdam, Rotterdam, the Netherlands, 4 Department of Intelligent Systems, Delft University of Technology, Delft, the Netherlands, 5 Quantitative Imaging Group, Faculty of Applied Sciences, Delft University of Technology, Delft, the Netherlands, 6 Department of Human Genetics, Leiden University Medical Center, Leiden, the Netherlands

Abstract

In small animal imaging studies, when the locations of the micro-structures of interest are unknown *a priori*, there is a simultaneous need for full-body coverage and high resolution. In MRI, additional requirements to image contrast and acquisition time will often make it impossible to acquire such images directly. Recently, a resolution enhancing post-processing technique called super-resolution reconstruction (SRR) has been demonstrated to improve visualization and localization of micro-structures in small animal MRI by combining multiple low-resolution acquisitions. However, when the field-of-view is large relative to the desired voxel size, solving the SRR problem becomes very expensive, in terms of both memory requirements and computation time. In this paper we introduce a novel *local* approach to SRR that aims to overcome the computational problems and allow researchers to efficiently explore both global and local characteristics in whole-body small animal MRI. The method integrates state-of-the-art image processing techniques from the areas of articulated atlas-based segmentation, planar reformation, and SRR. A proof-of-concept is provided with two case studies involving CT, BLI, and MRI data of bone and kidney tumors in a mouse model. We show that local SRR-MRI is a computationally efficient complementary imaging modality for the precise characterization of tumor metastases, and that the method provides a feasible high-resolution alternative to conventional MRI.

Editor: Gayle E. Woloschak, Northwestern University Feinberg School of Medicine, United States of America

Funding: This work was funded by Medical Delta (http://www.medicaldelta.nl/research/large-research-programs-and-initiatives/molecular-image-processing). A.K. also acknowledges support from the FP7 European Union Marie Curie IAPP Program, BRAINPATH, under grant number 612360. The funders had no role in study design, data collection and analysis, decision to publish, or preparation of the manuscript.

Competing Interests: The authors have declared that no competing interests exist.

* Email: b.p.f.lelieveldt@lumc.nl

⑨ These authors contributed equally to this work.

¶ OD, AK, EP, and PK are co-first authors on this work.

Introduction

In pre-clinical small animal research on complications of cancer, imaging modalities like bioluminescence (BLI), CT, and MRI are conventionally used. Such imaging techniques allow non-invasive studies on the metastatic behavior of tumors [1]. BLI gives an indication of metastatic tumor growth anywhere in the body (*e.g.* bones, liver, and lungs), but the spatial resolution is not sufficient to distinguish between lesions located in close proximity to each other and to actually localize all individual metastatic processes in an organ. CT gives excellent contrast in calcified tissue and can be used to study tumor-induced changes in the bone, but it is less suitable to image organs such as liver and lungs due to lack of soft tissue contrast. MRI is the preferred imaging modality for imaging liver and lung metastases as it gives sufficient anatomical detail and good contrast between the organs and

tumor masses. So, whereas BLI can be used to indicate the total tumor burden in an organ, MRI provides information on the location, size, and number of metastatic lesions in the organ. Since the location of the tumors is not known *a priori*, whole-body imaging is used, and CT, MRI, and BLI together aim to provide a comprehensive picture of the tumor and metastases development and spread in the entire body.

The sensitivity of MRI for small lesions is, however, relatively low compared to BLI, and the most robust pre-clinical protocols are still 2D MRI experiments with relatively thick slices. This slice thickness results in a large partial volume effect, making precise detection and localization of tumors difficult, especially for early stage tumors and micro tumors [2]. Recently, a resolution enhancing post-processing technique called super-resolution reconstruction (SRR) has been demonstrated to improve visualization and localization of micro-structures in molecular MRI

[3,4]. SRR computes a high-resolution image by combining a number of low-resolution images with varying fields-of-view (FOV). In a metastatic disease model, however, the size of the object under investigation (the mouse/rat) can be very large relative to the size of the structures of interest (the tumors). When attempting to capture both global and local scales in an image, this translates into a large field-of-view at high image resolution, resulting in images of tens of millions of voxels. In such cases, solving the SRR problem becomes very expensive, in terms of both computation time and memory requirements. Exploring large data sets in this way calls for conceptual new-thinking.

In this study, we propose a novel approach to overcome the computational issues of whole-body SRR without sacrificing reconstruction quality. By integrating state-of-the-art methods from the areas of articulated atlas-based segmentation of whole-body small animal data [5–9], planar reformation [10], and SRR in MRI [3,11], we arrive at a novel localized approach to SRR that enables interactive global-to-local exploration of *e.g.* whole-body mouse MRI data while being computationally efficient. The idea is similar to that of well-known web-based geographical maps, where it is possible, from a global overview image, to zoom in on a detail of interest. Guided by user interaction or by registration to images of higher sensitivity, such as BLI, local volumes-of-interest (VOIs) can be identified in the low-resolution MR image and enhanced by SRR to show a higher level of detail.

Thus, the goals of this work are two-fold:

1. To provide an integrated, interactive platform for local super-resolution reconstruction of MRI whole-body mouse data.

2. To demonstrate in a proof-of-concept study that local SRR is a feasible method for improving visualization and localization of metastases in whole-body small animal imaging studies, where by feasibility we refer to the following two aspects:

a) *Image quality:* Does the local SRR method improve the visualization of small anatomical details over conventional imaging methods, under the condition that the number of low-resolution images used for the SRR is constrained by a total acquisition time compatible with *in vivo* experiments?

b) *Computational feasibility:* Can the local SRR computations be handled on a desktop machine in a close-to-real-time time frame?

In the following sections, we first introduce our approach to local SRR in MRI. We briefly describe its components (for details we refer to previously published work in which each of the components has been thoroughly validated) and present a phantom experiment that quantifies the ability of SRR to detect micro-structures. We validate our approach in two case studies with bone and kidney breast cancer metastases visualization and finally discuss the presented results.

Materials and Methods

Experimental mouse model and imaging

To test the SRR approach, BLI, CT, and MRI were acquired in a mouse model of metastasizing breast cancer. One female, *Balb/c nu/nu* mouse of 19.5 g was used. At 7–8 weeks of age, the mouse was injected with 4T1-luc2 [12,13] breast cancer cells (100 μl, 150,000 cells) into the left heart ventricle under 2% Isoflurane anesthesia.

After 2–3 weeks, BLI and CT scans were made *in vivo*. The anesthesia applied was Ketamine:RomPun:PBS (1:1:1), approxi-

mately 60 μl/20 g. This was followed by an *ex vivo* MRI scan. The mouse was euthanized to allow flexibility in the MRI experiments and test different acquisition parameters.

The mouse, in prone position, was taped to an in-house made PMMA holder that was used in all three scanners. BLI data was acquired using an IVIS 3D BLI Imaging system (Caliper Life Sciences, Alameda, CA). BLI images were taken from 8 positions around the animal with an exposure time of 10 s per image, allowing for 3D data reconstruction. One of the eight BLI images is presented in Figure 1.

CT data was acquired on a SkyScan 1076 *in vivo* microCT scanner (Aartselaar, Belgium) at a resolution of 35 μm. The acquisition was performed with a step size of 1.4° over a trajectory of 360° (Voltage = 49 kV, Current = 200 uA, Exposure time = 100 ms, Filter: AL. 0.5 mm, Frame averaging = 1).

Several strategies can be adopted when acquiring MR data for an SRR experiment. By acquiring the low-resolution slice stacks with rotational increments around either the frequency or the phase encoding direction, as introduced in [14], a more effective sampling of k-space is achieved than by shifting the low-resolution images by sub-pixel distances along the slice selection direction [3]. In this way, a whole-body scan of the *post mortem* mouse was acquired on a 7T Bruker Pharmascan system using a fast spin echo (FSE) sequence (TR = 5300 ms, TE = 53.2 ms, with N_{avg} = 4). The 2D slice stack consisted of 40 slices (0.5 mm thick), with a FOV of $70 \times 45 \times 20$ mm^3, and a resulting resolution of $0.125 \times 0.125 \times 0.5$ mm^3. The scan time per stack was 13 min. The slice stack was acquired at 24 angles with uniform increments of $180°/24 = 7.5°$ around the phase encoding direction. First results obtained using 24 low-resolution images were published in [9]. In this study, we performed SRR on subsets of two and four low-resolution images. In the subset of two images, the angular increment between them was $180°/2 = 90°$ and in the subset of four images it was $180°/4 = 45°$.

Animal experiments were approved by the local committee for animal health, ethics and research of Leiden University Medical Center.

Integrated, Interactive Local SRR Reconstruction

The local SRR method integrates a series of processing and analysis steps, which depend on the available complementary data (CT, BLI, *etc.*) and vary in their level of user interaction. The overview of the presented method can be seen in the flowchart

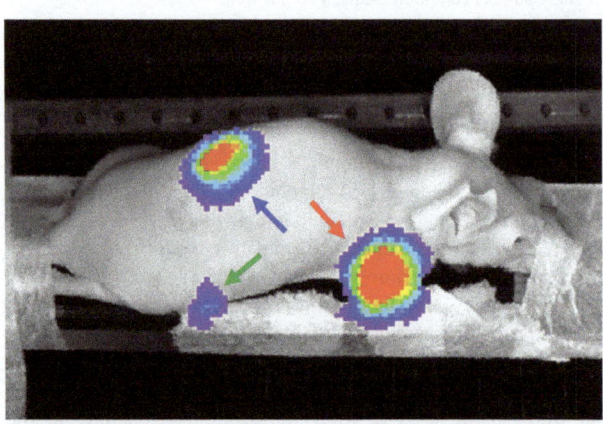

Figure 1. A BLI photographic image of the mouse acquired to validate the proposed approach. The arrows indicate the different tumor locations: humerus (red), femur (green), kidney (blue).

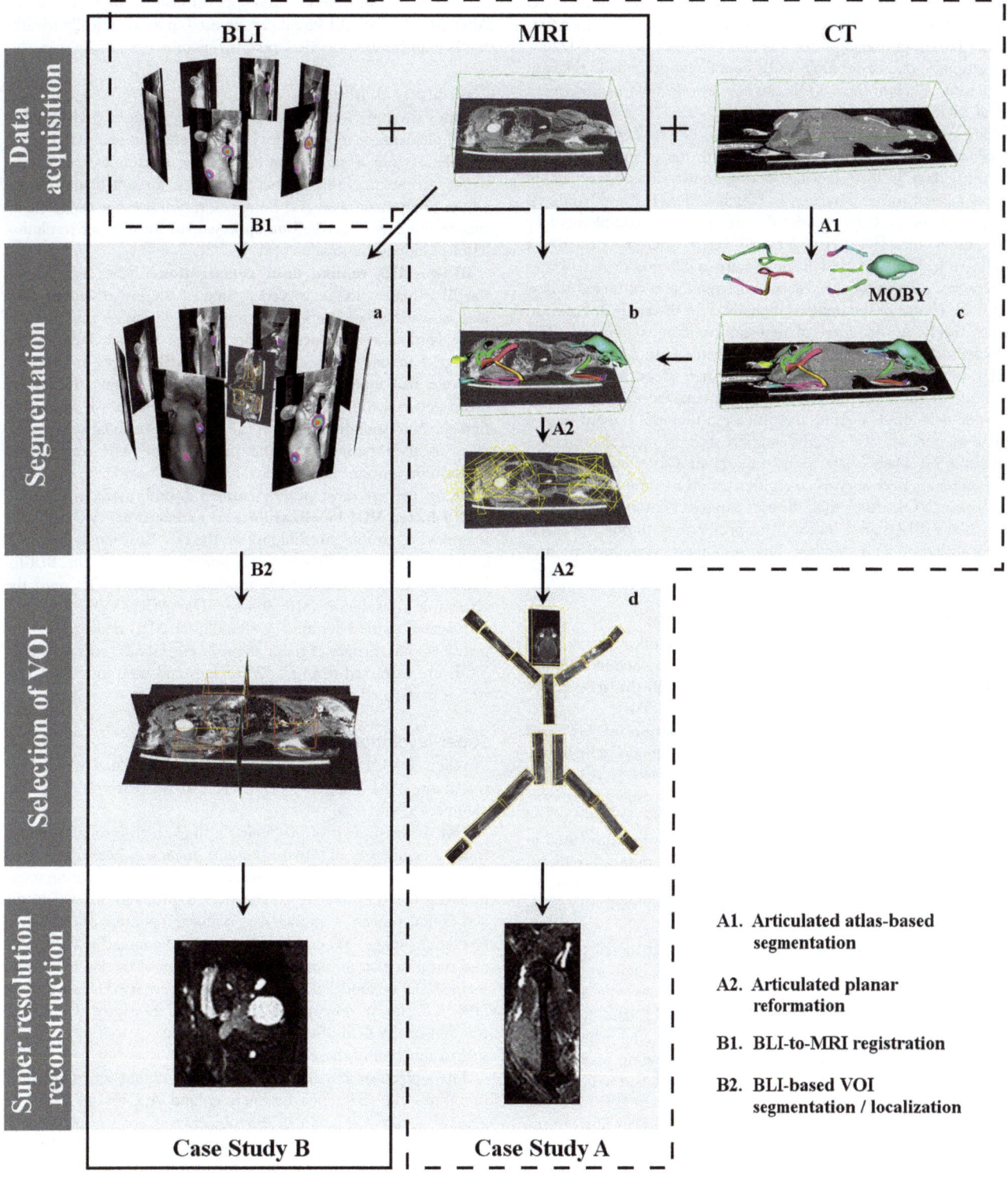

Figure 2. Overview of the integrated, interactive local SRR of MRI mouse data applied to two case studies. Case Study A: After rigidly registering CT to MRI, articulated atlas-based segmentation is performed (A1). Subsequently, articulated planar reformation is applied to the segmented MRI, and the data is visualized in the standardized atlas space (A2). The user can now interactively select any bone of interest guided by the BLI images for SRR reconstruction. A high-resolution SRR image of the humerus with a tumor is presented. **Case Study B:** BLI+MRI mouse data are first co-registered (B1) to define the VOIs (B2) using the BLI. A VOI is interactively selected for performing SRR. A high-resolution SRR image of the kidney with metastases is presented.

depicted in Figure 2. First, within a set of low-resolution MRI images, potential VOIs are identified. In our approach, this step is either based on user input or it is automated, as described below. Its output is one or multiple VOIs containing potentially relevant structures. Each of these VOIs can now be selected for subsequent local SRR.

The methods for segmentation and selection of VOIs are highly specific to the biological problem and to the available complementary data. In the following, we present two situations typical in small animal tumor imaging, in which BLI+CT (Case Study A) and BLI only (Case Study B) are used as complementary modalities to MRI (see Figure 2). Each situation presents a different level of automation and requires a different degree of user interaction. The way the relevant information is extracted differs with the choice of the imaging modalities for the study at hand. In Case Study A, the level of user intervention is minimal. The whole-body mouse is automatically segmented using an articulated atlas. Guided by the BLI, the user can then select the VOIs with tumors for further SRR reconstruction, visualize the results side-by-side with the CT data, and, in case a tumor is present near a bone on one side of the body, compare it to the contralateral side, where most likely there is no tumor. In Case Study B, user interaction is necessary to co-register the BLI to the MRI data to define the VOIs. After that, the user can select among the VOIs in which the BLI signal indicate the presence of tumors for SRR reconstruction and further high-resolution visualization and analysis.

Case Study A: MRI+CT+BLI

This case study was set up to explore the applicability of local SRR-MRI to image bone metastases as a complementary modality to CT, BLI and conventional MRI. In this section, we describe our approach to super-resolution bone MRI.

Articulated atlas-based bone segmentation of CT and MRI mouse data. First, rigid registration of the CT scan to one of the low-resolution MR images was performed [7,15]. Rigid registration was sufficient in this case because the mouse was fixated in the same animal bed during all imaging procedures and during transport between scanners. The bones were segmented in the CT image using the articulated MOBY mouse atlas [6,16] (Figure 2.c). The fully automated segmentation approach presented in [5] was used for this purpose. To deal with the large articulations between bones and/or bone groups, the registration of the atlas to the CT data used a hierarchical model tree. To begin with, a coarse alignment of the MOBY atlas to the CT skeleton was performed. This was followed by the stepwise alignment of the individual atlas bones to the CT data, using the ICP algorithm [17]: we started with the skull, after which each bone was accurately registered to the corresponding bone in the data. Given the CT-to-MR registration parameters, the transform obtained in the segmentation of the whole-body CT data was propagated to the MR. Figures 2.(b, c) show the atlas fitted to the CT and MRI datasets, respectively; see [5] for more details.

Articulated planar reformation of MRI data. Using the obtained transformations between each bone in the atlas and the low-resolution MR image, articulated planar reformation [10] can be applied to map the labeled data into a standardized atlas space. This method automatically creates for each bone a VOI, which is based on a principal component analysis of the bone shape. By constructing the VOIs in this manner, the final reformatted images are aligned with the principal axes of the bones [10].

(Interactive) selection of VOIs. Upon segmentation and reformation, the user is presented with a global view of the segmented bones; see Figure 2.d. From this view, the user can choose bones of interest and perform local SRR on them. Alternatively, the BLI-signal can be used to automatically identify VOIs with tumors for SRR reconstruction.

Case Study B: MRI+BLI

This case study was set up to explore the value of SRR-MRI as a complementary modality to BLI and conventional MRI when CT data is not available for establishing anatomical correspondence. In practice, this is usually the case for soft tissue tumors, where bone metastases and bone resorption are not expected. In this section, we describe our approach to local super-resolution MRI of kidney tumors.

BLI-to-MRI mouse data registration. After acquisition, the BLI images are registered to one of the low-resolution MR images using a landmark-based approach [7,15]. A minimum of three landmarks is selected. The location of each landmark is indicated in one of the low-resolution MR images and in two separate BLI images at different angulations. Using the known angle between the two BLI images, back-projection is applied to find the corresponding point in the three-dimensional space. This point is then paired with the point in the MR image, and registration is performed. Typical landmarks include the snout and limbs as they are most easily identified in both modalities.

BLI-based VOI localization and extraction. VOIs can be identified by simple thresholding on the raw BLI signal. Once the coordinates of the VOIs in world space are known, the BLI-to-MRI registration transform is used to map the VOIs onto the chosen low-resolution MR image. The MRI VOIs are then propagated to the remaining low-resolution MRI images using the transform parameters of these acquisitions. Finally, corresponding VOIs are extracted from all LR images and used for SRR. This step is performed automatically.

Super-resolution reconstruction

When a VOI has been selected and propagated to all low-resolution MRI images, local SRR can be performed on that volume.

SRR is the process of producing a single high-resolution image from a sequence of low-resolution images, where each low-resolution image transforms and samples the high-resolution scene in a distinct fashion. It is an inverse problem in which the acquisition process is modeled as a linear operator on the high-resolution image. When the high-resolution image is vectorized and put into a large vector $\mathbf{x}$, the acquisition of the low-resolution image k can be modeled as $\mathbf{y}_k = \mathbf{A}_k\mathbf{x}+\mathbf{n}_k$, where $\mathbf{n}$ is Gaussian noise [18]. The linear operator $\mathbf{A}_k$ models the transform due to the rotation of the field-of-view of the kth image as well as the point spread function of the acquisition.

The objective in SRR is to find an $\mathbf{x}$ that simultaneously minimizes the difference between $\mathbf{y}_k$ and $\mathbf{A}_k\mathbf{x}$ for all k [3]. In general, a direct solution of this objective is not feasible since it involves many operations with all $\mathbf{A}_k \in \mathcal{R}^{n \times m}$, where n and m are the number of voxels in the reconstruction ($\mathbf{x}$) and in a low-resolution image ($\mathbf{y}_k$), respectively. Instead, the reconstruction is obtained by iterative methods such as the conjugate gradient method. In this study, we apply the method described in [11], which uses the conjugate gradient method to solve the Tikhonov-regularized least-squares problem and implements $\mathbf{A}$ and $\mathbf{A}^T$ by an affine transformation scheme that minimizes aliasing and spectral distortion. The SRR method is extended with a bias-field correction step removing inhomogeneity differences between the images caused by variations in coil sensitivity.

Phantom validation study

To quantitatively evaluate the performance of SRR with respect to detection of micro tumors, we designed a phantom experiment in which micro tumors were simulated by fluorescent micro beads, and imaged using a very similar acquisition protocol to the one described in "Experimental mouse model and imaging" section. In the following we describe the phantom, the imaging setup, and our quantification method in full detail.

Different-sized clusters of fluorescent beads were immersed in agar and used to simulate the micro metastases. Fluorescence imaging (FLI) was used instead of BLI (Figure 3.i), and a 3D

gradient echo (GE) sequence was used as the gold standard (Figure 3.a). The use of this sequence was possible due to the low proton density of the fluorescent beads. The SRR results were quantitatively compared to that of the interpolated single low-resolution image and the 3D GE.

Phantom preparation. Red fluorescent polyethylene microspheres with a diameter of 150–180 nm (UVPMS-BR-0.995, Cospheric LCC, Santa Barbara, CA, USA) were left overnight in 2 ml 1‰ Tween (Sigma-Aldrich, St. Louis, MO, USA) in a 2 ml reaction vial (Eppendorf, Hamburg, Germany) on a roller bank in

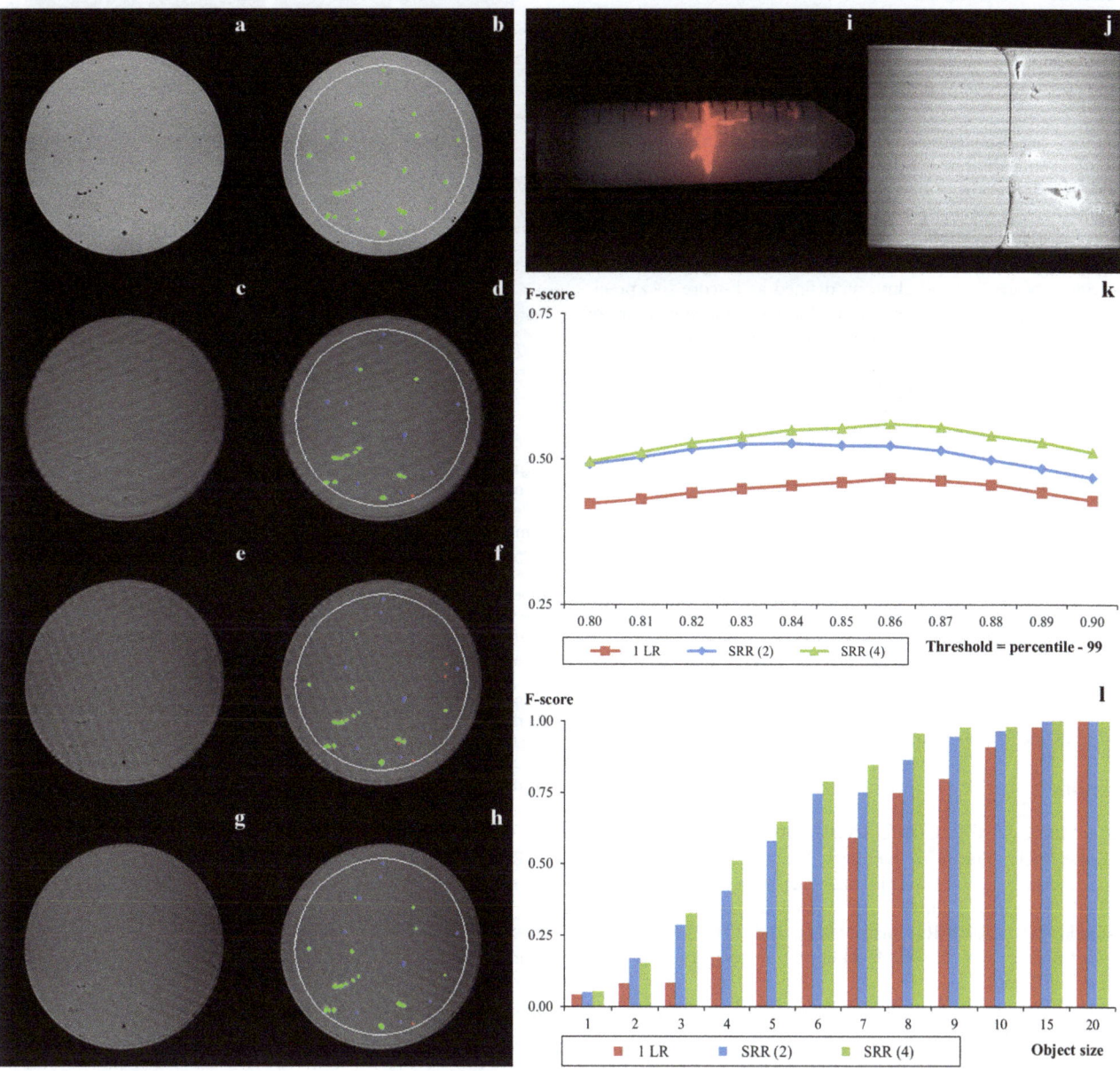

Figure 3. Phantom experiment. (a, c, e, g) One transversal slice from the 3D GE image (gold standard), single low-resolution (1 LR), SRR (2), and SRR (4) reconstructions respectively. (b, d, f, h) The same slice with the boundary of the region used for quantification (white) and detected objects (green, red, and blue; all regions occupied by segmented objects have been dilated with one pixel for better visualization). Green color indicates true positive detections based on the high-quality GE scan, red—false positives, and blue—false negatives (note that several visually missing objects were detected on other slices, hence they are not highlighted as false negatives on the shown slice). (i) FLI image of the phantom. (j) One coronal slice from the 1 LR image. (k) Detection performance in terms of the F-score of different reconstruction methods as functions of the threshold on the bottom-hat image. (l) F-score as function of object size for optimal threshold on each of the reconstructed volumes.

a concentration of 250 mg particles per ml in order to get single particles in suspension.

Approximately 25 ml 2% agar (Sigma-Aldrich) was poured into a 50 ml conic centrifuge tube (Sigma-Aldrich) and left at room temperature to cool down. Small volumes (10–20 µl) of microsphere suspension were carefully pipetted underneath the agar surface after the agar polymerization started, but before the agar gel was completely set. The rest of the tube was filled with 2% agar after the initial 25 ml agar polymerized (Figure 3.i).

Data acquisition. FLI of the phantom was performed using the IVIS Spectrum (PerkinElmer, Waltham, MA, USA) using the $\lambda_{ex} = 430$ nm and $\lambda_{em} = 600$ nm filters (Figure 3.i).

Four low-resolution MRI views of the phantom, rotated 45° with respect to each other, were acquired with a protocol very similar to the one described in the "Experimental mouse model and imaging" section: 64 slices, in plane resolution 0.1305×0.1305 mm^2, slice thickness 0.52 mm and a FOV $33 \times 33 \times 33$ mm^3. In addition, high-quality GE image of the phantom was acquired with the same resolution as the low-resolution images and used as the gold standard.

Object detection. The SRR images using 1, 2, and 4 low-resolution volumes (labeled 1 LR, SRR (2), and SRR (4) respectively) were calculated as explained in the "Super-resolution reconstruction" section. F-score of the detected objects (separate individual beads or bead clusters), defined as F-score = 2×precision×recall/(precision+recall) was used as quantitative measure of the quality of the three reconstructed volumes. The objects were detected by using a bottom-hat filter with a structuring element in the form of a 5×5 square, followed by thresholding and extraction of connected components [19]. Initially, multiple thresholds were defined as an intensity percentile of the corresponding bottom-hat map, and tested on the LR image, the SRR images, and the gold standard GE image; see Figure 3.k. For each data set, the threshold maximizing the F-score was chosen as the optimal one. In this analysis, objects located close to the boudary of the phantom were disregarded to exclude possibility of incorrect detection in this region due to reconstruction artifacts.

Hardware and Software platforms

The experiments described in the sections above were performed on a 2.80 GHz Intel Xeon with 12 GB of RAM Windows Workstation. The described registration, segmentation, and SRR algorithms were implemented in MATLAB R2009b.

Results

Case Study A: MRI+CT+BLI (bone tumors)

Local SRR images of the right femur and humerus with metastases were reconstructed at different levels of quality using 2 and 4 low-resolution images and compared with a single low-resolution (1 LR) MRI image, BLI, and CT. In addition, reconstruction times of individual bones were compared with that of the entire mouse.

On BLI (Figure 1), three distinct signal areas were observed, the smallest one at the position of the right femur (green arrow). The user therefore manually selected the right femur for SRR of the MRI data, using 2 or 4 low-resolution images for the reconstruction: SRR (2) and SRR (4) respectively; see Figure 4. The arrows in the BLI and the SRR (2) and SRR (4) images point to a tumor adjacent to the medial chondyle. This tumor is neither visible in the CT image, nor in the low-resolution image. When using 2 low-resolution images for SRR, the image quality increases, and the tumor becomes discernible. Using 4 low-resolution images further improves the visibility of the tumor and its margins.

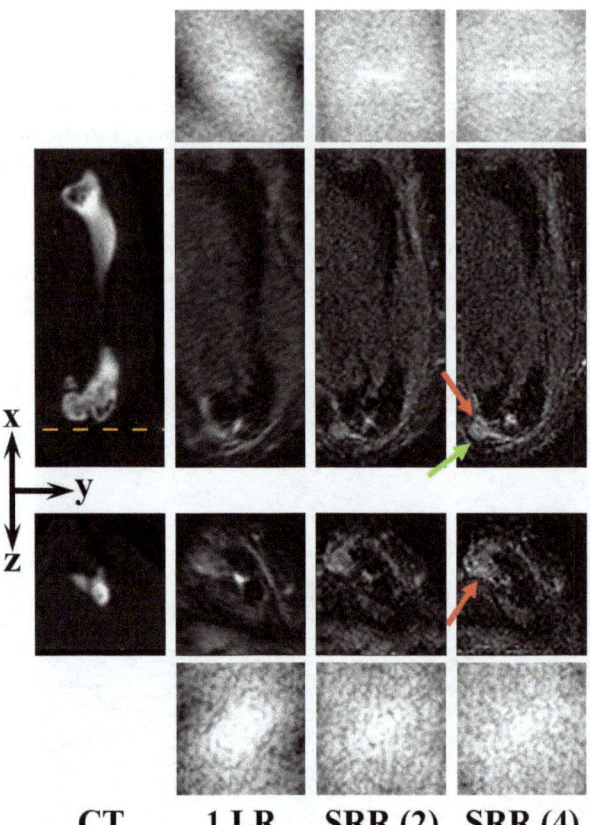

CT   1 LR   SRR (2)   SRR (4)

Figure 4. Right femur. From left to right: a CT scan, a single low-resolution image (1 LR), and SRR reconstructions, each based on a different number of low-resolution images. Two orthogonal slices of the same VOI are shown to illustrate the effect of the SRR in a 3D volume. The orange dashed line approximately indicates where the *yz*-slice (3rd row) intersects the *xy*-slice (2nd row). The red arrows points to the (micro) tumor in the knee. The green arrow points to a location outside the tumor, at which recovery of the fine details is obvious: the margins of the tumor are clearly delineated. The CT and all the MR images are shown in the coordinate system associated with the principal axes of the bone, and the low-resolution volume is resampled to isotropic resolution beforehand. Image contrast on the MRI images was increased for visualization purposes. For all MR images the corresponding frequency spectra up to the Nyquist frequency of the reconstruction volume are shown, above and beneath the *xy*-slices and the *yz*-slices, respectively, demonstrating enhanced high-frequency content.

BLI also showed a high intensity area at the location of the right humerus (Figure 1, red arrow). The tumor is not visible on CT (Figure 5). The single low-resolution image does show the tumor, but, due to the relatively thick slices, the tumor margins are blurred, particularly in the transverse plane. As before, the image quality improves when using more low-resolution images, showing a clear delineation of the tumor, with SRR (4) being sharper and less noisy than SRR (2).

To assert that SRR produced an actual resolution enhancement, frequency spectra were produced by applying a windowed Fourier transform to the shown MRI slices. The resolution enhancing effect in Figures 4 and 5 is clear: when more images are used for reconstruction, the spectrum of the SRR image contains more high-frequency content than the low-resolution images.

Table 1 shows how the SRR reconstruction times scale approximately linearly with the size of the low-resolution dataset. Since a single low-resolution image of the entire mouse contains

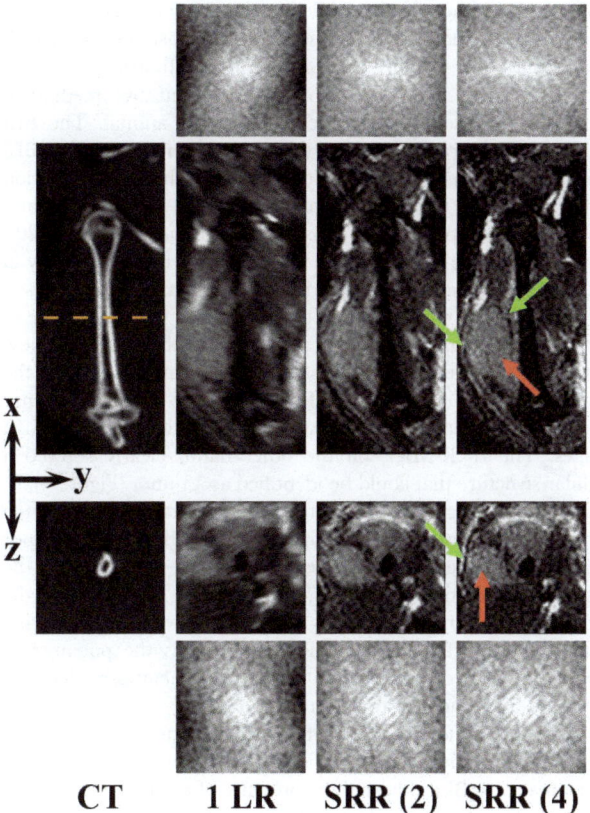

x

y

z

| CT | 1 LR | SRR (2) | SRR (4) |

Figure 5. Right humerus. From left to right: a CT scan, a single low-resolution image (1 LR), and SRR reconstructions, each based on a different number of low-resolution images. Two orthogonal slices of the same VOI are shown to illustrate the effect of the SRR in a 3D volume. The orange dashed line approximately indicates where the yz-slice (3rd row) intersects the xy-slice (2nd row). The red arrows point to the tumor. The green arrows point to some of the locations where recovery of the fine details is the most noticeable. The CT and all the MR images are shown in the coordinate system associated with the principal axes of the bone, and the low-resolution volume is resampled to isotropic resolution beforehand. Image contrast on the MRI images was increased for visualization purposes. For all MR images the corresponding frequency spectra up to the Nyquist frequency of the reconstruction volume are shown, above and beneath the xy-slices and the yz-slices, respectively, demonstrating enhanced high-frequency content.

approximately 20 million voxels, and a typical VOI contains around 250,000 voxels, we accelerate the reconstruction by

approximately a factor 80. From the table, it also follows that the SRR times scale approximately linearly with the number of low-resolution images used. While the entire mouse takes more than 40 minutes to reconstruct using 4 low-resolution images, a VOI can be reconstructed within 1–2 minutes.

The segmentation and selection of VOIs steps described above each take less than a minute to perform.

Case Study B: MRI+BLI (kidney tumors)

BLI showed a single high signal intensity around the area of the right kidney (Figure 1, blue arrow). Local SRR images of this area were reconstructed at different levels of quality and compared with a single low-resolution MRI image and BLI. Figure 6 shows orthogonal slices of the kidney for the different image types (a single low-resolution image, and SRR on 2 and 4 low-resolution images). On the BLI in Figure 1, the spatial resolution is too low to determine whether multiple tumors are present, but on MRI one large possibly cancerous lesion and several small suspected lesions can be detected. Most of these are readily detectable on the low-resolution image. However, the lesions appear blurred and cannot be clearly delineated. In such images, the smallest lesions are lost due to partial volume effects, but will be recovered in the SRR (2) or SRR (4) images. The high 3D resolution of the SRR scans also shows that most of these suspected lesions are located in the renal cortex and medulla, whereas the renal pelvis is relatively clean. Again, we asserted the resolution enhancement due to SRR by producing frequency spectra of the shown images.

Phantom quantification

A comparison of Figure 3.i and Figure 3.j clearly shows that it is impossible to distinguish the different clusters of beads (simulated micro tumors) using FLI due to its limited spatial resolution. It is, however, possible to distinguish the clusters using MRI.

From the plots shown in Figure 3.k, it follows that detection on both SRR volumes is, in general, much better in comparison with the interpolated 1 LR volume. SRR (4) exhibits consistently better object detection in comparison with SRR (2) and 1 LR.

Figure 3.l illustrates detection scores on each reconstructed volume as a function of the object size. Performing this analysis with increasing object size threshold shows an increasing trend for the detection score on all volumes, with perfect detection rates for all three volumes on objects larger than 20 voxels. This analysis shows that SRR greatly improves detection of small objects. Moreover, using more LR images for reconstruction results in higher detection rates, where the quality improvement is attributed to better performance on small objects.

Table 1. SRR times in seconds for each reconstructed right bone and the whole-body of the mouse, using 2 and 4 low-resolution images.

	2 low-resolution	4 low-resolution
Femur	56	98
Tibia-Fibula	38	75
Pelvis	79	151
Sternum	31	63
Humerus	48	83
Ulna-Radius	41	78
Whole-Body	1282	2479

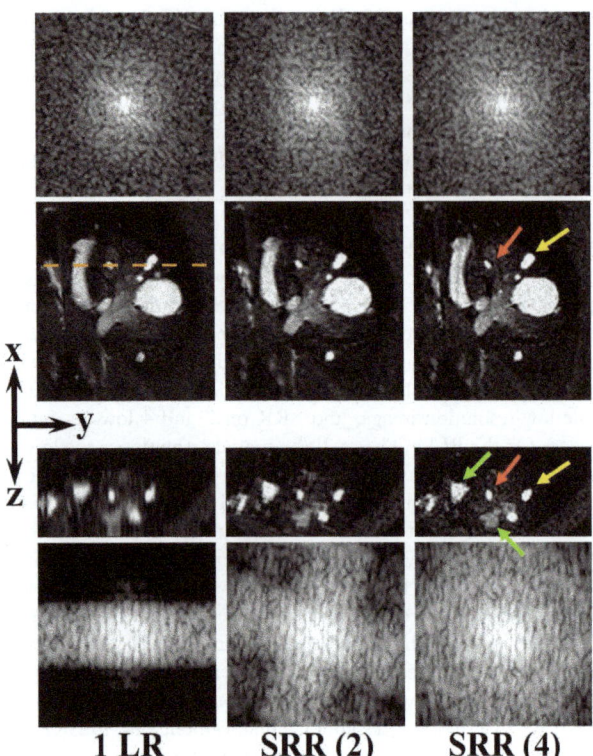

1 LR   SRR (2)   SRR (4)

Figure 6. Right kidney. From left to right: a single low-resolution image (1 LR), and SRR reconstructions, each based on a different number of low-resolution images. The red and yellow arrows point to two different tumors. Two orthogonal slices of the same VOI are shown to illustrate the effect of the SRR in a 3D volume. The green arrows point to other locations where the improvement in image quality is particularly noticeable. The orange dashed line approximately indicates where the yz-slice (3rd row) intersects the xy-slice (2nd row). In all the MR images, the xy-view is the in-plane direction of the scans. Note that the metastatic lesion seen in the BLI image (Figure 1, blue arrow) actually consists of numerous lesions as shown on MRI scans. For the low-resolution image, the selected views are resampled to isotropic resolution and the image contrast on the MRI images was increased for visualization purposes. For all MR images the corresponding frequency spectra up to the Nyquist frequency of the reconstruction volume are shown, above and beneath the xy-slices and the yz-slices, respectively, demonstrating enhanced high-frequency content.

Discussion

In this paper we have presented a proof-of-concept study as a first step towards real-time, interactive local SRR-MRI. While the approach can be applied in many biomedical imaging settings, where both global and local scales are relevant, we have chosen to explore our method in the context of bone and kidney metastases in mice. In the following, we discuss the results of the study and deliberate on potential challenges as well as advantages of the method.

Relevance to tumor research and other biological applications

Conventionally, bone resorption and metastases in soft tissues (such as kidney, lung, and liver) are visualized using BLI+CT and BLI+MRI, respectively. In this study, we have explored the value of adding SRR-MRI to improve soft tissue tumor detection. We have shown in two case studies how an integrated approach, combining state-of-the-art technologies from the area of image processing with the use of multiple imaging modalities, can be used to detect and study bone and soft tissue metastases with much greater sensitivity than by the conventional methods.

In Case Study A, we saw how BLI is a sensitive method to visualize luciferase-positive tumors in a living animal. The BLI signal intensity is proportional to the size of a tumor mass, and BLI can thus be used to give a rough estimate of both size and location of the lesion. In the case of bone metastases, the location and subsequent bone pathology are usually determined using CT [20]. However, in Case Study A there was no visible bone pathology in the CT scan. When local SRR-MRI guided by the BLI signal was performed, these images provided the location, size, and shape of tumors in the limbs of the animal and confirmed that these metastases were, indeed, soft tissue tumors located outside of the bone. In the low-resolution MRI images of the femur, the tumor could not have been identified without the guidance of the BLI images. The SRR-MRI, on the other hand, clearly showed a nodular structure that could be identified as a tumor (Figure 4). In the humerus images, which contain a large tumor outside of the bone, it can be appreciated how the delineation of the tumor boundary becomes much sharper in the SRR-MRI than in the single low-resolution MR image (see Figure 5; note that the improvement in image quality is especially noticeable when using a high zooming factor). The method thus has the potential to support detailed quantitative studies of *e.g.* metastases development and assessment of treatment response.

In Case Study B of kidney metastases, CT was not used, as this modality gives insufficient soft tissue contrast without the use of contrast agents. BLI indicated the presence of a cancerous lesion in or around the kidney (Figure 1, blue arrow). MRI revealed numerous independent metastases in the kidney (Figure 6), which is not possible with BLI alone due to its limited spatial resolution. Moreover, SRR-MRI allows the researcher to not only distinguish, but also to clearly delineate different tumors in close proximity. This cannot be achieved with conventional MRI, as illustrated in Figure 6 and evaluated quantitatively on phantom data. SRR-MRI can thus provide added value in studies where the number of metastases is an important parameter and where experimental treatment is used to intervene with the metastatic process. For instance, a researcher can differentiate between renal, adrenal, and peri-renal cancerous lesions with SRR-MRI but not with BLI.

BLI remains the preferred standard measurement for active tumor size as the signal originates only from living cells and not from a necrotic core or cells killed by a certain treatment. Light, however, only has a limited penetration in bone, which, in turn, can mask the BLI signal coming from small tumors that grow inside it, making these tumors appear smaller than they actually are. Having an MRI dataset, in which the tumor can be identified and clearly measured, helps overcoming these limitations.

An additional point to be made is the possibility to use BLI with SRR-MRI as an alternative for the CT anatomical reference, particularly in longitudinal studies where the repeated exposure to radiation in a CT scan may become a confounding factor or cause adverse effects [21].

Apart from oncology, the presented work flow may be of value in many research areas that requires whole-body examination for local ((sub-) slice-thickness sized) effects. Examples are the homing of labeled stem cells after systemic injection, or imaging of systemic inflammatory diseases.

Post mortem to in vivo SRR-MRI

In this study, we have applied our approach to *post mortem* MRI data. However, we have well-founded reasons to assume that our results translate to *in vivo* MRI imaging, because the acquisition protocol used in these experiments is compatible with *in vivo* mouse imaging. The main difference that can be expected between *ex vivo* and *in vivo* acquisitions is the presence of motion. Motion-induced artifacts are reduced by fast low-resolution acquisitions and accurate subsequent registrations. While accurate non-rigid registration of soft tissue structures, such as liver and kidney, may be possible, SRR is expected to be most successful for relatively rigid structures, such as the brain, bone, and tissue surrounding bone: cases in which rigid registration will yield accurate alignment of the low-resolution images. In [3], we showed SRR reconstructions of an *in vivo* mouse brain, and several studies have validated the assumption of accurate motion estimation in applications of SRR in fetal brain MRI [22,23].

Interactive local SRR

One of the contributions of this work has been the development of an approach that integrates recent progress in the areas of articulated atlas-based segmentation of whole-body small animal data, planar reformation, and SRR in MRI into a novel localized approach to SRR that enables global-to-local exploration of *e.g.* whole-body mouse MRI data. Together with the preliminary results first published in [9], we have provided a global solution to three possible scenarios that takes into account the availability of complementary data: (*i*) only MRI is available [9], (*ii*) MRI+BLI is available, (*iii*) MRI+CT+BLI is available. From first to last scenario, the proposed approach decreases in the required level of user interaction to segment the data into possible VOIs. Depending on the biological problem, the more complementary data available, the higher the level of automation of the approach and the more data can be provided for the user to explore, *i.e.*: in the approach of Case Study B (MRI+BLI), the user can choose only among VOIs in which BLI signal is present for a subsequent SRR reconstruction. Alternatively, (if CT is available) the user can select any bone for the SRR reconstruction and thus compare left with right, a bone with a tumor with the same bone without a tumor on the contralateral side, *etc*. Naturally, the more complementary data available in a study, the more information one can extract. Thus, while in (*i*) only MRI information is available, in (*iii*) one can fully integrate the information provided by the BLI (which quickly locates tumor growth and indicates tumor burden) together with the anatomical information provided by the CT (used to study tumor-induced changes in the bone—bone resorption) and the soft tissue information provided by MRI (which can provide the information about the size and the number of metastases).

Image quality vs imaging time

A major constraint when applying SRR in small animal MRI is the limited acquisition time that *in vivo* experiments allow. Each of the low-resolution images takes a certain amount of time to acquire and acquisition of multiple such images may quickly exceed the time during which a mouse can be kept sedated. It was shown in [3] that relatively few images are necessary to achieve significant improvements in the image quality. In this study, we have limited the number of low-resolution images to four, with a total acquisition time of 52 minutes – a realistic acquisition time for *in vivo* experiments. If the experimental setting allows it, the number of low-resolution images used can be extended at the expense of additional acquisition time. This will have some positive effect on the resolution. For an optimal coverage of k-space, the number of low-resolution images should be $\lceil \pi/2 \times F \rceil$, where F is the anisotropy factor, *i.e.*, the slice thickness relative to the in-plane resolution. In our case, that would mean using 7 low-resolution images. Using more than this number of low-resolution images will not have a significant impact on the resolution, but will increase the SNR slightly (for an in-depth study of these trade-offs, we refer the reader to [3,4]).

The major advantage of SRR in small-animal MRI is that it enables obtaining isotropic images in scenarios where T2-weighted image contrast is desired, requiring long repetition times and therefore long scan times, particularly for a 3D acquisition. By combining a small number of relatively fast thick-slice acquisitions with SRR, an isotropic resolution close to the original in-plane resolution is obtained. For comparison, direct acquisition of a 3D fast spin echo image with the same resolution and acquisition parameters would take about 28 hours and thus is infeasible. Alternatively, accelerating the 3D acquisition to similar scan times by reducing TR and increasing the echo train length leads to severe blurring at high field strength due to the relatively fast T2 decay. The proposed SRR solution would also be suitable on advanced acquisition schemes for high-field abdominal imaging. For instance, using SRR in combination with a self-navigated acquisition scheme like PROPELLER should provide high-resolution 3D T2-weighted contrast at high fields while reducing motion artifacts [24,25].

Reconstruction times

For large datasets, the SRR method is limited by the memory available on the computer. For the conjugate gradient solver, up to 5 data structures, each the size of the final reconstructed image, and 2 additional data structures, each the size the total low-resolution data, must be kept in memory simultaneously. For large 3D data sets, this soon becomes very difficult to achieve, even on a high-performance desktop computer. The interactive approach to locally reconstruct VOIs presented here, allows overcoming the time and memory limitations of the SRR technique. However, as shown in Table 1, the mean time for the best quality SRR result, *i.e.*, using 4 low-resolution images, is still in the order of minutes—91.3 s. The mean time for SRR using 2 low-resolution images is 48.8 s. These results are still far from the real-time target for this approach. Since the results presented here were acquired on a MATLAB implemented prototype, the computation times will decrease by re-implementing the algorithm in a C/C++ and GPU combination.

Conclusions

By combining a number of state-of-the-art image processing techniques, we have enabled a global-to-local exploration of whole-body mouse MRI. We have shown that the SRR-MRI is a valuable complementary modality in studies of tumor metastases. Using only a few low-resolution images, and a total acquisition time compatible with *in vivo* experiments, we have reconstructed SRR MR images from which detailed information about soft tissue metastases, not available in conventional imaging modalities, can be inferred. This cannot be obtained from direct MR acquisition within a feasible acquisition time.

Author Contributions

Conceived and designed the experiments: OD AK EP PK TJAS CWGML LvdW EM BPFL. Analyzed the data: OD AK EP PK TJAS LvdW BPFL. Contributed reagents/materials/analysis tools: OD AK EP PK TJAS DHJP LvdW. Wrote the paper: OD AK EP PK TJAS LvdW. Developed the Interactive Local SRR of MRI Whole-Body Mouse Data tool: OD AK EP PK. Performed the Interactive Local SRR experiments: OD AK EP PK. Performed the experiments with the animal and phantom and acquired the data: TJAS LvdW. Discussed the results and commented on the manuscript: OD AK EP PK TJAS DHJP CWGML CPB WJN LvdW EM BPFL.

References

1. Snoeks TJ, Khmelinskii A, Lelieveldt BPF, Kaijzel EL, Löwik CWGM (2011) Optical advances in skeletal imaging applied to bone metastases. Bone 48(1): 106–114.
2. Gauvain KM, Garbow JR, Song SK, Hirbe AC, Weilbaecher K (2005) MRI detection of early bone metastases in B16 mouse melanoma models. Clinical & Experimental Metastasis 22: 403–411.
3. Plenge E, Poot DHJ, Bernsen M, Kotek G, Houston G, et al. (2012) Super-resolution methods in MRI: can they improve the trade-off between resolution, signal-to-noise ratio, and acquisition time? Magn Reson Med 68(6): 1983–1993.
4. Poole DS, Plenge E, Poot DHJ, Lakke EA, Niessen WJ, et al. (2014) Three-dimensional inversion recovery manganese-enhanced MRI of mouse brain using super-resolution reconstruction to visualize nuclei involved in higher brain function. NMR Biomed 27(7): 749–759.
5. Baiker M, Milles J, Dijkstra J, Henning TD, Weber AW, et al. (2010) Atlas-based whole-body segmentation of mice from low-contrast Micro-CT data. Med Image Anal 14(6): 723–737.
6. Khmelinskii A, Baiker M, Kaijzel EL, Chen XJ, Reiber JHC, et al. (2011) Articulated whole-body atlases for small animal image analysis: construction and applications. Mol Imaging Biol 13(5): 898–910.
7. Kok P, Dijkstra J, Botha CP, Post FH, Kaijzel EL, et al. (2007) Integrated visualization of multi-angle bioluminescence imaging and micro CT. Proc SPIE Medical Imaging 65091U:1–10.
8. Khmelinskii A, Baiker M, Chen XJ, Reiber JHC, Henkelman RM, et al. (2010) Atlas-based organ & bone approximation for ex-vivo μMRI mouse data: a pilot study. Proc IEEE Intl Symp on Biomedical Imaging 1197–1200.
9. Khmelinskii A, Plenge E, Kok P, Dzyubachyk O, Poot DHJ, et al. (2012) Super-resolution reconstruction of whole-body MRI mouse data: an interactive approach. Proc IEEE Intl Symp on Biomedical Imaging 1723–1726.
10. Kok P, Baiker M, Hendriks EA, Post FH, Dijkstra J, et al. (2010) Articulated planar reformation for change visualization in small animal imaging. IEEE Trans Vis Comput Gr 16(6): 1396–1404.
11. Poot DHJ, Van Meir V, Sijbers J (2010) General and efficient super-resolution method for multi-slice MRI. Proc 13th MICCAI: Part I, 615–622.
12. Kim JB, Urban K, Cochran E, Lee S, Ang A, et al. (2010) Non-invasive detection of a small number of bioluminescent cancer cells in vivo. PLoS ONE 5(2): e9364.
13. Bolin C, Sutherland C, Tawara K, Moselhy J, Jorcyk CL (2012) Novel mouse mammary cell lines for in vivo bioluminescence imaging (BLI) of bone metastasis. Biol Proced Onlne 14(6) doi:10.1186/1480-9222-14-6.
14. Shilling RZ, Robbie TQ, Bailloeul T, Mewes K, Mersereau RM, et al. (2009) A super-resolution framework for 3-D high-resolution and high-contrast imaging using 2-D multislice MRI. IEEE Trans Med Imaging 28(5): 633–644.
15. CVP website. Available: http://graphics.tudelft.nl/pkok/CVP/. Accessed 2012 Nov 30.
16. Segars WP, Tsui BMW, Frey EC, Johnson GA, Berr SS (2004) Development of a 4D digital mouse phantom for molecular imaging research. Mol Imag Biol 6(3): 149–159.
17. Besl PJ, McKay ND (1992) A method for registration of 3D shapes. IEEE Trans Pattern Anal 14(2): 239–256.
18. Gudbjartsson H, Patz S (1995) The Rician distribution of noisy MRI data. Magn Reson Med 34(6): 910–914.
19. Smal I, Loog M, Niessen WJ, Meijering E (2010). Quantitative comparison of spot detection methods in fluorescence microscopy. IEEE Trans Med Imaging 29(2): 282–301.
20. Baiker M, Snoeks TJA, Kaijzel EL, Que I, Dijkstra J, et al. (2012) Automated bone volume and thickness measurements in small animal whole-body microCT data. Mol Imaging Biol 14(4): 420–430.
21. Hindorf C, Rodrigues J, Boutaleb S, Rosseau J, Govignon A, et al. (2010) Total absorbed dose to a mouse during microPET/CT imaging. Eur J Nucl Med Mol Imaging 37(Suppl 2): S274.
22. Rousseau F, Kim K, Studholme C, Koob M, Dietemann JL (2010) On super-resolution for fetal brain MRI. Proc 13th MICCAI: Part II, 355–362.
23. Gholipour A, Estroff J, Warfield S (2010) Robust super-resolution volume reconstruction from slice acquisitions: Application to fetal brain MRI. IEEE Trans Med Imaging 29(10): 1739–1758.
24. Teh I, Golay X, Larkman DJ (2010) PROPELLER for motion-robust imaging of in vivo mouse abdomen at 9.4 T. NMR Biomed 23(9): 1077–1086.
25. Pandit P, Qi Y, Story J, King KF, Johnson GA (2010) Multishot PROPELLER for high-field preclinical MRI. Magn Reson Med 64(1): 47–53.

19

A Statistical Parametric Mapping Toolbox Used for Voxel-Wise Analysis of FDG-PET Images of Rat Brain

Binbin Nie[1]⦾, Hua Liu[1]⦾, Kewei Chen[2,3,4,5], Xiaofeng Jiang[6], Baoci Shan[1]*

1 Key Laboratory of Nuclear Analysis Techniques, Beijing Engineering Research Center of Radiographic Techniques and Equipment, Institute of High Energy Physics, Chinese Academy of Sciences, Beijing, China, **2** Banner Alzheimer's Institute, Banner Good Samaritan Positron Emission Tomography Center, Phoenix, Arizona, United States of America, **3** Department of Mathematics and Statistics, Arizona State University, Tempe, Arizona, United States of America, **4** Department of Radiology, University of Arizona, Tucson, Arizona, United States of America, **5** Arizona Alzheimer's Consortium, Phoenix, Arizona, United States of America, **6** School of Public Health and Family Medicine, Capital Medical University, Beijing, China

Abstract

Purpose: PET (positron emission tomography) imaging researches of functional metabolism using fluorodeoxyglucose (^{18}F-FDG) of animal brain are important in neuroscience studies. FDG-PET imaging studies are often performed on groups of rats, so it is desirable to establish an objective voxel-based statistical methodology for group data analysis.

Material and Methods: This study establishes a statistical parametric mapping (SPM) toolbox (plug-ins) named spmratIHEP for voxel-wise analysis of FDG-PET images of rat brain, in which an FDG-PET template and an intracranial mask image of rat brain in Paxinos & Watson space were constructed, and the default settings were modified according to features of rat brain. Compared to previous studies, our constructed rat brain template comprises not only the cerebrum and cerebellum, but also the whole olfactory bulb which made the later cognitive studies much more exhaustive. And with an intracranial mask image in the template space, the brain tissues of individuals could be extracted automatically. Moreover, an atlas space is used for anatomically labeling the functional findings in the Paxinos & Watson space. In order to standardize the template image with the atlas accurately, a synthetic FDG-PET image with six main anatomy structures is constructed from the atlas, which performs as a target image in the co-registration.

Results: The spatial normalization procedure is evaluated, by which the individual rat brain images could be standardized into the Paxinos & Watson space successfully and the intracranial tissues could also be extracted accurately. The practical usability of this toolbox is evaluated using FDG-PET functional images from rats with left side middle cerebral artery occlusion (MCAO) in comparison to normal control rats. And the two-sample t-test statistical result is almost related to the left side MCA.

Conclusion: We established a toolbox of SPM8 named spmratIHEP for voxel-wise analysis of FDG-PET images of rat brain.

Editor: Jonathan A. Coles, Glasgow University, United Kingdom

Funding: This work was supported by grants from National Basic Research Program of China (973 Program) (2013CB835100), the National Natural Science Foundation of China (81201147 and 91232713) and the Xie Jialin Foundation of IHEP (3546370U2). All these funders support this study. In detail, 2013CB835100 support the modal construction and data collection of the MCAO group, 81201147 and 91232713 support the data collection of the group for template construction, 3546370U2 support the data collection of the group for intracranial mask image evaluation. The funders had no role in study design, data collection and analysis, decision to publish, or preparation of the manuscript.

* Email: shanbc@ihep.ac.cn

⦾ These authors contributed equally to this work.

Introduction

PET (positron emission tomography) imaging techniques of functional metabolism using fluorodeoxyglucose (^{18}F-FDG) have been increasingly used for the investigation of human brain functions in normal and diseased individuals [1–3]. Complementary to human brain studies, animal experiments are important for pathogenesis research, therapeutic efficacy evaluation, and drug development, for it allows transverse comparisons between different brain regions or between different rats, and longitudinal follow-up. While numbers of small-animal FDG-PET imaging studies are performed on groups of rodents, how to analyze images

for efficient interpretation of physiological significance is a pivotal problem to be solved. In ^{18}F-FDG imaging studies of human brain, the statistical parametric mapping (SPM, Wellcome Department of Cognitive Neurology, London, UK) is one of the most popular software for image analysis voxel-by-voxel. Groups of human brain images can be statistical analyzed in SPM objectively and automatically, which is also desirable in rodent studies.

In order to eliminate individual differences in voxel-wise analysis, the spatial normalization should be performed primarily, in which a standard template is the reference target image. Because of the relatively large difference in spatial resolution between MRI (magnetic resonance imaging) and FDG-PET images of small animals, automated image co-registration of FDG-PET data with MRI templates is difficult. Therefore, the established MRI template [4–6] could not be used in FDG-PET studies of rat brain. Casteels et al. [7] has first constructed an FDG-PET template of rat brain in Paxinos & Watson space [8] used for spatial normalization. The introduction of their template has accelerated a number of FDG-PET studies in rats [9,10]. However, we noted that this template do not include the olfactory bulb of rat. As implied in some important researches recently, there is a close association between olfactory dysfunction and cognitive impairment [11–16]. Therefore, the olfactory bulb is necessary not only in olfaction study but also in cognitive study, which should be included in template image of rat brain. In addition, in Casteels' study [7], only ten female rats ranged from 13 to 34 weeks old were used for the template construction. Hence, in order to improve the group representation of the template for both male and female rats, and to better account for the brain variability due to aging process, our current work will include rats with more balanced male/female ratio (twelve male and twelve female adult rats) and narrower age range (10~13 wk old).

The extracranial tissues were unwanted in imaging data analysis. Recently, the intracranial tissues of each rat are usually traced out manually [5,7], which is subjective, labor-intensive and time-consuming. In the human, the extracranial tissues could be automatically removed by an intracranial mask after spatial normalization, of which idea could also be used in rat brain studies. Therefore, in this study, an intracranial mask corresponding to our constructed FDG-PET template will be established to remove extracranial tissues of individual images automatically after spatial normalization.

Furthermore, the assignment of anatomical location to functional effects is critical in the interpretation physiological significance of statistical result of voxel-wise analysis. For anatomical localization, an atlas space is prerequisite, such as the Tailarach space for human brain studies [17]. In rat brain studies, the stereotaxic coordinates by Paxinos & Watson [18] is one of the most widely used. Previously, several groups established digital coordinates [5,7] or atlas image [4,6] for anatomical localization. However, only a digital atlas is not enough for functional location. It is prerequisite to standardize the template into the atlas space [5,7]. When the FDG-PET template is fitted into the Paxinos & Watson space, functional effects could be precisely allocated to anatomical structures, which could also be used to define the uptake in the structures [10].

To align the template into the atlas space, Schweinhardt et al. [5] used the landmark-based linear registration techniques with forty-nine homologous anatomical landmarks, which performed successfully in structural MRI template. In FDG-PET studies of rat brain, Rubins et al. [19] registered FDG-PET images to a synthetic FDG-PET target image which was constructed from atlas-derived VOI (voxel of interest) images using rigid body transformation, which has only six anatomical regions. Casteels et al. [7] standardized the functional template into the Paxinos space via the MRI template [5] using linear transformation method based on the mutual information maximization algorithm in SPM2. However, because the template image and the atlas are constructed from different subjects, only linear transformation is not sufficient to standardize the template into the atlas space. In order to combine both linear and non-linear transformation method in co-registration of the template and the atlas, Coello et al. [10] constructed synthetic FDG-PET image from MRI image, by segmenting the MRI image into white matter (WM) and

gray matter (GM) and then conducting a weighted sum of the GM and WM maps. Thus, an individual FDG-PET image can be standardized into the Paxinos & Watson space while it was spatially normalized to the synthetic FDG-PET template. However, the spatial resolution of the synthetic FDG-PET image with only two resolvable regions is too low. Therefore, in our study, in order to improve the co-registration accuracy, six main anatomy structures, all of which could be identified in the FDG-PET template according to the voxel intensity ranges and locations, will be defined from an atlas image [4] in Paxinos & Watson space [18] to construct a synthetic FDG-PET image. Then, both linear and non-linear transformation method will be employed to standardize the FDG-PET canonical brain into the Paxinos & Watson space [18] via the synthetic FDG-PET image.

With the introduction above, the current study is designed to establish a voxel-wise analysis method of FDG-PET images of rat brain. In detail, an FDG-PET rat brain template, comprised cerebrum, cerebellum, olfactory bulb and extracranial tissues, will be constructed which is used for spatial normalization of individual rat brain images. An intracranial mask image in the FDG-PET template space will be constructed for extracranial tissues automatic removing. The FDG-PET template will be standardized into the Paxinos & Watson space for the localization of functional investigation. Finally, the constructed template sets are compiled as a SPM8 toolbox (plug-ins) named spmratIHEP. Moreover, to evaluate the usefulness of the toolbox implemented in SPM8, we analyze the data from rats with left side middle cerebral artery occlusion (MCAO) and those without. The spmratIHEP toolbox is available by contacting the corresponding author at shanbc@ihep. ac.cn.

Materials and Methods

2.1. Animals and data acquisition

Twenty-four Sprague-Dawley (SD) rats of either sex, 10~13 weeks old, weight 350 g±20 g, were used for template construction. A further ten similar rats were used for evaluation of spatial normalization and removal of extracranial tissues. Voxel-wise analysis of brain images was done on male SD rats, 9~11 weeks old; weight 300 g±20 g; 9 underwent left side middle cerebral artery occlusion (MCAO) and 8 were healthy controls. Intraluminal occlusion of the middle cerebral artery (MCA) was accomplished using a modification of the Longa technique [20–22]. Under an operating microscope, the left common carotid artery (CCA), external carotid artery (ECA), and internal carotid artery (ICA) were exposed through a midline incision. The vagus nerve was carefully preserved as far as possible. After proximal CCA was ligated, a 3-0 uncoated monofilament nylon suture with rounded tip (2634,Beijing Sunbio Biotech Co., Ltd. China) was inserted from the lumen of the distal CCA and advanced into the ICA, approximately 18±0.5 mm beyond the bifurcation until mild resistance indicated that the tip was lodged in the anterior resistance cerebral artery, thus blocking blood flow to the middle cerebral artery. All the rats were deprived of food for 12–15 h before ^{18}F-FDG injection, but had access to drinking water at all time [23].

^{18}F-FDG was prepared at PET center of China PLA General Hospital. For each rat, ^{18}F-FDG (18.5 MBq/100 g of body weight) was administered via tailvein injection without anesthesia. Then the rats were kept in their cages and placed in a room with minimal ambient noise for the ^{18}F-FDG uptake. The uptake period was 40 min for maximization of ^{18}F-FDG uptake in the brain [24]. Then the rats were anesthetized with isoflurane

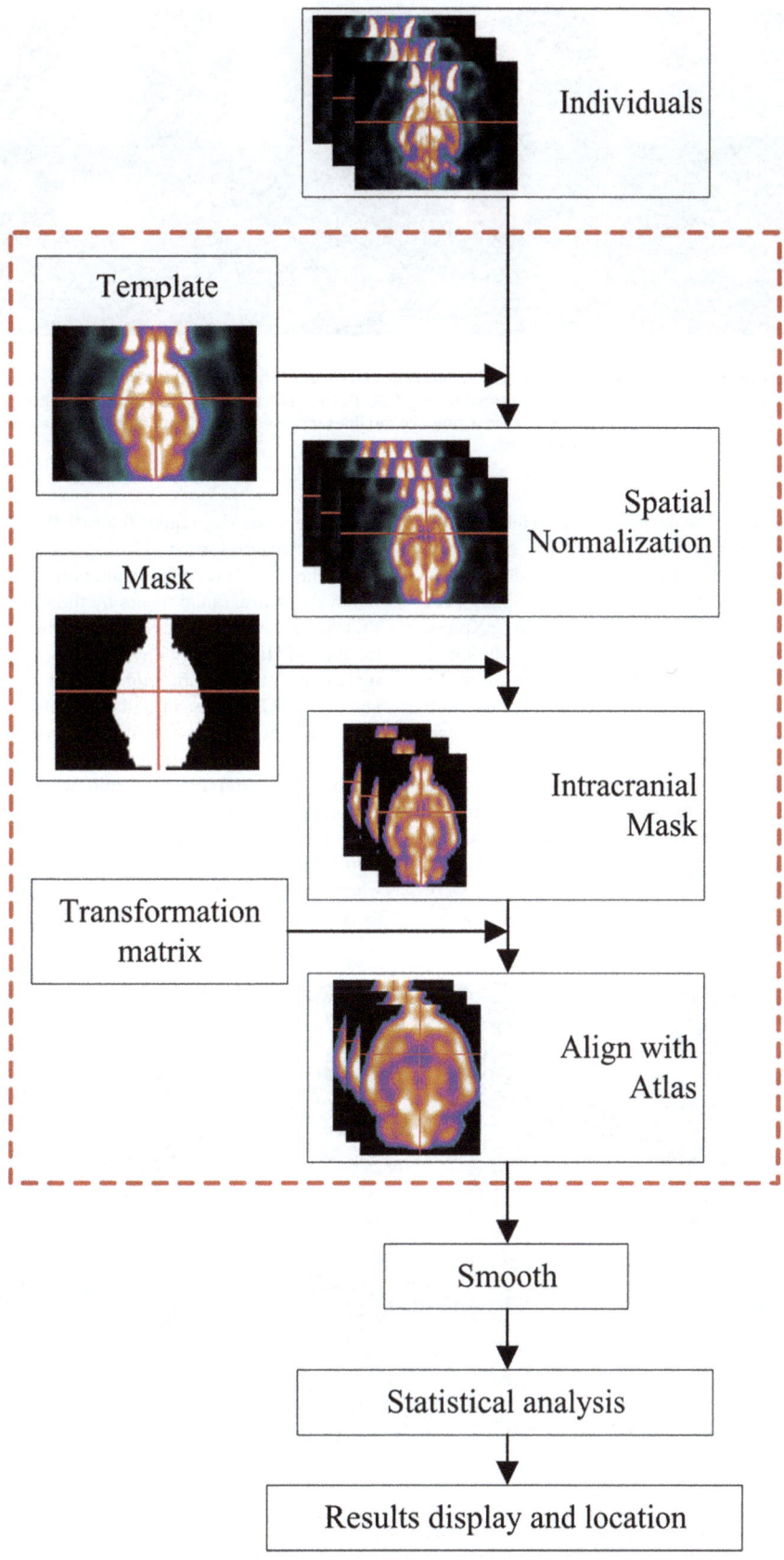

Figure 1. Schematic representation of the data analysis procedure in the spmratIHEP. The procedures of spatial normalization showed in the red dashed pane could be accomplished automatically in this toolbox.

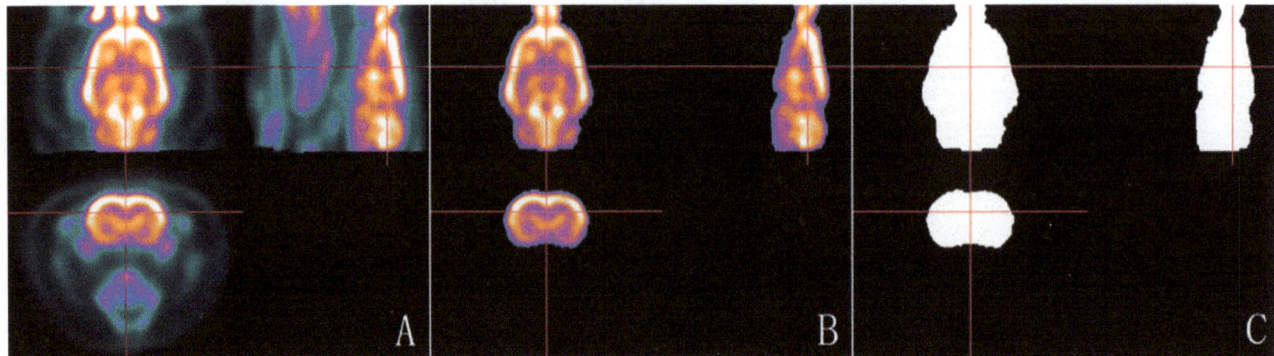

Figure 2. The constructed rat brain template. (A) Axial, sagittal and coronal views of the standard FDG-PET template with extracranial tissues in Paxinos space; (B) axial, sagittal and coronal views of the corresponding FDG-PET canonical brain; and (C) axial, sagittal and coronal views of the corresponding intracranial mask image in Paxinos space. The cross point of red lines represent the origin point D3V. The origin point was the same in the images of template, canonical brain and intracranial mask.

inhalation anesthesia (2% in 100% oxygen; IsoFlo: Hebei Jiumu Phama, ltd, China) using a nose cone.

For the twenty-four rats used in template construction, FDG-PET imaging was performed at the PET center of China PLA General Hospital in MicroPET/CT imaging system (eXplore Vista-CT, GE, USA), of which the radial spatial resolution is 1.0 mm full-width at half-maximum (FWHM) at the centre of the field of view (FOV). During FDG-PET scan, all the rats were anesthetized with isoflurane (the same as described above) and placed in the scanner with a plastic stereotactic head holder in prone position on the scanner bed. And the rat brain was centered in the FOV to perform a static acquisition of 10 minutes. Images were subsequently reconstructed using 3D ordered set expectation maximization (3D-OSEM) algorithm. Corrections for dead time, decay, attenuation, random coincidences and scattering were applied. Images were reconstructed on a $175 \times 175 \times 61$ matrix, where the voxel size equals $0.39 \times 0.39 \times 0.77$ mm. All scans were saved as Analyze format.

For the ten rats used for evaluation of spatial normalization and removal of extracranial tissues by the spmratIHEP toolbox, FDG-PET images were acquired on a micro PET system (E-plus166, Institute of High Energy Physics, CAS, China), of which the radial spatial resolution is 1.67 mm FWHM at the centre of the FOV. During FDG-PET scan, all the rats were anesthetized with isoflurane (the same as described above) and placed in the scanner with a plastic stereotactic head holder in prone position on the scanner bed. And the rat brain was centered in the FOV to perform a static acquisition of 30 minutes. Images were subsequently reconstructed using Filtered Back projection (FBP) algorithm. Images were reconstructed on a $128 \times 128 \times 63$ matrix, where the voxel size equals $0.5 \times 0.5 \times 1$ mm. All scans were saved as Analyze format.

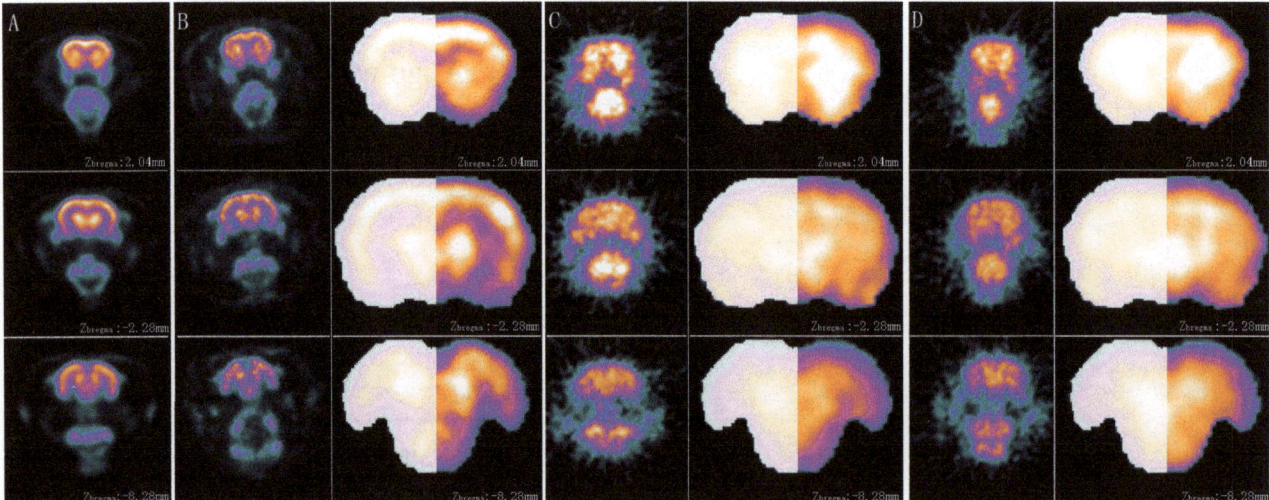

Figure 3. The extraction results. Panel A shows three planes from the standard FDG-PET template of rat brain, whose coordinates were Z_{bregma} 2.04 mm, Z_{bregma} −2.28 mm and Z_{bregma} −8.28 mm separately. Panel B shows the extraction result of a rat which is randomly selected from dataset obtained for template construction. Panel C and Panel D show the extraction results of two rats which are randomly selected for dataset obtained for the intracranial brain extraction evaluations. The original image of individual is shown on the left of Panels B, C, D separately. The extracted intracranial tissue of individual is shown on the right of Panels B, C, D separately, of which the left half shows the intracranial mask image superimposing on the extracted canonical brain and the right half shows the extracted canonical brain. The intracranial mask image is presented as a binary image with 25% transparency, while the extracted canonical brain is presented as a background.

Table 1. Volumetric and spatial correspondence measures between manually traced out intracranial tissues from three experts, of which the result is shown as 'the mean value ± standard deviation'.

	JS (%)	RV (%)	FP (%)	FN (%)
Rat1	91.24±0.94	1.10±0.48	4.38±0.43	4.38±1.09
Rat2	89.77±1.52	6.68±4.60	4.13±3.52	6.10±5.02
Rat3	87.09±2.82	8.93±7.47	6.45±6.31	6.45±6.29

JS (%): Jaccard similarity (the optimal value is 100%);
RV (%): The relative error on volume (the optimal value is 0%);
FP (%): The proportions of false-positive (the optimal value is 0%);
FN (%): The proportions of false-negative (the optimal value is 0%).

The nine rats with MCAO and eight ones without were used for evaluation of this toolbox spmratIHEP for its capacity for functional localization. Twenty-four hours after operation, FDG-PET images were acquired on Siemens Inveon PET (Siemens Medical Solutions), of which the radial spatial resolution is 1.4 mm FWHM at the centre of the FOV. During FDG-PET scan, all the rats were anesthetized with isoflurane (the same as described above) and placed in the scanner with a plastic stereotactic head holder in prone position on the scanner bed. And the rat brain was centered in the FOV to perform a static acquisition of 20 minutes. Images were subsequently reconstructed using FBP algorithm. Corrections for dead time, decay, attenuation, random coincidences and scattering were applied. Images were reconstructed on a 128×128×159 matrix, where the voxel size equals 1.4×1.4×0.79 mm. All scans were saved as Analyze format.

All experiments were performed with the approval of the Animal Care and Use Committee of the Chinese Academy of Sciences and conformed to named international guidelines on the ethical use of animals.

2.2. Template construction

2.2.1. Construction of an average template image. The FDG-PET rat brain template image with the extracranial tissues was created using SPM8. All of the 24 images included in this study were inspected and were found equally of high quality in terms of the image contrast, noise level, and resolution. Firstly, the voxel size of all the brain images of 24 rats were adjusted to [1 1 1.8], which was scaled up in the Analyze header by the factor of 4 to better approximate human dimensions [5]. Then, the images were manually sheared to roughly remove voxels of the body and background by MRIcro [25]. Afterwards, the average template image was created recursively by registering [26–28] and averaging. In detail, one of these 24 rat brains was selected as the initial brain template. Each rat brain image was spatially normalized to this initial rat brain template, using the affine transformation and subsequent non-linear warping algorithm [29] implemented in SPM8.

The 24 spatially normalized images were averaged to create a new template. The mean squared residual difference between the old and new templates was computed. The mean squared residual difference is defined as in Eq. (1).

$$\frac{\sqrt{(imgf_1 - imgs_1)^2 + (imgf_2 - imgs_2)^2 + \cdots + (imgf_n - imgs_n)^2}}{n} \quad (1)$$

where $imgf$ and $imgs$ are the initial and the new target images respectively, the subscript i is the running voxel position index (ordered as 1, 2, … n as a 1D vector) in the image matrix, and n is the total number of voxels. Then the original 24 images were recursively registered to the new average target image. A newer average target image was created from the newly registered images. And the mean squared residual difference was subsequently computed between the current target image and the previous one. This procedure, including registration, averaging and computing the mean squared residual difference, was repeated until the latest mean residual squared difference was stabilized (less than 5% in this current study) [4]. And the latest average target image was our final average image with extracranial tissue.

2.2.2. Creation of canonical brain and intracranial mask. The canonical brain was created by extracting intracranial voxels from the average template image constructed above. We adopted the global histogram threshold method to exclude voxels outside the rat brain. The threshold was determined by Otsu's criterion [30], which maximizes the between-class variance to get the optimal global threshold value. Prior to determining the threshold, a rectangular bounding box containing the intracranial tissue was defined straightforwardly for each slice with two mouse

Table 2. Volumetric and spatial correspondence measures between three manually traced out and automatically extracted intracranial tissues, of which the result is shown as 'the mean value ± standard deviation'.

	JS (%)	RV (%)	FP (%)	FN (%)
Rat1	91.50±7.36	4.41±3.91	6.31±5.49	2.19±1.92
Rat2	91.74±7.16	1.45±2.04	4.63±4.18	3.63±3.26
Rat3	92.59±6.42	0.10±0.10	3.72±3.22	3.69±3.20

JS (%): Jaccard similarity (the optimal value is 100%);
RV (%): The relative error on volume (the optimal value is 0%);
FP (%): The proportions of false-positive (the optimal value is 0%);
FN (%): The proportions of false-negative (the optimal value is 0%).

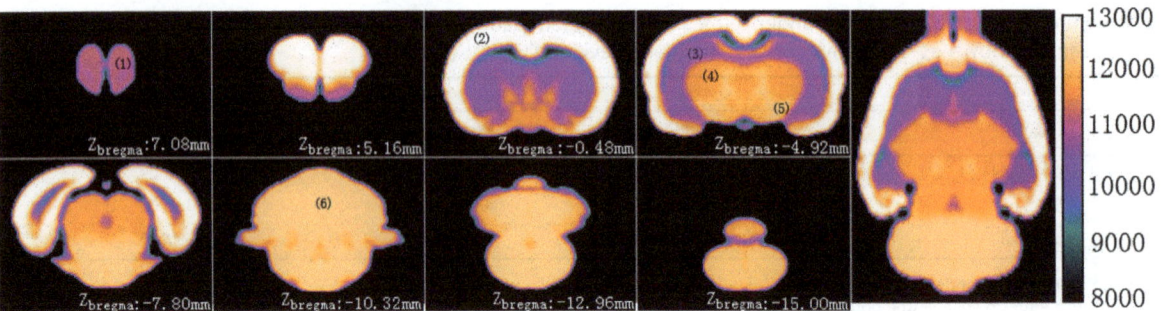

Figure 4. The constructed synthetic FDG-PET images from atlas images in Paxinos & Watson space. It was shown in pseudo-color scaled and the color-bar stands for the intensity of each voxel in synthetic FDG-PET image. The six main anatomy structures were labeled, in which (1) stands for the olfactory bulb, (2) stands for the cortex, (3) stands for the hippocampi, (4) stands for the mesencephalon, (5) stands for the thalamus and (6) stands for the cerebellar.

clicks for the upper left and lower right vertices in MRIcro [25]. And voxels outside the bounding box of the rat brain were removed (assigned zero intensity). Similarly, smaller rectangles over left and right eyes were drawn separately to remove the eyeballs. Finally, the intracranial portion of the image including the olfactory could be identified by collecting the non-zero voxels whose intensities were greater than the global histogram threshold obtained by Otsu's criterion [30].

Moreover, this extracted canonical brain was processed by binarization transformation to create an intracranial mask image in the standard template space. The origin point of the canonical brain and intracranial mask was the same with the template. Thus, after normalizing to the FDG-PET template, the extracranial tissues of individuals could be automatically removed by this intracranial mask image.

2.2.3. Construction of synthetic PET image. In this study, the paired rat brain structural MRI template and digital atlas in Paxinos & Watson space we constructed before [4] were used for functional effects localization, which comprised from the anterior part of olfactory bulb (z_{bregma} +7.56 mm) to the posterior part of cerebellum (z_{bregma} −15.72 mm). In order to co-register the canonical FDG-PET brain with the MRI structural template and atlas, we created a low-resolution synthetic PET image from the atlas [4]. For this purpose, the 624 regions were merged into six main anatomy structures, all of which could be identified in the FDG-PET template according to the voxel intensity ranges and locations. These 6 anatomy structures included olfactory bulb, cortex, hippocampi, thalamus, mesencephalon and cerebellar. Voxels within each of these 6 regions over the pseudo FDG-PET image were assigned the mean intensity value over the corresponding part in the FDG-PET template. Finally, this synthetic FDG-PET image was further smoothed using an isotropic Gaussian kernel of $2 \times 2 \times 4$ mm^3 FWHM to smooth the juncture of the neighboring segmented parts.

2.2.4. Co-registration of the canonical brain with the atlas in Paxinos & Watson space. The synthetic FDG-PET image was chosen as the target image. The SPM intensity-based affine transformation algorithm and subsequent non-linear warping algorithm was employed to co-register the canonical brain with this target atlas image [31], and the same transformation matrix was applied to the average template image and mask image. At this point, the co-registered template image, canonical brain and mask image were in Paxinos space, which consist the final standard template set. Finally, the origin point of the template set coordinate space was positioned at dorsal 3rd ventricle (D3V).

2.3. Construction of the SPM8 plug-ins toolbox named spmratIHEP

In order to analyze rat brain images with less manual manipulation, we constructed a SPM8 plug-ins toolbox named spmratIHEP using MATLAB. Because of the differences between human brain and rat brain, the processing methods and parameter settings in SPM8 must be modified according to the feature of rat brain FDG-PET imaging, which were described in detail as below.

Firstly, spatial normalization is prerequisite in voxel-wise analysis to eliminate individual differences. In order to use the available affine transformation and subsequent non-linear warping algorithm in SPM8, the voxel size of individual brain images was scaled up in the Analyze header by a factor to better approximate human dimensions, which will not affect any interpretation of the statistical results of rat brain.

Then, the constructed FDG-PET template and intracranial mask of rat brain took replacement of the human brain. And the default parameter settings of spatial normalization were adjust according to the feature of rat brain, that the bounding box was adjust to [−150 −180 −126; 150 60 72], the voxel size was adjust to [1 1 1.8] after zooming and the affine regularization was adjust to 'average sized template'. Moreover, the image matrix of intracranial rat brain images after spatial normalization was sheared to [120 80 98] automatically to cut off the background.

Smoothing was used to improve the signal-to-noise ratio in SPM, in which the Gaussian kernel was adjust to $2 \times 2 \times 4$ mm^3 FWHM, which was approximately two times of the spatial resolution of rat brain after zooming [7].

Finally, in order to display the statistical results of rat brain in Paxinos & Watson space, the definition of coordinates of rat brain took replacement of the human brain. The accurate location of the maximum FDG changes was modified according to the Paxinos & Watson space, in which the x-axis is negative to the left from the midline and positive to the right, the y-axis is positive to the ventral direction relative to the dorsal, and the z-axis is positive to the olfactory bulb direction relative to the bregma and negative to the cerebellum direction. Moreover, a new projection figure of rat brain was created to show the projection of overall blob regions, and a MRI T2-weighted (MRI T2WI) structural image of a single rat brain in Paxinos & Watson space was prepared to show the three-dimensional view of a blob region.

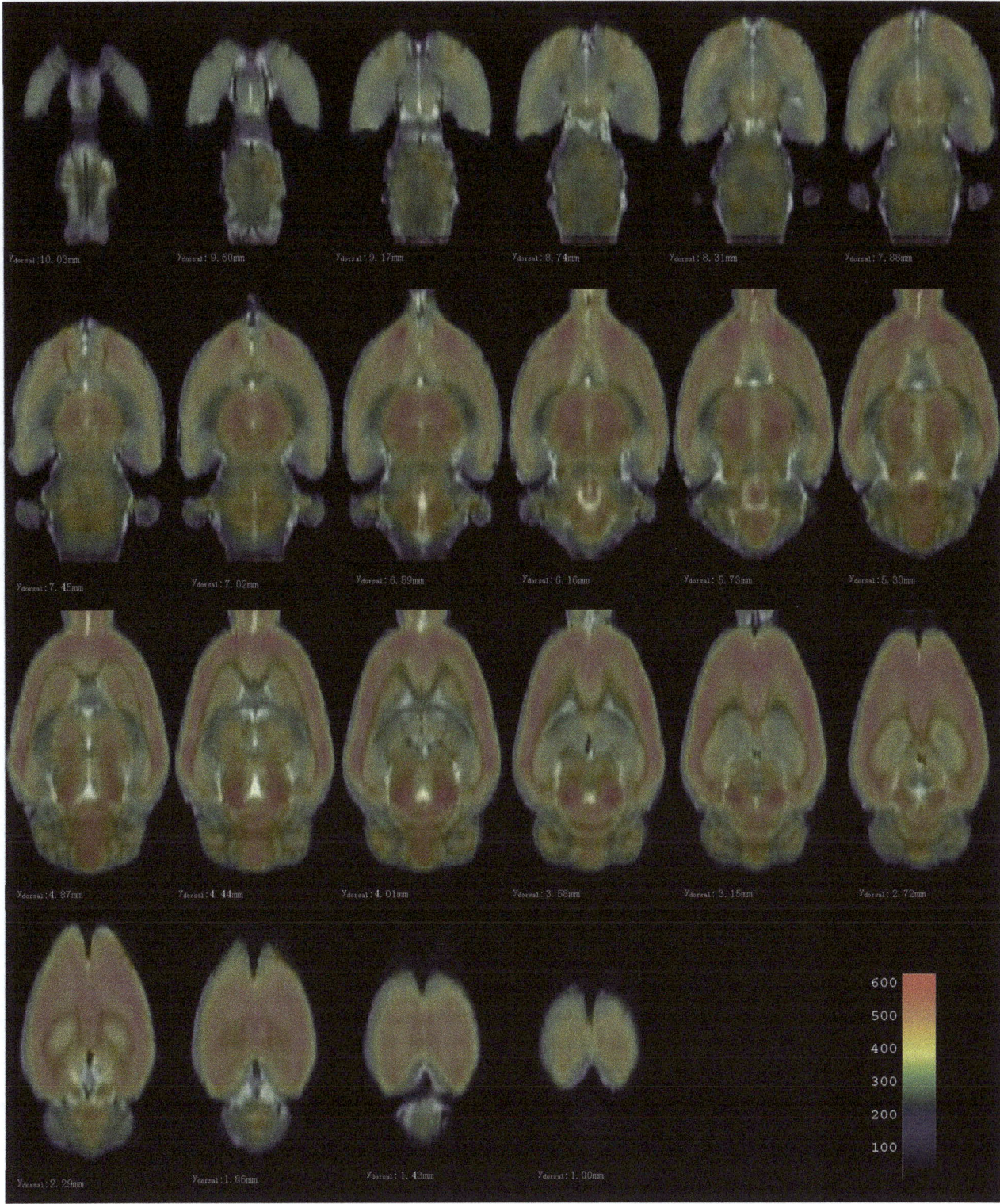

Figure 5. Superimposing the co-registered FDG-PET canonical brain on the MRI T2WI structural canonical brain in Paxinos & Watson space. The co-registered FDG-PET canonical brain is presented with translucency and pseudo-color scaled. The MRI T2WI canonical brain is presented in gray-scale as a background. The color-bar stands for the intensity of each voxel in FDG-PET canonical brain, which is not translucent.

Table 3. The statistical result of two sample t-test between the MCAO and healthy controls.

Cluster number	K_E	P_{FWE_corr}	Max_T	Max_Z	Peak coordinates (mm) x	y	z
1	2992	0.006	10.79	5.63	−5	7	−7
		0.008	10.55	5.58	−4	5	−4
2	52	0.013	10.14	5.48	−3	6	3

Cluster number: the number of clusters with consecutive voxels with a significant decrease in FDG signal, which is assigned sequentially and artificially. The second line of Cluster 1 which contains large number of contiguous voxels refers to the other significant point in this Cluster.

K_E: the size of a cluster, in which the number such as 2992 stands for the voxel numbers in the cluster;

P_{FWE_corr}: the maximum confidence level in each cluster;

Max_T: the maximum t-value in each cluster;

Max_Z: the maximum Z-value in each cluster;

Peak coordinates (mm): the coordinates of the maximum point in Paxinos & Watson space;

x: the x-axis, which is negative to the left from the midline and positive to the right;

y: the y-axis, which is positive to the ventral direction relative to the dorsal;

z: the z-axis, which is positive to the olfactory bulb direction relative to the bregma and negative to the cerebellum direction.

2.4. Data analysis of MCAO rat model in the spmratIHEP toolbox

The analysis of MCAO rat model images was performed using our spmratIHEP toolbox to evaluate its practical use. Firstly, the body tissues and background of individual images were manually removed using MRIcro [25] and the origin of the image was repositioned at D3V which is corresponding to the standard FDG-PET template in Paxinos space. Then, the data sets were analyzed in the spmratIHEP automatically as described in the flowchart of Fig. 1. In detail, the FDG-PET images of MCAO rat model and healthy controls were preprocessed as described below. (1) Spatially normalize the individual images of rat brain into Paxinos & Watson space, comprising scaling up the voxel size in the Analyze header by the factor of 4, registering to the FDG-PET template, subsequently removing extracranial tissues via the intracranial image, shearing the matrix to cut off the background. (2) Smooth the normalized images by a Gaussian kernel of $2 \times 2 \times 4$ mm^3 FWHM.

Then, the preprocessed images were analyzed based on the framework of the general linear model (GLM). Two-sample t-test was performed to identify the difference of FDG signals between the rats with MCAO and the healthy controls, in which proportional scaling and intensity normalization was applied to account for global confounds. Finally, the brain regions with significant FDG changes in rats with MCAO were yielded based on a voxel-level height threshold of $p < 0.05$ (FWE corrected) and a cluster-extent threshold of 50 voxels.

Results

3.1. The constructed template set in Paxinos space

The constructed template set in Paxinos space was shown in Fig. 2, matrix size $300 \times 240 \times 110$, voxel size $1 \times 1 \times 1.8$ mm^3 after zooming. This template set was consisted of the standard FDG-PET template with extracranial tissues (Fig. 2A), the corresponding canonical brain (Fig. 2B) and the mask image (Fig. 2C). The original point was on D3V, as the cross point of red lines shown in Fig. 2.

3.2. Spatial normalization and extracranial tissue removing of the individual images

To illustrate the successful use of the intracranial mask image in removing non-brain tissues automatically, both datasets obtained for template construction and spatial normalization evaluations were used. The individual images from both datasets were spatially normalized in spmratIHEP. The extraction of three randomly chosen rats result was shown in Fig. 3, of which one was from the group for template construction (Fig. 3B) and the other two were from the group obtained by E-plus166 system of IHEP (Fig. 3C and Fig. 3D). Moreover, for quantitatively evaluation, three experts, who are the co-authors of this paper (Hua Liu, Xiaofeng Jiang and Baoci Shan), were invited to manually extract the brain tissues from individual FDG-PET images from both two datasets separately by the software ImageJ (Image Processing and Analysis in Java) (http://rsbweb.nih.gov/ij). Then, four volumetric and spatial correspondence measures, Jaccard similarity (JS) [32,33], the relative error on volume (RV), the proportions of false-positive (FP), and false-negative (FN) [4,34,35], were calculated between manually traced out intracranial tissues from three experts, and the manually traced out and automatically extracted intracranial brain volumes. The details of these measures are listed as below.

The Jaccard similarity was defined as in Eq.(2), of which the optimal value is 100%.

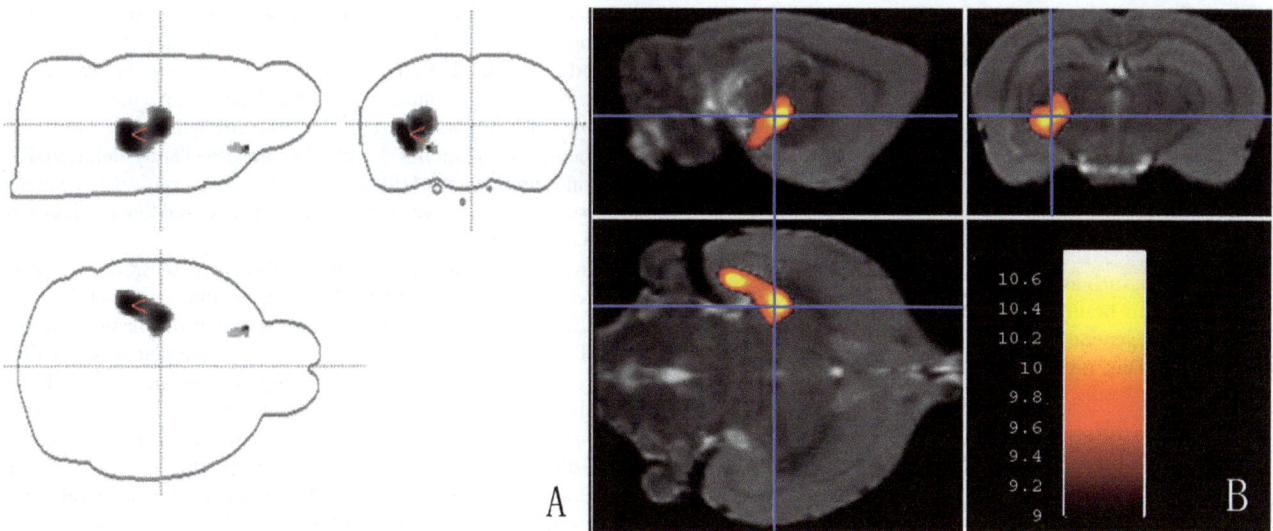

Figure 6. The result of two-sample t-test between the MCAO and healthy controls. (A) The projection of all the blobs were shown in a figure of rat brain, in which the red vees point to the global maximal t-value. (B) The display of the statistical result overlaid on axial, sagittal and coronal views of a structural single brain in Paxinos & Watson space, which is the three-dimensional illustration of one blob. And the color bar stands for the t-value of each significant voxel in Paxinos & Watson space.

$$JS = \frac{N\_voxels\{R \cap E\}}{N\_voxels\{R \cup E\}} \times 100\% \qquad (2)$$

Where N_voxels stands for the number of voxels, R stands for the reference image and E stands for the image to be evaluated.

The relative error on volume was defined as in Eq.(3), of which the optimal value is 0%.

$$RV = 2 \cdot \frac{|N\_voxels\{E - R\}|}{N\_voxels\{E + R\}} \times 100\% \qquad (3)$$

Where N_voxels stands for the number of voxels, R stands for the reference image and E stands for the image to be evaluated.

The proportions of false-positive was defined as in Eq.(4), of which the optimal value is 0%.

$$FP = \frac{N\_voxels\{E - (R \cap E)\}}{N\_voxels\{R \cup E\}} \times 100\% \qquad (4)$$

Where N_voxels stands for the number of voxels, R stands for the reference image and E stands for the image to be evaluated.

The proportions of false-negative was defined as in Eq.(5), of which the optimal value is 0%.

$$FN = \frac{N\_voxels\{R - (R \cap E)\}}{N\_voxels\{R \cup E\}} \times 100\% \qquad (5)$$

Where N_voxels stands for the number of voxels, R stands for the reference image and E stands for the image to be evaluated.

The calculated results are given in Table 1 and Table 2 separately. As we can see from Table 1 and Table 2, although these two datasets were reconstructed using different reconstruc-tion algorithms and had different spatial resolutions, the intracra-nial tissue could be extracted successfully by the intracranial mask.

3.3. Co-registration of the FDG-PET canonical brain to the atlas

The strategy we proposed to co-register the FDG-PET rat brain template with the atlas via synthetic FDG-PET image worked well. The pseudo FDG-PET with six major structures is shown in Fig. 4. This image was only used as a target image for co-registering the FDG-PET template.

For qualitatively evaluation, the co-registered FDG-PET canonical brain is overlaid on the MRI T2WI structural canonical brain which has already standardized into Paxinos & Watson space in our prior study [4], as shown in Fig. 5. As seen in Fig. 5, the rat brain canonical brain was successfully standardized into the Paxinos space. As illustrated in Figure 5, the FDG-PET canonical brain has been standardized into the atlas space very well.

3.4. Data analysis of MCAO rat model in spmratIHEP toolbox

The analysis of MCAO rat model images was performed using our spmratIHEP toolbox to evaluate its practical use. The statistical result that brain regions with significant FDG declined in rats with MCAO was shown in a projection figure (Fig. 6A) and fused on structural slices of rat brain in Paxinos & Watson space (Fig. 6B). Meanwhile, the quantitative information of the statistical result was listed in Table 3, in which the 'Cluster number' stands for the number of brain regions with significant FDG declined, the 'K_E' stands for the voxel numbers in each cluster, the 'P_{FWE_coor}' stands for the maximum confidence level in each cluster, the 'Max_T' stands for the maximum t-value in each cluster, the 'Max_Z' stands for the maximum Z-value in each cluster, the 'Peak coordinates (mm)' stands for the coordinates of the maximum point in Paxinos space. These regions are exclusively related to the left side MCA.

Discussion

In the current study, we established a SPM8 plug-ins toolbox named spmratIHEP for voxel-wise analysis of FDG-PET images of rat brain, in which an FDG-PET template and an intracranial mask image of rat brain in Paxinos & Watson space [4,18] were constructed, and the default settings were modified according to the feature of rat brain.

For voxel-based statistical analysis of functional images, all the individual images should be primarily normalized into one common space, such as the MNI (Montreal Neurological Institute) space in human brain studies. And the standard brain template performs as a general criterion in spatial normalization. In our study, to spatially normalizing individual rat brain images, an FDG-PET rat brain template was iteratively created from 24 healthy adult rats. Because there are minor differences in anatomical structures between healthy ones [7], our created FDG-PET rat brain template could be a group representation of SD rat brain. Furthermore, because there is a close association between olfactory dysfunction and cognitive impairment [14–16], our constructed FDG-PET template comprised not only the cerebrum and cerebellum, but also the whole olfactory bulb, which made the later cognitive studies much more exhaustive.

How to locate the anatomical regions of functional effects in statistical results is important in voxel-wise analysis. In physiological significance location, the brain atlas also called stereotaxic coordinates corresponding to the template space provides detailed anatomical information for functional results, such as the Tailarach coordinates for human brain studies [17]. In this study, one of the most popular atlases in rat brain studies, the stereotaxic coordinates established by Paxinos & Watson [18], was used for functional effects location, based on which our group has constructed the digital atlas and corresponding MRI T2WI

structural canonical brain in Paxinos & Watson space [4]. The technique of synthetic FDG-PET was employed [10,19] to standardize the FDG-PET canonical brain into the Paxinos & Watson space. As illustrated in the Result part, the FDG-PET canonical brain was standardized into the atlas space very well. Although the anatomical structures are excellently delineated in Paxinos and Watson [18], the accuracy of anatomical coordinates for statistical result was millimeter because of the low resolution of FDG-PET imaging.

In addition, to evaluate the performance of spmratIHEP in voxel-wise analysis of FDG-PET images, nine rats with left side MCAO and eight healthy controls, acquired on Siemens Inveon PET which differs from the one imaging for template construction, were enrolled in this study. The data preprocessing and voxel-wise analyzing of these two groups were all performed automatically in spmratIHEP based on SPM8. As illustrated in the Result part, the statistical result was almost related to the left side MCA. Therefore, our constructed toolbox performed well in rat brain imaging data analyzing in SPM8.

In conclusion, demonstrating its adequacy and practical usage in SPM environment, we reported the constructed FDG-PET rat brain template in the stereotaxic coordinate space of the Paxinos and Watson rat brain atlas. We believe it will be helpful to streamline the neuroimaging data analyses for rat brain images from the pre-processing stage to the reports of the statistical inference results.

Author Contributions

Conceived and designed the experiments: BBN. Performed the experiments: HL XFJ. Analyzed the data: BBN. Contributed reagents/materials/analysis tools: BBN HL XFJ. Wrote the paper: BBN KWC BCS.

References

1. Zimmer L, Luxen A (2012) PET radiotracers for molecular imaging in the brain: past, present and future. NeuroImage 61: 363–370.
2. Huang YC, Hsu CC, Huang P, Yin TK, Chiu NT, et al. (2011) The changes in brain metabolism in people with activated brown adipose tissue: a PET study. NeuroImage 54: 142–147.
3. Jagust WJ, Bandy D, Chen K, Foster NL, Landau SM, et al. (2010) The Alzheimer's Disease Neuroimaging Initiative positron emission tomography core. Alzheimers Dement 6: 221–229.
4. Nie B, Chen K, Zhao S, Liu J, Gu X, et al. (2013) A rat brain MRI template with digital stereotaxic atlas of fine anatomical delineations in paxinos space and its automated application in voxel-wise analysis. Human Brain Mapping 34: 1306–1318.
5. Schweinhardt P, Fransson P, Olson L, Spenger C, Andersson JL (2003) A template for spatial normalisation of MR images of the rat brain. Journal of Neuroscience Methods 129: 105–113.
6. Schwarz AJ, Danckaert A, Reese T, Gozzi A, Paxinos G, et al. (2006) A stereotaxic MRI template set for the rat brain with tissue class distribution maps and co-registered anatomical atlas: application to pharmacological MRI. NeuroImage 32: 538–550.
7. Casteels C, Vermaelen P, Nuyts J, Van Der Linden A, Baekelandt V, et al. (2006) Construction and evaluation of multitracer small-animal PET probabilistic atlases for voxel-based functional mapping of the rat brain. J Nucl Med 47: 1858–1866.
8. Paxinos G, Watson C (1982) The rat brain in stereotaxic coordinates 2nd edition. Sydney: Academic Press.
9. Buiter HJ, van Velden FH, Leysen JE, Fisher A, Windhorst AD, et al. (2012) Reproducible Analysis of Rat Brain PET Studies Using an Additional [(18)F]NaF Scan and an MR-Based ROI Template. International Journal of Molecular Imaging 2012: 580717.
10. Coello C, Hjornevik T, Courivaud F, Willoch F (2011) Anatomical standardization of small animal brain FDG-PET images using synthetic functional template: experimental comparison with anatomical template. Journal of Neuroscience Methods 199: 166–172.
11. Schiffman SS, Graham BG, Sattely-Miller EA, Zervakis J, Welsh-Bohmer K (2002) Taste, smell and neuropsychological performance of individuals at familial risk for Alzheimer's disease. Neurobiology of Aging 23: 397–404.

12. Li W, Howard JD, Gottfried JA (2010) Disruption of odour quality coding in piriform cortex mediates olfactory deficits in Alzheimer's disease. Brain 133: 2714–2726.
13. Wong KK, Muller ML, Kuwabara H, Studenski SA, Bohnen NI (2010) Olfactory loss and nigrostriatal dopaminergic denervation in the elderly. Neuroscience Letters 484: 163–167.
14. Peters JM, Hummel T, Kratzsch T, Lotsch J, Skarke C, et al. (2003) Olfactory function in mild cognitive impairment and Alzheimer's disease: an investigation using psychophysical and electrophysiological techniques. The American Journal of Psychiatry 160: 1995–2002.
15. Devanand DP, Michaels-Marston KS, Liu X, Pelton GH, Padilla M, et al. (2000) Olfactory deficits in patients with mild cognitive impairment predict Alzheimer's disease at follow-up. The American Journal of Psychiatry 157: 1399–1405.
16. Schubert CR, Carmichael LL, Murphy C, Klein BE, Klein R, et al. (2008) Olfaction and the 5-year incidence of cognitive impairment in an epidemiological study of older adults. Journal of the American Geriatrics Society 56: 1517–1521.
17. Talairach P, Tournoux J (1988) A stereotactic coplanar atlas of the human brain. Stuttgart: Thieme.
18. Paxinos G, Watson C (2005) The rat brain in stereotaxic coordinates 5th edition. New York: Academic Press.
19. Rubins DJ, Melega WP, Lacan G, Way B, Plenevaux A, et al. (2003) Development and evaluation of an automated atlas-based image analysis method for microPET studies of the rat brain. NeuroImage 20: 2100–2118.
20. Longa EZ, Weinstein PR, Carlson S, Cummins R (1989) Reversible middle cerebral artery occlusion without craniectomy in rats. Stroke; a Journal of Cerebral Circulation 20: 84–91.
21. Minematsu K, Li L, Fisher M, Sotak CH, Davis MA, et al. (1992) Diffusion-weighted magnetic resonance imaging: Rapid and quantitative detection of focal brain ischemia. Neurology 42: 235–240.
22. Kuge Y, Minematsu K, Yamaguchi T, Miyake Y (1995) Nylon monofilament for intraluminal middle cerebral artery occlusion in rats. Stroke 26: 1655–1658.
23. Fueger BJ, Czernin J, Hildebrandt I, Tran C, Halpern BS, et al. (2006) Impact of animal handling on the results of 18F-FDG PET studies in mice. J Nucl Med 47: 999–1006.
24. Matsumura A, Mizokawa S, Tanaka M, Wada Y, Nozaki S, et al. (2003) Assessment of microPET performance in analyzing the rat brain under different

types of anesthesia: comparison between quantitative data obtained with microPET and ex vivo autoradiography. NeuroImage 20: 2040–2050.

25. Friston KJ, Ashburner J, Frith CD, Pline J-B, Heather JD, et al. (1995a) Spatial registration and normalization of images. Human Brain Mapping 2: 89–165.

26. Ashburner J, Friston KJ (1999) Nonlinear spatial normalization using basis functions. Human Brain Mapping 7: 254–266.

27. Zhilkin P, Alexander ME (2004) Affine registration: a comparison of several programs. Magnetic Resonance Imaging 22: 55–66.

28. Friston KJ, Ashburner JT, Kiebel SJ, Nichols TE, Penny WD (2007) Statistical parametric mapping: The analysis of functional brain images. London: Academic Press.

29. Jaccard P (1912) The distribution of the flora in the alpine zone. New Phytol 11: 37–50.

30. Murugavel M, Sullivan JM Jr (2009) Automatic cropping of MRI rat brain volumes using pulse coupled neural networks. NeuroImage 45: 845–854.

31. Chupin M, Mukuna-Bantumbakulu AR, Hasboun D, Bardinet E, Baillet S, et al. (2007) Anatomically constrained region deformation for the automated segmentation of the hippocampus and the amygdala: Method and validation on controls and patients with Alzheimer's disease. NeuroImage 34: 996–1019.

32. Rodionov R, Chupin M, Williams E, Hammers A, Kesavadas C, et al. (2009) Evaluation of atlas-based segmentation of hippocampi in healthy humans. Magnetic Resonance Imaging 27: 1104–1109.

33. Nie B, Hui J, Wang L, Chai P, Gao J, et al. (2010) Automatic method for tracing regions of interest in rat brain magnetic resonance imaging studies. J Magn Reson Imaging 32: 830–835.

34. Chupin M, Mukuna-Bantumbakulu AR, Hasboun D, Bardinet E, Baillet S, et al. (2007): Anatomically constrained region deformation for the automated segmentation of the hippocampus and the amygdala: Method and validation on controls and patients with Alzheimer's disease. NeuroImage 34(3): 996–1019.

35. Rodionov R, Chupin M, Williams E, Hammers A, Kesavadas C, et al. (2009): Evaluation of atlas-based segmentation of hippocampi in healthy humans. Magnetic resonance imaging 27(8): 1104–1109.

20

CT-Based Attenuation Correction in I-123-Ioflupane SPECT

Catharina Lange[1], Anita Seese[2], Sarah Schwarzenböck[3], Karen Steinhoff[2], Bert Umland-Seidler[4], Bernd J. Krause[3], Winfried Brenner[1], Osama Sabri[2], Jens Kurth[3☉¶], Swen Hesse[2☉¶], Ralph Buchert[1*☉¶]

1 Department of Nuclear Medicine, Charité – Universitätsmedizin Berlin, Berlin, Germany, 2 Department of Nuclear Medicine, Universitätsklinikum Leipzig, Leipzig, Germany, 3 Department of Nuclear Medicine, Universitätsmedizin Rostock, Rostock, Germany, 4 GE Healthcare Buchler GmbH & Co. KG, Munich, Germany

Abstract

Purpose: Attenuation correction (AC) based on low-dose computed tomography (CT) could be more accurate in brain single-photon emission computed tomography (SPECT) than the widely used Chang method, and, therefore, has the potential to improve both semi-quantitative analysis and visual image interpretation. The present study evaluated CT-based AC for dopamine transporter SPECT with I-123-ioflupane.

Materials and methods: Sixty-two consecutive patients in whom I-123-ioflupane SPECT including low-dose CT had been performed were recruited retrospectively at 3 centres. For each patient, 3 different SPECT images were reconstructed: without AC, with Chang AC and with CT-based AC. Distribution volume ratio (DVR) images were obtained by scaling voxel intensities using the whole brain without striata as reference. For assessing the impact of AC on semi-quantitative analysis, specific-to-background ratios (SBR) in caudate and putamen were obtained by fully automated SPM8-based region of interest (ROI) analysis and tested for their diagnostic power using receiver-operator-characteristic (ROC) analysis. For assessing the impact of AC on visual image reading, screenshots of stereotactically normalized DVR images presented in randomized order were interpreted independently by two raters at each centre.

Results: CT-based AC resulted in intermediate SBRs about half way between no AC and Chang. Maximum area under the ROC curve was achieved by the putamen SBR, with negligible impact of AC (0.924, 0.935 and 0.938 for no, CT-based and Chang AC). Diagnostic accuracy of visual interpretation also did not depend on AC.

Conclusions: The impact of CT-based versus Chang AC on the interpretation of I-123-ioflupane SPECT is negligible. Therefore, CT-based AC cannot be recommended for routine use in clinical patient care, not least because of the additional radiation exposure.

Editor: Qinghui Zhang, University of Nebraska Medical Center, United States of America

Funding: These authors have no support or funding to report.

Competing Interests: One of the authors, Bert Umland-Seidler, is employee of GE Healthcare Buchler GmbH & Co. KG. However, there are no competing interests arising from this relationship.

* Email: ralph.buchert@charite.de

☉ These authors contributed equally to this work.

¶ These authors are senior authors on this work

Introduction

Single photon emission computed tomography (SPECT) with I-123-labelled cocaine ligands for the presynaptic dopamine transporter (DAT) is widely used for the diagnosis of Parkinsonian syndromes and for differentiation between Alzheimer's and Lewy body disease [1–8]. It is also used for monitoring progression of presynaptic dopaminergic degeneration [9]. The interpretation of DAT SPECT is based on visual evaluation of the images supported by semi-quantitative analysis [10–16] both of which are affected by photon attenuation in the head [17].

There are several methods for attenuation correction (AC) in brain SPECT. The most widely used method, proposed by Chang [18], is based on post-processing of images reconstructed without attenuation correction. However, this method has three limitations. First, delineation of the outer contour of the head is required which is prone to errors in case of both manual and automatic threshold-based methods [19]. Second, Chang's method assumes a uniform attenuation coefficient throughout the whole head which is an approximation only. Third, it is an approximation even if the actual attenuation coefficient is uniform. It is strictly correct only for a point source (at least in its non-iterative form).

Errors associated with these limitations of the Chang AC might be avoided by modelling attenuation within the reconstruction process using the correct attenuation map, for example measured by low-dose x-ray computed tomography (CT). Whereas CT-based AC has become standard in positron emission tomography (PET) of the brain, it is not widely used in brain SPECT, despite the increasing availability of dual-modality SPECT/CT systems. CT-based AC could provide more accurate AC than the Chang method and, therefore, has the potential to improve both semi-quantitative analysis and visual interpretation of DAT SPECT.

The aim of the present study was to compare CT-based AC and Chang AC in dopamine transporter SPECT with N-ω-fluoropropyl-2β-carbomethoxy-3β-(4-I-123-iodophenyl)nortropane (I-123-ioflupane). The impact of the AC method was assessed on both semi-quantitative analysis and visual evaluation of the SPECT images by independent readers blinded for clinical information.

Materials and Methods

1. Phantom studies

SPECT/CT of an anthropomorphic phantom for quantitative SPECT and PET imaging of the striatum (Striatal Phantom, Alderson, Radiology Support Devices Inc., Long Beach, CA, USA) was performed at each of 3 centers (Berlin, Leipzig, Rostock). The striata were filled symmetrically with about 40 kBq/ml I-123 solution. The background was filled with about 5 kBq/ml. Actual activity concentrations in striatum and background were determined by measuring aliquots in a well counter.

2. Subjects

The study included 62 patients who had received SPECT with I-123-ioflupane including low-dose CT in clinical routine patient care for the diagnosis of a Parkinsonian syndrome (Berlin n = 21, Leipzig n = 22 and Rostock n = 19). Consecutive patients were included at each centre without any further inclusion or exclusion criteria.

3. Ethics statement

The protocol of this retrospective study had been approved by the Ethics Committee at Rostock University Medical Centre (reference number A 2013-0144) and the Ethics Committee at Charité University Medical Centre Berlin (reference number EA1/326/13). The protocol complied with the Declaration of Helsinki. All patients had given written consent for retrospective analyses of their data.

4. SPECT imaging

SPECT imaging including low-dose CT had been performed with a Symbia T6 dual-head SPECT/CT system equipped with low energy high resolution parallel-hole collimators at each centre. The acquisition protocol, based on procedure guidelines for I-123-labelled dopamine transporter ligands and the ENC-DAT study [11,20,21], was the same at each centre except for small differences in the energy window at the I-123 peak and the two additional energy windows for scatter correction (SC; energy windows in keV: Berlin [141.66, 173.14], [130.64 141.66], [173.14, 182.58], Leipzig: [147.07, 170.93], [123.22, 147.07], [170.93, 194.77], Rostock: [140.91, 172.91], [129.95, 140.91], [172.23, 181.62]). These differences were taken into account by adjustment of the weight factors during scatter correction (s. below).

Patients did not use medication or drugs known to strongly interact with I-123-ioflupane SPECT [22,23]. 150 to 200 MBq I-123-ioflupane were injected intravenously as a slow bolus after blocking the thyroid gland by oral administration of perchlorate. SPECT imaging was started between 3 and 4 hours post injection. The rotation radius was adjusted for each patient so that collimator-patient distance was as small as possible. The duration of the SPECT acquisition was 30 minutes (step-and-shoot mode, matrix 128×128, angular range 180°, angular sampling 3°, zoom

1.23). A low-dose CT was performed immediately after the SPECT (130 keV, 50 mAs, 3 mm slice thickness).

The anonymized raw data from all centres were transferred to one centre (Berlin) for centralized image reconstruction and processing. Transversal images were reconstructed using the 3D ordered-subset expectation-maximisation algorithm 'Flash-3D' provided by the Siemens scanner software (15 subsets and 6 iterations) [24–26]. Flash-3D allows CT-based AC, uniform AC according to Chang and no AC. Spatial resolution in the reconstructed images was about 8 mm full-width-at-half-maximum, voxel size was $3.9 \times 3.9 \times 3.9$ mm^3.

For conversion of Hounsfield units to linear attenuation coefficients (LAC) in CT-based AC, the narrow-beam LAC of $\mu = 0.148$ cm^{-1} was assumed for soft tissue, because SC using the triple energy window approach implemented in the scanner software was applied in all cases [27]. In order to achieve best comparability between Chang and CT-based AC, Chang AC was performed with the same LAC, i.e. $\mu = 0.148$ cm^{-1}. For Chang AC, the threshold-based automatic delineation of the head contour implemented in the system software was used. The threshold was optimized in each individual patient so that the best match with the outer contour of the scalp was obtained according to visual inspection.

Image reconstruction without AC, with CT-based AC and Chang AC for each patient resulted in a total of 3 • 62 = 186 SPECT images.

5. Data evaluation

The impact of the AC method was assessed on both semi-quantitative analysis and visual evaluation of the SPECT images.

5.1. Impact on semi-quantitative analysis. For semi-quantitative assessment of DAT availability, the I-123-ioflupane SPECT image of each individual patient was stereotactically normalized into the anatomical space of the Montreal Neurological Institute (MNI) using the normalization tool of the freely available Statistical Parametric Mapping software package SPM (version SPM8, Wellcome Trust Centre for Neuroimaging, Institute of Neurology, UCL, London, UK) [28] and a custom-made tracer-specific template (Fig. 1). The stereotactically normalized I-123-ioflupane uptake image was scaled to the 75th percentile of the voxel intensities in the whole brain without striata as reference region (Fig. 1), i.e. the intensity value of each voxel was divided by the 75th percentile of the voxel intensities in the reference region [29]. The voxel intensity of the scaled SPECT image represents the distribution volume ratio (DVR) as semi-quantitative measure for local DAT availability.

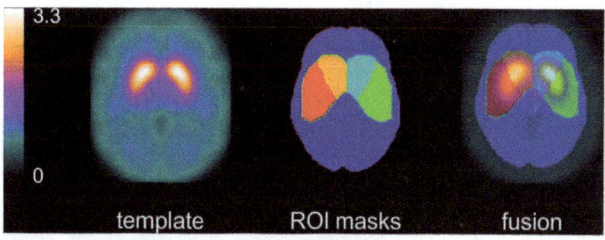

Figure 1. Custom-made I-123-ioflupane template. Transversal slice (**left**). ROIs for left/right caudate and putamen used for hottest voxel analysis, and ROI for the reference region used for intensity scaling, all defined in MNI space (**middle**). The union of caudate and putamen ROI was used as ROI for the whole striatum. Fusion image (**right**).

The DVRs in caudate and putamen were obtained by 'hottest voxel analysis' in large predefined ROIs for left/right caudate and left/right putamen in MNI space (Fig. 1). The number of hottest voxels to be averaged was fixed to a total volume of 5 ml for the caudate and 10 ml for the putamen. The DVR of the whole striatum was obtained by averaging over the 15 ml hottest voxels in the union of the caudate and the putamen ROI. DVRs were converted to specific binding ratios (SBR) according to the formula $SBR = DVR - 1$. The SBR may be considered an estimate of the nondisplaceable binding potential and, therefore, to be proportional to the density of DAT available for binding of I-123-ioflupane [30].

Caudate-to-putamen ratio ($= SBR_{caudate}/SBR_{putamen}$) and left/right asymmetry ($asym(\%) = 200 \cdot abs[(SBR_{left} - SBR_{right})/(SBR_{left}+SBR_{right})]$) were considered in addition to SBRs.

5.2. Impact on visual scoring. For retrospective visual interpretation of the SPECT images, a pdf document was prepared with 186 pages, one page for each SPECT image (Fig. 2 a). The SPECT images were anonymized and presented in randomized order. To guarantee comparable display conditions, the upper threshold of the colour table was adjusted separately for each AC method. For Chang AC, the upper threshold of the colour table was set to 5.50. For CT-based AC, the upper threshold of the colour table was scaled by the DVR of the caudate (mean over left and right hemisphere) averaged over all patients, i.e. $threshold(CT) = avgDVR(CT)/avgDVR(Chang) \cdot threshold(Chang)$, analogously for no AC. The lower threshold of the colour table was set to one-tenth of the upper threshold in all cases.

Visual scoring of DAT availability was performed on a patient base referring to Benamer et al. [31] using the following 5-score:

– 'normal': clear delineation of the whole striatum on both sides, some minor global reduction of tracer uptake is allowed as well as some minor left/right asymmetry ('only big effects indicate pathology')

– 'reduced type 1': distinct reduction in the putamen in one hemisphere ('big' effect), the striatum in the other hemisphere still more or less normal

– 'reduced type 2': distinct reduction in both putamina, still some uptake in the caudate nuclei

– 'reduced type 3': essentially no uptake in both striata

– 'reduced other': clear reduction of tracer uptake, but the pattern does not match type 1, 2 or 3. This category was added to the Benamer scheme in order to account for atypical patterns, for example due to vascular pathology

The examples shown in Fig. 2 b were provided to the raters.

The certainty with respect to the differentiation between normal and reduced (including all types of reduction) was scored in addition to DAT availability. A 5-score was used ranging from 1 = 'very sure' to 5 = 'very unsure'.

Image quality was scored from 1 = 'very good' to 5 = 'very bad' using the anatomical delineation of the striata and the level of statistical noise in the background as criteria.

Visual scoring was performed by two independent raters at each of the 3 centres (image quality in Leipzig only). In addition, the two raters at each centre reached a consensus with respect to DAT availability in those cases in which they had disagreed.

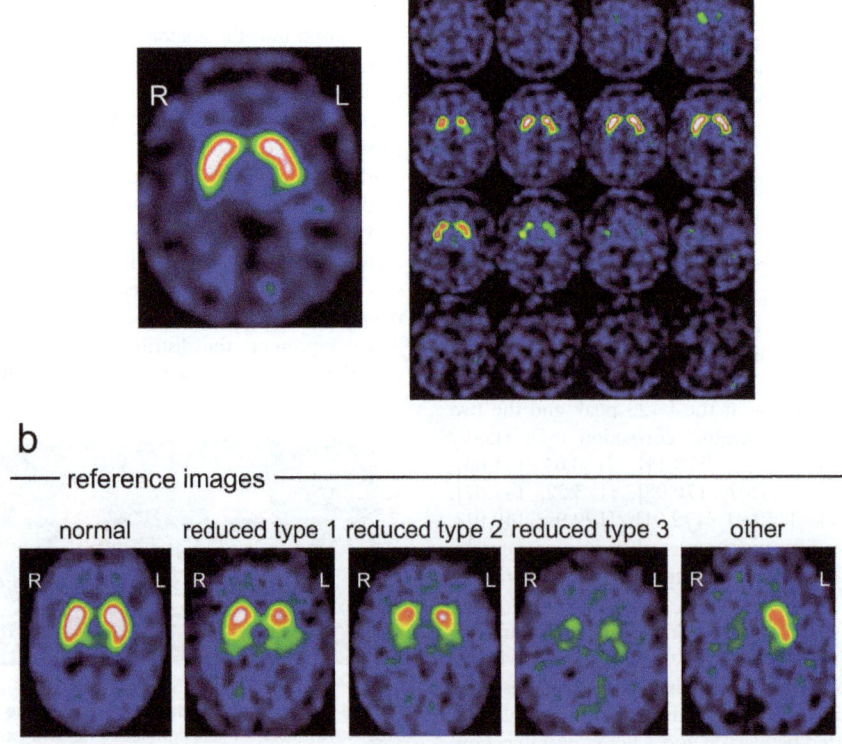

Figure 2. Example page from the pdf document for visual scoring. The pdf document comprised one page for each I-123-ioflupane SPECT image showing a 12 mm thick slab (**a, left**) and 4x4 slices of 4 mm thickness (**a, right**). Example I-123-ioflupane SPECTs used as reference images for the visual scoring (**b**).

Table 1. Results of the semi-quantitative analysis of the phantom studies.

| centre | method | actual SBR | measured SBR | | measured/actual SBR (%)[a] |
			left	right	
Berlin	no AC	5.47	2.30	2.09	40.1
	CT-based	5.47	2.55	2.37	45.0
	Chang	5.47	2.88	2.62	50.3
Leipzig	no AC	5.74	2.57	2.36	42.9
	CT-based	5.74	2.92	2.53	47.5
	Chang	5.74	3.04	2.88	51.6
Rostock	no AC	5.19	2.36	2.40	45.9
	CT-based	5.19	2.60	2.64	50.5
	Chang	5.19	2.85	2.86	55.0
mean	no AC				43.0±2.9
	CT-based				47.6±2.8
	Chang				52.3±2.4

The specific-to-background ratio (SBR) was measured using the same whole striatum ROIs as in the patient studies (Fig. 1).
[a]measured SBR: mean over left and right hemisphere.

6. Statistical methods

Statistics were performed with IBM SPSS Statistics (version 21, IBM Corp., Armonk, NY, USA).

Concerning the results of the semi-quantitative analysis, the effect of the AC method on the SBRs, left/right asymmetries and caudate-to-putamen ratio was first assessed by Bland-Altman plots [32]. Then the impact of AC on the diagnostic power of the semi-quantitative parameters was tested using receiver-operator characteristic (ROC) analysis. The classification of DAT availability in the written report in the patient's file served as gold standard (22 patients with normal DAT availability, 40 patients with reduced DAT availability). The area under the ROC curve (AUC) was used as performance measure. Multiple binary logistic regression (forward conditional) was performed to analyze the diagnostic power of combinations of SBR, asymmetry and caudate-to-putamen ratio. Only the putamen SBR was included in the multiple regression analysis, since there was a strong correlation between caudate and putamen SBR (Pearson correlation coefficient = 0.87, p = 0.000, Chang AC) so that it was not advisable to include both as independent parameters. The putamen SBR was selected, because it showed higher diagnostic power than the caudate SBR in the univariate ROC analyses.

Concerning the results of the visual reading, inter-rater agreement was quantified by Cohen's unweighted κ [33], both for the full 5-score for DAT availability and the binary score derived from the 5-score by subsuming 'reduced type 1, 2, 3' and 'reduced other' into one single category 'reduced'. Agreement was assessed between the 6 raters and between the 3 consensus scores. Diagnostic accuracy of the visual scoring was characterized by the % agreement with the gold standard.

The effect of the AC method on the certainty in differentiation between normal and reduced DAT availability as well as on image quality was tested by the general linear model for repeated measures. The DAT availability (normal or reduced) according to the report was added to the model as within-subject factor.

Potential covariates such as age or body mass index were not taken into account [34].

Results

1. Impact on semi-quantitative analysis

Results of the semi-quantitative analysis of the phantom and patient studies are summarized in Table 1 and Table 2, respectively.

In the phantom studies, the actual SBR was strongly underestimated in all cases, by about 57%, 52% and 48% with no, CT-based and Chang AC (Table 1), i.e. CT-based AC resulted in intermediate SBRs about half way between no AC and Chang AC.

The latter was confirmed in the patient studies (Table 2, Fig. 3). Chang AC resulted in an overestimation of the caudate SBR compared to CT-based AC that was increasing with increasing SBR (Fig. 3 a). The mean difference (CT-based – Chang) was −0.445±0.188 (one sample t-test for zero mean: p<0.0005). The mean difference of the putamen SBR was −0.117±0.100 (p< 0.0005). The mean difference of left/right asymmetry in the caudate was 1.66±4.94% (p=0.011), in the putamen 0.41±7.16% (p=0.652), and in the whole striatum 1.60±4.79% (p=0.011). The mean difference of the caudate-to-putamen ratio was −0.15±0.15 (p<0.0005).

Univariate analysis of variance with the SBR (minimum over both hemispheres) as dependent variable and region of interest (caudate, putamen), DAT status (normal or reduced according to the written report in the patient's file) and centre (Berlin, Leipzig, Rostock) as fixed factors revealed highly significant effects of the region of interest and DAT status (both p<0.0005), whereas there was no centre effect, independent of the AC method.

ROC curves for the differentiation between reduced and normal DAT availability by the SBRs are shown in Fig. 4. The putamen provided larger AUC than the caudate. The impact of AC on the AUC was very small: AUC for the caudate 0.892 versus 0.886 versus 0.887, and for the putamen 0.924 versus 0.935 versus 0.938 for no AC, CT-based AC and Chang AC, respectively. Asymmetries and caudate-to-putamen ratio provided less diagnostic power than the SBR (AUC ≤0.875).

The binary regression model included only the putamen SBR (minimum over both hemispheres). The asymmetry of the SBR in

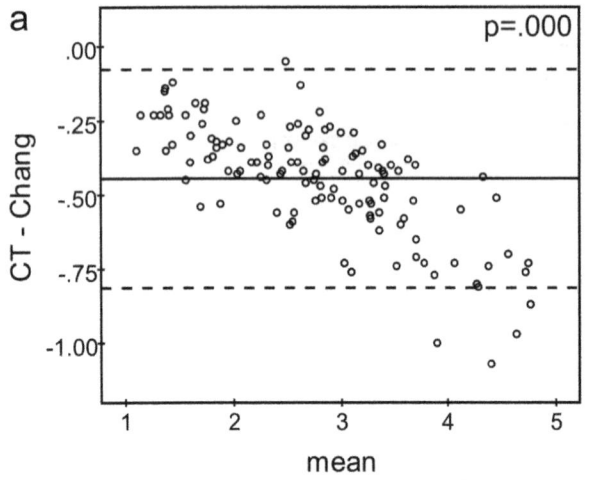

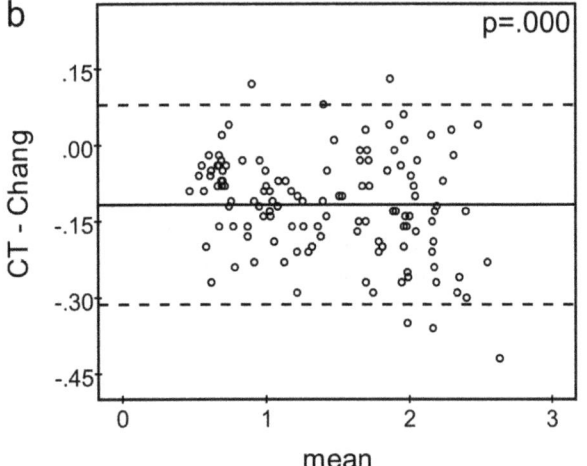

Figure 3. Bland-Altman plots comparing the SBR of the caudate (a) and the putamen (b) between CT-based and Chang AC (SBRs of both hemispheres were included independently, i.e. n = 124). Different scales were chosen for abscissae and ordinates in **a** and **b** for display purposes. The horizontal continuous line represents the mean difference, the dashed lines indicate the 95% confidence interval. The given p-value corresponds to the one-sample t-test for zero mean.

the whole striatum and the caudate-to-putamen ratio (maximum over both hemispheres) were not included, independent of the AC method (asymmetry: $p \geq 0.415$, caudate-to-putamen ratio: $p \geq 0.179$). The number of false classified patients was 8 for no AC and 9 for both CT-based and Chang AC.

2. Impact on visual scoring

Inter-rater agreement of the visual scoring of DAT availability was higher (i) for the consensus scores compared to the scores of individual raters and (ii) for the binary score compared to the 5-score for DAT availability (Table 3). The impact of the AC method was very small (Table 3).

Percent agreement of the visual score for DAT availability between CT-based and Chang AC was $81.5 \pm 7.9\%$ for the full 5-score and $92.7 \pm 2.7\%$ for the binary differentiation between normal and reduced DAT availability (averaged over the 6 individual raters). The consensus scores of the two raters at each centre showed very similar agreement of $83.3 \pm 6.5\%$ for the 5-score and $91.4 \pm 0.9\%$ for the binary decision. Diagnostic accuracy averaged over all raters was $81.7 \pm 3.2\%$, $81.5 \pm 4.9\%$ and $79.6 \pm 1.7\%$ for no AC, CT-based and Chang AC, respectively. Diagnostic accuracy of the consensus was $83.3 \pm 1.9\%$, $83.9 \pm 1.6\%$ and $79.6 \pm 2.5\%$.

The AC method had no significant effect on the raters' certainty in the differentiation between reduced and normal DAT availability (p = 0.922). However, there was a significant effect of the status of DAT availability: the certainty of the visual scoring was lower in patients with normal DAT availability (score averaged over all raters and all AC methods: 2.40 ± 0.83 versus 1.24 ± 0.60 in patients with normal and reduced DAT availability, $p < 0.0005$).

Image quality appeared slightly reduced without AC (score = 2.36 ± 0.54), but very similar for the two AC methods (2.16 ± 0.44 and 2.22 ± 0.53 for CT-based and Chang AC, p = 0.393).

Discussion

The present study compared CT-based AC and Chang AC for dopamine transporter SPECT with I-123-ioflupane with respect to both semi-quantitative and visual analysis. The same reconstruction algorithm with the same parameter settings was used with both AC methods in order to simplify the interpretation of observed differences in reconstructed images (as effects of AC), in contrast to most previous studies which used Chang AC with

Table 2. Results of the semi-quantitative analysis of the patient studies.

	reduced DAT availability (n = 40)			normal DAT availability (n = 22)		
	no AC	CT-based	Chang	no AC	CT-based	Chang
SBR caudate	1.85±0.75	2.03±0.71	2.42±0.83	3.01±0.51	3.15±0.54	3.67±0.65
SBR putamen	0.80±0.41	0.96±0.44	1.07±0.46	1.64±0.21	1.89±0.26	2.00±0.25
SBR striatum	1.33±0.57	1.51±0.57	1.78±0.65	2.36±0.35	2.54±0.39	2.91±0.45
caudate-to-putamen ratio	2.67±0.84	2.37±0.61	2.53±0.64	1.93±0.30	1.75±0.23	1.91±0.28
asymmetry caudate (%)	15.17±11.95	14.92±12.19	12.59±10.82	7.06±6.14	6.95±5.53	6.52±5.87
Asymmetry putamen (%)	23.28±24.18	20.50±15.81	18.82±16.84	9.11±7.91	7.15±7.81	9.06±8.29
asymmetry striatum (%)	15.92±12.94	15.43±11.58	13.35±10.65	5.65±5.13	6.00±4.55	5.28±5.15

Given are mean values ±1 standard deviation (minimum over both hemispheres for the SBRs, maximum over both hemispheres for the caudate-to-putamen ratio). Subjects were categorized as 'reduced' or 'normal' DAT availability according to the written report in the patient's file.

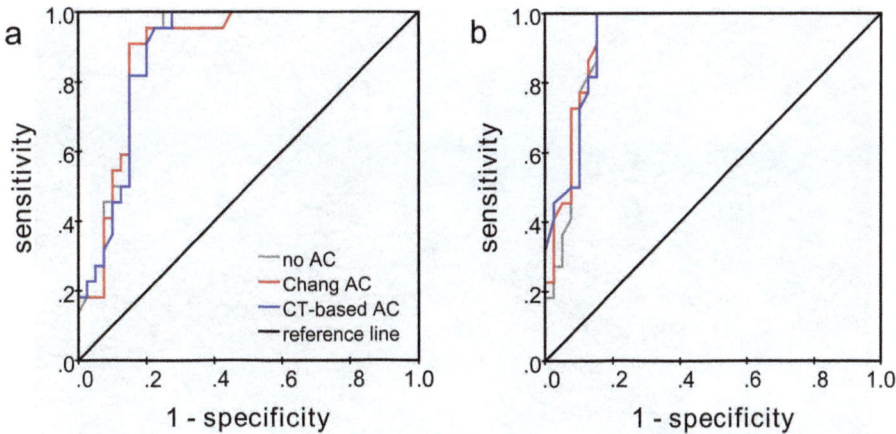

Figure 4. ROC curves for the differentiation between reduced and normal DAT availability by the SBR of the caudate (a) and the putamen (b) (minimum over both hemispheres).

filtered backprojection whereas CT-based AC was implemented within an iterative reconstruction algorithm [24–26]. It is well known that the reconstruction algorithm itself, in this case iterative reconstruction versus filtered backprojection, has an impact on the SPECT images. In the present study, the 3D ordered-subset expectation-maximisation algorithm 'Flash-3D' was used with the same number of subsets (15) and iterations (6) in all cases. This might have introduced a systematic effect not directly related to AC, since the speed of convergence of iterative reconstruction depends on whether attenuation is modelled or not. However, this effect is expected to be rather small in the present setting and, therefore, was neglected.

Concerning the results of the semi-quantitative analysis in the present study, CT-based AC resulted in intermediate SBRs about half way between no AC and Chang AC. However, the differences were rather small. For example, the increase of the SBR of the whole striatum by CT-based AC compared to no AC was only about 12% in the phantom studies (Table 1). This is explained by the fact that (i) the effect of photon attenuation is considerably smaller in I-123-ioflupane SPECT than in brain PET, due to the shorter path length to be covered by the single photon in SPECT compared to the total path length of both photons in PET which overcompensates the higher attenuation coefficient in SPECT, and that (ii) the effect of attenuation cancels to some extent during the computation of the SBRs as uptake ratios.

The phantom studies demonstrated strong underestimation of the actual SBR between about 48% (Chang AC) and about 57% (no AC) in the reconstructed SPECT images. Simulation showed that this can be explained by partial volume effects to large extent (Fig. 5). The effect of photon attenuation is rather small compared to the partial volume effects.

Assuming that iterative reconstruction modelling attenuation using the CT-based attenuation map provides more accurate correction of photon attenuation in the brain than Chang AC, the latter being based on a strongly simplified model, the results of the present study suggest that Chang AC overestimates attenuation of photons originating from the striatum relative to the attenuation of photons from the reference region. To some extent this might be explained by the use of the narrow-beam LAC $\mu = 0.148$ cm^{-1} for both Chang and CT-based AC, which might be too large, if scatter correction is incomplete. However, Chang AC resulted in larger SBRs than CT-based AC even with LAC as low as $\mu = 0.10$ cm^{-1} (LAC for CT-based AC fixed at $\mu = 0.148$ cm^{-1}). Warwick and co-workers also found larger SBRs in dopamine transporter SPECT with Chang AC than with CT-based AC, at least in the patient scans included in their study [35]. Rajeevan et al. evaluated non-uniform AC based on transmission imaging for I-123-β-CIT and concluded that both non-uniform and uniform AC provide a small improvement of semi-quantitative analysis compared to no AC [36].

The effect of the AC method on left/right asymmetry was small (Table 2). This can be explained by the definition of left/right asymmetry as the difference of SBRs within a ROI and its mirror ROI. Effects of AC cancel, because attenuation characteristics are essentially the same in both hemispheres. The effect on the caudate-putamen ratio was also small, which is explained by similar arguments.

Concerning the diagnostic value of the considered semi-quantitative parameters, the putamen SBR provided the best differentiation between normal and reduced DAT availability (with the written report in the patient's file as gold standard) [37]. The effect of AC was again negligible.

Table 3. Cohen's unweighted κ (mean ±1 standard deviation) for inter-rater agreement of visual scoring of DAT availability.

| | individual raters | | | consensus scores | | |
| | (15 pairs of raters) | | | (3 pairs of consensi) | | |
	no AC	CT-based	Chang	no AC	CT-based	Chang
5-score	0.71±0.11	0.70±0.10	0.72±0.09	0.80±0.14	0.78±0.04	0.80±0.06
binary score	0.73±0.13	0.77±0.12	0.76±0.11	0.90±0.05	0.82±0.02	0.81±0.06

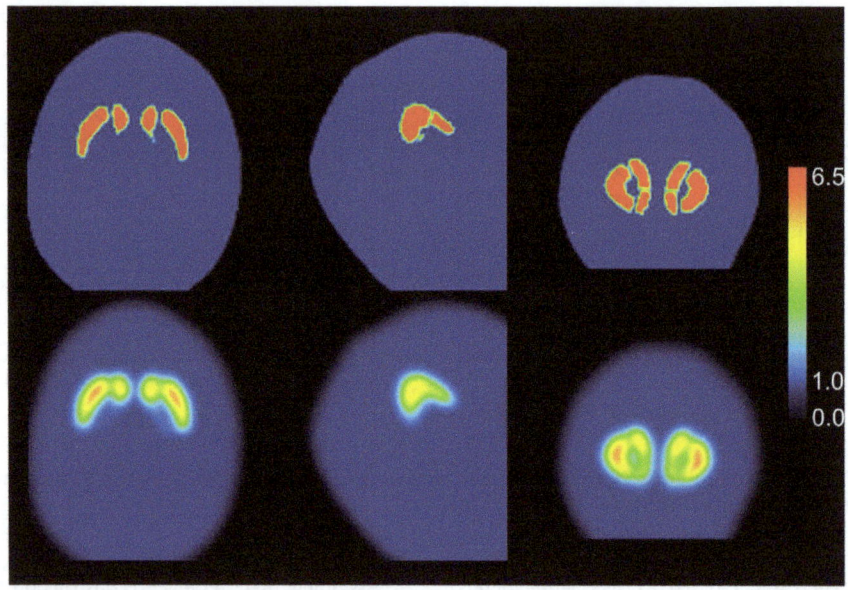

Figure 5. SPECT underestimates the true activity concentration in small structures such as the striatum and its substructures due to the limited spatial resolution in the reconstructed SPECT image (partial volume effect, PVE). In order to estimate the extent of underestimation in the present study, the reconstructed spatial resolution was estimated on the basis of a line source measurement using the same acquisition and reconstruction protocol as in the measurements of the striatal phantom and the patients included in the present study (no AC). Spatial resolution was found to be about 8 mm full-width-at-half-maximum (FWHM). Then a high-resolution CT of the striatal phantom was segmented manually (top row; from left to right: transversal, sagittal and coronal slice). Voxel values in the striatum were set to 6.5, voxel values in the background to 1.0 in order to simulate the actual SBR of about 5.5 in the phantom studies (Table 1). Then the segmented CT image was smoothed with a 3-dimensional Gaussian kernel with 8 mm FWHM to simulate the PVE in SPECT (bottom row). ROI analysis of the smoothed image resulted in a striatal SBR of 3.2 which underestimates the actual SBR of 5.5 by about 42%.

The lack of an impact of AC on the diagnostic power of I-123-ioflupane SPECT was confirmed by the results of the visual interpretation of the SPECT images. Neither the scores of the 6 individual raters nor the consensus scores obtained at each centre showed an effect of AC on their diagnostic value. This finding is in agreement with the results of Bienkiewicz and colleagues who

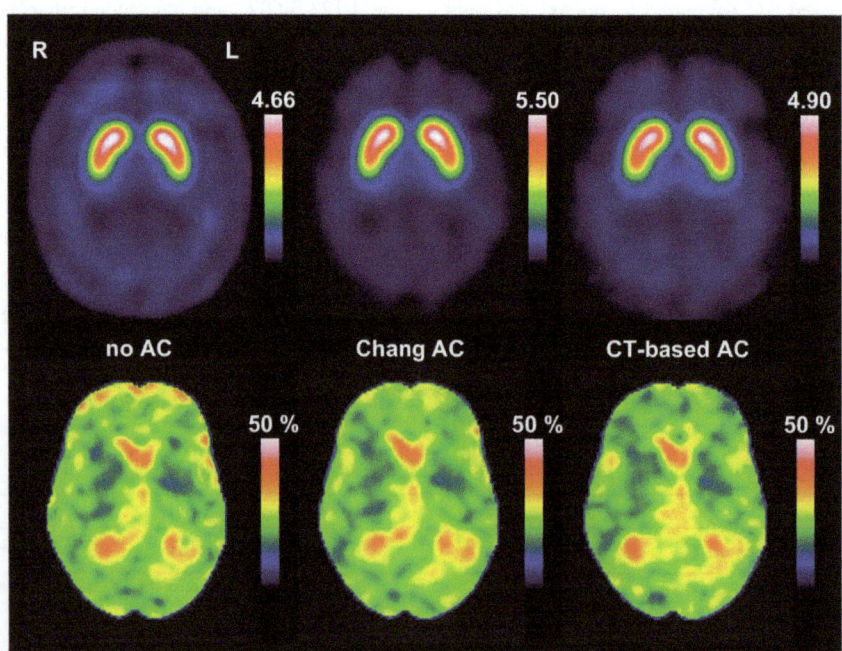

Figure 6. Image quality. Slab of 12 mm thickness of the scaled, stereotactically normalized I-123-ioflupane SPECT averaged over all patients with normal DAT availability (**top**). Slab displaying the coefficient of variation (%) of the DVR over all patients with normal DAT availability (**bottom**).

compared Chang AC (with filtered backprojection) and CT-based AC (with iterative OS-EM reconstruction) in I-123-ioflupane SPECT with respect to visual evaluation by a single reader and found no sigificant effect [38].

Agreement of the retrospective binary consensus score with the classification of DAT availability in the written report ranged between 79.6% and 83.3%, which appears rather low. The most frequent discrepancy was that a scan which had been classified as normal in the written report was scored as reduced in the retrospective visual analysis, indicating somewhat more sensitive reading in the restrospective analysis. This might be explained, at least in part, by the fact that only anonymized SPECT images were provided for the restrospective visual reading (Fig. 2), whereas clinical data and semi-quantitative analysis of the I-123-ioflupane uptake had been available in addition to the SPECT images for the classification in the written report in the patient's file. Furthermore, retrospective visual reading was based on a standardized documentation page presenting exactly the same slices in each individual patient with a fixed, predefined colortable (Fig. 2), whereas there is variation of slice orientation and colortable in visual analysis of SPECT images in clinical routine.

In addition to accuracy, stability is an important attribute of any diagnostic procedure in clinical routine patient care. In case of radionuclide imaging, variability in the interpretation of the images between different readers is most likely the limiting factor rather than variability of tracer uptake between different scans of the same patient [39]. The present study demonstrated very good to excellent inter-rater agreement of visual reading, particularly for the binary differentiation between normal and reduced DAT availability, which is more relevant clinically than grading the reduction of DAT availability using the 5-score based on Benamer et al. [31]. Inter-rater agreement in this study was comparable to results reported by Kahraman and colleagues [40]. The effect of AC on inter-rater agreement was negligible (Table 3).

AC also had no impact on the certainty of visual differentiation between normal and reduced DAT availability. Only the status of DAT availability had an effect: the certainty was significantly higher in patients with reduced DAT availability than in patients with normal DAT availability, as direct consequence of the instruction given to the raters to interpret the SPECT images conservatively, as in clinical routine patient care where it is important to keep the rate of false positive results low.

Finally, the method for AC, i.e. CT-based versus Chang, also had no significant effect on image quality. Image quality appeared slightly worse without AC, most likely because of apparently increased tracer uptake outside the brain which somewhat complicates the identification of the brain (Fig. 6).

The following limitations of the present study should be noted. First, the diagnosis in the original report was used as gold standard for the evaluation of diagnostic accuracy, because a final clinical diagnosis based on follow-up was not available. However, we do not consider this as a major limitation, since the gold standard mainly affects the absolute value of the diagnostic accuracy. Relative diagnostic accuracy is much less affected. The statement that the impact of attenuation correction (with versus without) and the impact of the AC method (CT-based versus Chang) on diagnostic accuracy is negligible, therefore, is not affected. In addition, semi-quantitative analyses (Bland-Altman plots) as well as percent agreement, certainty and image quality according to the visual reading are also not affected by the gold standard.

Second, Chang attenuation correction is a post reconstruction method, i.e. the correction is performed by voxelwise multiplication of the SPECT image reconstructed without attenuation correction with a correction image calculated for a constant attenuation coefficient within the head contour according to Chang [18]. Now, the simplified μ map consisting in a constant value within the head contour might also be used for modelling attenuation within the iterative reconsruction instead of the attenuation map derived from the low-dose CT. It would be interesting to check whether this approach further reduces the difference of SBRs between CT-based AC and AC based on a uniform μ map. However, whereas there might be an effect on absolute values of SBRs, we do not expect an effect on diagnostic value of I-123-ioflupane SPECT, because there is already no difference between CT-based AC and post reconstruction Chang AC with respect to diagnostic value.

Conclusion

CT-based attenuation correction was compared with Chang attenuation correction with respect to its impact on the diagnostic accuracy of visual and semi-quantitative analysis as well as on inter-rater variability of visual image interpretation in I-123-ioflupane SPECT. These measures are more relevant in clinical routine patient care than absolute quantitative accuracy, as the objective is the discrimination between healthy and diseased state rather than accurate measurement of the density of dopamine transporters (for example in fmol/ml).

The impact of CT-based attenuation correction on the visual interpretation and the diagnostic value of semi-quantitative analysis of I-123-ioflupane SPECT was found to be negligible. Therefore, CT-based attenuation correction cannot be recommended for routine use, not least because of the additional radiation exposure caused by the low-dose CT.

Author Contributions

Conceived and designed the experiments: CL BUS BJK WB OS JK SH RB. Performed the experiments: AS SS KGS BUS CL. Analyzed the data: CL BUS JK SH RB AS SS KGS. Contributed reagents/materials/analysis tools: CL RB BUS JK SH AS SS KGS. Contributed to the writing of the manuscript: CL RB. Approved final manuscript: CL BUS JK SH RB AS SS KGS WB OS BJK.

References

1. Booij J, Speelman JD, Horstink MW, Wolters EC (2001) The clinical benefit of imaging striatal dopamine transporters with [123I]FP-CIT SPET in differentiating patients with presynaptic parkinsonism from those with other forms of parkinsonism. Eur J Nucl Med 28: 266–272.
2. Hesse S, Oehlwein C, Meyer PT, Roessler A, Tietze F, et al. (2003) Is there a role for I-123-FP-CIT SPECT in the management of suspected Parkinson's disease? Journal of Nuclear Medicine 44: 234p-235p.
3. Innis RB, Seibyl JP, Scanley BE, Laruelle M, Abi-Dargham A, et al. (1993) Single photon emission computed tomographic imaging demonstrates loss of striatal dopamine transporters in Parkinson disease. Proc Natl Acad Sci U S A 90: 11965–11969.
4. Tatsch K, Poepperl G (2013) Nigrostriatal dopamine terminal imaging with dopamine transporter SPECT: an update. J Nucl Med 54: 1331–1338.

5. Van Laere K, Everaert L, Annemans L, Gonce M, Vandenberghe W, et al. (2008) The cost effectiveness of 123I-FP-CIT SPECT imaging in patients with an uncertain clinical diagnosis of parkinsonism. Eur J Nucl Med Mol Imaging 35: 1367–1376.
6. Varrone A, Halldin C (2010) Molecular imaging of the dopamine transporter. J Nucl Med 51: 1331–1334.
7. Walker Z, Costa DC, Walker RW, Shaw K, Gacinovic S, et al. (2002) Differentiation of dementia with Lewy bodies from Alzheimer's disease using a dopaminergic presynaptic ligand. J Neurol Neurosurg Psychiatry 73: 134–140.
8. Garibotto V, Montandon ML, Viaud CT, Allaoua M, Assal F, et al. (2013) Regions of interest-based discriminant analysis of DaTSCAN SPECT and FDG-PET for the classification of dementia. Clin Nucl Med 38: e112–117.
9. Gamez J, Lorenzo-Bosquet C, Cuberas-Borros G, Carmona F, Badia M, et al. (2014) Progressive Presynaptic Dopaminergic Deterioration in Huntington

Disease: A [123I]-FP-CIT SPECT Two-Year Follow-Up Study. Clin Nucl Med 39: e227–228.

10. Booij J, Habraken JB, Bergmans P, Tissingh G, Winogrodzka A, et al. (1998) Imaging of dopamine transporters with iodine-123-FP-CIT SPECT in healthy controls and patients with Parkinson's disease. J Nucl Med 39: 1879–1884.

11. Darcourt J, Booij J, Tatsch K, Varrone A, Vander Borght T, et al. (2010) EANM procedure guidelines for brain neurotransmission SPECT using (123)I-labelled dopamine transporter ligands, version 2. Eur J Nucl Med Mol Imaging 37: 443–450.

12. Koch W, Radau PE, Hamann C, Tatsch K (2005) Clinical testing of an optimized software solution for an automated, observer-independent evaluation of dopamine transporter SPECT studies. J Nucl Med 46: 1109–1118.

13. Soderlund TA, Dickson JC, Prvulovich E, Ben-Haim S, Kemp P, et al. (2013) Value of semiquantitative analysis for clinical reporting of 123I-2-beta-carbomethoxy-3beta-(4-iodophenyl)-N-(3-fluoropropyl)nortropane SPECT studies. J Nucl Med 54: 714–722.

14. Tatsch K, Poepperl G (2012) Quantitative approaches to dopaminergic brain imaging. Q J Nucl Med Mol Imaging 56: 27–38.

15. Zubal IG, Early M, Yuan O, Jennings D, Marek K, et al. (2007) Optimized, automated striatal uptake analysis applied to SPECT brain scans of Parkinson's disease patients. J Nucl Med 48: 857–864.

16. Cuberas-Borros G, Lorenzo-Bosquet C, Aguade-Bruix S, Hernandez-Vara J, Pifarre-Montaner P, et al. (2011) Quantitative evaluation of striatal I-123-FP-CIT uptake in essential tremor and parkinsonism. Clin Nucl Med 36: 991–996.

17. Soret M, Koulibaly PM, Darcourt J, Hapdey S, Buvat I (2003) Quantitative accuracy of dopaminergic neurotransmission imaging with (123)I SPECT. J Nucl Med 44: 1184–1193.

18. Chang LT (1978) Method for Attenuation Correction in Radionuclide Computed Tomography. Ieee Transactions on Nuclear Science 25: 638–643.

19. Zaidi H, Hasegawa B (2003) Determination of the attenuation map in emission tomography. J Nucl Med 44: 291–315.

20. Tossici-Bolt L, Dickson JC, Sera T, de Nijs R, Bagnara MC, et al. (2011) Calibration of gamma camera systems for a multicentre European (1)(2)(3)I-FP-CIT SPECT normal database. Eur J Nucl Med Mol Imaging 38: 1529–1540.

21. Varrone A, Dickson JC, Tossici-Bolt L, Sera T, Asenbaum S, et al. (2013) European multicentre database of healthy controls for [123I]FP-CIT SPECT (ENC-DAT): age-related effects, gender differences and evaluation of different methods of analysis. Eur J Nucl Med Mol Imaging 40: 213–227.

22. Booij J, Kemp P (2008) Dopamine transporter imaging with [(123)I]FP-CIT SPECT: potential effects of drugs. Eur J Nucl Med Mol Imaging 35: 424–438.

23. Borghammer P, Knudsen K, Danielsen E, Ostergaard K (2014) False-positive 123I-FP-CIT scintigraphy and suggested dopamine transporter upregulation due to chronic modafinil treatment. Clin Nucl Med 39: e87–88.

24. Dickson JC, Tossici-Bolt L, Sera T, Erlandsson K, Varrone A, et al. (2010) The impact of reconstruction method on the quantification of DaTSCAN images. Eur J Nucl Med Mol Imaging 37: 23–35.

25. Koch W, Hamann C, Welsch J, Popperl G, Radau PE, et al. (2005) Is iterative reconstruction an alternative to filtered backprojection in routine processing of dopamine transporter SPECT studies? Journal of Nuclear Medicine 46: 1804–1811.

26. Winz OH, Hellwig S, Mix M, Weber WA, Mottaghy FM, et al. (2012) Image quality and data quantification in dopamine transporter SPECT: advantage of 3-dimensional OSEM reconstruction? Clin Nucl Med 37: 866–871.

27. Ichihara T, Ogawa K, Motomura N, Kubo A, Hashimoto S (1993) Compton Scatter Compensation Using the Triple-Energy Window Method for Single-Isotope and Dual-Isotope Spect. Journal of Nuclear Medicine 34: 2216–2221.

28. Frackowiak RSJ, Friston KJ, Frith CD, Dolan RJ, Price CJ, et al, editors (2004) Human Brain Function. San Diego: Academic Press.

29. Buchert R, Berding G, Wilke F, Martin B, von Borczyskowski D, et al. (2006) IBZM tool: a fully automated expert system for the evaluation of IBZM SPECT studies. Eur J Nucl Med Mol Imaging 33: 1073–1083.

30. Innis RB, Cunningham VJ, Delforge J, Fujita M, Gjedde A, et al. (2007) Consensus nomenclature for in vivo imaging of reversibly binding radioligands. J Cereb Blood Flow Metab 27: 1533–1539.

31. Benamer HTS, Patterson J, Grosset DG, Booij J, de Bruin K, et al. (2000) Accurate differentiation of parkinsonism and essential tremor using visual assessment of [I-123]-FP-CIT SPECT imaging: The [I-123]-FP-CIT study group. Movement Disorders 15: 503–510.

32. Bland JM, Altman DG (1986) Statistical Methods for Assessing Agreement between Two Methods of Clinical Measurement. Lancet 1: 307–310.

33. Cohen J (1960) A Coefficient of Agreement for Nominal Scales. Educational and Psychological Measurement 20: 37–46.

34. van de Giessen E, Hesse S, Caan MW, Zientek F, Dickson JC, et al. (2013) No association between striatal dopamine transporter binding and body mass index: a multi-center European study in healthy volunteers. Neuroimage 64: 61–67.

35. Warwick JM, Rubow S, du Toit M, Beetge E, Carey P, et al. (2011) The Role of CT-Based Attenuation Correction and Collimator Blurring Correction in Striatal Spect Quantification. Int J Mol Imaging 2011: 195037.

36. Rajeevan N, Zubal IG, Ramsby SQ, Zoghbi SS, Seibyl J, et al. (1998) Significance of nonuniform attenuation correction in quantitative brain SPECT imaging. J Nucl Med 39: 1719–1726.

37. Oh M, Kim JS, Kim JY, Shin KH, Park SH, et al. (2012) Subregional patterns of preferential striatal dopamine transporter loss differ in Parkinson disease, progressive supranuclear palsy, and multiple-system atrophy. J Nucl Med 53: 399–406.

38. Bienkiewicz M, Gorska-Chrzastek M, Siennicki J, Gajos A, Bogucki A, et al. (2008) Impact of CT based attenuation correction on quantitative assessment of DaTSCAN ((123)I-Ioflupane) imaging in diagnosis of extrapyramidal diseases. Nucl Med Rev Cent East Eur 11: 53–58.

39. Sadik M, Suurkula M, Hoglund P, Jarund A, Edenbrandt L (2008) Quality of planar whole-body bone scan interpretations–a nationwide survey. Eur J Nucl Med Mol Imaging 35: 1464–1472.

40. Kahraman D, Eggers C, Holstein A, Schneider C, Pedrosa DJ, et al. (2012) 123I-FP-CIT SPECT imaging of the dopaminergic state. Visual assessment of dopaminergic degeneration patterns reflects quantitative 2D operator-dependent and 3D operator-independent techniques. Nuklearmedizin 51: 244–251.

21

Contourlet Textual Features: Improving the Diagnosis of Solitary Pulmonary Nodules in Two Dimensional CT Images

Jingjing Wang[1,2], Tao Sun[1,2], Ni Gao[1,2], Desmond Dev Menon[3,4], Yanxia Luo[1,2], Qi Gao[1,2], Xia Li[1,5], Wei Wang[1,2,3], Huiping Zhu[1,2], Pingxin Lv[6], Zhigang Liang[7], Lixin Tao[1,2], Xiangtong Liu[1,2], Xiuhua Guo[1,2]*

1 School of Public Health, Capital Medical University, Beijing, China, 2 Beijing Municipal Key Laboratory of Clinical Epidemiology, Beijing, China, 3 School of Medical Sciences, Edith Cowan University, Perth, Australia, 4 School of Exercise and Health Sciences, Edith Cowan University, Perth, Australia, 5 Department of Epidemiology & Public Health, University College Cork, Cork, Ireland, 6 Department of Radiology, Beijing Chest Hospital, Capital Medical University, Beijing, China, 7 Department of Radiology, Xuanwu Hospital, Capital Medical University, Beijing, China

Abstract

Objective: To determine the value of contourlet textural features obtained from solitary pulmonary nodules in two dimensional CT images used in diagnoses of lung cancer.

Materials and Methods: A total of 6,299 CT images were acquired from 336 patients, with 1,454 benign pulmonary nodule images from 84 patients (50 male, 34 female) and 4,845 malignant from 252 patients (150 male, 102 female). Further to this, nineteen patient information categories, which included seven demographic parameters and twelve morphological features, were also collected. A contourlet was used to extract fourteen types of textural features. These were then used to establish three support vector machine models. One comprised a database constructed of nineteen collected patient information categories, another included contourlet textural features and the third one contained both sets of information. Ten-fold cross-validation was used to evaluate the diagnosis results for the three databases, with sensitivity, specificity, accuracy, the area under the curve (AUC), precision, Youden index, and *F*-measure were used as the assessment criteria. In addition, the synthetic minority over-sampling technique (SMOTE) was used to preprocess the unbalanced data.

Results: Using a database containing textural features and patient information, sensitivity, specificity, accuracy, AUC, precision, Youden index, and *F*-measure were: 0.95, 0.71, 0.89, 0.89, 0.92, 0.66, and 0.93 respectively. These results were higher than results derived using the database without textural features (0.82, 0.47, 0.74, 0.67, 0.84, 0.29, and 0.83 respectively) as well as the database comprising only textural features (0.81, 0.64, 0.67, 0.72, 0.88, 0.44, and 0.85 respectively). Using the SMOTE as a pre-processing procedure, new balanced database generated, including observations of 5,816 benign ROIs and 5,815 malignant ROIs, and accuracy was 0.93.

Conclusion: Our results indicate that the combined contourlet textural features of solitary pulmonary nodules in CT images with patient profile information could potentially improve the diagnosis of lung cancer.

Editor: Konradin Metze, University of Campinas, Brazil

Funding: Natural Science Fund of China (serial no.: 81172772) and the Natural Science Fund of Beijing (serial nos.: 4112015 and 7131002). The funders had no role in study design, data collection and analysis, decision to publish, or preparation of the manuscript.

Competing Interests: The authors have declared that no competing interests exist.

* Email: guoxiuh@ccmu.edu.cn

Introduction

Lung cancer is a disease characterized by uncontrolled cell division in the tissues of the lung, and is the most common cause of cancer-related death in men and women worldwide [1]. The presence of lung cancer often appears as a solitary pulmonary nodule (SPN) as well as other lung lesions. An SPN is a single, spherical, well-circumscribed, radiographically opaque object that measures up to 3 cm in diameter and is completely surrounded by aerated lung tissue [2]. The definitive diagnosis of lung cancer is based on histological examination, which is usually performed by bronchoscopy or computed tomography- (CT)-guidance. Individuals who show the presence of these observations often have a low

five-year survival rate (about 15%) [3]. CT technology, a useful computer aided diagnosis tool used in lung cancer detection, is used to screen and forecast patients with solitary pulmonary nodules (SPNs). With the low-dose CT screening, a 20% reduction of mortality was shown in lung cancer cases [4].

Morphological characteristics, such as: nodule size, density, and margins shown in CT slices, coupled with demographic characteristics, such as: gender, age, and smoking history, amongst other characteristics are used to differentiate between benign and malignant SPNs [5]. There are several studies that have evaluated the use of different combinations of these characteristics in prediction models in attempts to increase the accuracy of spotting

Table 1. Description of the data.

Diagnosis		Cases	(%)	ROIs	(%)
Benign		84	100.0	1454	100.0
	Tuberculosis	28	33.3	496	34.1
	Inflammatory pseudotumor	15	17.9	265	18.2
	Hamartoma	20	23.8	367	25.2
	Pulmonary interstitial edema	2	2.4	34	2.3
	Sclerosing hemangioma	12	14.3	189	13.0
	Clear cell tumor	2	2.4	31	2.1
	Chondroma	5	6.0	72	5.0
Malignant		252	100.0	4845	100.0
	Adenocarcinoma	183	72.6	3443	71.1
	Squamous cell carcinoma	45	17.9	887	18.3
	Adenosquamous carcinoma	18	7.1	379	7.8
	Malignant carcinoid tumor	6	2.4	136	2.8

potential malignant nodules. Using some of these features, Gould et al. [6] established a logistic regression based clinical prediction model to estimate the pre-test probability of malignancy in patients with SPNs, with a model accuracy of 0.79 in its area under the curve of receiver operating characteristic. Li et al. [7] also established a mathematical model to predict malignancy of SPNs, with a higher accuracy rate (0.888) compared to the Mayo model and VA group model. Although these studies obtained good results, textural features such as entropy, correlation, energy, homogeneity, etc. which are considered vital components were omitted from their research. Way et al. [8] used a fully automated system to extract image features to differentiate malignant and benign lung nodules on CT scans, in combination with morphological and demographic features. Zhu et al. [9] on the other hand used 25 features selected from 67 features, extracted by a feature extraction procedure to establish SVM-based classifier. Research by Wu et al. [10] used two GLCM based textural features and two radiological features as determined by non-linear regression to build a back propagation artificial neural network diagnosis model. Sun et al. [2] used a dataset including 476 textural features extracted by curvelet, three demographic parameters and nine morphological features to establish a support vector machine (SVM) prediction model.

The choice of methods used to extract textural features, have also established their importance in this process. Dettor et al. [11] and Meselhy et al. [12] found that the curvelet transform yielded better results in image processing than previous methods. Inspired by curvelet, Do and Vetterli [13] developed the contourlet transform, which allows for differences and flexibility in the number of directions permitted at each scale compared to other multiscale directional systems. In this study, a contourlet was used to extract textural features as a trial and SVM, which was more suitable for CT texture analysis than the other six models in previous studies [14], used to predict lung cancer. The aim of this study was to determine the value of contourlet textural features by comparing the diagnostic effect of datasets combining textural features and patient information, with datasets containing only patient information or textural features.

Methods

Ethics Statement

This study was performed with ethics approval (Ethics Committee of Xuanwu Hospital, Capital Medical University, Approval Document NO. [2011] 01). Written consent was given by the patients.

Survey of patient information

The data were obtained from Chaoyang Hospital and Beijing Chest Hospital in Beijing, which is part of a cross-sectional study established in 2009 [14]. Seven demographic parameters (age, gender, smoking habits, tuberculosis history, dust history, genetic disease and tumour history) were obtained from medical histories of patients. In addition, twelve morphological features of the pulmonary nodules (calcification, cavitation, density, ground-glass, lobulation, lymph node status, margin, vacuoles, pleural indentation, pleural fluid, diameter, and substantial changes) reported by experienced radiologists for the patients were also included in this study. The distributions of age and diameter were continuous. In gender, 1 represented female, 0 represented male while for the other variables, 1 represented yes, and 0 represented no. The patient inclusion/exclusions decision was based on the results of the final diagnoses where the final diagnosis of malignant cases was confirmed by an operation or biopsy, while benign cases were determined either pathologically or after a 2-year minimum follow-up by patients. Morphological features in two dimensional CT images were obtained by eight radiologists and conflicts in the final interpretation of the CT images were resolved through consensus discussion. All of the nineteen variables were utilized as patient information data categories.

Feature extraction strategies

A total of 6,299 regions of interest (ROIs) were acquired from 336 patients, with 1,454 benign ROIs from 84 patients (50 male, 34 female) and 4,845 malignant ROIs from 252 patients (150 male, 102 female). These details are listed in Table 1.

CT scans were obtained using a 64-slice helical CT scanner (GE/Light speed ultra System CT99, USA) with a tube voltage of 120 kV and a current of 200 mA [10]. The reconstruction interval

Table 2. The performance of each kind of textural features.

Textural features	Sensitivity	Specificity	Youden	AUC	Accuracy	Precision	F
Correlation	0.69	0.55	0.24	0.63	0.65	0.82	0.75
Cluster tendency	0.81	0.29	0.10	0.53*	0.68	0.77	0.79
Difference-entropy	0.63	0.52	0.15	0.58	0.60	0.80	0.70
Difference-mean	0.67	0.48	0.15	0.57	0.63	0.79	0.73
Energy	0.81	0.38	0.19	0.60	0.70	0.80	0.80
Entropy	0.66	0.55	0.21	0.62	0.63	0.81	0.73
Homogeneity	0.73	0.45	0.18	0.59	0.66	0.80	0.76
IDM	0.66	0.54	0.19	0.60	0.63	0.81	0.73
Inertia	0.67	0.57	0.24	0.63	0.65	0.82	0.74
Mean	0.68	0.43	0.11	0.53*	0.62	0.78	0.73
MP	0.68	0.54	0.21	0.61	0.64	0.81	0.74
SD	0.53	0.62	0.15	0.59	0.55	0.81	0.64
Sum-mean	0.82	0.29	0.10	0.52*	0.68	0.77	0.80
Sum-entropy	0.58	0.62	0.19	0.63	0.59	0.82	0.68

Abbreviation used: AUC, the least area under the curve; IDM, Inverse difference moment; MP, Maximum probability; SD, Standard deviation; F, F_measure;
*P>0.05.

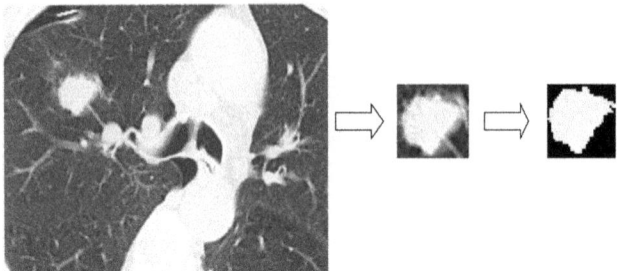

Figure 1. Image segmentation using gray level threshold algorithm.

and reconstruction thickness for routine scanning were 0.625 mm. The kernel was a B31f/B70 type and the data were reconstructed using a 512×512 matrix [15].

All of the pulmonary nodules in CT images were segmented manually to obtain a region of interest (ROI) and the textural features were extracted by contourlet from each ROI. Figure 1 shows an example of image segmentation. The ROI was obtained

from CT image by a rectangular box, which covered the whole ROI at the smallest area. Subsequently Region Grow Algorithm, a popular tool for image segmentation, was used to remove any background pixels, such as muscle and blood vessels. Using a validated contourlet transform method [13], a filter bank structure capable of proficiently working with piecewise smooth images with smooth contours. Fourteen kinds of textural features were extracted. These included entropy, mean, correlation, energy, homogeneity, standard deviation, maximum probability, inverse difference moment, cluster tendency, inertia, sum-mean, difference-mean, sum-entropy, and difference-entropy [16]. The contourlet transform process included two steps: a Laplacian pyramid (LP) and a directional filter bank (DFB). The LP was first used to capture point discontinuities and the DFB subsequently used to link point discontinuities into linear structures [17]. In this study, 48 sub-bands were chosen, resulting in 672 textural features calculated. The differences of textual features between benign and malignant group were subsequently analyzed. The comparative evaluation of each kind of textural features and the results are shown in Table 2. The least areas under the curve (AUC) obtained from cluster tendency, mean, sum-mean were 0.53, 0.53 and 0.52 respectively with P values not smaller than 0.05, while P values of

Table 3. Distribution of seven demographic parameters: benign and malignant cases.

Variables	Benign	Malignant	Statistic	P
Gender				
N (missing)	84 (0)	252 (0)	0.00	1.0000
Female (%)	34 (40.48)	102 (40.48)		
Male (%)	50 (59.52)	150 (59.52)		
Smoking habits				
N (missing)	84 (0)	252 (0)	26.78	<0.0001
Yes (%)	24 (28.57)	154 (61.11)		
No (%)	60 (71.43)	98 (38.89)		
Age				
N (missing)	84 (0)	252 (0)	3.45	0.0006
Mean (std)	54.10 (13.57)	59.90 (12.68)		
Median (Q1, Q3)	57 (46.5,63)	61 (53,69.5)		
Min~Max	21~80	25~83		
Tuberculosis history				
N (missing)	84 (0)	252 (0)	1.13	0.2869
Yes (%)	6 (7.14)	15 (5.95)		
No (%)	78 (92.86)	237 (94.05)		
Tumor hisory				
N (missing)	84 (0)	252 (0)	1.13	0.2869
Yes (%)	3 (3.57)	17 (96.75)		
No (%)	81 (96.43)	235 (93.25)		
Genetic disease				
N (missing)	84 (0)	252 (0)	-	0.5760
Yes (%)	0 (0)	3 (1.19)		
No (%)	84 (0)	249 (98.81)		
Dust history				
N (missing)	84 (0)	252 (0)	0.05	0.8255
Yes (%)	1 (1.19)	6 (2.38)		
No (%)	83 (98.81)	246 (97.62)		

Table 4. Distribution of twelve morphological features: benign and malignant cases.

Variables	Benign	Malignant	Statistic	P
Lymphadenectasis				
N (Missing)	84 (0)	252 (0)	10.32	0.0013
No (%)	73 (86.90)	174 (69.05)		
Yes (%)	11 (13.10)	78 (30.95)		
Uniform density				
N (Missing)	84 (0)	252 (0)	0.04	0.8455
Yes (%)	31 (36.90)	96 (38.10)		
No (%)	53 (63.10)	156 (61.90)		
Substantial changes				
N (Missing)	84 (0)	252 (0)	0.04	0.8345
No (%)	9 (10.71)	25 (9.92)		
Yes (%)	75 (89.29)	227 (90.08)		
Ground-glass				
N (Missing)	84 (0)	252 (0)	0.01	0.9045
No (%)	78 (92.86)	233 (92.46)		
Yes (%)	6 (7.14)	19 (7.54)		
Spiculation				
N (Missing)	84 (0)	252 (0)	0.05	0.8304
No (%)	23 (27.38)	66 (26.19)		
Yes (%)	61 (72.62)	186 (73.81)		
Lobulation				
N (Missing)	84 (0)	252 (0)	0.29	0.5929
No (%)	20 (23.81)	53 (21.03)		
Yes (%)	64 (76.19)	199 (78.97)		
Vacuoles				
N (Missing)	84 (0)	252 (0)	2.38	0.1227
No (%)	66 (78.57)	216 (85.71)		
Yes (%)	18 (21.43)	36 (14.29)		
Calcification				
N (Missing)	84 (0)	252 (0)	0.52	0.4704
No (%)	77 (91.67)	224 (88.89)		
Yes (%)	7 (8.33)	28 (11.11)		
Cavitation				
N (Missing)	84 (0)	252 (0)	1.71	0.1909
No (%)	78 (92.86)	221 (87.70)		
Yes (%)	6 (7.14)	31 (12.30)		
Pleural indentation				
N (Missing)	84 (0)	252 (0)	0.45	0.5021
No (%)	54 (64.29)	172 (68.25)		
Yes (%)	30 (35.71)	80 (31.75)		
Pleural fluid				
N (Missing)	84 (0)	252 (0)	0.01	0.9157
No (%)	76 (90.48)	227 (90.08)		
Yes (%)	8 (9.52)	25 (9.92)		
Diameter				
N (Missing)	84 (0)	252 (0)	4.50	<0.0001
Mean (Std)	1.80 (0.68)	2.22 (0.73)		
Median (Q1~Q3)	1.8 (1.2~2.3)	2.3 (1.7~2.7)		

Table 5. The performance of classifier in different nodule size.

Groups	Sensitivity	Specificity	Youden	Accuracy	AUC	Precision	F_measure
A	0.77	0.62	0.38	0.69	0.70*	0.67	0.71
B	0.92	0.65	0.57	0.83	0.73	0.84	0.88
C	0.93	0.43	0.36	0.86	0.65	0.90	0.92
A+B	0.92	0.66	0.58	0.83	0.74	0.83	0.87

Abbreviation used: AUC, the least area under the curve; A, nodules within the 7 to 10 millimeters; B, nodules within the 11 to 20 millimeters; C, nodules within the 21 to 30 millimeters;
*P>0.05.

other textural features were smaller than 0.05. All the textual features between benign and malignant group were analyzed to determine their differences. Table S1 displays the ones with P value smaller than 7.4e-5.

Data analysis

In our study, a support vector machine (SVM), which is a popular machine learning technique, established by recent studies in this field, was used in pattern recognition and classification in various research fields [18–20]. Developed for binary (two-class) classification problems, it can efficiently perform a non-linear classification using what is called a kernel function, implicitly mapping inputs into high-dimensional feature spaces. In this study, the Gaussian radial basis function kernel (Eq. 1) was chosen as the kernel function and 10-fold cross validation was used to access the datasets with and without, contourlet-based textural features.

$$k(x,y) = \exp\left(-\frac{\|x-y\|^2}{2\sigma^2}\right) \quad (1)$$

The original training data included images of 1,454 benign ROIs and 4,845 malignant ROIs, with a ratio of malignant to benign cases of 3, which were not balanced. The synthetic minority over-sampling technique (SMOTE) was used to preprocess the data, which was one of over-sampling method [21]. The purpose of applying this method is to generate a balanced dataset by generating new examples of minority class using the nearest k (which is set to 5 in SMOTE) neighbors of these cases while under-sampling majority class examples.

Assessment criteria

Five indicators were calculated to evaluate the results using three datasets, including sensitivity, specificity, accuracy, Yonden index and precision. Additionally, the area under the curve (AUC) was calculated to establish the received operation characteristic (ROC), and malignant rate (Eq. 2) was used as variable to draw an ROC curve.

Malignant rate

$$= \frac{Number\ of\ malignant\ images\ of\ one\ case\ by\ model}{Total\ number\ of\ images\ of\ one\ case} \quad (2)$$

The F-measure (F), typically used in machine learning, was also calculated to measure the quality of the binary classifications as expressed by

$$F = \frac{(\beta^2+1) * \frac{T_p}{T_p+F_p} * \frac{T_p}{T_p+F_n}}{\beta^2 * \frac{T_p}{T_p+F_p} + \frac{T_p}{T_p+F_n}} \quad (3)$$

where T_p refers to the number of malignant nodules correctly classified as malignant and F_n indicates the number of malignant nodules wrongly classified as benign; T_n represents the number of benign nodules correctly classified as benign and F_p indicates the number of benign nodules wrongly classified as malignant. The F-measure is a measure of the accuracy of a test and when β is selected as 1, it can be interpreted as a weighted average of sensitivity and precision, with its best value occurring at 1 and worst at 0.

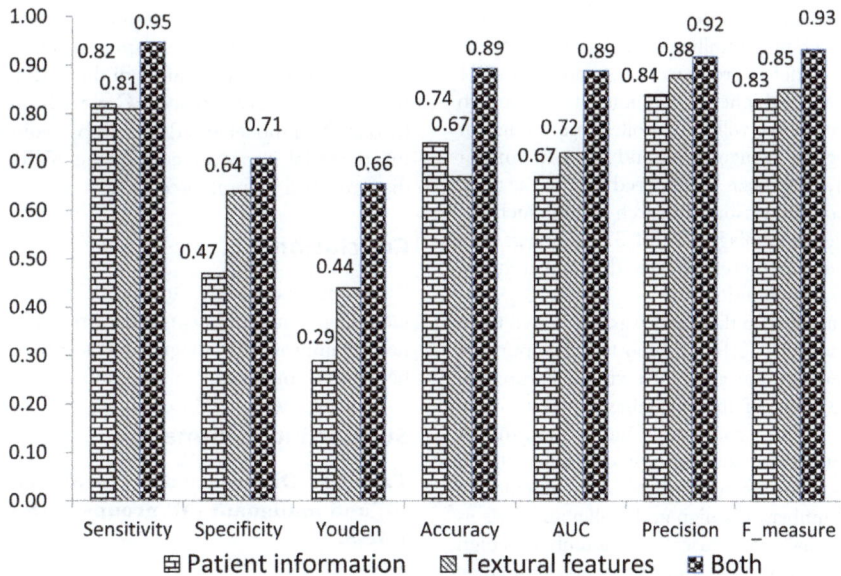

Figure 2. Results of three datasets run through the support vector machine.

Results

The distribution of demographic parameters between benign and malignant cases is shown in Table 3, with the distribution of twelve morphological features displayed in Table 4. Table 5 shows comparative evaluations of textural features in different nodule sizes, which are 7 to 10 millimeters (group A, 26 cases), 11 to 20 millimeters (group B, 129 cases) and 21 to 30 millimeters (group C, 181 cases). As AUC obtained from group A was 0.70 with a P value of 0.073 which was not smaller than 0.05, we combined group A and group B, with its results also shown in Table 5. Three datasets, one comprising the seven demographic parameters and twelve morphological features, the second with only contourlet-based textural features, and the third one containing both, were used as input data to establish three separate SVM prediction models, respectively. Through ten-fold cross validation, seven indicators, including sensitivity, specificity, accuracy, AUC, precision, Youden index, and F-measure, were calculated to compare the three datasets, which were shown in Figure 2. Using the SMOTE as a pre-processing procedure, new data including the contourlet-based textural features, seven demographic parameters and twelve morphological features were generated, resulting in final data containing observations of 5,816 benign ROIs and 5,815 malignant ROIs. Accuracy based on ten-fold cross validation for balanced data were 93.3%.

Discussion

Lung cancer, the most common cancer-related death worldwide, accounted for 28% and 26% of all cancer deaths among men and women, respectively in the United States [22,23] and has also been ranked first amongst causes of mortality involving malignant neoplasms in China [24]. This study is aimed at using textural features extracted by contourlet, incorporated with patient information, with the intention of establishing an SVM model, that will better assist in discerning between malignant and benign pulmonary nodules in the diagnosis of lung cancer as opposed to utilizing demographic and morphological indicators or nodule textural features alone. When combined with textural features, the accuracy rate improved from 0.74 to 0.89, with sensitivity and

specificity showing a 0.13% and 0.24% improvement respectively. A meta-analysis [25] showed a pooled sensitivity of 0.57 (95% confidence interval, 0.49 to 0.66) for CT scanning in lung cancer. The sensitivity in this study was also improved after combining with the textural features (from 0.82 to 0.95), along with other assessment criteria, including F-measure which is used in machine learning. In addition to comparing results between datasets constructed from only textual features and one containing both, the study also reinforced the need for greater patient information to improve the diagnosis of lung cancer.

The top 4 textural features that attained better Youden index, were inertia, correlation, maximum probability and entropy, while the top 4 acquainted with sensitivity were sum-mean, cluster tendency, energy and homogeneity, and the top 4 for specificity were sum-entropy, standard deviation, inertia and correlation. In our study, we were unable to identify one particular textural feature acquainted with both better sensitivity as well as better specificity that could be utilized in combination to produce an overall relatively higher sensitivity and specificity.

A contourlet transform is a multi-directional, multi-scale transform used in medical imaging [26,27]. It uses elongated basis functions with different aspects to capture smooth contours in images. For images in DICOM format, the contourlet data provided the algorithm with more efficiency and robustness against the effect of noise compared to other transforms [28], and as such this was our justification for using it to extract the textural features required for this study. To determine which size of nodules were more suitable for the 48 subbands of textural features extracted by contourlet, comparative evaluations of textural features in different nodule sizes were added. These included nodules within the 7 to 10 millimeters group, those within the 11 to 20 millimeters group and nodules that fell within the 21 to 30 millimeters groups. Nodules within the 11 to 20 millimeters group achieved relatively better results as indicated by their AUC values while AUC obtained from 7 to 10 millimeters group was 0.70 with P value of 0.073 which was not smaller than 0.05, we combined to 7 to 20 millimeters group, with performance of classifier did not change so much with 11 to 20 millimeters group. One reason may be that the 48 subbands of textural features extracted by contourlet were more suitable for pulmonary nodules smaller than 20 millimeters, especially 11 to 20 millimeters. Another may be that the cases in 7 to 10 millimeters group were not enough and 21 to 30 millimeters group had the highest malignant rate (28 benign cases vs 153 malignant cases). We will try to collect more data for further exploration, especially benign cases and cases in smaller size. In addition, SVM, has been considered to be a good algorithm for classification in various research fields, such as: clinical form analysis [29], cancer diagnosis [30–32], subtle gesture recognition [33], *etc.* and was therefore utilised to differentiate between lung cancer and benign lesions.

In this study, the accuracy rate in this study was not shown to be better than some previous studies [2,10,14] reported. The purpose of this study was to determine the value of textural features by comparing the predictive effect of three databases, whose input data were raw data without pre-processing. One of the limiting factors was that data required for such a study can only rely on cases obtained from hospitals. As such, there is a difficulty in obtaining a comparable number of benign and malignant cases as there is a propensity for malignant cases to outnumber benign ones. The malignant cases from our study were approximately three times as frequent as benign ones. This could have contributed to the poor specificity obtained. In this study, the SMOTE, an over-sampling method, was used as the pre-processing procedure to balance the data. The original training data was balanced with a ratio of malignant to benign cases of 1:1 and the classification performance (accuracy) of the prediction model improved from 0.89 to 0.93. Thus, the SMOTE is a useful method to account for unbalanced data and can improve the capability of the models. The reasons why it performed better may be that SMOTE can improve the accuracy of classifiers for a minority class as it is an over-sampling approach in which the minority class is over-sampled by creating "synthetic" examples rather than by over-sampling with replacement [34]. However, it should be noted that in introducing synthesized examples, there is also a possibility that the application of SMOTE might have introduced an overestimation of the performance metrics [35] and further studies are required. Comparisons between the diagnosis by our SVM model and diagnosis by radiologists are on-going and the potential improvements of the SVM model to lung cancer diagnosis will be presented later.

Conclusion

Combined contourlet textural features with patient information including demographic parameters and morphological features helped improve the diagnostics accuracy of discerning between benign and malignant solitary pulmonary nodules.

Supporting Information

Table S1 Difference of textural features between benign (B) and malignant (M) groups with P value smaller than 7.4e-5.

Acknowledgments

The authors thank the doctors from the Department of Radiology, Chaoyang Hospital and Beijing Chest Hospital, for their assistance with data acquisition.

Author Contributions

Conceived and designed the experiments: XG. Performed the experiments: JW XG. Analyzed the data: TS JW XG DM. Contributed reagents/materials/analysis tools: JW TS NG DM YL QG X. Li WW HZ PL ZL LT X. Liu XG. Wrote the paper: JW TS NG DM YL QG X. Li WW HZ PL ZL LT X. Liu XG.

References

1. Qu X, Huang X, Yan W, Wu L, Dai K (2012) A meta-analysis of (1)(8)FDG-PET-CT, (1)(8)FDG-PET, MRI and bone scintigraphy for diagnosis of bone metastases in patients with lung cancer. Eur J Radiol 81: 1007–1015.

2. Sun T, Zhang R, Wang J, Li X, Guo X (2013) Computer-aided diagnosis for early-stage lung cancer based on longitudinal and balanced data. PLoS One 8: e63559.

3. Collins LG, Haines C, Perkel R, Enck RE (2007) Lung cancer: diagnosis and management. Am Fam Physician 75: 56–63.

4. Aberle DR, Adams AM, Berg CD, Black WC, Clapp JD, et al. (2011) Reduced lung-cancer mortality with low-dose computed tomographic screening. N Engl J Med 365: 395–409.

5. Paslawski M, Krzyzanowski K, Zlomaniec J, Gwizdak J (2004) Morphological characteristics of malignant solitary pulmonary nodules. Ann Univ Mariae Curie Sklodowska Med 59: 6–13.

6. Gould MK, Ananth L, Barnett PG (2007) A clinical model to estimate the pretest probability of lung cancer in patients with solitary pulmonary nodules. Chest 131: 383–388.

7. Li Y, Chen KZ, Wang J (2011) Development and validation of a clinical prediction model to estimate the probability of malignancy in solitary pulmonary nodules in Chinese people. Clin Lung Cancer 12: 313–319.

8. Way TW, Sahiner B, Chan HP, Hadjiiski L, Cascade PN, et al. (2009) Computer-aided diagnosis of pulmonary nodules on CT scans: improvement of classification performance with nodule surface features. Med Phys 36: 3086–3098.

9. Zhu Y, Tan Y, Hua Y, Wang M, Zhang G, et al. (2010) Feature selection and performance evaluation of support vector machine (SVM)-based classifier for differentiating benign and malignant pulmonary nodules by computed tomography. J Digit Imaging 23: 51–65.

10. Wu H, Sun T, Wang J, Li X, Wang W, et al. (2013) Combination of radiological and gray level co-occurrence matrix textural features used to distinguish solitary pulmonary nodules by computed tomography. J Digit Imaging 26: 797–802.

11. Dettori L, Semler L (2007) A comparison of wavelet, ridgelet, and curvelet-based texture classification algorithms in computed tomography. Comput Biol Med 37: 486–498.

12. Meselhy Eltoukhy M, Faye I, Belhaouari Samir B (2010) A comparison of wavelet and curvelet for breast cancer diagnosis in digital mammogram. Comput Biol Med 40: 384–391.

13. Do MN, Vetterli M (2005) The contourlet transform: an efficient directional multiresolution image representation. IEEE Trans Image Process 14: 2091–2106.

14. Sun T, Wang J, Li X, Lv P, Liu F, et al. (2013) Comparative evaluation of support vector machines for computer aided diagnosis of lung cancer in CT based on a multi-dimensional data set. Comput Methods Programs Biomed 111: 519–524.

15. Wang JJ, Wu HF, Sun T, Li X, Wang W, et al. (2013) Prediction models for solitary pulmonary nodules based on curvelet textural features and clinical parameters. Asian Pac J Cancer Prev 14: 6019–6023.

16. Wang H, Guo XH, Jia ZW, Li HK, Liang ZG, et al. (2010) Multilevel binomial logistic prediction model for malignant pulmonary nodules based on texture features of CT image. Eur J Radiol 74: 124–129.

17. Lazrag H, Naceur MS (2012) Combination of the Level-Set Methods with the Contourlet Transform for the Segmentation of the IVUS Images. Int J Biomed Imaging 2012: 439597.

18. Abrishami V, Zaldivar-Peraza A, de la Rosa-Trevin JM, Vargas J, Oton J, et al. (2013) A pattern matching approach to the automatic selection of particles from low-contrast electron micrographs. Bioinformatics.

19. Yang HX, Feng W, Wei JC, Zeng TS, Li ZD, et al. (2013) Support vector machine-based nomogram predicts postoperative distant metastasis for patients with oesophageal squamous cell carcinoma. Br J Cancer.

20. Fang YH, Chiu YF (2013) A novel support vector machine-based approach for rare variant detection. PLoS One 8: e71114.

21. Blagus R, Lusa L (2013) SMOTE for high-dimensional class-imbalanced data. BMC Bioinformatics 14: 106.

22. Siegel R, Naishadham D, Jemal A (2013) Cancer statistics, 2013. CA Cancer J Clin 63: 11–30.

23. Kovalchik SA, Tammemagi M, Berg CD, Caporaso NE, Riley TL, et al. (2013) Targeting of low-dose CT screening according to the risk of lung-cancer death. N Engl J Med 369: 245–254.

24. He J, Gu D, Wu X, Reynolds K, Duan X, et al. (2005) Major causes of death among men and women in China. N Engl J Med 353: 1124–1134.

25. Toloza EM, Harpole L, McCrory DC (2003) Noninvasive staging of non-small cell lung cancer: a review of the current evidence. Chest 123: 137S–146S.

26. Swaminathan A, Ramapackiam SS, Thiraviam T, Selvaraj J (2013) Contourlet transform-based sharpening enhancement of retinal images and vessel extraction application. Biomed Tech (Berl) 58: 87–96.

27. Al-Azzawi N, Sakim HA, Abdullah AK, Ibrahim H (2009) Medical image fusion scheme using complex contourlet transform based on PCA. Conf Proc IEEE Eng Med Biol Soc 2009: 5813–5816.

28. Rahimi F, Rabbani H (2011) A dual adaptive watermarking scheme in contourlet domain for DICOM images. Biomed Eng Online 10: 53.

29. Strauss J, Peguero AM, Hirst G (2013) Machine learning methods for clinical forms analysis in mental health. Stud Health Technol Inform 192: 1024.

30. Filipczuk P, Fevens T, Krzyzak A, Monczak R (2013) Computer-Aided Breast Cancer Diagnosis Based on the Analysis of Cytological Images of Fine Needle Biopsies. IEEE Trans Med Imaging.

31. Wang H, Huang G (2011) Application of support vector machine in cancer diagnosis. Med Oncol 28 Suppl 1: S613–618.

32. Gopinath B, Shanthi N (2013) Support Vector Machine based diagnostic system for thyroid cancer using statistical texture features. Asian Pac J Cancer Prev 14: 97–102.

33. Naik GR, Kumar DK, Jayadeva (2010) Hybrid independent component analysis and twin support vector machine learning scheme for subtle gesture recognition. Biomed Tech (Berl) 55: 301–307.

34. Chawla N, Bowyer K, Hall L, Kegelmeyer W (2002) SMOTE: synthetic minority over-sampling technique. J Artif Intell Res 6: 321–357.

35. Exarchos K, Carpeggiani C, Rigas G, Exarchos T, Vozzi F, et al. (2014) A Multiscale Approach for Modeling Atherosclerosis Progression. IEEE J Biomed Health Inform.

22

3′-Deoxy-3′-[^{18}F]-Fluorothymidine PET Imaging Reflects PI3K-mTOR-Mediated Pro-Survival Response to Targeted Therapy in Colorectal Cancer

Eliot T. McKinley[1,2,3]**, Ping Zhao**[1]**, Robert J. Coffey**[3,4]**, M. Kay Washington**[3,4,5]**, H. Charles Manning**[1,2,4,6,7,8]*

1 The Vanderbilt University Institute of Imaging Science (VUIIS), Vanderbilt University Medical School, Nashville, TN, United States of America, **2** Department of Biomedical Engineering, Vanderbilt University Medical School, Nashville, TN, United States of America, **3** Department of Medicine, Vanderbilt University Medical School, Nashville, TN, United States of America, **4** Department of Vanderbilt Ingram Cancer Center, Vanderbilt University Medical School, Nashville, TN, United States of America, **5** Department of Pathology, Vanderbilt University Medical School, Nashville, TN, United States of America, **6** Department of Radiology and Radiological Sciences, Vanderbilt University Medical School, Nashville, TN, United States of America, **7** Department of Neurosurgery, Vanderbilt University Medical School, Nashville, TN, United States of America, **8** Department of Chemical and Physical Biology, Vanderbilt University Medical School, Nashville, TN, United States of America

Abstract

Biomarkers that predict response to targeted therapy in oncology are an essential component of personalized medicine. In preclinical treatment response studies that featured models of wild-type *KRAS* or mutant *BRAF* colorectal cancer treated with either cetuximab or vemurafenib, respectively, we illustrate that [^{18}F]-FLT PET, a non-invasive molecular imaging readout of thymidine salvage, closely reflects pro-survival responses to targeted therapy that are mediated by PI3K-mTOR activity. Activation of pro-survival mechanisms forms the basis of numerous modes of resistance. Therefore, we conclude that [^{18}F]-FLT PET may serve a novel and potentially critical role to predict tumors that exhibit molecular features that tend to reflect recalcitrance to MAPK-targeted therapy. Though these studies focused on colorectal cancer, we envision that the results may be applicable to other solid tumors as well.

Editor: Chunming Liu, University of Kentucky, United States of America

Funding: Research funding: R25 CA136440, K25 CA127349, P50 CA128323, P50 CA095103, R25 CA092043, R01 CA140628, RC1 CA145138, R01 CA046413, P30 DK058404, The Kleberg Foundation. The funders had no role in study design, data collection and analysis, decision to publish, or preparation of the manuscript.

Competing Interests: The authors have declared that no competing interests exist.

* Email: henry.c.manning@vanderbilt.edu

Introduction

With increased ability to rapidly and inexpensively characterize the genetic basis of an individual patient's tumor, personalized therapies are rapidly becoming widespread in oncology. Landmark examples of the success of personalized medicine in oncology include the use of vemurafenib to treat $^{V600E}BRAF$ melanoma [1] and trastuzumab to treat *HER2* overexpressing breast cancers [2]. With an increasing reliance on molecularly targeted therapies, there remains an equally critical challenge to develop and validate specific biomarkers that reflect target inhibition, pathway inactivation, and predict overall clinical response. Most biomarkers utilized in oncology studies require tissue sampling which is highly susceptible to sampling error and bias due to heterogeneity. Serum-based biomarkers lack the ability to directly visualize the tumor and demonstrate that the measured effect is directly the result of tumor response. Non-invasive imaging circumvents these limitations and offers major advantages over traditional biomarkers. Of the imaging modalities available clinically, the sensitivity and the ability to readily produce biologically active molecules bearing positron-emitting isotopes makes positron emission tomography (PET) one of the most attractive modalities for detecting tumors and profiling biological responses to therapy.

Our laboratory has studied the biological basis of 3′-deoxy-3′[18F]-fluorothymidine ([^{18}F]-FLT) accumulation in tumors [3–6] and other diseased tissue [7]. A thymidine analog, [^{18}F]-FLT

was originally developed to serve as a non-invasive measure of cellular proliferation, with obvious utility in oncology [8,9] by reporting on the thymidine salvage pathway that provides DNA precursors to dividing cells. Upon cellular internalization, [^{18}F]-FLT is phosphorylated in a reaction catalyzed by the cytosolic enzyme thymidine kinase 1 (TK1) and trapped in the cell. TK1 activity is closely correlated with DNA synthesis and tends to be diminished in quiescent cells. [^{18}F]-FLT has been widely studied as a marker of treatment response in a spectrum of tumor types and treatments both in the pre-clinical and clinical settings [10]. However, it is important to note that unlike more generalizable proliferation markers, such as Ki67, [^{18}F]-FLT PET reflects proliferative indices to variable and potentially unreliable extents [6,11]. [^{18}F]-FLT-PET cannot discriminate moderately proliferative, thymidine salvage-driven tumors from those of highly proliferative tumors that rely primarily upon *de novo* thymidine synthesis. Despite a lack of correlation with proliferation in some circumstances, we envisioned that TK1 levels, and thus [^{18}F]-FLT PET, could reflect other potentially important molecular events associated with response to therapy.

Using preclinical models of colorectal cancer we demonstrate two circumstances where [^{18}F]-FLT PET does not correlate with proliferation, but rather reflects PI3K-mTor mediated pro-survival responses to targeted therapy. In these settings, [^{18}F]-FLT PET was discordant 2-deoxy-2-[^{18}F]fluoro-D-glucose ([^{18}F]-FDG) PET, the most widely utilized tracer in clinical oncology, which was not sensitive to mTOR- or PI3K-pathway activity. Cetuximab mediated inhibition of MAPK activity in a wild-type *KRAS* cell line model and vemurafenib-mediated inhibition of BRAF in a *V600E BRAF* mutant cell line model had no effect on [18F]-FLT PET unless PI3K-mTOR was subsequently attenuated pharmacologically or *via* genetic silencing. Overall, these studies demonstrate a novel role for [18F]-FLT PET as a means to predict tumors that resist MAPK inhibition through PI3K-mTOR activation in colorectal cancer and potentially other solid tumors.

Materials and Methods

Cell lines and mouse models

All studies were approved by the Vanderbilt University Institutional Animal Care and Use Committee and all efforts were made to minimize animal suffering. DiFi human cells were a gift from Dr. Bruce Boman [12] and COLO 205 cells were obtained from ATCC (CCL-222). DiFi human colorectal cancer cells were grown in Dulbecco's modified Eagle's medium (DMEM) and COLO 205 cells were grown in RPMI (Cellgro) with 10% fetal bovine serum, (Atlanta biologicals), 1% penicillin and streptomycin (GIBCO) at 37°C and 5% CO_2. C225 was obtained from the Vanderbilt Pharmacy, PLX4032 and PLX4720 were synthesized as described [13], PP242 was obtained from Sigma Aldrich, and BEZ235 from Selleck Chem. Stock solutions of each drug were prepared and aliquoted to achieve final drug concentrations for *in vitro* studies.

For *in vivo* studies, cell line xenografts were generated in athymic nude mice (Harlan) as described [3] and treatment began when volume reached approximately 150 mm³. For treatment of DiFi xenografts, saline vehicle, 20 mg/kg, or 40 mg/kg cetuximab were administered i.p. every third day. PET imaging of DiFi xenograft bearing mice was conducted 7 days after the initiation of treatment, 24 hours following the third treatment. For COLO 205 xenografts, mice were treated with DMSO vehicle, 60 mg/kg PLX4720, or 40 mg/kg BEZ235 daily by oral gavage (100 μL total volume). PET imaging of COLO 205 xenograft bearing mice was conducted 4 days after the initiation of treatment, approximately 24 hours following the third treatment. Mice were sacrificed immediately following completion of PET imaging.

siRNA methods

Raptor (L-004107-00) and random sequence (D-001810-01) siRNA reagents were obtained from Thermo Scientific. siRNA was transfected into DiFi cells using the DharmaFect transfection kit (Thermo Scientific) as per manufacturer's instructions. In short, 500,000 DiFi cells were plated into each well of a 6-well plate. After 24 hours, siRNA was added to the appropriate wells. After 48 hours, saline vehicle, 0.5 μg/mL or 5.0 μg/mL C225 were added to the appropriate wells. After a further 24 hours, cells were harvested for Western blotting and qRT-PCR as described below.

Radiopharmaceutical synthesis

[18F]-FLT was prepared in a two-step, one-pot reaction as described [4,14]. [18F]-FLT was obtained with average radiochemical purity of 98.3% and specific activity ≥345.5 TBq/mmol. [18F]-FDG was synthesized in the Vanderbilt University Medical Center Radiopharmacy and distributed by PETNET. The average radiochemical purity of the product was 98.5% and specific activity was more than 37 TBq/mmol.

Small-animal imaging

Small-animal PET imaging was performed using a dedicated microPET scanner (Concorde Microsystems Focus 220). Mice were maintained under 2% isofluorane anesthesia in oxygen at 2 L/min and kept warm via a circulating water heating pad for the duration of the PET scan. For [18F]-FLT PET imaging animals were administered 7.4–9.3 MBq (200–250 μCi) intravenously. Animals were allowed free access to food and water during a 40 minute uptake period, followed by anesthetization and a 20 minute image acquisition. For [18F]-FDG PET imaging, mice were fasted for approximately 6 h prior to imaging and warmed in a heated (31°C) chamber for 1 h prior to [18F]-FDG injection and during the uptake period to minimize brown fat uptake of [18F]-FDG. Mice were administered 7.4–9.3 MBq of [18F]-FDG intravenously and allowed free access to water during a 50 minute uptake period followed by a 10 min PET acquisition.

PET data were reconstructed using OSEM3D/MAP. The resulting three-dimensional reconstructions had an x-y voxel size of 0.474 mm and inter-slice distance of 0.796 mm. ASIPro software (Siemens) was used to manually draw three-dimensional regions of interest in the tumor volume. Tumor samples were immediately collected following [18F]-FLT-PET and flash frozen in liquid nitrogen. [18F]-FLT uptake was quantified as the percentage of the injected dose per gram of tissue (%ID/g) by dividing the ROI activity by the injected dose and multiplying by 100.

Immunoblotting

For *in vitro* studies, cells were lysed with CelLytic M (Sigma Aldrich), centrifuged at 16,000 rpm for 15 minutes at 4°C, and the supernatant removed prior to measurement of protein concentration by bicinchoninic acid (BCA) assay (Thermo Scientific). For *in vivo* studies, fresh frozen tissue was homogenized in CelLytic MT (Sigma Aldrich) lysis buffer, centrifuged at 16,000 rpm for 15 minutes at 4°C, and the supernatant removed prior to measurement of protein concentration by BCA assay. Prior to resolution by electrophoresis, 20–40 μg of protein from each sample was loaded into 7.5–12% SDS PAGE gels and transferred to PVDF membranes (PerkinElmer). Membranes were blocked overnight at 4°C in tris-buffered saline 0.1% Tween-20 (TBST) containing 5% w/v nonfat dry milk powder. Subsequently, membranes were interrogated with antibodies obtained from Cell Signaling Technology unless noted to p-ERK 1/2 Thr202/Tyr204 (#4370), ERK 1/2 (#4372), TK1 (Abcam, #57757), p27 (#3686), p-AKT Ser473 (#4060), p-AKT Thr308 (#4056), AKT (#4685), p-rpS6 Ser236/236 (#4858), rpS6 (#2217), p-4EBP1 Thr37/46 (#2855), p-MEK Ser217/221 (#9154), MEK (#9126), DUSP6 (#3058), β-actin (#4970), β-tubulin (Novus Biologicals, #NB600-936). Membranes were probed for 1 hour at room temperature in TBST with 3% bovine serum albumin (BSA). Membranes were subsequently incubated for 1 hour at room temperature with horseradish peroxidase-conjugated secondary antibody (Jackson ImmunoResearch) diluted 1:5000 in TBST containing 3% BSA. Western Lightning Plus-ECL (PerkinElmer) was used for chemiluminescent detection on a Xenogen IVIS 200.

Immunohistochemistry (IHC)

Animals were sacrificed and tumor samples were collected immediately following PET imaging, then subsequently fixed in 10% formalin for 24 hours. Tissues were then transferred to 70% ethanol prior to paraffin embedding. Tissues were sectioned (5 μm thickness) and stained for p-rpS6 (Cell Signaling, #4858, 1:100 primary dilution), p-AKT Ser473 (Cell Signaling, #4060, 1:100 primary dilution), Ki67 (Dako, #M7240, 1:100 primary dilution), p27 (Dako, #M7203, 1:100 primary dilution). Briefly, the tissue

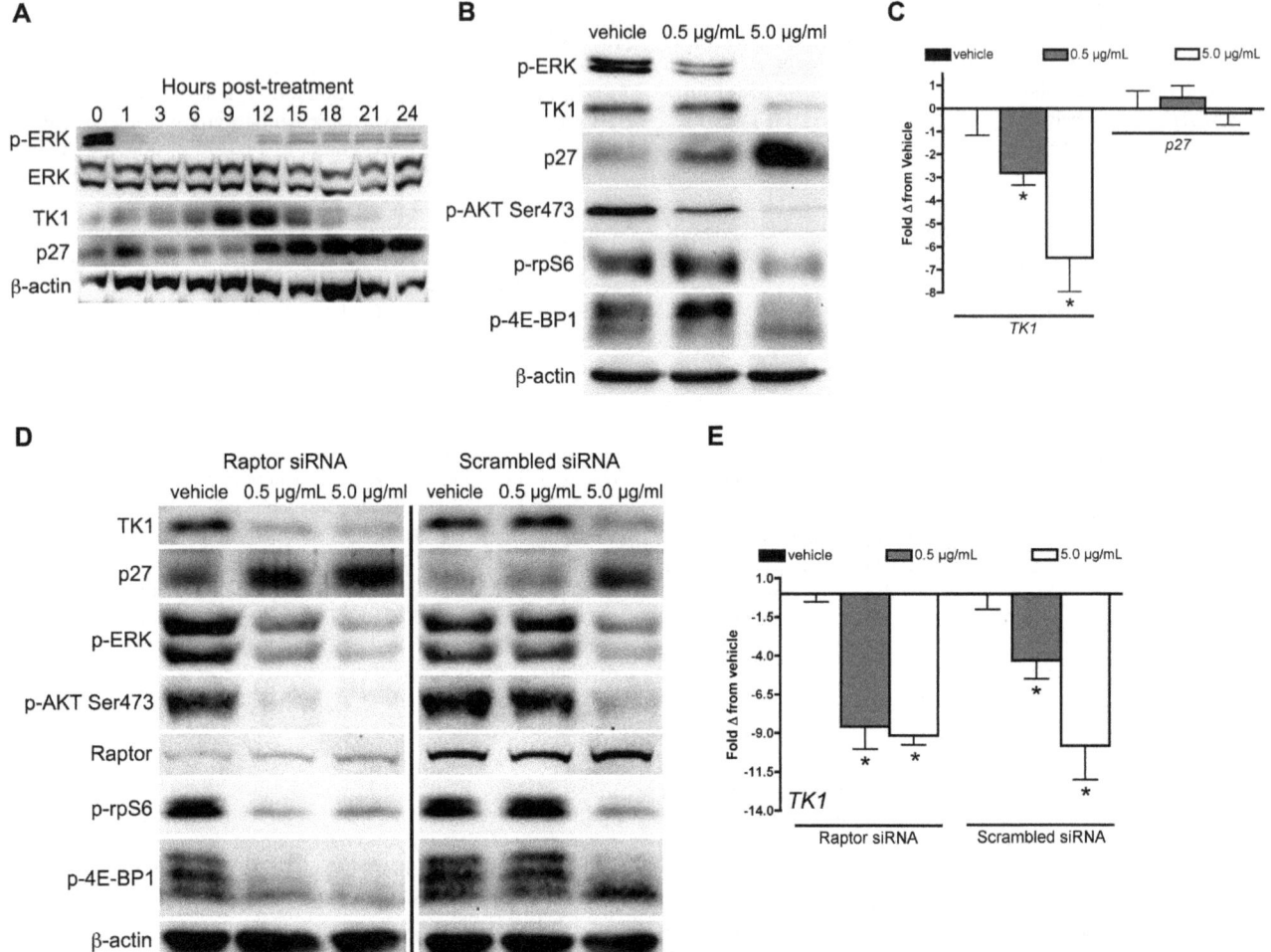

Figure 1. Diminished TK1 protein levels correlate with attenuation of mTOR-PI3K pathway activity and upregulation of p27. (A) Western blot of DiFi cell lysates following cetuximab exposure (5 μg/mL) resulted in rapid attenuation of downstream MAPK targets including p-ERK, which remained well-below baseline levels to 24 hours. Paradoxically, TK1 protein levels increased from 1–12 hours until p27 protein levels rose, at which time TK1 fell bellow baseline. **(B)** DiFi cells treated with either 0.5 μg/mL or 5.0 μg/mL cetuximab resulted in a 50% reduction and full attenuation of p-ERK protein levels, respectively at 24 hours. At 0.5 μg/mL TK1 levels were unaffected despite a modest rise in p27 protein levels. However, 5.0 μg/mL cetuximab resulted in greatly decreased TK1 with a large increase in p27 protein levels. PI3K-mTOR activity, as measured by p-AKT Ser473, p-rpS6, and p-4E-BP1, was either maintained or elevated at 0.5 μg/mL cetuximab but was attenuated at 5.0 μg/mL cetuximab. **(C)** qRT-PCR analysis showed *TK1* mRNA was significantly reduced at 0.5 μg/mL (p = 0.0279) and 5.0 μg/mL (p = 0.0186), while no change in *p27* mRNA levels was observed at either dose. **(D)** Silencing mTORC1 facilitated upregulation of p27 and attenuated TK1 protein levels at 0.5 μg/mL cetuximab without affecting the anti-MAPK activity effects of cetuximab. Levels of p-AKT Ser473, p-rpS6, and p-4E-BP1 were reduced at 0.5 μg/mL cetuximab exposure with Raptor knockdown but not in scrambled siRNA control. **(E)** As evidence of the functionality of p27, *TK1* mRNA levels were similarly reduced at 0.5 μg/mL and 5.0 μg/mL with Raptor knockdown.

samples were de-paraffinized, rehydrated, and antigen retrieval was performed using citrate buffer (ph 6.0) solution for 15 minutes at 105°C followed by a 10 minute bench cool down. The samples were then treated with 3% hydrogen peroxide to eliminate endogenous peroxidase activity. The sections were subsequently blocked with a serum-free protein blocking reagent for 20 minutes. Primary antibody detection was accomplished using the following system: The tissue sections were incubated at room temperature for 60 minutes at the noted dilutions followed by a 30 minute incubation utilizing the Envision + System-HRP Labeled Polymer detection method (Dako, Carpinteria, CA). Staining was completed after incubation with a 3,3'-Diaminobenzidine substrate-chromogen solution. Tissue slides were imaged at 40x magnification and manually scored to determine the percentage of positive cells per high power field.

qRT-PCR

RNA was collected by using RNeasy as suggested by supplier (QIAGEN). Both cDNA and realtime PCR experiments were carried out by using iScript cDNA synthesis kit and iQ SYBR Green Supermix (BIO-RAD) by supplier instruction. Amplifications were performed in a BIO-RAD CFX96 Real-Time System for 40 cycles. Data was acquired by Bio-Rad CFX Manager software and fold changes were analyzed as described by Schefe et al [15]. Human TK1 (5'-AATCAGCTGCATTAACCTGCCCAC-3' forward; 5'-ATCACCAGGCACTTGTACTGAGCA-3' reverse), human P27 (5'-AGCAATGCGCAGGAATAAGGAAGC-3' forward; 5'-TACGTTTGACGTCTTCTGAGGCCA-3' reverse) were obtained from Integrated DNA Technologies.

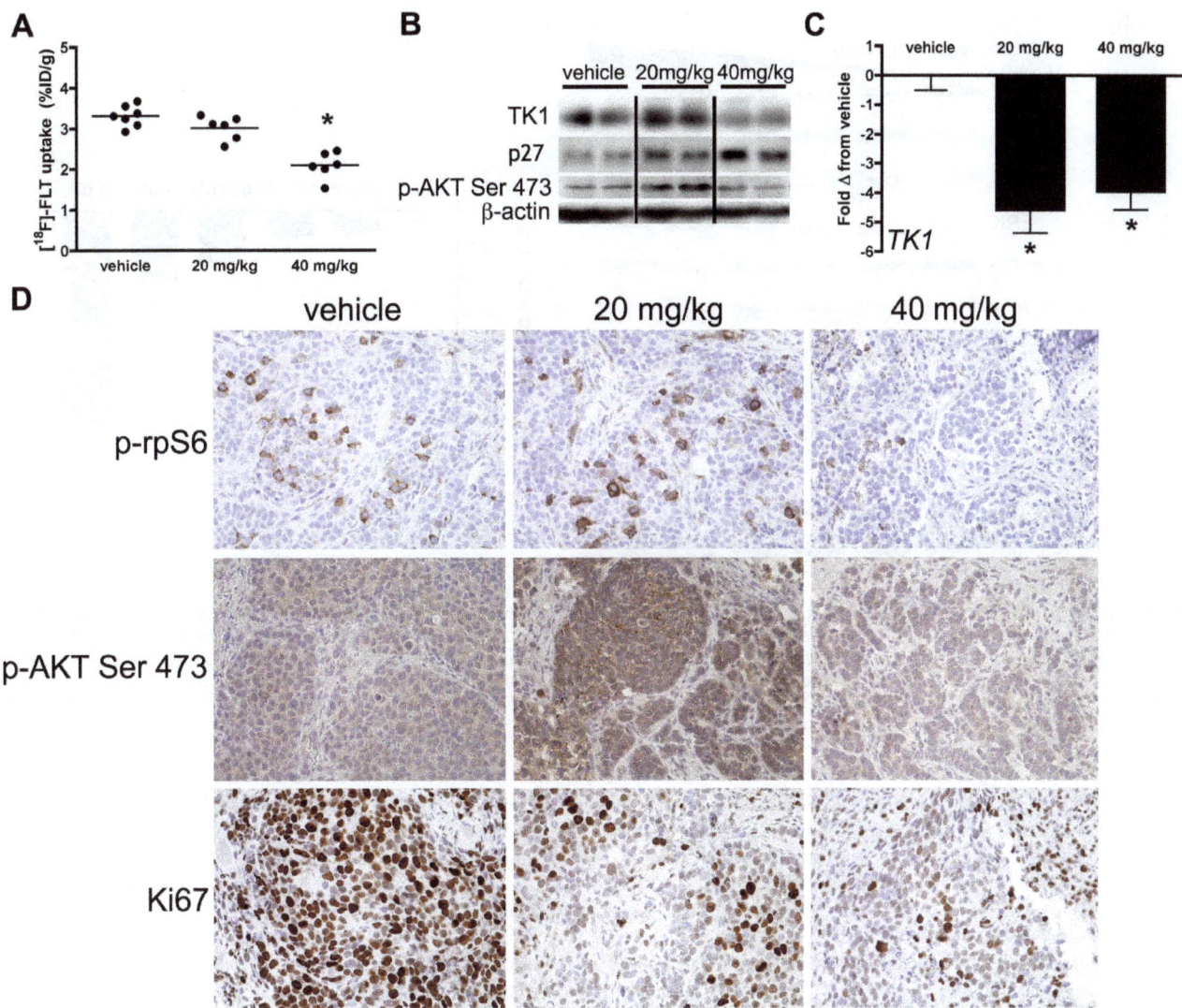

Figure 2. [18F]-FLT PET reflects inhibition of PI3K-mTOR activity in cetuximab-treated DiFi xenografts. DiFi tumor xenografts were imaged on day 7 of 20 mg/kg or 40 mg/kg cetuximab treatment regimens. (**A**) [18F]-FLT PET was only reduced in DiFi xenografts treated at the 40 mg/kg level (p = 0.0012). (**B**) Western blot analysis of tissues harvested immediately after imaging confirmed that TK1 protein levels were only decreased at the 40 mg/kg dose level. Increased p27 protein levels were observed at the 40 mg/kg dose levels. Increased p-AKT Ser473 protein levels were observed at the 20 mg/kg dose level. (**C**) Similar to *in vitro* observations, *TK1* mRNA was significantly reduced at both 20 mg/kg (p = 0.0009) and 40 mg/kg (p = 0.0001) dose levels. (**D**) IHC analysis of p-rpS6 and p-AKT Ser473 showed slightly elevated staining levels at 20 mg/kg. However, both markers were greatly reduced at 40 mg/kg. Ki67 immunoreactivity was reduced at both levels of cetuximab exposure.

Statistical Analysis

Statistical significance of data was evaluated using the non-parametric Wilcoxon Rank Sum (Mann-Whitney U) tests using the GraphPad Prism 4 software package. Differences were considered statistically significant if p<0.05.

Results

Regulation of TK1 following EGFR blockade in wild-type *KRAS* colorectal cancer cells

Previously, we showed that imaging readouts of EGFR occupancy and apoptosis, but not [18F]-FLT PET, predicted response to cetuximab in DiFi cell line xenografts that express wild-type KRAS and exhibit EGFR amplification [3,12]. Therefore, in this study, we first sought to elucidate the relationships between EGFR blockade with cetuximab and TK1 regulation.

Initially, we used cultured DiFi cells to evaluate the temporal relationship between cetuximab exposure and p-ERK, TK1, and p27 protein levels over 24 hours (**Fig. 1A**). As expected, p-ERK levels were almost immediately attenuated, showing a dramatic reduction within the first hour of cetuximab exposure (5.0 µg/mL), and remaining well-below baseline levels for up to 24 hours. Paradoxically, TK1 levels increased following cetuximab exposure, which peaked at 12 hours, and then rapidly declined to below baseline levels. Protein levels of the cell cycle inhibitor p27 rose dramatically and plateaued by 12 hours. The inverse relationship between TK1 and p27 protein levels implicated p27 as a key determinant of TK1 regulation in DiFi cells.

To further evaluate the relationships between MAPK pathway inhibition, TK1 regulation, and p27, DiFi cells were exposed to two concentrations (0.5 µg/mL and 5.0 µg/mL) of cetuximab for 24 hours (**Fig. 1B**). At 0.5 µg/mL, TK1 protein levels were

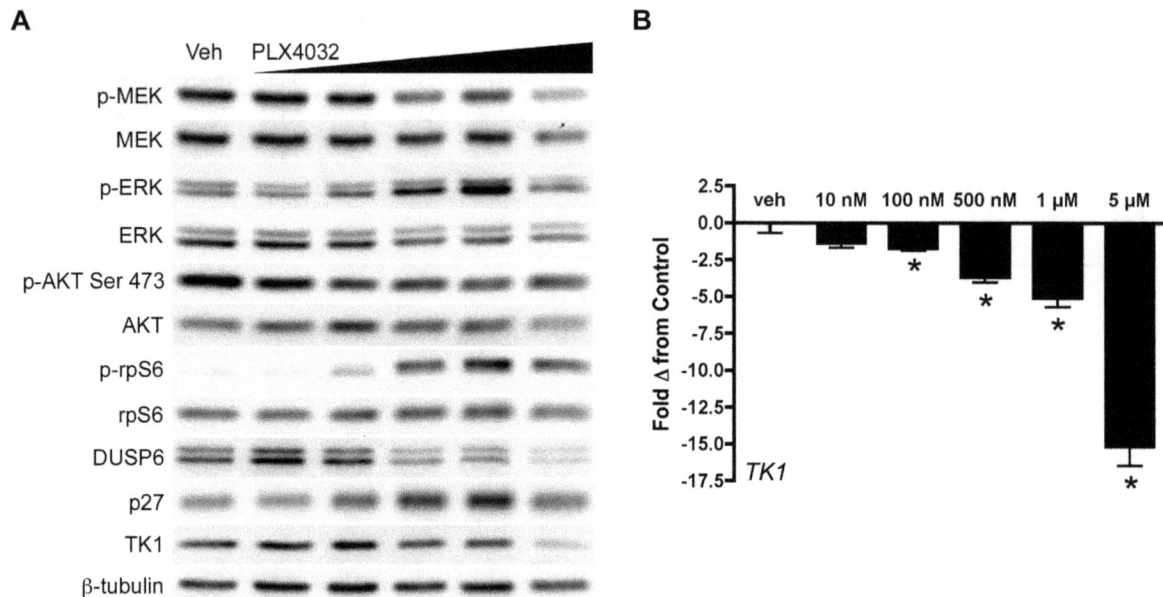

Figure 3. TK1 protein levels do not reflect p-ERK attenuation following inhibition of [V600E]BRAF inhibition in COLO 205 cells. COLO 205 cells were collected 48 hours of PLX 4032 exposure at 10 nM, 100 nM, 500 nM, 1 μM, or 5 μM. (**A**) Western blot analysis demonstrated target inhibition of p-MEK despite increased p-ERK levels. PI3K-mTOR signaling was elevated in a PLX 4032-dependent manner as exhibited by a steady rise in p-rpS6 levels. The ERK-phosphatase DUSP6 decreased in conjunction with mTOR signaling and was inversely proportional to p-ERK levels. A slight increase in p27 levels were observed concomitantly with only modest changes in TK1 levels, except at the highest dose of PLX4032. (**B**) Decreased *TK1* mRNA levels were observed at all drug concentrations above 10 nM ($p < 0.05$).

unaffected despite modestly elevated p27 and an approximately 50% reduction of p-ERK and p-AKT Ser473. Conversely, the 5.0 μg/mL level of exposure resulted in dramatically attenuated TK1 levels. Similar to the time course study, reduced TK1 correlated with a robust increase in p27. Additionally, complete attenuation of p-ERK and p-ATK Ser473 was observed at 5.0 μg/mL. In contrast to protein, *TK1 mRNA* tended to follow p-ERK levels more directly (**Fig. 1C**), which is not surprising given *TK1*'s dependence on E2F transcription [16], a downstream product of MAPK activity. Interestingly, *p27* mRNA was unaffected by cetuximab exposure, suggesting that elevated p27 protein levels stemmed from inhibition of downstream targets that affect post-transcriptional modification of p27, with AKT typically being one of these [17]. To determine if TK1 protein levels observed at 0.5 μg/mL levels of exposure were maintained through increased translational efficiency, we measured p-rpS6 and p-4E-BP1 levels, both products of pro-translational PI3K-mTOR activity (**Fig. 1B**). We found p-rpS6 levels to be attenuated only at the highest concentration of cetuximab. Furthermore, p-4E-BP1 levels were elevated at the lower concentration of cetuximab, suggesting increased potential for translation at the ribosomal cap [18]. Taken together with the *TK1* mRNA levels, these results may suggest that translational efficiency of TK1 at the lower level of cetuximab exposure that likely proceed through activation of mTOR.

Silencing mTOR-PI3K activity facilitates cetuximab-mediated attenuation of TK1 levels in DiFi cells

To explore the role of mTOR on TK1 regulation in this context, we silenced mTOR using siRNA to Raptor, an essential member of the functional mTOR Complex 1 (mTORC1) [19]. In the absence of mTORC1 activity, TK1 protein levels were attenuated at both 0.5 μg/mL and 5.0 μg/mL concentrations of

cetuximab, without an obvious effect on MAPK pathway activity (**Fig. 1D**). As expected, Raptor silencing resulted in greater cetuximab-mediated attenuation of p-AKT Ser473 and p-rpS6 as well as blocking phosphorylation of 4E-BP1. In addition to attenuated TK1 protein levels, mTORC1 inactivation resulted in increased p27 protein levels that appeared to be at least partially responsible for *TK1* transcriptional regulation at the lowest level of cetuximab exposure (**Fig. 1E**). Interestingly, as observed previously, the rise in p27 protein levels was itself not a product of increased *p27* transcription (**Fig. S1**). These results suggest that mTOR activation imparts its effect on TK1 through downstream effectors such as AKT and ERK through post-translational modification and degradation of cell cycle inhibitors, including p27 [17]. As evidence of this, mTORC1 inhibition in conjunction with EGFR blockade led to a profound reduction of TK1 protein levels not observable with cetuximab exposure alone at the lower concentration.

[18F]-FLT PET reflects inhibition of PI3K-mTOR activity in cetuximab treated DiFi cell line xenografts *in vivo*

We subsequently imaged DiFi xenograft-bearing mice with [18F]-FLT PET following cetuximab treatment (20 mg/kg or 40 mg/kg) or saline vehicle. In agreement with our previous studies [3], similar [18F]-FLT accumulation was observed in xenografts treated with vehicle or 20 mg/kg cetuximab. Increasing the dosage of cetuximab to 40 mg/kg resulted in diminished [18F]-FLT accumulation (**Fig. 2A**). Diminished TK1 protein levels were observed at the 40 mg/kg dosage relative to vehicle- and 20 mg/kg cetuximab-treated tumors (**Fig. 2B**). Similar to *in vitro* studies, diminished TK1 protein levels correlated with elevated p27 protein, but not *p27* mRNA levels (**Fig. S2**). Additionally, p-AKT Ser473 tumor protein levels were increased at the 20 mg/kg dose compared to both vehicle and 40 mg/kg cetuximab. TK1 protein

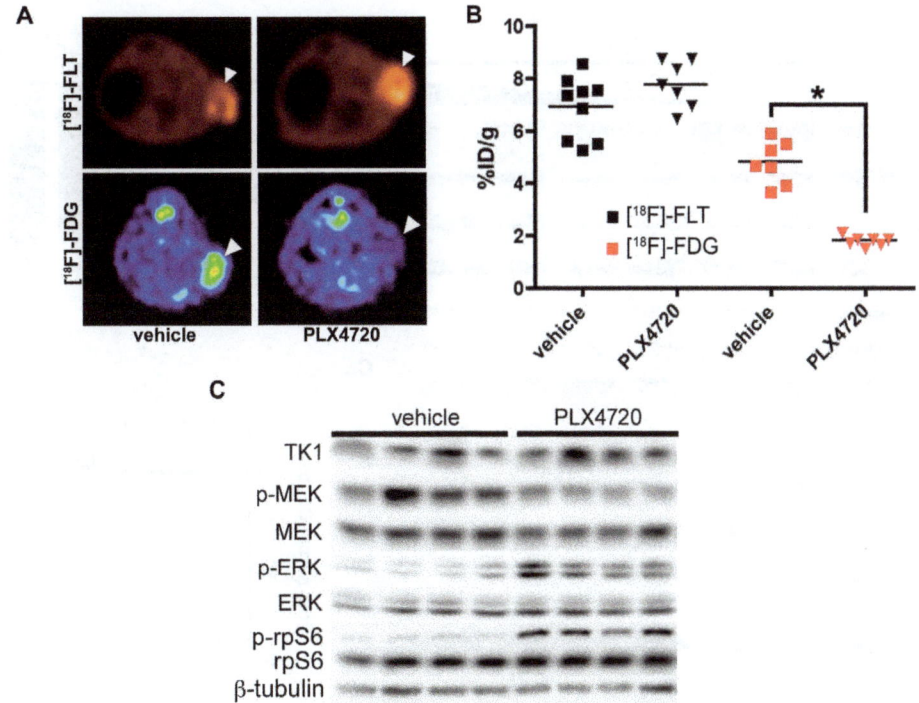

Figure 4. PLX4720 exposure does not affect [¹⁸F]-FLT PET in COLO 205 xenografts, despite evidence of target inhibition and diminished [¹⁸F]-FDG uptake. (A) Representative transverse [¹⁸F]-FLT and [¹⁸F]-FDG PET images acquired after three daily treatments with vehicle or 60 mg/kg PLX4720 (tumor indicated by arrowhead). (B) Quantification of PET data illustrated similar [¹⁸F]-FLT uptake in vehicle-treated and PLX4720-treated tumors. Unlike [¹⁸F]-FLT PET, PLX4720 exposure elicited a significant reduction in [¹⁸F]-FDG uptake (p = 0.0006). (C) Western blot analysis of vehicle- and PLX4720-treated tumor tissue confirmed that PLX4720 had no effect on TK1 protein levels in agreement with [¹⁸F]-FLT PET. Target inhibition as measured by p-MEK levels was observed. However, similar to *in vitro* studies, PLX4720-treated COLO 205 xenografts exhibited elevated p-ERK and p-rpS6 protein levels relative to vehicle controls.

levels were unaffected by the lower dosage of cetuximab, despite significantly reduced *TK1* mRNA (**Fig. 2C**), which was reduced relative to vehicle-treated controls at both levels of cetuximab exposure. IHC of imaging-matched xenograft tissues illustrated that PI3K-mTOR activity, as measured by p-rpS6 and p-AKT Ser473 levels, was inhibited at the highest cetuximab exposure (**Fig. 2D, Fig. S3**). Interestingly, Ki67 was reduced at both levels of cetuximab exposure (**Fig 2D, Fig. S4**), suggesting that [¹⁸F]-FLT PET was decoupled from standard measures of proliferation at the lower dosage. While [¹⁸F]-FLT PET appeared to be sensitive to PI3K-mTOR activity, [¹⁸F]-FDG PET imaging was not sensitive to this phenomenon. We observed reduced [¹⁸F]-FDG uptake relative to vehicle controls at both levels of cetuximab exposure (**Fig. S5**). Overall, these results suggest that [¹⁸F]-FLT PET provides unique information regarding mTOR signaling that is not captured by [¹⁸F]-FDG PET or standard measures of proliferation, such as Ki67 IHC.

TK1 protein levels do not reflect ᵛ⁶⁰⁰ᴱBRAF inhibition in COLO 205 cells

Analogous to the DiFi model treated with cetuximab, we evaluated relationships between target inhibition, downstream effectors, and TK1 levels in a ᵛ⁶⁰⁰ᴱBRAF expressing cell line, COLO 205, treated with a selective ᵛ⁶⁰⁰ᴱBRAF inhibitor (**Fig. 3**). PLX4032 exposure for 48 hours led to concentration-dependent inhibition of p-MEK levels. Paradoxically, p-ERK levels were increased in a concentration-dependent manner, except at the highest dose (5 µM) (**Fig. 3A**). The mismatch between p-MEK and p-ERK was not observed at exposure durations of 2 hours

(**Fig. S6**) or 24 hours (**Fig. S7**). While p-AKT Ser473 levels were only moderately reduced with PLX4032 exposure at 48 hours, we observed a concentration-dependent increase in p-rpS6 that correlated with the increase in p-ERK. Concomitantly increased p-rpS6 and diminished DUSP6 levels suggested that the increase in p-ERK was at least partially resulted from diminished phosphatase activity that was likely related to mTOR activation [20]. PLX4032 exposure led to a modest increase in p27 protein levels. TK1 levels were increased slightly at lower PLX4032 concentrations and unchanged from vehicle at higher levels of exposure, except for the highest concentration (5 µM). Surprisingly, *TK1* mRNA levels appeared to be more closely associated with inhibition of p-MEK and, unlike TK1 protein levels, were reduced in an essentially concentration-dependent manner (**Fig. 3B**).

[¹⁸F]-FLT PET, but not [¹⁸F]-FDG PET, reflects elevated mTOR activity and correlates with a lack of p-ERK inhibition in PLX4720-treated COLO 205 xenografts

Mice bearing COLO 205 xenografts were treated daily with 60 mg/kg PLX4720 for 4 days and imaged with [¹⁸F]-FLT PET or [¹⁸F]-FDG PET (**Fig. 4**). In agreement with *in vitro* studies showing that BRAF inhibition had little effect on TK1 levels in COLO 205 cells, treatment with PLX4720 had little effect on [¹⁸F]-FLT PET imaging. Conversely, [¹⁸F]-FDG PET was significantly reduced in similarly treated cohorts (**Fig. 4B**). In agreement with imaging, TK1 levels of PLX4720-treated xenografts were similar to vehicle-treated controls. Also similar to *in vitro* studies, we found elevated p-ERK levels and p-rpS6 levels in

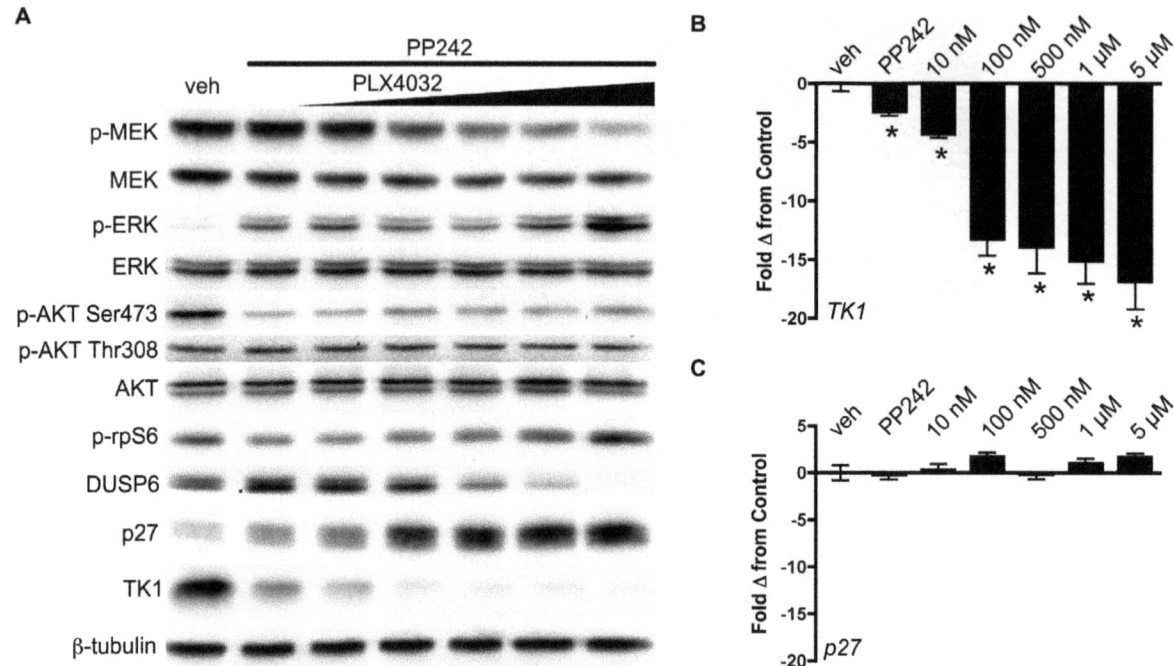

Figure 5. Combined [V600E]BRAF and mTOR inhibition results in transcriptional control of TK1 protein levels in COLO 205 cells. (A) Western blot of COLO 205 cells treated with PP242 (250 nM) and increasing PLX4032. Similar to single agent PLX4032, p-MEK, but not p-ERK, was inhibited in a PLX4032-dependent manner. Consistent with mTORC1/mTORC2 inhibition, p-AKT Ser473, but not p-AKT Thr308, was inhibited. Unlike single agent PLX4032, which resulted in concentration-dependent activation of p-rpS6, combined treatment maintained p-rpS6 levels at essentially baseline levels except at the highest PLX4032 concentration. Similarly, DUSP6 levels were inversely related to p-ERK protein levels. With combined mTOR and [V600E]BRAF blockade, p27 and TK1 protein levels were inversely correlated and dramatically affected by PLX4032 exposure. **(B)** Similarly, *TK1* mRNA was significantly reduced at PLX4032 concentrations as low as 10 nM. **(C)** Despite elevated p27 protein levels, *p27* mRNA was unaffected by combined mTOR-[V600E]BRAF inhibition.

PLX4720 treated xenografts relative to vehicle-treated controls, despite inhibition of the BRAF effector, p-MEK.

Regulation of TK1 following mTOR or dual PI3K-mTOR inhibition and [V600E]BRAF inhibition in COLO 205 cells

To examine mTOR's role in TK1 regulation following [V600E]BRAF inhibition, cultured COLO 205 cells were treated

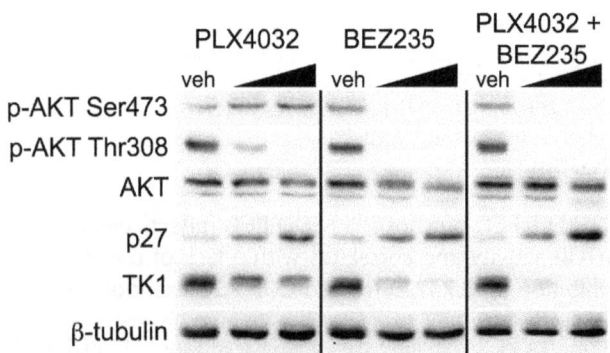

Figure 6. Dual pathway inhibition regulates TK1 protein levels and results in greater p27 protein levels than single agents alone. Single agent PLX4032 resulted in activation of p-AKT Ser473 following 24 hours of exposure at two concentrations (100 nM, 1 μM). The addition of the dual PI3K/mTOR inhibitor BEZ235 blocks p-AKT Ser473 activation and resulted in a greater increase in p27 protein levels and diminished TK1 protein levels.

concomitantly with 250 nM pp242, a selective mTORC1/mTORC2 inhibitor [21] and increasing concentrations of PLX4032 for 48 hours (**Fig. 5**). Adding PP242 had little effect on PLX4032-dependent inhibition of p-MEK, yet effectively blocked activation of p-AKT at Ser473 and blunted the previously observed activation of p-rpS6 caused by PLX4032 exposure (compare to **Fig. 3A**). However, mTOR blockade was insufficient to attenuate p-ERK or p-AKT Thr308 levels in a PLX4032-dependent manner, nor to completely attenuate p-rpS6 levels (**Fig. 5A**). As with single agent *in vitro* studies, p-rpS6 activation correlated with a slight attenuation of DUSP6 levels and a slight elevation of p-ERK at higher PLX4032 concentrations. Nonetheless, combined inhibition of p-AKT Ser473 and p-MEK resulted in dramatically decreased TK1, at both the protein and mRNA level. In the presence of elevated p27, *TK1* mRNA levels fell dramatically, with significant reductions observed at PLX4032 concentrations as low as 10 nM (**Fig. 5A**). Furthermore, suggesting that AKT activity was responsible for post-translational modification and degradation of p27, in the presence of p-AKT Ser473 inhibition, p27 protein was dramatically elevated but *p27* mRNA was not (**Fig. 5C**).

Given that combined [V600E]BRAF-mTOR inhibition was insufficient to attenuate p-rpS6, and coupled with the observation that PI3K activity and downstream signaling has been proposed as a mechanism of resistance to BRAF inhibition in colorectal cancer [22] and melanoma [23,24], we evaluated the effects of dual PI3K-mTOR inhibition in COLO 205 cells in conjunction with [V600E]BRAF inhibition (**Fig. 6**). COLO 205 cells were treated with either PLX4032, BEZ235, a small molecule dual inhibitor of PI3K

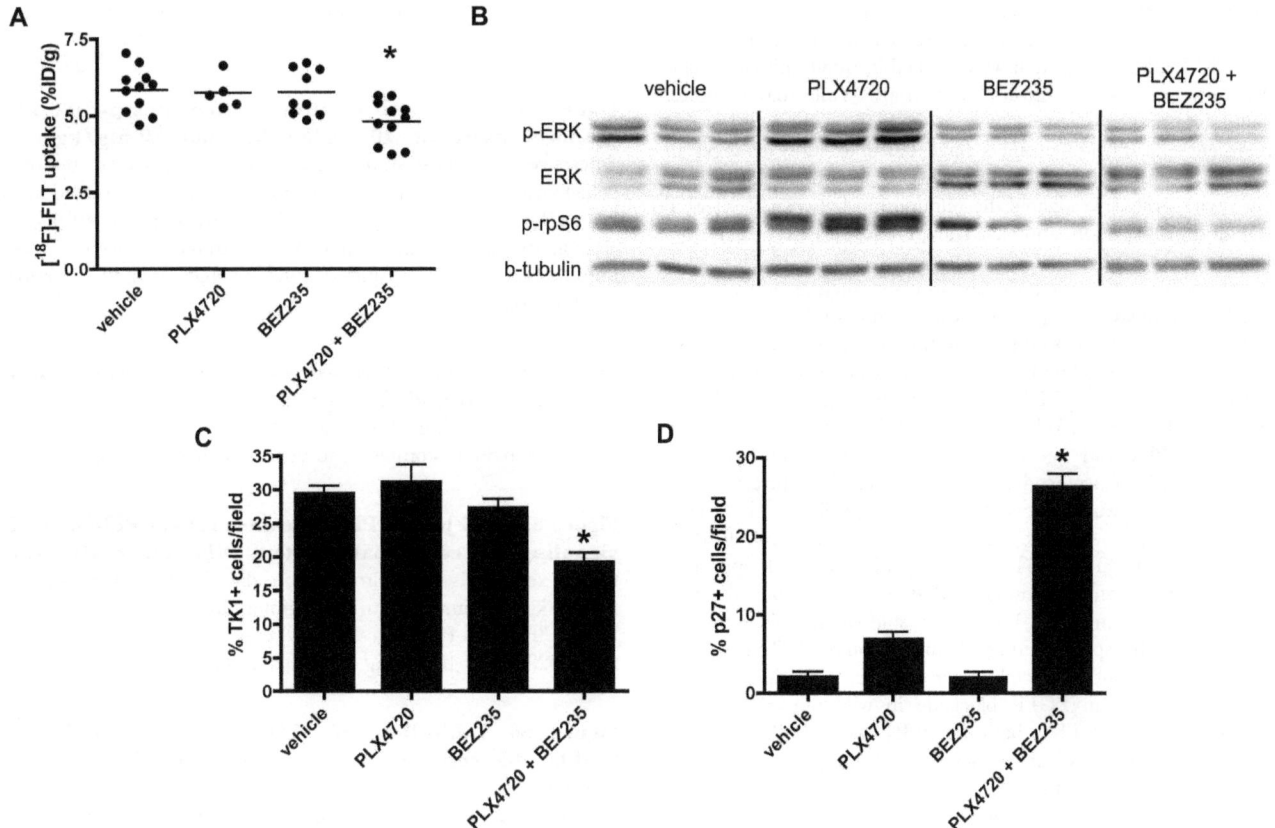

Figure 7. [18F]-FLT PET reflects BEZ235-dependent inhibition of PI3K/mTOR activity in PLX4720 treated COLO 205 xenografts. Xenograft-bearing mice were imaged with [18F]-FLT PET on treatment day 4. (**A**) [18F]-FLT uptake was diminished in the combination treatment cohort relative to vehicle (p = 0.0087), but not single agent PLX4720- or BEZ235-treated cohorts. (**B**) Western blot of xenograft tissue harvested immediately following imaging illustrated elevated p-ERK and p-rpS6 levels in PLX4720-treated mice. Combining PLX4032 with BEZ235 resulted in reduced p-ERK and p-rpS6 protein levels. (**C**) TK1 levels, as measured by IHC, were reduced only in the combination treatment group in agreement with [18F]-FLT PET. (**D**) Consistent with *in vitro* studies, diminished TK1 levels, and consequently [18F]-FLT PET, correlated with elevated p27 that was elevated only in the combination treated group.

and mTOR [25], or the combination for 24 hours. Indeed, inhibiting both mTOR activity, as measured by p-AKT Ser473, and PI3K activity, as measured by p-AKT Thr308, in the presence of PLX4032 resulted in greater p27 protein levels and decreased TK1 protein levels. These results prompted our evaluation of this combination *in vivo*.

[18F]-FLT PET reflects inhibition of PI3K-mTOR activity in PLX4720-treated xenografts

To explore the effects of dual PI3K-mTOR inhibition on [18F]-FLT PET *in vivo*, we treated COLO 205 xenograft bearing mice daily with either vehicle, PLX4720, BEZ235, or in combination, and imaged the mice on treatment day 4. Strikingly, only the combination cohort exhibited decreased [18F]-FLT PET relative to vehicle-treated controls or single agent-treated cohorts (**Fig. 7A**). Western blot analysis of imaging-matched xenograft tissue revealed the anticipated increase of p-ERK levels and p-rpS6 levels in PLX4720 treated mice (**Fig. 7B**). However, combination treatment with PLX4720 and BEZ235 led to an overall reduction of p-ERK and p-rpS6 levels compared to vehicle-treated controls. In agreement with imaging, TK1 protein levels were reduced in the combination group only (**Fig. 7C**), although Ki67 immunoreactivity was reduced for all treatment

groups relative to the vehicle-treated cohort (**Fig. S8**). Importantly, and agreement with *in vitro* studies, combination treatment led to a significant increase in p27 protein levels, but not mRNA levels, compared to vehicle and single agent cohorts (**Fig. 7D**, **Fig. S9**). These results suggest that the primary determinant of reduced [18F]-FLT PET in this setting was inhibition of V600EBRAF and PI3K-mTOR activity in conjunction with the rise in p27 protein levels.

Discussion

Imaging biomarkers to both predict early response to targeted therapy was well as to predict resistance to treatment response are essential components of personalized medicine in oncology. Current clinical means of assessing treatment response by imaging are based upon the Response Evaluation Criteria in Solid Tumors (RECIST) guidelines [26]. Based upon changes in tumor size, RECIST does not take advantage of cellular and molecular information now available through contemporary imaging methodologies. As cellular and molecular changes can occur within hours of treatment and may precede changes in tumor volume, newer criteria, such as PERCIST [27], recognize the potential utility of [18F]-FDG PET to predict early response. However, as [18F]-FDG uptake in tissue reflects a broad range of metabolic processes, a more specific marker of cellular proliferation may better assess treatment response in targeted therapy [28].

[^{18}F]-FLT has been extensively studied in small animal models of treatment response and in clinical trials. While many studies, including our own, have shown [^{18}F]-FLT to be sensitive to treatment efficacy [4,5], others have failed to show changes in [^{18}F]-FLT tumor uptake despite effective treatment [3,29]. We have extensively investigated the relationship between [^{18}F]-FLT PET and proliferation, and have shown that [^{18}F]-FLT PET does not necessarily reflect proliferation directly [6]. [^{18}F]-FLT PET exhibits sensitivity to vital cellular processes such as activation of signaling pathways, as we demonstrate in this study.

In the context of EGFR inhibition in a wild-type KRAS colorectal cancer cell line we show that a lack of TK1 attenuation, and thus similar [^{18}F]-FLT PET, in treated xenografts reflected PI3K-mTOR activity. Where PI3K-mTOR activity was elevated, [^{18}F]-FLT PET did not reflect target inhibition and did not correlate with pharmacodynamic response. In contrast, when mTOR activity was abrogated, either genetically or pharmacologically, TK1 levels were attenuated, which, in turn, lead to decreased [^{18}F]-FLT PET. Here, [^{18}F]-FLT PET provides clinically important information that is unavailable through [^{18}F]-FDG PET imaging. We further studied this phenomenon in a different therapeutic setting, the inhibition of ^{V600E}BRAF in a ^{V600E}BRAF mutant colorectal cancer cell line. While inhibition of mTOR signaling in EGFR blockade in wild-type KRAS was sufficient to control TK1, both the PI3K and mTOR pathways served to maintain TK1 protein levels by transcriptional and post-translational mechanisms during pro-survival signaling during ^{V600E}BRAF inhibition. As such, [^{18}F]-FLT PET may aid the elucidation of the mechanisms of resistance to targeted therapies which are relevant in colorectal cancer [30], and potentially other solid tumors such as melanoma [31].

In many cases tumors may initially respond to targeted therapy only to recur with more aggressive phenotypes, notably as after ^{V600E}BRAF inhibition in melanoma [31–33]. It is therefore important clinically to detect activation of resistance pathways and to predict possible recurrence. This study demonstrates that [^{18}F]-FLT may serve as an early PET biomarker that may be sensitive to activation of pro-survival mechanisms that may predict tumors that are more likely to resist treatment and ultimately may be more prone to recurrence. It is notable that [^{18}F]-FDG PET was insufficient to observe the activity of the pro-survival signals detected by [^{18}F]-FLT PET. Therefore, we envision a new role for [^{18}F]-FLT PET in the setting of predicting response to targeted therapy.

Supporting Information

Figure S1 Elevated p27 protein levels observed following cetuximab exposure in DiFi cells are not transcriptionally induced. No statistically significant change in *p27* was observed in DiFi cells treated with raptor siRNA or scrambled RNA when treated with either 0.5 μg/mL or 5.0 μg/mL cetuximab.

Figure S2 Elevated p27 protein levels observed following cetuximab treatment in DiFi xenografts are not transcriptionally induced. No statistically significant change in *p27* levels was observed in DiFi xenografts treated with either

20 mg/kg or 40 mg/kg cetuximab relative to vehicle-treated xenografts.

Figure S3 Cetuximab treatment attenuates p-rpS6 immunoreactivity at 40 mg/kg but not 20 mg/kg. No difference in p-rpS6 immunoreactivity was observed between vehicle-treated controls and DiFi tumor xenografts treated with 20 mg/kg cetuximab (p = 0.9743). When treated with 40 mg/kg cetuximab, DiFi tumor xenografts exhibit reduced p-rpS6 immunoreactivity compared to vehicle-treated tumors (p = 0.0334).

Figure S4 Cetuximab treatment attenuates Ki67 immunoreactivity at both 20 mg/kg and 40 mg/kg. Ki67 IHC was reduced at both 20 mg/kg (p<0.0001) and 40 mg/kg (p< 0.0001) cetuximab compared to vehicle-treated controls.

Figure S5 [^{18}F]-FDG PET does not reflect PI3K-mTOR signaling in cetuximab-treated DiFi xenografts DiFi tumor xenografts were imaged on day 7 of a 20 mg/kg or 40 mg/kg cetuximab treatment regimen. In contrast to [^{18}F]-FLT PET, [^{18}F]-FDG PET was similarly reduced at both the 20 mg/kg (p = 0.0286) and 40 mg/kg (p = 0.0286) dose levels.

Figure S6 Inhibition of MAPK-pathway activity in COLO 205 cells following exposure to PLX4032 for 2 hours. ^{V600E}BRAF downstream effectors p-MEK and p-ERK were similarly inhibited following 2 hours PLX4032 exposure.

Figure S7 Relative inhibition of ^{V600E}BRAF downstream effectors following 24 hour exposure of PLX4032 in COLO 205 cells. Cells were collected at 24 hours following treatment with 10 nM, 100 nM, 500 nM, 1 μM, or 5 μM PLX4032.

Figure S8 Ki67 is reduced in COLO 205 xenografts treated with PLX4720, BEZ235, as well as the combination. Ki67 immunostaining was significantly reduced in all treatment regimens in COLO 205 xenografts (p<0.0001) compared to vehicle-treated xenografts.

Figure S9 *p27* mRNA is not affected by PLX4720, BEZ235, or combination treatment in COLO 205 tumors. No change in *p27* mRNA levels was observed in any treatment regimen compared to vehicle-treated xenografts.

Acknowledgments

The authors wish to thank Saffet Guleryuz, Nathan J. Mutic, Jinping Xie, Md. Imam Uddin, M. Noor Tantawy, George Wilson, Clare Osborne, and R. Adam Smith for experimental support.

Author Contributions

Conceived and designed the experiments: ETM HCM RJC. Performed the experiments: ETM PZ. Analyzed the data: ETM HCM MKW. Wrote the paper: ETM HCM.

References

1. Bollag G, Hirth P, Tsai J, Zhang J, Ibrahim PN, et al. (2010) Clinical efficacy of a RAF inhibitor needs broad target blockade in BRAF-mutant melanoma. Nature 467: 596–9.

2. Vogel CL, Cobleigh MA, Tripathy D, Gutheil JC, Harris LN, et al. (2002) Efficacy and safety of trastuzumab as a single agent in first-line treatment of HER2-overexpressing metastatic breast cancer. J Clin Oncol 20: 719–26.

3. Manning HC, Merchant NB, Foutch AC, Virostko JM, Wyatt SK, et al. (2008) Molecular imaging of therapeutic response to epidermal growth factor receptor blockade in colorectal cancer. Clin Cancer Res 14: 7413–22.

4. Shah C, Miller TW, Wyatt SK, McKinley ET, Olivares MG, et al. (2009) Imaging biomarkers predict response to anti-HER2 (ErbB2) therapy in preclinical models of breast cancer. Clin Cancer Res 15: 4712–21.

5. McKinley ET, Smith RA, Zhao P, Fu A, Saleh SA et al. (2013) 3'-Deoxy-3'-18F-Fluorothymidine PET Predicts Response to V600EBRAF-Targeted Therapy in Preclinical Models of Colorectal Cancer. J Nucl Med 54: 424–30.

6. McKinley ET, Ayers GD, Smith RA, Saleh SA, Zhao P, et al. (2013) Limits of [18F]-FLT PET as a Biomarker of Proliferation in Oncology. 8(3): e58938. doi:10.1371/journal.pone.0058938.

7. McKinley ET, Smith RA, Tanksley JP, Washington MK, Walker R, et al. (2012) [18F]FLT-PET to predict pharmacodynamic and clinical response to cetuximab therapy in Menetrier's disease. Ann Nucl Med 26: 757–63.

8. Shields AF, Grierson JR, Dohmen BM, Machulla HJ, Stayanoff JC, et al. (1998) Imaging proliferation in vivo with [F-18]FLT and positron emission tomography. Nat Med 4: 1334–6.

9. Barthel H, Cleij MC, Collingridge DR, Hutchinson OC, Osman S, et al. (2003) 3'-deoxy-3'-[18F]fluorothymidine as a new marker for monitoring tumor response to antiproliferative therapy in vivo with positron emission tomography. Cancer Res 63: 3791–8.

10. Soloviev D, Lewis D, Honess D, Aboagye E. (2012) [(18)F]FLT: an imaging biomarker of tumour proliferation for assessment of tumour response to treatment. Eur J Cancer 48: 416–24.

11. Zhang C, Yan Z, Li W, Kuszpit K, Painter CL, et al. (2012) [(18)F]FLT-PET imaging does not always "light up" proliferating tumor cells. Clin Cancer Res 18: 1303–12.

12. Olive M, Untawale S, Coffey RJ, Siciliano MJ, Wildrick DM, et al. (1993) Characterization of the DiFi rectal carcinoma cell line derived from a familial adenomatous polyposis patient. In Vitro Cell Dev Biol 29A: 239–48.

13. Buck JR, Saleh S, Imam Uddin M, Manning HC. (2012) Rapid, microwave-assisted organic synthesis of selective V600EBRAF inhibitors for preclinical cancer research. Tetrahedron Lett 53: 4161–5.

14. Choi SJ, Kim JS, Kim JH, Oh SJ, Lee JG, et al. (2005) [F-18]3'-deoxy-3'-fluorothymidine PET for the diagnosis and grading of brain tumors. Eur J Nucl Med Mol Imaging 32: 653–9.

15. Schefe JH, Lehmann KE, Buschmann IR, Unger T, Funke-Kaiser H. (2006) Quantitative real-time RT-PCR data analysis: current concepts and the novel "gene expression's CT difference" formula. J Mol Med 84: 901–10.

16. Ogris E, Rotheneder H, Mudrak I, Pichler A, Wintersberger E. (1993) A binding site for transcription factor E2F is a target for trans activation of murine thymidine kinase by polyomavirus large T antigen and plays an important role in growth regulation of the gene. J Virol 67: 1765–71.

17. Liang J, Zubovitz J, Petrocelli T, Kotchetov R, Connor MK, et al. (2002) PKB/Akt phosphorylates p27, impairs nuclear import of p27 and opposes p27-mediated G1 arrest. Nat Med 8: 1153–60.

18. Pause A, Belsham GJ, Gingras AC, Donze O, Lin TA, et al. (1994) Insulin-dependent stimulation of protein synthesis by phosphorylation of a regulator of 5'-cap function. Nature 371: 762–7.

19. Kim DH, Sarbassov DD, Ali SM, King JE, Latek RR, et al. (2002) mTOR interacts with raptor to form a nutrient-sensitive complex that signals to the cell growth machinery. Cell 110: 163–75.

20. Bermudez O, Marchetti S, Pages G, Gimond C. (2008) Post-translational regulation of the ERK phosphatase DUSP6/MKP3 by the mTOR pathway. Oncogene 27: 3685–91.

21. Feldman ME, Apsel B, Uotila A, Loewith R, Knight ZA, et al. (2009) Active-Site Inhibitors of mTOR Target Rapamycin-Resistant Outputs of mTORC1 and mTORC2. PLoS Biol 7(2): e1000038. doi:10.1371/journal.pbio.1000038.

22. Mao M, Tian F, Mariadason JM, Tsao CC, Lemos R et al. (2013) Resistance to BRAF Inhibition in BRAF-Mutant Colon Cancer Can Be Overcome with PI3K Inhibition or Demethylating Agents. Clin Cancer Res 19: 657–67.

23. Villanueva J, Vultur A, Lee JT, Somasundaram R, Fukunaga-Kalabis M, et al. (2010) Acquired resistance to BRAF inhibitors mediated by a RAF kinase switch in melanoma can be overcome by cotargeting MEK and IGF-1R/PI3K. Cancer Cell 18: 683–95.

24. Villanueva J, Vultur A, Herlyn M. (2011) Resistance to BRAF Inhibitors: Unraveling Mechanisms and Future Treatment Options. Cancer Res 71: 7137–40.

25. Maira SM, Stauffer F, Brueggen J, Furet P, Schnell C, et al. (2008) Identification and characterization of NVP-BEZ235, a new orally available dual phosphatidylinositol 3-kinase/mammalian target of rapamycin inhibitor with potent in vivo antitumor activity. Mol Cancer Ther 7: 1851–63.

26. Eisenhauer EA, Therasse P, Bogaerts J, Schwartz LH, Sargent D, et al. (2009) New response evaluation criteria in solid tumours: revised RECIST guideline (version 1.1). Eur J Cancer 45: 228–47.

27. Wahl RL, Jacene H, Kasamon Y, Lodge MA. (2009) From RECIST to PERCIST: Evolving Considerations for PET response criteria in solid tumors. J Nucl Med 50 Suppl 1: 122S–50S.

28. Shields AF. (2003) PET imaging with 18F-FLT and thymidine analogs: promise and pitfalls. J Nucl Med 44: 1432–4.

29. Katz SI, Zhou L, Ferrara TA, Wang W, Mayes PA, et al. (2011) FLT-PET may not be a reliable indicator of therapeutic response in p53-null malignancy. Int J Oncol 39: 91–100.

30. Corcoran RB, Ebi H, Turke AB, Coffee EM, Nishino M, et al. (2012) EGFR-mediated re-activation of MAPK signaling contributes to insensitivity of BRAF mutant colorectal cancers to RAF inhibition with vemurafenib. Cancer Discov 2: 227–35.

31. Solit DB, Rosen N. (2011) Resistance to BRAF inhibition in melanomas. N Engl J Med 364: 772–4.

32. Nazarian R, Shi H, Wang Q, Kong X, Koya RC, et al. (2010) Melanomas acquire resistance to B-RAF(V600E) inhibition by RTK or N-RAS upregulation. Nature 468: 973–7.

33. Wagle N, Emery C, Berger MF, Davis MJ, Sawyer A, et al. (2011). Dissecting therapeutic resistance to RAF inhibition in melanoma by tumor genomic profiling. J Clin Oncol 29: 3085–96.

23

Feasibility Study of Dual Energy Radiographic Imaging for Target Localization in Radiotherapy for Lung Tumors

Jie Huo[1], Xianfeng Zhu[1], Yang Dong[2], Zhiyong Yuan[2], Ping Wang[2]*, Xuemin Wang[1], Gang Wang[1], Xin-Hua Hu[3], Yuanming Feng[1,2,4]*

1 Department of Biomedical Engineering, Tianjin University, Tianjin, China, 2 Department of Radiation Oncology, Tianjin Cancer Hospital, Tianjin, China, 3 Department of Physics, East Carolina University, Greenville, North Carolina, United States of America, 4 Department of Radiation Oncology, East Carolina University, Greenville, North Carolina, United States of America

Abstract

Purpose: Dual-energy (DE) radiographic imaging improves tissue discrimination by separating soft from hard tissues in the acquired images. This study was to establish a mathematic model of DE imaging based on intrinsic properties of tissues and quantitatively evaluate the feasibility of applying the DE imaging technique to tumor localization in radiotherapy.

Methods: We investigated the dependence of DE image quality on the radiological equivalent path length (EPL) of tissues with two phantoms using a stereoscopic x-ray imaging unit. 10 lung cancer patients who underwent radiotherapy each with gold markers implanted in the tumor were enrolled in the study approved by the hospital's Ethics Committee. The displacements of the centroids of the delineated gross tumor volumes (GTVs) in the digitally reconstructed radiograph (DRR) and in the bone-canceled DE image were compared with the averaged displacements of the centroids of gold markers to evaluate the feasibility of using DE imaging for tumor localization.

Results: The results of the phantom study indicated that the contrast-to-noise ratio (CNR) was linearly dependent on the difference of EPL and a mathematical model was established. The objects and backgrounds corresponding to ΔEPL less than 0.08 are visually indistinguishable in the bone-canceled DE image. The analysis of patient data showed that the tumor contrast in the bone-canceled images was improved significantly as compared with that in the original radiographic images and the accuracy of tumor localization using the DE imaging technique was comparable with that of using fiducial makers.

Conclusion: It is feasible to apply the technique for tumor localization in radiotherapy.

Editor: Masaru Katoh, National Cancer Center, Japan

Funding: The authors have no support or funding to report.

Competing Interests: The authors have declared that no competing interests exist.

* Email: fengyu@ecu.edu (YF); wangping@tjmuch.com (PW)

Introduction

As a method for tissue discrimination, dual energy (DE) imaging has been shown to be of good performance in thoracic [1], cardiac [2] and mammographic [3] imaging applications. In DE imaging the acquired images are combined to effectively separate an imaged object into distinct component images of specific tissue types or tissue-selection for generating high contrast images of targeted structures, which can be applied to improve tumor detection for diagnostic interpretation.

Planar kilovoltage (kV) imaging plays an important role in image guidance in radiation therapy (RT) systems, such as CyberKnife (Accuray, Inc., Sunnyvale, CA), ExacTrac (Brainlab AG, Feldkirchen, Germany) and others. It operates by acquiring two radiographs of the patient's anatomy in the treatment room at two different beam angles in real-time and comparing them with pre-generated digitally reconstructed radiographs (DRRs) from the computed tomography (CT) image data used in the RT planning. This procedure is designed to monitor the position variation of the

patient's anatomy in the CT coordinate frame [4]. The projection of three dimensional (3D) structures into a two dimensional (2D) image can result in obscuration of the structure of interest such as a lung nodule by overlying structures such as the ribs, which has been identified as a major limiting factor in the detection of lung nodules in radiographs [5].

As DE imaging could provide tissue-selecting images by eliminating the overlying structures, it could bring potential benefits of improved tumor localization if DE imaging can be applied using the kV image guidance unit. Additionally, tumor localization without implanted metallic or radio frequency fiducials may eliminate a number of problems such as pneumothorax and hemorrhage [6]. Previous studies have explored the optimization of DE image acquisition parameters including kVp combinations [7], differential beam filtration and dose allocation [8] based on different image quality metrics such as contrast-to-noise ratio (CNR) [9], signal-to-noise ratio (SNR) [4], signal difference to noise ratio (SDNR) [10] and detectability index [11]. However, much more remains to be investigated quantitatively on the attenuation of x-ray as a function of the properties of the intervening tissues (such as atomic composition, mass density and thickness) in additional to the photon energy [12]. Enhanced discrimination of targeted structures such as tumor tissues through optimized DE imaging can only be achieved through a clear understanding of the effects of intrinsic tissue properties.

The purpose of this report was to quantify the effects of intrinsic tissue properties on tissue discrimination in DE images and to investigate the feasibility of applying the technique in radiotherapy image guidance systems such as the CyberKnife. We first derived the mathematical model for generating bone-canceled images. Then we conducted experimental studies with two phantoms to quantitatively analyze the influence of intrinsic tissue properties (represented by EPL) on the CNR of the image. Finally we applied the DE imaging technique to 10 lung cancer patients to evaluate the accuracy for tumor localization by comparing the results with that using the existing method of implanted fiducial markers.

Materials and Methods

1. Modeling of bone-canceled image

DE imaging exploits differences in the photoelectric and Compton cross sections of different type of tissues in the object as x-ray photon energy varies [13]. Since the photoelectric absorption is dependent sensitively on atomic number, bony structures with high calcium concentration present different image contrast in the high energy (HE) radiograph from that in the low energy (LE) radiograph. Therefore, tissue-selecting image can be obtained by combining the two radiographs of different energies. A common algorithm for DE image reconstruction, derived from the Beer–Lambert law, is to apply a weighted log-subtraction scheme [1]. If we assume that an object consists of bone, lung tissue and other soft tissues, the transmitted intensities of x-ray beams at two different energies of HE and LE can be written as

$$I^L = I_0^L \exp[-(\mu_{Bone}^L t_{Bone} + \mu_{Soft-tissue}^L t_{Soft-tissue} + \mu_{Lung}^L t_{Lung})] \quad (1a)$$

$$I^H = \\ I_0^H \exp[-(\mu_{Bone}^H t_{Bone} + \mu_{Soft-tissue}^H t_{Soft-tissue} + \mu_{Lung}^H t_{Lung})] \quad (1b)$$

where L and H denote LE and HE, respectively, I_0 and I are the intensities of incident and transmitted x-ray beams, μ_{Bone}, $\mu_{Soft-tissue}$, and μ_{Lung} are the linear attenuation coefficients of bone, soft-tissue, and lung tissue respectively, and t_{Bone}, $t_{Soft-tissue}$, and t_{Lung} are the thicknesses of bone, soft-tissue, and lung tissue respectively. Because of the linear relationship with the transmitted intensities, the grey-level values of pixels in a HE or LE image can be expressed by Eq. (1) except a proportional constant.

A "bone-canceled" DE image can be calculated from a pair of HE and LE images as the following,

$$P_{Bone-canceled}^{DE} = \ln(I^H) - w_s \ln(I^L) \quad (2)$$

where $w_s = \mu_{Bone}^H / \mu_{Bone}^L$ is the ratio of the bone attenuation coefficients to the HE beam and to the LE beam used as a weighting coefficient. In practice, because of the difference of imaging systems (such as difference in beam filtration and spectrum of energy, etc.), the calculated value of w_s is not necessarily the ideal value for a specific DE imaging study. In this study, we set up w_s from 0.05 to 1 with a step size of 0.05 in the calculation of bone-canceled DE images and chose the optimized

value to best eliminate the bony structures in the DE images. Substituting the I^L and I^H given by Eq. (1a) and (1b) into Eq. (2), one can derive the bone-canceled image as

$$P_{Bone-canceled}^{DE} = \ln(I_0^H) - w_s \ln(I_0^L) - t_{Lung}(\mu_{Lung}^H - w_s\mu_{Lung}^L) \\ - t_{soft-tissue}(\mu_{Soft-tissue}^H - w_s\mu_{Soft-tissue}^L) \quad (3)$$

For the concerned energy range of diagnostic imaging, the x-ray interaction with tissues is dominated by photoelectric absorption and Compton scattering. Attenuation coefficient can therefore be decomposed into two components as given by the following approximate form [14],

$$\mu(E) \approx \rho_e(C_p Z^{3.8}/E^{3.2} + f_{KN}(E)) \quad (4)$$

where $\rho_e C_p Z^{3.8}/E^{3.2}$ provides the photoelectric absorption coefficient with a fitting parameter of $C_p = 9.8 \times 10^{-24}$, photon energy E in keV [14] and Z as the effective atomic number while the Klein-Nishina function $f_{KN}(E)$ yields the electronic cross section of Compton scattering which depends only on E with ρ_e as the electron density. Combining Eq. (3) with Eq. (4) leads to Eq. (5).

$$P_{Bone-canceled}^{DE} = \ln(I_0^H) - w_s \ln(I_0^L) - (t_{Soft-tissue}\rho_{eSoft-tissue} \\ + t_{Lung}\rho_{eLung})\{[f_{KN}(E^H) - w_s f_{KN}(E^L)] \\ + [1/(E^H)^{3.2} - w_s/(E^L)^{3.2}]C_p(Z_{Water})^{3.8}\} \quad (5)$$

Here, we used Z_{Water} to replace $Z_{Soft-tissue}$ and Z_{Lung} due to the following fact. Given the definition of effective atomic number as $Z = (\sum w_i Z_i^{3.5})^{1/3.5}$, with w_i as the weight fraction of the element i of atomic number Z_i [15], the effective atomic number of soft-tissue and lung tissue can be found as 7.5666 and 7.5881, respectively, which are close to Z_{Water} at 7.6843 [16]. To correlate the grey-level values of pixels in the bone-canceled image with the characteristics of the tissues that the x-ray photons transport through, a parameter of radiological equivalent path length (EPL) is used which is usually defined as the summed products of the thickness Δd_i of a bone-excluding tissue component i and the ratio of electron density of the tissue component to that of water ρ_{ei} as given by Eq. (6).

$$EPL = \sum_i \Delta d_i \rho_{ei} \quad (6)$$

Hence, Eq. (5) can be simplified with EPL,

$$P_{Bone-canceled}^{DE} = \ln(I_0^H) - w_s \ln(I_0^L) - \rho_{eWater} \cdot EPL\{[f_{KN}(E^H) \\ - w_s f_{KN}(E^L)] + [1/(E^H)^{3.2} \\ - w_s/(E^L)^{3.2}]C_p(Z_{Water})^{3.8}\} \quad (7)$$

where EPL accounts for the accumulated equivalent path length that x-ray photons pass through except the tissue to be canceled, i.e., bone.

The model expressed in Eq. (7) correlates the grey-level values of pixels in the bone-canceled image with the characteristics of bone-excluding tissues in terms of the EPL and the photon energies clearly. Therefore, the dependence of the image quality on the tissue properties expressed by EPL and image acquisition parameters can be quantitatively analyzed.

2. Evaluation of image quality

The visibility of targeted structures in a radiograph is largely dependent upon the absolute signal difference and the noise in the image, which can be related to the parameter CNR as defined below,

$$CNR = (\overline{P_{object}} - \overline{P_{background}})/[0.5(\sigma_{object} + \sigma_{background})] \quad (8)$$

where $\overline{P_{object}}$ is the averaged grey-level values of pixels in an object region, and $\overline{P_{background}}$ is the averaged grey-level values of pixels in an adjacent background region. σ_{object} is the standard deviation (SD) of grey-level values in an object region, and $\sigma_{background}$ is the SD of grey-level values in an adjacent background region, which are calculated as the root-mean-square of the grey-level variance for all pixels in the regions respectively. CNR was used in this study for the quantitative evaluation of bone-canceled image quality.

3. Phantom study

We employed two phantoms to investigate the influence of the EPL on the DE image quality. HE and LE radiographs of the phantoms were acquired with the kV radiographic imaging unit of a CyberKnife system (G3, Version 7.1.1). The x-ray detector of the unit has a 20×20 cm^2 field of view (FOV) with a 392 µm pixel size. The geometry of the imaging unit is shown in Figure 1.

Two elliptic cylinder phantoms, a chest phantom (Model 002LFC, CIRS, Norfolk, VA) and an Xsight Lung Tracking (XLT) phantom (Model 18023, CIRS), were used to assess the impacts of the tissue EPL on the quality of bone-canceled image. The first phantom has dimensions of $30 \times 20 \times 30$ cm^3 and

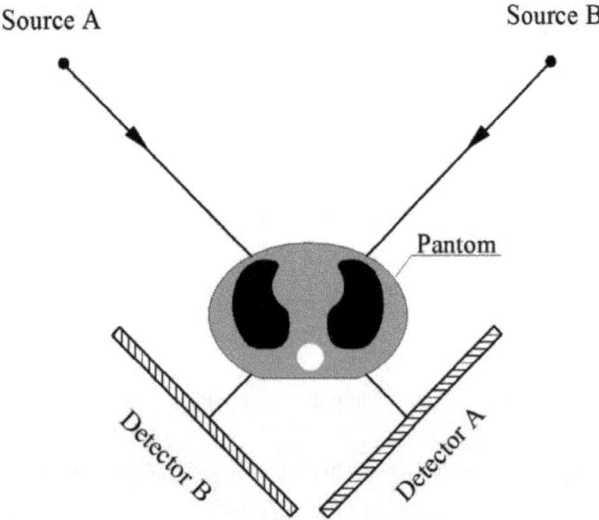

Figure 1. Geometric schematic of the radiographic imaging unit. The imaging system uses 2 diagnostic X-ray sources (Source A and Source B) mounted on the ceiling and paired with 2 flat panel detectors (Detector A and Detector B) with the same source-to-detector distance (SDD) of 3 m to acquire real-time digital radiographic images of the patient. The patient is imaged at 45 degree LAO (left anterior oblique) and RAO (right anterior oblique) angles to facilitate target localization in the 3D space.

simulates the structure of human chest consisting of three tissue equivalent components mimicking soft tissue (water), lung, and bone of which the relative electron densities are 1.002, 0.207, and 1.506, respectively. The second one has an elliptic cylinder configuration with dimensions of $30 \times 20 \times 18$ cm^3 and tissue-equivalent inserts mimicking cortical bone, lung, soft tissue, and a tumor, of which the relative electron densities are 1.782, 0.207, 1.002, and 1.028, respectively.

According to the published data [8], optimal DE image quality can be achieved with the beam energy combination of 120 kVp and 60 kVp for HE and LE images respectively. With this combination, the milliampere seconds (mAs) were set at 7.5 and 90 for the HE and LE images respectively in our phantom study for obtaining optimal image quality and avoiding overheating of the x-ray tubes during the image acquisition. The bone-canceled images of the chest phantom were obtained by combining the HE and LE images according to Eq. (2). In order to quantify the quality of bone-canceled images with CNRs, twelve ROIs of 12 pixels × 12 pixels in each bone-canceled image were identified with six as the object regions and six as the background regions. Each ROI was divided into 9 sub-areas for the calculation of mean value and SD of CNR. Then the CNRs were calculated using Eq. (8) to quantitatively analyze the impact of EPL. The EPL difference between an object region and a background region normalized by the averaged EPL level of the two regions (ΔEPL) was derived and the correlation between the CNR and ΔEPL was established and tested by evaluating the agreement of the calculated relationship between ΔEPL and CNR among the two different phantoms.

The EPL of each ROI is the averaged value of the region and was calculated according to the method described in the next section.

4. Calculation of EPL

EPL calculation was performed in the volumes of objects represented by their 3D CT image data sets. We used the ray tracing algorithm [17] to track the exact radiological path by propagating the incident x-ray photons through an object's 3D voxels. Following steps were used in the calculation of EPL. First, the 3D volume of a calibration phantom with known electron densities (Model 062, CIRS, Norfolk, VA) was reconstructed from the CT image data acquired with a Brilliance Big Bore CT simulator (Philips, Cleveland, OH) at 120 kVp and 400 mAs. This allowed us to build a look-up table to correlate the electron density of the object with the CT numbers in the 3D image sets acquired by the same scanner. The next step was to identify all voxels on the trajectories of x-ray photons propagating through a study phantom, the XLT or chest phantom, from source to the corresponding pixels of a flat panel detector placed behind the phantom. Once the voxels were identified we could retrieve the electron density values of these voxels from the look-up table based on their CT numbers and distinguish the bony structures at the same time. Finally, the values of EPL on the photon trajectories were summed by integrating along the path excluding bones since they were performed on the bone-canceled images.

5. Feasibility study with patient data

Image data from 10 patients with lung cancers who underwent SBRT with the CyberKnife system were used with the approval of the Ethics Committee of Tianjin Cancer Hospital (#2013-10) and the patients' written consents. Before including a patient in the study, tumor movement range due to respiratory motion was evaluated with fluoroscopic imaging first to minimize the effect of motion artifacts. Patients with tumor movement ranges of less than

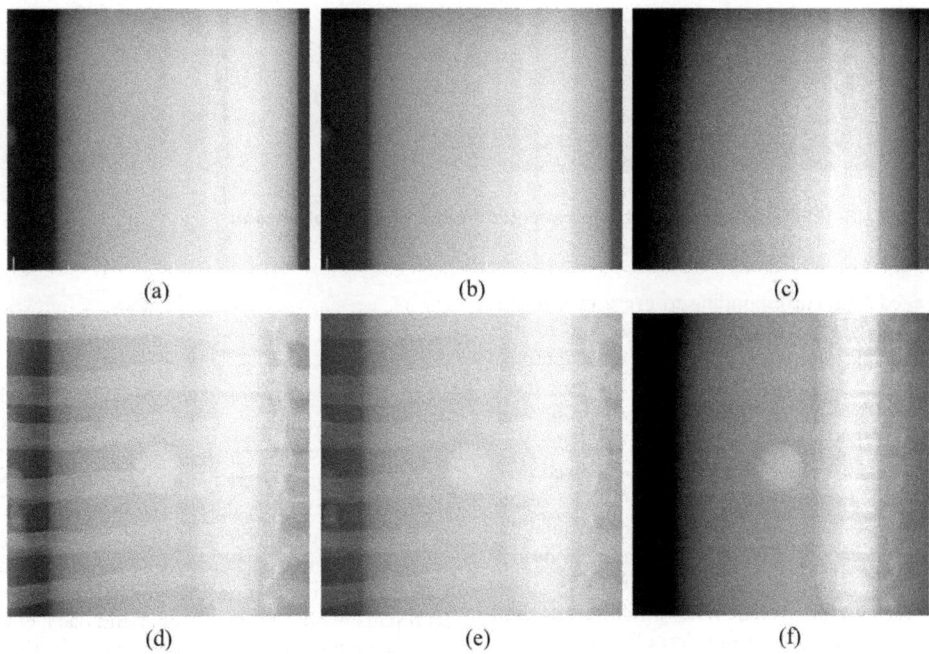

Figure 2. Radiographic images of chest phantom. (a), (b), and (c) are the images of chest phantom at 60 kVp, 120 kVp, and the bone-canceled image by combining (a) and (b), respectively. (d), (e), and (f) are the images of XLT phantom at 60 kVp, 120 kVp, and the bone-canceled image by combining (d) and (e), respectively.

12 mm in a respiration cycle were selected and then trained for holding their body still and exercising shallower breathing before the image acquisition. Radiographic images of HE and LE were obtained sequentially during the radiation delivery at the same phases of respiration which was guaranteed by the synchrony respiratory tracking system. We also chose to only include patients who had nodule size ≥ 10 mm in diameter as the identification of small nodules is still problematic for DE imaging [18]. Image data from 10 patients were selected. Each patient had at least three gold fiducial markers implanted before their CT simulation for treatment planning. And the maximum displacement of the tumors was checked with the markers to be ≤ 0.23 mm between the HE and LE images at the same phases of respiration.

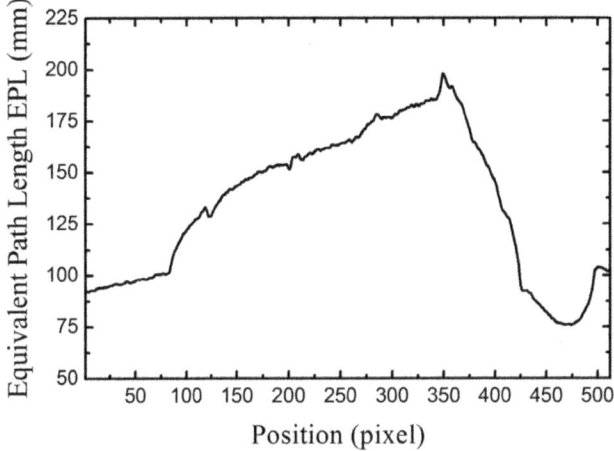

Figure 3. Averaged EPL per pixel column in the bone-canceled image of chest phantom.

The DRRs generated with the simulation CT image data for the image guidance of the treatment were used for comparison in the study, which carried the projected gross tumor volume (GTV) contours delineated in the CT images by an experienced radiation oncologist. HE and LE images (120 kVp, 100 mA, 75 ms and 60 kVp, 250 mA, 150 ms) were acquired with the image guidance unit before the start of treatment. Then bone-canceled images were obtained using the above discussed method and the GTVs were delineated in the bone-canceled images using an algorithm for automatically detecting pulmonary nodules in chest x-ray images [19]. The averaged displacement of the gold marker centroids between in the DRR and in the bone-canceled image was used as the reference for the GTV position variance analysis for each patient. The difference between the variation of the centroid of the delineated GTV in the DRR and in the bone-canceled image and the averaged variation of gold marker centroids in the two image sets was used to quantify the accuracy and evaluate the feasibility of the proposed DE imaging method for GTV localization. To quantitatively evaluate the improvement of tumor contrast, CNRs of the tumors in the radiographs at LE and HE, and in the bone-canceled DE images were calculated respectively using the same method as described in Section 2.3.

Statistical analysis was performed with GraphPad Prism 6 (GraphPad Software, Inc., La Jolla, CA). A 2-sided Student's t-test was used to compare the displacement between fiducial centroids and the GTV centroids, and evaluate the improvement of CNR of tumors with the DE imaging technique. A p-value of less than or equal to 0.05 was regarded as statistically significant.

Results

1. Influence of ΔEPL on CNR

Figures 2(a) and 2(b) show the planar x-ray images of the chest phantom at 60 kVp and 120 kVp, respectively, and Figure 2 (c) is the bone-canceled image calculated from these two images.

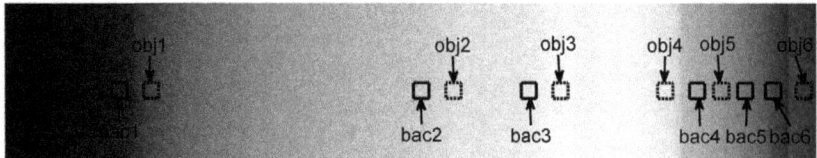

Figure 4. ROIs used in CNR-ΔEPL analysis of the bone-canceled image of chest phantom.

Figure 3 is the averaged EPL corresponding to every column in the image (512 columns) which was calculated according to the method described above. By comparing Figure 2(c) and Figure 3, it can be observed that the EPL is proportional to the grey-level value of the corresponding pixel, which corroborates with the model expressed in Eq. (7). Measurement of CNR in Figure 2(c) and data fitting using the linear-least-squares method showed that a linear relationship exists between CNR and ΔEPL. The result was evaluated with the parameter of coefficient of determination R^2, which indicates how well measured data fit a statistical model and ranges from 0 to 1 with 1 indicating a perfect fit. The evaluation yielded a very high R^2 value (0.99), which means that the CNR in bone-canceled image as a function of ΔEPL can be expressed by Eq. (9). Figure 4 plots the CNR against ΔEPL, the dots represent measured data and the solid line is the modeled result.

$$CNR = 22.35 \times \Delta EPL + \delta \qquad (9)$$

Because of noise, CNR can fluctuate in DE image for tissue trajectories with same EPL which is represented by δ in Eq. (9). Figure 2 (d) and (e) show the planar x-ray images of the XLT phantom acquired at 60 kVp and 120 kVp, respectively, and Figure 2(f) is the bone-canceled image. The CNR dependence on ΔEPL as expressed in Eq. (9) was also verified with the XLT phantom with the slope given by 23.29 and the difference was 4.2% between the two phantoms. Therefore, for the image guidance unit, the correlation of CNR with ΔEPL can be written as

$$CNR = k \times \Delta EPL + \delta \qquad (10)$$

where k is a system parameter with value around 22.8 and equal to the averaged value of the slope for the two phantoms.

Figure 4 presents the bone-canceled image with ROIs of the chest phantom selected for the CNR calculation, and the corresponding CNR values are indicated in Figure 5. The squares in dash line are the object ROIs (marked as obj) while the ones in solid line are the background ROIs (marked as bac). By visual inspection, one can find that the visual differences between the ROI pairs of obj2 and bac2, obj3 and bac3, obj5 and bac5 cannot be observed; the visual differences between the ROI pairs of obj1 and bac1, obj4 and bac4, obj6 and bac6 can be observed. And the smallest observable difference in the image is between the pair of obj6 and bac6, of which the CNR is 2.57±0.34 (Mean ± SD). According to Figure 5, when CNR = 2.91 (2.57+0.34), ΔEPL is 0.08, therefore, when ΔEPL is greater than 0.08, the difference between the object and the background in the bone-canceled image can be discriminated. In comparison, objects and backgrounds corresponding to ΔEPL less than 0.08 are visually indistinguishable.

2. Study with patient data

Figure 6 shows the DRRs, radiographic images and bone-canceled images of one of the patients. Calculation of CNR for the tumors showed that the mean value and SD of CNR of the 10 tumors was 5.22±2.96 in LE images, 7.43±3.33 in HE images and 8.29±3.56 in DE images, respectively. The p-value was 0.16 for the CNR in HE images versus in LE images, 0.01 for the CNR in DE images versus in LE images, and 0.03 for the CNR in DE images versus in HE images, respectively. This indicates that tumor contrast in the bone-canceled images is improved significantly as compared with those in the original planar radiographic images. The GTVs in the DRRs were projected from the planning RT data which were delineated and confirmed by an experienced radiation oncologist. And the contours in the radiographs were delineated with the automatic tumor detection algorithm as discussed above. Using the displacement of GTV centroid to represent the variation of tumor location, we compared the displacements of the fiducial centroids and the GTV centroids. The results are shown in Table 1. With a 2-sided Student's t-test, we found the p-value was 0.53 indicating that the variation measured by the two methods does not exhibit significant difference.

Discussion

Dual-energy imaging technique holds promise to provide valuable information for improving target or tumor localization. However, its implementation as a practical clinical tool requires a clear understanding of the underlying mechanism for optimizing the image acquisition process and quality assurance. Specifically

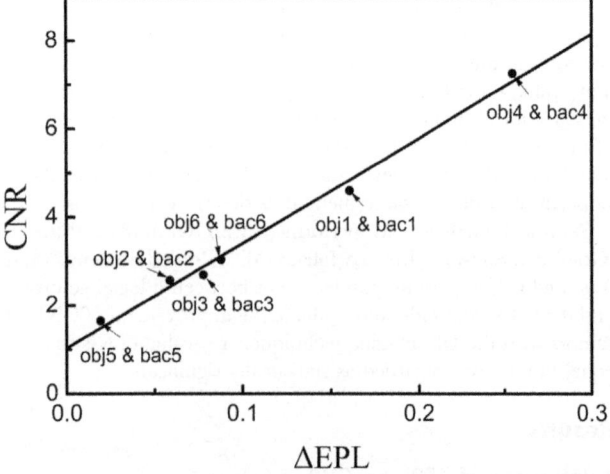

Figure 5. CNR versus ΔEPL in the bone-canceled image of chest phantom.

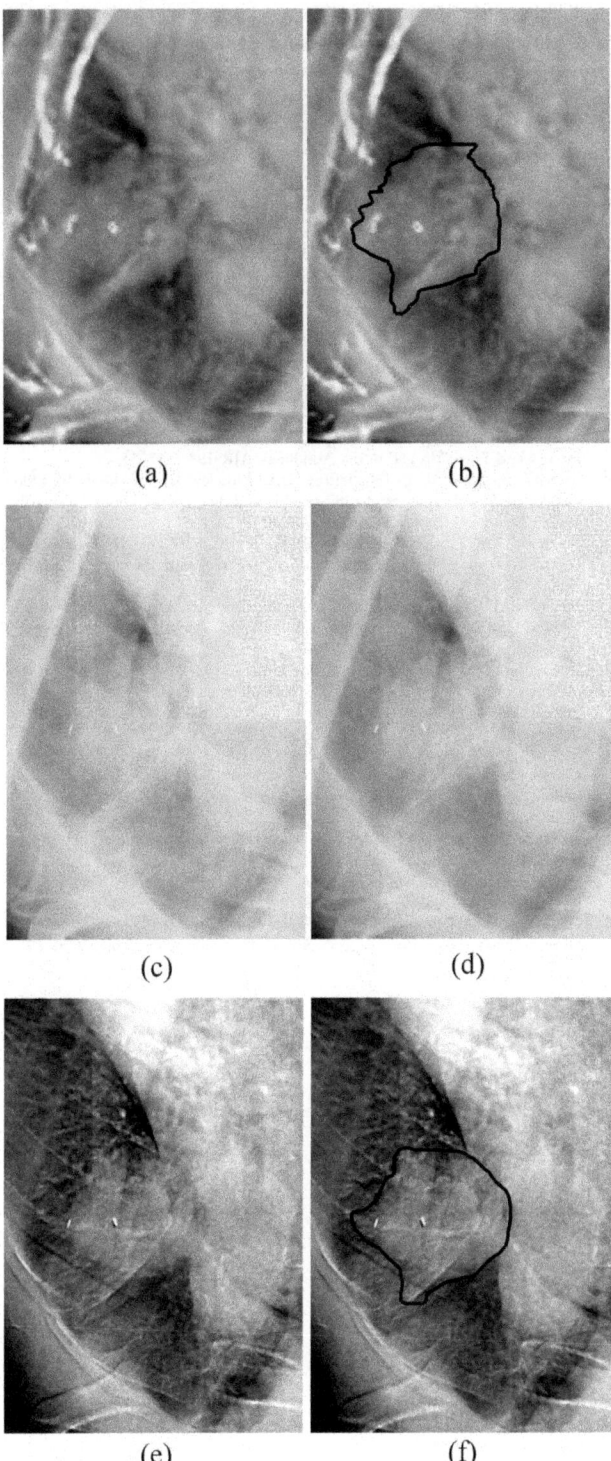

(a)   **(b)**

(c)   **(d)**

(e)   **(f)**

Figure 6. DRRs and radiographs of a patient. (a) DRR of a patient, (b) DRR with the projected GTV contour, (c) radiograph at LE, (d) radiograph at HE, (e) bone-canceled image by pairing two original radiographs, and (f) bone-canceled image with the GTV contour automatically segmented.

Table 1. Displacements of GTV centroids and fiducial markers.

Patient	D[a] of GTV centroids (mm)	D[a] of fiducials (mm)
1	4.22	4.22
2	6.36	4.36
3	5.63	3.05
4	6.67	6.06
5	9.37	7.82
6	6.09	6.63
7	1.11	0.40
8	15.03	11.94
9	3.11	3.15
10	2.81	2.50
Mean[b]	6.04	5.10
SD[c]	3.93	3.26

[a]D: Displacement.
[b]Mean: mean value.
[c]SD: standard deviation.

derived an expression for the image contrast CNR in terms of EPL which allows quantification of the target localization in a DE image.

Previously published studies focused mainly on the effect of phantom size on the quality of image. For example, Kappadath et al. employed a phantom consisting of different aluminum strips to simulate calcifications and breast-tissue-equivalent materials to evaluate the CNR in tissue-canceled DE images under the conditions of different strip thicknesses or glandular ratios [9]. The results showed that the CNR increases with increasing aluminum strip thickness and decreases with increasing glandular ratio in DE image, which is consistent with our results. However, the strip thickness used in that study differs from the realistic clinical situations. In contrast we utilized the anthropomorphic phantoms and the EPL to study the influence of intrinsic tissue properties with of improved clinical relevance. Although the qualitative relationship between EPL and CNR agrees with previous studies, the values of CNR obtained in our study differ because of the large variation in the imaging systems. As the image quality is influenced by detector performance such as the modulation transfer function (MTF), the noise-power spectrum (NPS), and the noise-equivalent quanta (NEQ), the image quality of different imaging system and CNR can vary widely. Therefore, it is necessary to calibrate the CNR-ΔEPL curve according to the specifications of each imaging system.

Finally, we would like to point out that the feasibility study with data of 10 patients has indicated that the tumor in the bone-canceled image as shown in Figure 6 can be easily seen with higher contrast than those in the planar radiographs. We expect that the DE imaging technique has the potential as a powerful tool for tumor localization. There are other advanced image processing methods and imaging techniques, such as rib suppression method [20] or MRI, which could provide similar image quality or superior soft tissue discrimination. But the feasibility for tumor localization in radiotherapy treatment with these advanced methods yet to be quantitatively evaluated.

one needs to quantitatively characterize the intrinsic tissue properties to accurately assess the discrimination of targets. For this purpose, we have analyzed the DE imaging process and

Conclusion

CNR is linearly dependant on ΔEPL in bone-canceled DE images and the relationship can be shown with a mathematical model as given by Eq. (10). The contrast for tumors in the bone-canceled images is improved significantly as compared with the one in the planar radiographic images and the accuracy of tumor localization using the DE imaging technique has been demonstrated to be comparable with that of using fiducial makers. Therefore, it is feasible to apply the technique for tumor localization in radiotherapy. Comprehensive clinical study with more patient data to model DE image quality with intrinsic tissue properties for tumor localization is ongoing and the results will be presented after completion of the study.

Author Contributions

Conceived and designed the experiments: JH YF PW. Performed the experiments: YD ZY PW. Analyzed the data: JH YF XW XZ GW. Wrote the paper: JH XH YF. Final approval of the version to be published: YF.

References

1. Sabol JM, Avinash GB, Nicolas F, Claus BEH, Zhao J, et al. (2001) The development and characterization of a dual-energy subtraction imaging system for chest radiography based on CsI: Tl amorphous silicon flat-panel technology. Proc. SPIE 2001: 399–408.
2. Ducote JL, Xu T, Molloi S. (2007) Dual-energy cardiac imaging: an image quality and dose comparison for a flat-panel detector and x-ray image intensifier. Phys. Med Biol 52(1):183–96.
3. Arvanitis CD, Speller R. (2009) Quantitative contrast-enhanced mammography for contrast medium kinetics studies. Phys Med Biol 54(20):6041–64.
4. Murphy MJ, Adler JR, Bodduluri M, Dooley J, Forster K, et al. (2000) Image-guided radiosurgery for the spine and pancreas. Comput Aided Surg 5(4):278–88.
5. Samei E, Flynn MJ, Eyler WR. (1999) Detection of subtle lung nodules: relative influence of quantum and anatomic noise on chest radiographs. Radiology 213(3):727–34.
6. Collins BT, Erickson K, Reichner CA, Collins SP, Gagnon GJ, et al. (2007) Radical stereotactic radiosurgery with real-time tumor motion tracking in the treatment of small peripheral lung tumors. Radiat Oncol 2(39): 2(39), 717X–2.
7. Williams DB, Siewerdsen JH, Tward DJ, Paul NS, Dhanantwari AC, et al. (2007) Optimal kVp selection for dual-energy imaging of the chest: Evaluation by task-specific observer preference tests. Med Phys 34(10):3619–25.
8. Shkumat NA, Siewerdsen JH, Dhanantwari AC, Williams DB, Richard S, et al. (2007) Optimization of image acquisition techniques for dual-energy imaging of the chest. Med Phys 34(10):3904–15.
9. Kappadath SC, Shaw CC. (2004) Quantitative evaluation of dual-energy digital mammography for calcification imaging. Phys Med Biol 49(12):2563–76.
10. Carton AK, Ullberg C, Lindman K, Acciavatti R, Francke T, et al. (2010) Optimization of a dual-energy contrast-enhanced technique for a photon-counting digital breast tomosynthesis system: I. A theoretical model. Med Phys 37(11):5896–5907.
11. Richard S, Siewerdsen JH. (2006) Optimization of dual-energy imaging systems using generalized NEQ and imaging task. Med Phys 34(1):127–39.
12. Yeh BM, Shepherd JA, Wang ZJ, Teh HS, Hartman R, et al. (2009) Dual-Energy and Low-kVp CT in the Abdomen. AJR 193(1):47–54.
13. Richard S, Siewerdsen JH, Jaffray DA, Moseley DJ, Bakhtiar B. (2005) Generalized DQE analysis of radiographic and dual-energy imaging using flat-panel detectors. Med Phys 32(5):1397–413.
14. Lehmann LA, Alvarez RE, Macovski A, Brody WR, Pelc NJ, et al. (1981) Generalized image combinations in dual KVP digital radiography. Med Phys 8(5):659–67.
15. Bazatova M, Carrier JF, Beautieu L, Verhaegen F. (2008) Tissue segmentation in Monte Carlo treatment planning: A simulation study using dual-energy CT images. Radiother Oncol 86(1):93–98.
16. International Commission on Radiation Units and Measurements. (1989) Tissue substitutes in radiation dosimetry and measurement. ICRU Report 44.
17. Siddon RL. (1985) Fast calculation of exact radiological path for a three-dimensional CT array. Med Phys 12(2):252–55.
18. Szucs-Farkas Z, Patak MA, Yuksel-Hatz S, Ruder T, Vock P. (2008) Single-exposure dual-energy subtraction chest radiography: Detection of pulmonary nodules and masses in clinical practice. Eur Radiol 18(1):24–31.
19. Schilham AMR, van Ginneken B, Loog M. (2006) Computer-aided diagnosis system for detection of lung nodules in chest radiographs with an evaluation on a public database. Med Image Anal 10(2):247–58.
20. Szucs-Farkas Z, Schick A, Cullmann JL, Ebner1 L, Megyeri B et al (2013) Comparison of Dual-Energy Subtraction and Electronic Bone Suppression Combined With Computer-Aided Detection on Chest Radiographs: Effect on Human Observers' Performance in Nodule Detection. AJR 200(5):1006–13.

24

^{99m}Tc-3P$_4$-RGD$_2$ Scintimammography in the Assessment of Breast Lesions: Comparative Study with ^{99m}Tc-MIBI

Qingjie Ma[1♥], Bin Chen[1♥], Shi Gao[1], Tiefeng Ji[1], Qiang Wen[1], Yan Song[1], Lei Zhu[2], Zheli Xu[1], Lin Liu[1]*

1 China-Japan Union Hospital, Jilin University, Changchun, China, 2 State Key Laboratory of Molecular Vaccinology and Molecular Diagnostics & Center for Molecular Imaging and Translational Medicine, School of Public Health, Xiamen University, Xiamen, China

Abstract

Purpose: To compare the potential application of ^{99m}Tc-3P-Arg-Gly-Asp (^{99m}Tc-3P$_4$-RGD$_2$) scintimammography (SMM) and ^{99m}Tc-methoxyisobutylisonitrile (^{99m}Tc-MIBI) SMM for the differentiation of malignant from benign breast lesions.

Method: Thirty-six patients with breast masses on physical examination and/or suspicious mammography results that required fine needle aspiration cytology biopsy (FNAB) were included in the study. ^{99m}Tc-3P$_4$-RGD$_2$ and ^{99m}Tc-MIBI SMM were performed with single photon emission computed tomography (SPECT) at 60 min and 20 min respectively after intravenous injection of 738±86 MBq radiotracers on a separate day. Images were evaluated by the tumor to non-tumor localization ratios (T/NT). Receiver operating characteristic (ROC) curve analysis was performed on each radiotracer to calculate the cut-off values of quantitative indices and to compare the diagnostic performance for the ability to differentiate malignant from benign diseases.

Results: The mean T/NT ratio of ^{99m}Tc-3P$_4$-RGD$_2$ in malignant lesions was significantly higher than that in benign lesions (3.54±1.51 vs. 1.83±0.98, p<0.001). The sensitivity, specificity, and accuracy of ^{99m}Tc-3P$_4$-RGD$_2$ SMM were 89.3%, 90.9% and 89.7%, respectively, with a T/NT cut-off value of 2.40. The mean T/NT ratio of ^{99m}Tc-MIBI in malignant lesions was also significantly higher than that in benign lesions (2.86±0.99 vs. 1.51±0.61, p<0.001). The sensitivity, specificity and accuracy of ^{99m}Tc-MIBI SMM were 87.5%, 72.7% and 82.1%, respectively, with a T/NT cut-off value of 1.45. According to the ROC analysis, the area under the curve for ^{99m}Tc-3P$_4$-RGD$_2$ SMM (area = 0.851) was higher than that for ^{99m}Tc-MIBI SMM (area = 0.781), but the statistical difference was not significant.

Conclusion: ^{99m}Tc-3P$_4$-RGD$_2$ SMM does not provide any significant advantage over the established ^{99m}Tc-MIBI SMM for the detection of primary breast cancer. The T/NT ratio of ^{99m}Tc-3P$_4$-RGD$_2$ SMM was significantly higher than that of ^{99m}Tc-MIBI SMM. Both tracers could offer an alternative method for elucidating non-diagnostic mammograms.

Editor: Jason Mulvenna, Queensland Institute of Medical Research, Australia

Funding: This research was supported by the National Natural Science Foundation of China (NSFC) projects (51373144, 81271606 and 81201129), and Research Fund of Science and Technology Department of Jilin Province (201015185 and 201201041). The funders had no role in study design, data collection and analysis, decision to publish, or preparation of the manuscript.

Competing Interests: The authors have declared that no competing interests exist.

* Email: liulinjlu@163.com

♥ These authors contributed equally to this work.

Introduction

Breast cancer continues to be a major public health problem all over the world. The American Cancer Society estimates that there will be about 296,980 new cases of breast cancer in 2013, which is expected to account for 14% of female cancer deaths.

A realistic strategy for the reduction of breast cancer mortality rates and timely treatment is to detect the disease while it is still in an early stage.[1,2]. The most common screening method for early breast cancer is mammography, which is very sensitive in the detection of malignant breast disease. However in several groups of breast cancer patients, including those with fibroadenoma breasts, post implants, mastectomy or severe dysplasia, mammography has a low predictive value (20%–30%) and is not accurate, requiring patients to undergo histopathological examinations for a definitive diagnosis [3,4]. To improve diagnostic accuracy, new methods are being studied as alternatives to mammography. Over the last twenty years, Scintimammography (SMM) has been introduced as an adjunct modality to present imaging modalities for breast cancer imaging [5]. In addition to the imaging modality, several radiopharmaceuticals have also been investigated for diagnostic imaging procedures in patients with suspected breast cancer [6]. ^{18}F-fluorodeoxyglucose (FDG) positron emission tomography (PET) [7] is proven to be the most effective in detection of breast cancer for diagnosis, staging and restaging, but its use is limited by the high cost of equipment and lack of general availability, especially in developing countries. Alternatively, single photon emission computed tomography (SPECT) is more widely used with a much lower cost worldwide.

^{99m}Tc-methoxyisobutylisonitrile (^{99m}Tc-MIBI) is an important tracer for oncological applications and has been widely used in breast tumor imaging. However, this tracer originated from nuclear medicine for cardiac imaging and was not specifically designed for tumor imaging. The exact mechanism of uptake in breast cancer cells is still not entirely clear. It is reported that ^{99m}Tc-MIBI is concentrated in cancer cells by an energy-requiring transport mechanism, specifically by transmembrane electrical potentials, as well as by non-specific mechanisms, and the tracer is stored within the mitochondria [8].

It is well documented that integrin $\alpha v \beta 3$ plays a critical role in the regulation of tumor angiogenesis and metastasis [9,10]. The integrin is upregulated on activated endothelial cells and is highly expressed in tumor cells of various tumor types, including breast cancer [11,12]. Over the past decade, radiolabeled Arg-Gly-Asp (RGD) peptides and analogs that specifically target integrin $\alpha v \beta 3$ have been intensively investigated for noninvasive imaging of tumors in pre-clinical and clinical studies [13–19]. We previously developed the $\alpha v \beta 3$-specific tracer ^{99m}Tc-3P-Arg-Gly-Asp (^{99m}Tc-3P$_4$-RGD$_2$) for SPECT and already demonstrated that ^{99m}Tc-3P$_4$-RGD$_2$ SPECT allows specific imaging of $\alpha v \beta 3$ expression with high accuracy in detecting malignant solitary pulmonary nodules (SPNs), esophageal cancer, and malignant gliomas [20–22].

In this study, we compare the diagnostic value of ^{99m}Tc-3P$_4$-RGD$_2$ SMM with ^{99m}Tc-MIBI SMM for the detection of breast cancer by receiver operating characteristic (ROC) curve analysis.

Materials and Methods

Patients

Thirty-six patients with breast masses on physical examination and/or suspicious mammographic findings that required fine needle aspiration cytology biopsy (FNAB) were included in this study. The patient mean age was 41.9 ± 12.2 years (age range 22–65 years. All patients were referred for ^{99m}Tc-MIBI and ^{99m}Tc-3P$_4$-RGD$_2$ SMM on an individual basis. The time interval between the two imaging procedures was 3.2 ± 1.4 days. Finally, ^{99m}Tc-3P$_4$-RGD$_2$ and ^{99m}Tc-MIBI SMM results were compared with each other and with the final histopathological diagnosis. Inclusion and exclusion criteria for entry into the study are summarized in Table 1. This study was approved by the Ethics Committee of China-Japan Union Hospital of Jilin University. Informed written consent to participate in the SMM studies was obtained from all patients.

Scintimammography protocol

Radiolabeling and quality control procedures for 3P$_4$-RGD$_2$ were performed as described previously [20]. Both 3P$_4$-RGD$_2$ and MIBI (ShiHong Drug Development Center, Beijing, China) were radiolabelled with 738 ± 86 MBq ^{99m}technetium and thereafter

administered via a single intravenous bolus injection in the contralateral arm to the affected breast, followed by a 10 mL saline flush. The effective radiation dose to the body of ^{99m}Tc-3P$_4$-RGD$_2$ and ^{99m}Tc-MIBI were 2.89 ± 0.34 mSv and 5.83 ± 0.67 mSv, respectively [23,24]. ^{99m}Tc-3P$_4$-RGD$_2$ and ^{99m}Tc-MIBI SMM were performed at 60 min and 20 min after intravenous injection, respectively. Patients were in supine position with raised arms during imaging.

SPECT was performed using a double-head γ camera (Precedence, Philips Healthcare), equipped with low-energy parallel hole collimators. The matrix was 128×128 pixels, and the photopeak was centered at 140 keV with a symmetrical 20% window. Imaging with both radiotracers was performed using 6° angular steps in a 20 s time frame. Distance between the breast and detector was minimized.

Data analysis

Both ^{99m}Tc-3P$_4$-RGD$_2$ and ^{99m}Tc-MIBI SMM uptake were evaluated by semiquantitative analysis. Regions of interest (ROIs) were drawn around the tumor and an area of normal breast tissue in the same breast on lateral images and used to determine the tumor to non-tumor ratios (T/NT) of ^{99m}Tc-3P$_4$-RGD$_2$ and ^{99m}Tc-MIBI.

All numerical results are reported as mean values with standard deviations (SDs). Student's t test was used for statistical comparison of quantitative indices between the malignant and benign breast disease groups. The IBM SPSS Statistics19 software was used to determine cut-off values of quantitative indices in the detection of primary breast cancer. The incremental diagnostic value of quantitative indices analysis was performed using calculated areas under the curve (AUCs) in ROC analysis. Statistical significance was defined as $p < 0.05$.

Results

Samples for histological examination were obtained by surgery in 28 patients and by core needle biopsy in eight patients. Breast cancer was confirmed in 26 patients and resulted in a total of 28 cancer lesions with diameters ranging from 0.3 cm to 7.9 cm (mean $\pm$ SD: 2.86 ± 1.73 cm). Benign breast disease was found in 10 patients with a total of 11 benign lesions ranging in diameter from 0.4 cm to 6.5 cm (mean $\pm$ SD: 2.83 ± 1.91 cm). In this study, the yielding breast cancer prevalence was 71.8% (Table 2).

We observed high ^{99m}Tc-3P$_4$-RGD$_2$ uptake in breast cancer and low ^{99m}Tc-3P$_4$-RGD$_2$ uptake in benign lesions (Fig. 1A). In ^{99m}Tc-3P$_4$-RGD$_2$ SMM, the T/NT of breast cancer was 3.54 ± 1.51 and that of benign lesions was 1.83 ± 0.98. The difference was statistically significant ($p < 0.001$). Similarly in ^{99m}Tc-MIBI SMM, high MIBI uptake was observed in breast cancer while low MIBI uptake was detected in benign lesions

Table 1. Inclusion and exclusion criteria of study.

Inclusion Criteria	Exclusion Criteria
Female	Pregnancy
Not pregnant	Recurrent disease
Suspicious lesion of the breast	Pervious mastectomy
Recommendation for excision biopsy after mammography	Fine needle aspiration within 1 week prior to scintimammography
Informed consent from the patient	Previous chemotherapy
	Medically unstable patient (severe arrhythmia, heart failure or recent surgery)

Table 2. Scintimammography results versus final histopathological diagnosis of 36 patients.

Patient	Age (years)	Diameter (cm)	RGD (T/NT)	MIBI (T/NT)	Histopathological Diagnosis
1	58	2.8	4.55	2.70	Invasive ductal
2	43	4.2	2.81	1.90	Invasive lobular
3	26	0.6	1.31	1.02	Invasive ductal
4	52	3.2	3.51	1.70	DCIS
5	53	2.5	5.70	3.10	Invasive ductal
6	65	1.8	3.33	1.90	Invasive ductal
7	45	0.9	2.71	1.54	Invasive ductal
8	59	7.9/3.0	4.24/3.32	3.51/1.85	Invasive ductal/Invasive ductal
9	49	0.3	1.29	1.14	Invasive ductal
10	49	1.8	2.91	1.68	Invasive ductal
11	33	3.7	2.48	2.33	Invasive ductal
12	23	2.5	5.04	3.65	Invasive ductal
13	36	0.4	1.02	1.23	Invasive ductal
14	29	6.0	8.27	4.87	Invasive lobular
15	31	2.2	2.96	1.31	DCIS
16	56	4.2	3.82	2.08	Invasive ductal
17	41	3.5	5.62	4.21	Invasive mucinous
18	37	3.8	4.20	2.10	Invasive ductal
19	22	4.5	2.52	1.62	Invasive ductal
20	31	1.7/0.8	4.12/2.49	1.85/1.91	Invasive ductal/DCIS
21	39	4.1	3.34	2.17	Invasive ductal
22	61	1.2	3.40	3.74	Invasive ductal
23	46	3.3	2.99	1.61	Invasive mucinous
24	58	2.9	5.23	3.21	Invasive ductal
25	27	2.0	3.01	1.60	Invasive lobular
26	44	4.2	2.79	1.82	Invasive ductal
27	41	4.3	1.11	1.34	Fibroadenoma
28	28	2.1	4.47	2.58	Fibroadenoma with mastitis
29	31	6.5/0.7	1.92/1.32	1.26/1.10	Fibroadenoma/ductal ectasia
30	47	3.2	1.34	2.81	Fibroadenoma
31	29	1.8	1.43	1.37	Fibrocystic disease
32	54	5.2	2.31	1.22	Fibroadenoma
33	49	3.3	1.1	1.09	Fibroadenoma
34	37	1.2	1.85	1.69	Fibroadenoma
35	25	2.4	2.17	1.02	Fibrocystic disease
36	55	0.4	1.08	1.17	Ductal ectasia

DCIS: ductal carcinoma in situ.

(Fig. 1B). The T/NT of breast cancer was 2.86 ± 0.99 and that of benign lesions was 1.51 ± 0.61. The difference was statistically significant ($p < 0.001$).

^{99m}Tc-3P$_4$-RGD$_2$ SMM was false negative in 3 breast cancer of invasive ductal which was the same as ^{99m}Tc-MIBI SMM. The tumor size was 0.6 cm or smaller in the long axis diameter. One patient with ductal carcinoma in situ (DCIS) in the long axis diameter of 2.2 cm was clear detected by ^{99m}Tc-3P$_4$-RGD$_2$ SMM, but not with ^{99m}Tc-MIBI SMM (Fig. 2). ^{99m}Tc-MIBI SMM was false positive in 3 benign lesions. Of the false positive cases, two were fibroadenoma and one was fibroadenoma with mastitis. The fibroadenoma with mastitis was also false positive in ^{99m}Tc-3P$_4$-RGD$_2$ SMM (Fig. 3).

ROC analyses were performed to determine the optimal cut-off values of both ^{99m}Tc-3P$_4$-RGD$_2$ and ^{99m}Tc-MIBI SMM T/NT for the detection of malignant breast cancer. When a cut-off value was used based on the ROC analysis, the sensitivity, specificity and accuracy of ^{99m}Tc-3P$_4$-RGD$_2$ SMM were 89.3%, 90.9% and 89.7%, respectively (cutoff = 2.40 of T/NT), and those of ^{99m}Tc-MIBI SMM were 87.5%, 72.7% and 82.1%, respectively (cutoff = 1.46 of T/NT). The empirical ROC areas, which estimate the overall diagnostic performance, did not differ significantly among the two diagnostic analyses (Fig. 4). The value was 0.851 for ^{99m}Tc-3P$_4$-RGD$_2$ SMM and 0.781 for ^{99m}Tc-MIBI SMM.

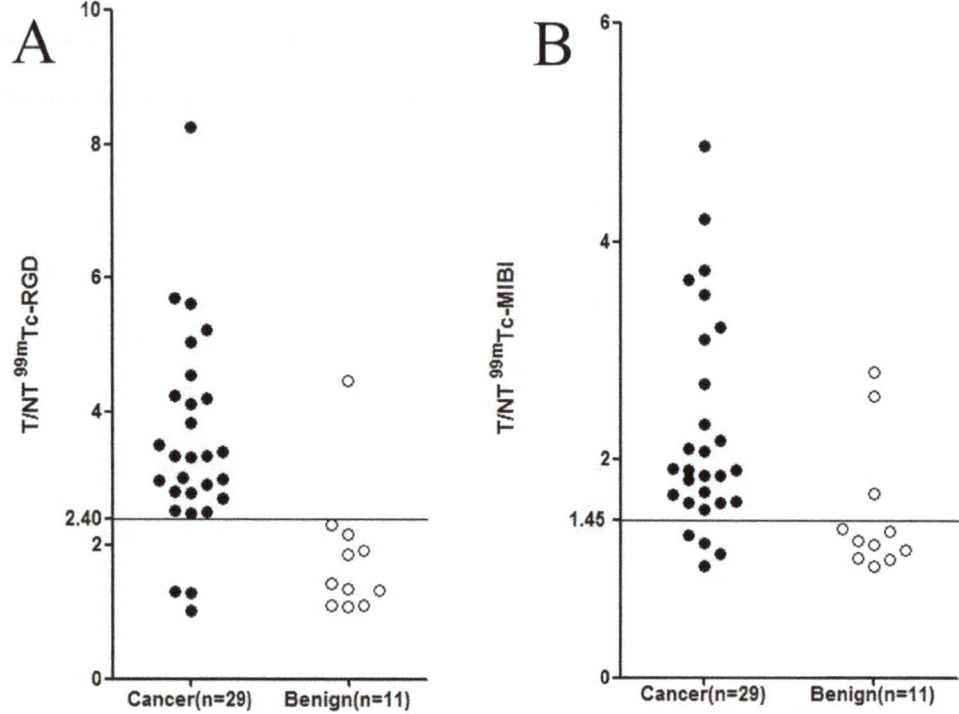

Figure 1. T/NT for ^{99m}Tc-RGD and ^{99m}Tc-MIBI in malignant and benign tumors. (A) The T/NT for ^{99m}Tc-RGD in breast cancer was significantly higher than that in benign lesions (p<0.001). (B) The T/NT for ^{99m}Tc-MIBI in breast cancer was significantly higher than that in benign lesions (p<0.001).

Discussion

Over the last twenty years, SMM has been proposed to be a complementary tool to mammography in the diagnosis of primary breast cancer [5]. An already widely used radiopharmaceutical, ^{99m}Tc-MIBI appears to be a suitable SMM scanning agent. Many publications have reported favorable sensitivity and specificity results, 84%–96% and 72%–94%, respectively, for ^{99m}Tc-MIBI scintigraphy in the diagnosis of breast cancer [25–32]. ^{99m}Tc-3P$_4$-RGD$_2$ is a new agent with a high affinity for the $\alpha v \beta 3$ integrin, a

receptor associated with angiogenesis. In our previous study, we found that ^{99m}Tc-3P$_4$-RGD$_2$ could accumulate in a variety of malignant lesions [20–22]. However, a comparative study between ^{99m}Tc-3P$_4$-RGD$_2$ and ^{99m}Tc-MIBI SMM has not been previously reported.

In this present study, to differentiate benign from malignant lesions, ROC analyses were performed to determine the optimal cut-off values of T/NT of ^{99m}Tc-3P$_4$-RGD$_2$ and ^{99m}Tc-MIBI SMM. When T/NT of 2.40 was used as a cut-off point, the

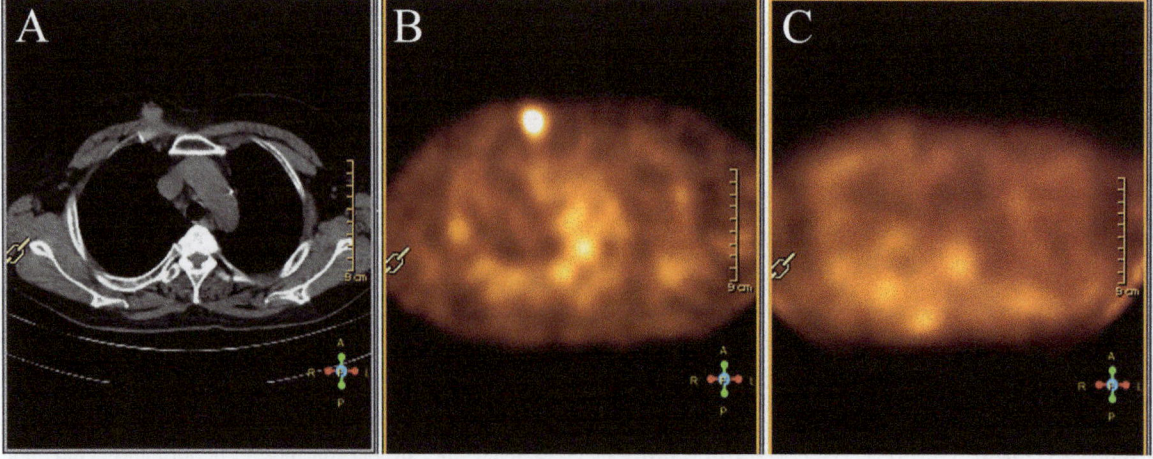

Figure 2. A 2.2 cm ductal carcinoma in situ of the right breast in a 31-year-old woman (Patient 15). (A) CT scan demonstrates a mass in the right breast. (B) ^{99m}Tc-3P$_4$-RGD$_2$ SMM demonstrates focal uptake of ^{99m}Tc-3P$_4$-RGD$_2$ in the tumor (T/NT = 2.96). (C) ^{99m}Tc-MIBI SMM demonstrates low uptake of ^{99m}Tc-MIBI in the tumor (T/NT = 1.31).

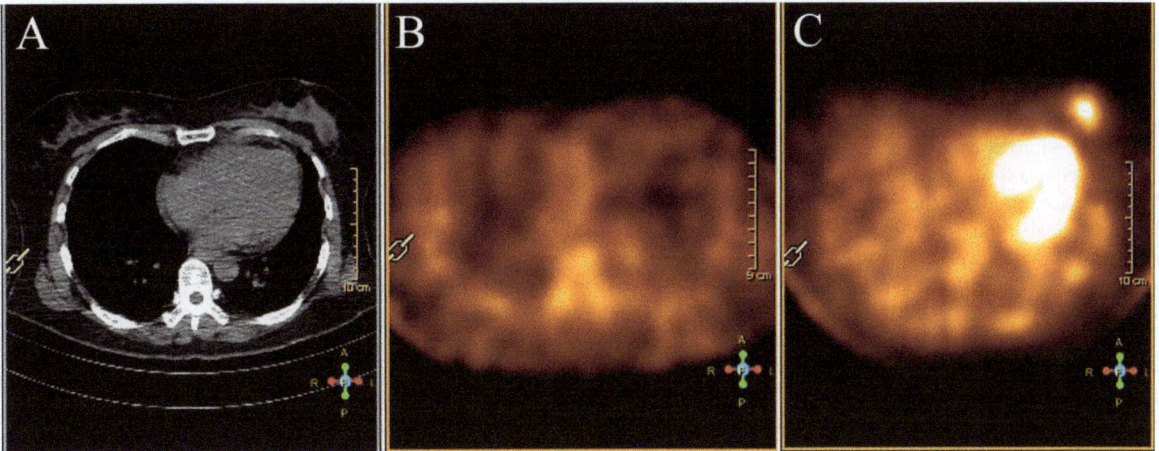

Figure 3. A 3.2 cm fibroadenoma of the left breast in a 47-year-old woman (Patient 30). (A) CT scan demonstrates a mass in the left breast. (B) ^{99m}Tc-3P$_4$-RGD$_2$ SMM demonstrates low uptake of ^{99m}Tc-3P$_4$-RGD$_2$ in the tumor (T/NT = 1.34). (C) ^{99m}Tc-MIBI SMM demonstrates focal uptake of ^{99m}Tc-MIBI in the tumor (T/NT = 2.81).

sensitivity, specificity and accuracy of ^{99m}Tc-3P$_4$-RGD$_2$ SMM were 89.3%, 90.9% and 89.7%, respectively. With a T/NT of 1.45 as a cut-off value, the same findings were 87.5%, 72.7% and 82.1% in ^{99m}Tc-MIBI SMM, respectively. The sensitivities reported in this study for ^{99m}Tc-3P$_4$-RGD$_2$ SMM are comparable with our previous reports; however the specificity is slightly higher than previous studies, which may be due to the low total number of benign breast lesions [20–22]. For ^{99m}Tc-MIBI SMM, the results reported here are comparable with those in previous studies

[25–32]. Although the sensitivity, specificity and accuracy of ^{99m}Tc-3P$_4$-RGD$_2$ SMM was slightly superior to that of ^{99m}Tc-MIBI SMM in this study, the difference was not statistically significant. The area under the curve of ^{99m}Tc-3P$_4$-RGD$_2$ SMM was slightly larger than that of ^{99m}Tc-MIBI SMM, although this difference was also not significant.

It is generally accepted that the detection sensitivity of SMM is much lower for small breast cancer lesions with a diameter less than 1 cm over larger lesions [29]. Data from a multicentre

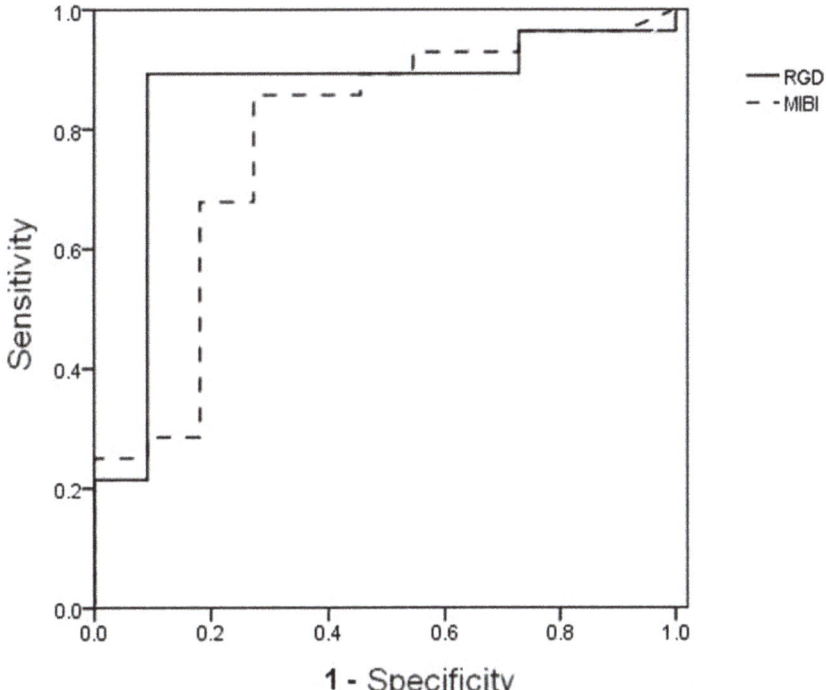

Figure 4. Comparison the sensitivity and specificity of ^{99m}Tc-3P$_4$-RGD$_2$ SMM and ^{99m}Tc-MIBI SMM. Comparison between ^{99m}Tc-3P$_4$-RGD$_2$ SMM and ^{99m}Tc-MIBI SMM in the differential diagnosis of breast cancer and benign lesions using ROC analysis (solid line: ^{99m}Tc-3P$_4$-RGD$_2$ SMM, dashed line: ^{99m}Tc-MIBI SMM). The area under the curve of both ^{99m}Tc-3P$_4$-RGD$_2$ SMM and ^{99m}Tc-MIBI SMM are 0.851 and 0.781, respectively. The difference was not significant.

European study showed a sensitivity of 26%–56% for lesions less than 1 cm [33]. Similarly in the present study, neither ^{99m}Tc-3P$_4$-RGD$_2$ nor ^{99m}Tc-MIBI was sufficient to visualize tumors in three patients having malignant lesions with diameters at 0.3 cm, 0.4 cm and 0.6 cm, respectively. The ^{99m}Tc-3P$_4$-RGD$_2$ and ^{99m}Tc-MIBI uptake in small lesions is considered to be underestimated due to partial volume effects from the relatively low spatial resolution of the SPECT device, though other factors such as the degree of radiopharmaceutical uptake by tumors and normal breast tissue may have contributed as well.

In one case of DCIS with a long axis diameter of 2.2 cm was false negative on ^{99m}Tc-MIBI SMM but not ^{99m}Tc-3P$_4$-RGD$_2$ SMM. Some reports state that ^{99m}Tc-MIBI SMM always showed a low sensitivity for detecting DCIS. Vassilios Papantoniou et al. [34] studied the diagnostic accuracy of ^{99m}Tc-MIBI SMM in 13 cases of DCIS and achieved a low sensitivity of 46%. Reinhard Obwegeser et al. [35] reported that ^{99m}Tc-MIBI SMM could not detect all four DCIS in their study. They conceived it may be due to the histological type of DCIS, which is known to show a lower density of tumor cells per square unit than invasive ductal carcinomas. Conversely, experimental studies using in vivo assays have shown that breast carcinoma in situ may be antigenic [36]. Sections stained for endothelial markers have shown increased vascularity around DCIS [37–39]. A more detailed study demonstrated two patterns of increased vascularity: cuffs of vessels close to the involved ducts and vessels diffusely arranged in the interductal stroma [40]. The true positive result with ^{99m}Tc-3P$_4$-RGD$_2$ SMM in this common malignant tumor may be an advantage of RGD targeting. Further studies with a larger patient population is needed to determine this issue.

Three of the 11 patients with fibroadenoma showed focal ^{99m}Tc-MIBI uptake, and one patient from this group who was diagnosed with fibroadenoma with severe mammitis on histopath-ological examination showed high focal tracer accumulation of ^{99m}Tc-3P$_4$-RGD$_2$. The false positive results obtained with ^{99m}Tc-MIBI in three fibroadenoma may be due to the high cellular activity associated in fibroadenoma. Previous studies have demonstrated that integrin $\alpha v \beta 3$ is preferentially expressed on several types of cancer cells including melanoma, glioma, and ovarian and breast cancer. However, because expression is very low in existing blood vessels and absent in normal tissue, the accumulation of ^{99m}Tc-3P$_4$-RGD$_2$ may be mainly due to its higher specificity [41–44]. As is known to all, inflammation was different from other benign lesions, always showed high cell density and vascularity, likely responsible for the increased uptake. Previous studies have also shown that the integrin $\alpha v \beta 3$ can exist on neutrophils, monocytes, and vascular smooth muscle cells [45], which can be the main reason for the false positive result using ^{99m}Tc-3P$_4$-RGD$_2$ SMM.

In conclusion, ^{99m}Tc-3P$_4$-RGD$_2$ SMM does not provide any significant advantage over the established ^{99m}Tc-MIBI SMM for differentiating breast lesions. The uptake of ^{99m}Tc-3P$_4$-RGD$_2$ in breast cancer was higher than that of ^{99m}Tc-MIBI. ^{99m}Tc-3P$_4$-RGD$_2$ seems to be more accurate than ^{99m}Tc-MIBI in the detection of DCIS and fibroadenoma. But with only a few patients, there was no statistically significant difference between ^{99m}Tc-3P$_4$-RGD$_2$ and ^{99m}Tc-MIBI SMM. Future studies will involve higher sample numbers.

Author Contributions

Conceived and designed the experiments: LL QM. Performed the experiments: QM BC SG TJ QW YS ZX. Analyzed the data: QM SG LZ LL. Contributed reagents/materials/analysis tools: QM LL. Wrote the paper: QM SG LZ LL.

References

1. Panel NIoHCD (2001) National Institutes of Health Consensus Development Conference statement: adjuvant therapy for breast cancer, November 1–3, 2000. Journal of the National Cancer Institute 93: 979–989.
2. Buscombe JR, Cwikla JB, Holloway B, Hilson AJ (2001) Prediction of the usefulness of combined mammography and scintimammography in suspected primary breast cancer using ROC curves. Journal of nuclear medicine : official publication, Society of Nuclear Medicine 42: 3–8.
3. Kopans DB (1992) The positive predictive value of mammography. AJR. American journal of roentgenology 158: 521–526.
4. Murphy IG, Dillon MF, Doherty AO, McDermott EW, Kelly G, et al. (2007) Analysis of patients with false negative mammography and symptomatic breast carcinoma. Journal of surgical oncology 96: 457–463.
5. Schillaci O, Danieli R, Romano P, Santoni R, Simonetti G (2005) Scintimammography for the detection of breast cancer.
6. Liberman M, Sampalis F, Mulder DS, Sampalis JS (2003) Breast cancer diagnosis by scintimammography: a meta-analysis and review of the literature. Breast cancer research and treatment 80: 115–126.
7. Soussan M, Orlhac F, Boubaya M, Zelek L, Ziol M, et al. (2014) Relationship between Tumor Heterogeneity Measured on FDG-PET/CT and Pathological Prognostic Factors in Invasive Breast Cancer. PloS one 9: e94017.
8. Tiling R, Tatsch K, Sommer H, Meyer G, Pechmann M, et al. (1998) Technetium-99m-sestamibi scintimammography for the detection of breast carcinoma: comparison between planar and SPECT imaging. Journal of nuclear medicine: official publication, Society of Nuclear Medicine 39: 849–856.
9. Hood JD, Cheresh DA (2002) Role of integrins in cell invasion and migration. Nature Reviews Cancer 2: 91–100.
10. Ruoslahti E (2002) Specialization of tumour vasculature. Nature Reviews Cancer 2: 83–90.
11. Desgrosellier JS, Cheresh DA (2010) Integrins in cancer: biological implications and therapeutic opportunities. Nature Reviews Cancer 10: 9–22.
12. Niu G, Chen X (2011) Why integrin as a primary target for imaging and therapy. Theranostics 1: 30.
13. Jia B, Liu Z, Zhu Z, Shi J, Jin X, et al. (2011) Blood Clearance Kinetics, Biodistribution, and Radiation Dosimetry of a Kit-Formulated Integrin $\alpha v \beta 3$-Selective Radiotracer 99mTc-3PRGD2 in Non-Human Primates. Molecular Imaging and Biology 13: 730–736.
14. Wang L, Shi J, Kim Y-S, Zhai S, Jia B, et al. (2008) Improving tumor-targeting capability and pharmacokinetics of 99mTc-labeled cyclic RGD dimers with PEG4 linkers. Molecular pharmaceutics 6: 231–245.
15. Beer AJ, Haubner R, Sarbia M, Goebel M, Luderschmidt S, et al. (2006) Positron emission tomography using [18F] Galacto-RGD identifies the level of integrin $\alpha v \beta 3$ expression in man. Clinical Cancer Research 12: 3942–3949.
16. Bach-Gansmo T, Danielsson R, Saracco A, Wilczek B, Bogsrud TV, et al. (2006) Integrin receptor imaging of breast cancer: a proof-of-concept study to evaluate 99mTc-NC100692. Journal of Nuclear Medicine 47: 1434–1439.
17. Kenny LM, Coombes RC, Oulie I, Contractor KB, Miller M, et al. (2008) Phase I trial of the positron-emitting Arg-Gly-Asp (RGD) peptide radioligand 18F-AH111585 in breast cancer patients. Journal of nuclear medicine 49: 879–886.
18. Liu Z, Jia B, Shi J, Jin X, Zhao H, et al. (2010) Tumor uptake of the RGD dimeric probe 99mTc-G3-2P4-RGD2 is correlated with integrin $\alpha v \beta 3$ expressed on both tumor cells and neovasculature. Bioconjugate chemistry 21: 548–555.
19. Bhojani MS, Ranga R, Luker GD, Rehemtulla A, Ross BD, et al. (2011) Synthesis and investigation of a radioiodinated F3 peptide analog as a SPECT tumor imaging radioligand. PloS one 6: e22418.
20. Qingjie M, Bin J, Bing J, Shi G, Tiefeng J, et al. (2011) Differential diagnosis of solitary pulmonary nodules using ^{99m}Tc-3P$_4$-RGD$_2$ scintigraphy. Eur J Nucl Med Mol Imaging 38: 2145–2152.
21. Gao S, Ma Q, Cui Q, Liu L, Zhou X, et al. (2013) A pilot study on yymTc-3PRGD2 scintigraphy in diagnosis of brain glioma. Nuclear Science and Techniques: 020301.
22. Gao S, Ma Q, Wen Q, Jia B, Liu Z, et al. (2013) 99mTc-3P4-RGD2 radiotracers for SPECT/CT of esophageal tumor. Nuclear Science and Techniques 24: 040302.
23. Guanghui C, Shi G, Tiefeng J, Qingjie M, Bing J, et al. (2012) Pharmacokinetics and radiation dosimetry of~(99m) Tc-3PRGD_2 in healthy individuals: A pilot study. Nuclear Science and Techniques 23: 349-349-354.
24. Mitchell D, Hruska CB, Boughey JC, Wahner-Roedler DL, Jones KN, et al. (2013) 99mTc-Sestamibi Using a Direct Conversion Molecular Breast Imaging System to Assess Tumor Response to Neoadjuvant Chemotherapy in Women With Locally Advanced Breast Cancer. Clinical nuclear medicine 38: 949–956.
25. Burak Z, Argon M, Memis A, Erdem S, Balkan Z, et al. (1994) Evaluation of palpable breast masses with 99Tcm-MIBI: a comparative study with

mammography and ultrasonography. Nuclear medicine communications 15: 604–612.

26. Khalkhali I, Mena I, Diggles L (1994) Review of imaging techniques for the diagnosis of breast cancer: a new role of prone scintimammography using technetium-99m sestamibi. European journal of nuclear medicine 21: 357–362.

27. Khalkhali I, Cutrone JA, Mena IG, Diggles LE, Venegas RJ, et al. (1995) Scintimammography: the complementary role of Tc-99m sestamibi prone breast imaging for the diagnosis of breast carcinoma. Radiology 196: 421–426.

28. Khalkhali I, Cutrone J, Mena I, Diggles L, Venegas R, et al. (1995) Technetium-99m-sestamibi scintimammography of breast lesions: clinical and pathological follow-up. Journal of nuclear medicine: official publication, Society of Nuclear Medicine 36: 1784–1789.

29. Palmedo H, Schomburg A, Grünwald F, Mallmann P, Krebs D, et al. (1996) Technetium-99m-MIBI scintimammography for suspicious breast lesions. Journal of nuclear medicine: official publication, Society of Nuclear Medicine 37: 626–630.

30. Taillefer R, Robidoux A, Lambert R, Turpin S, Laperrière J (1995) Technetium-99m-sestamibi prone scintimammography to detect primary breast cancer and axillary lymph node involvement. The Journal of nuclear medicine 36: 1758–1765.

31. Tiling R, Sommer H, Pechmann M, Moser R, Kress K, et al. (1997) Comparison of technetium-99m-sestamibi scintimammography with contrast-enhanced MRI for diagnosis of breast lesions. Journal of nuclear medicine: official publication, Society of Nuclear Medicine 38: 58–62.

32. Waxman A, Nagaraj N, Ashok G, Khan S, Yadegar J, et al. (1994) Sensitivity and specificity of TC-99M methoxy isonitrile (MIBI) in the evaluation of primary-carcinoma of the breast-comparison of palpable lesions with mammography. SOC NUCLEAR MEDICINE INC 1850 SAMUEL MORSE DR, RESTON, VA 20190-5316. pp. P22-22.

33. Scopinaro F, Schillaci O, Ussof W, Nordling K, Capoferro R, et al. (1996) A three center study on the diagnostic accuracy of 99mTc-MIBI scintimammography. Anticancer research 17: 1631–1634.

34. Papantoniou V, Tsiouris S, Mainta E, Valotassiou V, Souvatzoglou M, et al. (2004) Imaging in situ breast carcinoma (with or without an invasive component) with technetium-99m pentavalent dimercaptosuccinic acid and technetium-99m 2-methoxy isobutyl isonitrile scintimammography. Breast Cancer Research 7: R33.

35. Brem SS, Jensen HM, Gullino PM (1978) Angiogenesis as a marker of preneoplastic lesions of the human breast. Cancer 41: 239–244.

36. Obwegeser R, Berghammer P, Rodrigues M, Granegger S, Hohlagschwandtner M, et al. (1999) A head-to-head comparison between technetium-99m-tetrofosmin and technetium-99m-MIBI scintigraphy to evaluate suspicious breast lesions. European journal of nuclear medicine 26: 1553–1559.

37. Weidner N, Semple JP, Welch WR, Folkman J (1991) Tumor angiogenesis and metastasis—correlation in invasive breast carcinoma. New England Journal of Medicine 324: 1–8.

38. Bosari S, Lee AK, DeLellis RA, Wiley BD, Heatley GJ, et al. (1992) Microvessel quantitation and prognosis in invasive breast carcinoma. Human pathology 23: 755–761.

39. Schor A, Van Hoef M, Dhesi S, Howell A, Knox W (1993) Assessment of tumour vascularity as a prognostic factor in lymph node negative invasive breast cancer. European Journal of Cancer 29: 1141–1145.

40. Guidi AJ, Fischer L, Harris JR, Schnitt SJ (1994) Microvessel density and distribution in ductal carcinoma in situ of the breast. Journal of the National Cancer Institute 86: 614–619.

41. van der Flier A, Sonnenberg A (2001) Function and interactions of integrins. Cell and tissue research 305: 285–298.

42. Eliceiri B, Cheresh D (2000) Role of alpha v integrins during angiogenesis. Cancer journal (Sudbury, Mass.) 6: S245–249.

43. Carmeliet P (2000) Mechanisms of angiogenesis and arteriogenesis. Nature medicine 6.

44. Kuwano M, Fukushi J-i, Okamoto M, Nishie A, Goto H, et al. (2001) Angiogenesis factors. Internal medicine (Tokyo, Japan) 40: 565–572.

45. Horton MA (1997) The $\alpha v \beta 3$ integrin "vitronectin receptor". The international journal of biochemistry & cell biology 29: 721–725.

Permissions

The contributors of this book come from diverse backgrounds, making this book a truly international effort. This book will bring forth new frontiers with its revolutionizing research information and detailed analysis of the nascent developments around the world.

We would like to thank all the contributing authors for lending their expertise to make the book truly unique. They have played a crucial role in the development of this book. Without their invaluable contributions this book wouldn't have been possible. They have made vital efforts to compile up to date information on the varied aspects of this subject to make this book a valuable addition to the collection of many professionals and students.

This book was conceptualized with the vision of imparting up-to-date information and advanced data in this field. To ensure the same, a matchless editorial board was set up. Every individual on the board went through rigorous rounds of assessment to prove their worth. After which they invested a large part of their time researching and compiling the most relevant data for our readers.

The editorial board has been involved in producing this book since its inception. They have spent rigorous hours researching and exploring the diverse topics which have resulted in the successful publishing of this book. They have passed on their knowledge of decades through this book. To expedite this challenging task, the publisher supported the team at every step. A small team of assistant editors was also appointed to further simplify the editing procedure and attain best results for the readers.

Apart from the editorial board, the designing team has also invested a significant amount of their time in understanding the subject and creating the most relevant covers. They scrutinized every image to scout for the most suitable representation of the subject and create an appropriate cover for the book.

The publishing team has been an ardent support to the editorial, designing and production team. Their endless efforts to recruit the best for this project, has resulted in the accomplishment of this book. They are a veteran in the field of academics and their pool of knowledge is as vast as their experience in printing. Their expertise and guidance has proved useful at every step. Their uncompromising quality standards have made this book an exceptional effort. Their encouragement from time to time has been an inspiration for everyone.

The publisher and the editorial board hope that this book will prove to be a valuable piece of knowledge for researchers, students, practitioners and scholars across the globe.

List of Contributors

Jeremias Motte and Carina Ewering
Department of Neurology, University of Muenster Medical Center, Muenster, Germany

Florian Alten, Christoph R. Clemens and Nicole Eter
Department of Ophthalmology, University of Muenster Medical Center, Muenster, Germany

Nani Osada
Institution of Medical Informatics, University of Muenster, Muenster, Germany

Ella M. Kadas, Alexander U. Brandt and Timm Oberwahrenbrock
NeuroCure Clinical Research Center and Experimental and Clinical Research Center, Charité University Medicine Berlin and Max Delbrück Center for Molecular Medicine, Berlin, Germany

Friedemann Paul
NeuroCure Clinical Research Center and Experimental and Clinical Research Center, Charité University Medicine Berlin and Max Delbrück Center for Molecular Medicine, Berlin, Germany
Department of Neurology, Charité University Medicine Berlin, Berlin, Germany

Martin Marziniak
Department of Neurology, University of Muenster Medical Center, Muenster, Germany
Department of Neurology, Isar-Amper-Klinikum, Haar, Germany

Ireneusz P. Grudzinski
Department of Toxicology, Medical University of Warsaw, Faculty of Pharmacy, Warsaw, Poland

Karolina Jakoniuk-Glodala, Irena Chlipala-Nitek and Olgierd Rowinski
2nd Department of Clinical Radiology, Medical University of Warsaw, Warsaw, Poland Bartosz Kaczynski

Bartosz Kaczynski
Department of Medical Informatics and Telemedicine, Medical University of Warsaw, Warsaw, Poland

Andrzej Cieszanowski, Edyta Maj and Piotr Kulisiewicz
2nd Department of Clinical Radiology, Medical University of Warsaw, Warsaw, Poland Bartosz Kaczynski
Diagnostic Center, Medicover Hospital, Warsaw, Poland

Rebecca N. Preston-Campbell and Muhammad A. Parvaz
Department of Psychiatry, Friedman Brain Institute, Icahn School of Medicine at Mount Sinai, New York, New York, United States of America

Wei Zhu
Applied Mathematics and Statistics, SUNY, Stony Brook, New York, United States of America

Millard C. Jayne, Chris Wong, Dardo Tomasi and Nora D. Volkow
Laboratory of Neuroimaging, National Institute on Alcohol Abuse and Alcoholism, Bethesda, Maryland, United States of America

Joanna S. Fowler
Medical Department, Brookhaven National Laboratory, Upton, New York, United States of America

Nelly Alia-Klein, Scott J. Moeller and Rita Z. Goldstein
Department of Psychiatry, Friedman Brain Institute, Icahn School of Medicine at Mount Sinai, New York, New York, United States of America
Department of Neuroscience, Friedman Brain Institute, Icahn School of Medicine at Mount Sinai, New York, New York, United States of America

Gene-Jack Wang
Department of Psychiatry, Friedman Brain Institute, Icahn School of Medicine at Mount Sinai, New York, New York, United States of America
Laboratory of Neuroimaging, National Institute on Alcohol Abuse and Alcoholism, Bethesda, Maryland, United States of America

Masamichi Mineshita, Hirotaka Kida, Hiroshi Handa, Hiroki Nishine, Naoki Furuya, Seiichi Nobuyama, Takeo Inoue and Teruomi Miyazawa
Division of Respiratory and Infectious Diseases, Department of Internal Medicine, St. Marianna University School of Medicine, Kawasaki, Japan

Shin Matsuoka
Department of Radiology, St. Marianna University School of Medicine, Kawasaki, Japan

Yiming Wang and Fangxian Chai
Department of Psychiatry, Hospital Affiliated to Guiyang Medical University, Guiyang, Guizhou, China

Hongming Zhang
Department of Cardiology, The General Hospital of Jinan Military Region, Jinan, China

Xingde Liu
Department of Cardiology, Hospital Affiliated to Guiyang Medical University, Guiyang City, Guizhou, China

Fanying Chen
Mental Health Education And Counseling Center, Guiyang Medical University, Guiyang City, Guizhou, China

Songlin Tang
Department of Psychiatry, Hospital Affiliated to Guiyang Medical University, Guiyang, Guizhou, China
Department of Neurology, First People's Hospital of Shaoyang, Shaoyang, Hunan, China

Adrienne O'Neil
IMPACT Strategic Research Centre, School of Medicine, Deakin University, Geelong, Australia
School of Public Health and Preventive Medicine, Monash University, Melbourne, Australia

Alyna Turner
IMPACT Strategic Research Centre, School of Medicine, Deakin University, Geelong, Australia
Department of Psychiatry, The University of Melbourne, Parkville, Victoria, Australia
School of Medicine and Public Health, The University of Newcastle, Callaghan, New South Wales, Australia

Michael Berk
IMPACT Strategic Research Centre, School of Medicine, Deakin University, Geelong, Australia
School of Public Health and Preventive Medicine, Monash University, Melbourne, Australia
School of Medicine and Public Health, The University of Newcastle, Callaghan, New South Wales, Australia
Department of Psychiatry, Orygen Youth Health Research Centre, The University of Melbourne, Parkville, Victoria, Australia,
Florey Institute of Neuroscience and Mental Health, University of Melbourne, Parkville, Victoria, Australia

Bradley J. Beattie, Keith S. Pentlow, Joseph O'Donoghue and John L. Humm
Medical Physics, Memorial Sloan Kettering Cancer Center, New York, New York, United States of America

Daniela Muenzel, Alexander A. Fingerle, Simone Waldt, Edgar Bendik, Tina Zahel, Martin Dobritz, Ernst J. Rummeny and Peter B. Noël
Department of Radiology, Technische Universitaet Muenchen, Munich, Germany

Thomas Koehler
Philips Technologie GmbH, Innovative Technologies, Hamburg, Germany

Kevin Brown and Stanislav Žabic
Philips Healthcare, Cleveland, Ohio, United States of America

Armin Schneider
MITI - Minimal-invasive Interdisciplinary therapeutic intervention research group, Technische Universitaet Muenchen, Munich, Germany

Jui-Ting Hsu, Jung-Ting Ho and Heng-Li Huang
School of Dentistry, College of Medicine, China Medical University, Taichung, Taiwan

Ying-Ju Chen and Fu-Chou Cheng
Stem Cell Medical Research Center, Department of Medical Research, Taichung Veterans General Hospital, Taichung, Taiwan

Shun-Ping Wang
Department of Orthopaedics, Taichung Veterans General Hospital, Taichung, Taiwan

Jay Wu
Department of Biomedical Imaging and Radiological Science, China Medical University, Taichung, Taiwan

Ming-Tzu Tsai
Department of Biomedical Engineering, Hungkuang University, Taichung, Taiwan

Gábor Szalóki, Ágnes Tóth, Zoltán Krasznai, Gábor Szabó and Katalin Goda
Department of Biophysics and Cell Biology, Faculty of Medicine, University of Debrecen, Debrecen, Hungary

Zoárd T. Krasznai
Department of Obstetrics and Gynecology, Faculty of Medicine, University of Debrecen, Debrecen, Hungary

Laura Vízkeleti and Margit Balázs
Department of Preventive Medicine, Faculty of Medicine, University of Debrecen, Debrecen, Hungary

Attila G. Szöllősi
Department of Physiology, Faculty of Medicine, University of Debrecen, Debrecen, Hungary

György Trencsényi, Imre Lajtos and Teréz Márián
Department of Nuclear Medicine, Faculty of Medicine, University of Debrecen, Debrecen, Hungary

István Juhász
Department of Dermatology, Faculty of Medicine, University of Debrecen, Debrecen, Hungary
Department of Surgery and Operative Techniques, Faculty of Medicine, University of Debrecen, Debrecen, Hungary

Lukas Ebner and Andreas Christe
Department of Radiology, Inselspital, University of Bern, Freiburgstrasse, Bern, Switzerland

Shiming Jiang
Department of Radiology, Nanchong Central Hospital of North Sichuan Medical College, Nanchong, Sichuan, P. R. China

Yi Wu and Shaoxiang Zhang
Institute of Computing Medicine, Third Military Medical University, Chongqing, P. R. China

Xiaoming Zhang
Sichuan Key Laboratory of Medical Imaging, Department of Radiology, Affiliated Hospital of North Sichuan Medical College, Nanchong, Sichuan, P. R. China

Zhulin Luo and Fuzhou Tian
Postdoctoral Workstation, the General Surgery Center of the Peoples' Liberation Army, Chengdu Army General Hospital, Chengdu, Sichuan, P. R. China

Haotong Xu
Postdoctoral Workstation, the General Surgery Center of the Peoples' Liberation Army, Chengdu Army General Hospital, Chengdu, Sichuan, P. R. China
Department of Radiology, Sichuan Provincial People's Hospital Supo, Chengdu, Sichuan, P. R. China

Christopher R. Tench and Cris S. Constantinescu
Division of Clinical Neurosciences, Clinical Neurology, University of Nottingham, Queen's Medical Centre, Nottingham, United Kingdom

Radu Tanasescu
Division of Clinical Neurosciences, Clinical Neurology, University of Nottingham, Queen's Medical Centre, Nottingham, United Kingdom
Department of Neurology, Neurosurgery, and Psychiatry, University of Medicine and Pharmacy Carol Davila Bucharest, Colentina Hospital, Bucharest, Romania

Dorothee P. Auer and William J. Cottam
Division of Clinical Neurosciences, Radiological and Imaging Sciences, University of Nottingham, Queen's Medical Centre, Nottingham, United Kingdom
ARUK National Pain Centre, University of Nottingham, Queen's Medical Centre, Nottingham, United Kingdom

Masahiro Miyake, Kenji Yamashiro, Yumiko Akagi-Kurashige, Akio Oishi, Akitaka Tsujikawa, Masanori Hangai and Nagahisa Yoshimura
Department of Ophthalmology and Visual Sciences, Kyoto University Graduate School of Medicine, Kyoto, Japan

Na-Young Shin, Kyung-eun Kim, Mina Park, Dong Joon Kim, Sung Jun Ahn and Ji Seung-Koo Lee
Department of Radiology, Severance Hospital, Yonsei University College of Medicine, Seoul, Korea

Young Dae Kim and Hoe Heo
Department of Neurology, Severance Hospital, Yonsei University College of Medicine, Seoul, Korea

Stefanie Nittka and Michael Neumaier
Institute for Clinical Chemistry, Medical Faculty Mannheim, University of Heidelberg, Mannheim, Germany

Marcel A. Krueger and Bernd J. Pichler
Department of Preclinical Imaging and Radiopharmacy, Werner Siemens Imaging Center, University of Tuebingen, Tuebingen, Germany

John E. Shively
Department of Immunology, Beckman Research Institute, City of Hope, Duarte, California, United States of America

Hanne Boll
Department of Neuroradiology, Medical Faculty Mannheim, University of Heidelberg, Mannheim, Germany

Fabian Doyon
Department of Surgery, Medical Faculty Mannheim, University of Heidelberg, Mannheim, Germany

Marc A. Brockmann
Department of Neuroradiology, Medical Faculty Mannheim, University of Heidelberg, Mannheim, Germany
Department of Diagnostic and Interventional Neuroradiology, University Hospital of the Rheinisch-Westfaehlische Technical University Aachen, Aachen, Germany

Michelle R. Ananda-Rajah
Infectious Diseases Unit, Alfred Health, Melbourne, Victoria, Australia

David Martinez
Computing and Information Systems, University of Melbourne, Melbourne, Victoria, Australia

Lawrence Cavedon
School of Computer Science and IT, RMIT University, Melbourne, Victoria, Australia

Monica A. Slavin and Karin A. Thursky
Victorian Infectious Diseases Service, Peter Doherty Centre, Melbourne, Victoria, Australia
Infectious diseases department, Peter MacCallum Cancer Institute, Melbourne, Victoria, Australia

Michael Dooley
Pharmacy Department, Alfred Health, Melbourne, Victoria, Australia
Faculty of Pharmacy & Pharmaceutical Science, Monash University, Melbourne, Victoria, Australia

Allen Cheng
Infectious Diseases Unit, Alfred Health, Melbourne, Victoria, Australia
Department of Epidemiology and Preventative Medicine, Monash University, Melbourne, Victoria, Australia

Huafeng Liu, Min Guo and Zhenghui Hu
State Key Laboratory of Modern Optical Instrumentation, Department of Optical Engineering, Zhejiang University, Hangzhou, China

Pengcheng Shi
B. Thomas Golisano College of Computing and Information Sciences, Rochester Institute of Technology, Rochester, New York, United States of America

Hongjie Hu
Department of Radiology, Sir Run Run Shaw Hospital, College of Medicine, Zhejiang University, Hangzhou, China

Wouter G. Wieringa and Gabija Pundziute
University of Groningen, University Medical Center Groningen, Department of Cardiology, Groningen, The Netherlands

Lennart Nilsson, Marcus Gjerde, Eva Swahn and Lena Jonasson
Department of Medical and Health Sciences, Linköping University, Linköping, Sweden
Department of Cardiology, Linköping University, Linköping, Sweden

Jan Engvall
Department of Medical and Health Sciences, Linköping University, Linköping, Sweden
Department of Clinical Physiology, Linköping University, Linköping, Sweden

Oleh Dzyubachyk, Thomas J. A. Snoeks and Clemens W. G. M. Löwik
Department of Radiology, Leiden University Medical Center, Leiden, the Netherlands

Esben Plenge and Erik Meijering
Departments of Radiology and Medical Informatics, Erasmus MC — University Medical Center Rotterdam, Rotterdam, the Netherlands

Artem Khmelinskii
Department of Radiology, Leiden University Medical Center, Leiden, the Netherlands
Percuros B.V., Enschede, the Netherlands

Peter Kok, Charl P. Botha and Boudewijn P. F. Lelieveldt
Department of Radiology, Leiden University Medical Center, Leiden, the Netherlands
Department of Intelligent Systems, Delft University of Technology, Delft, the Netherlands

Dirk H. J. Poot and Wiro J. Niessen
Departments of Radiology and Medical Informatics, Erasmus MC — University Medical Center Rotterdam, Rotterdam, the Netherlands
Quantitative Imaging Group, Faculty of Applied Sciences, Delft University of Technology, Delft, the Netherlands

Louise van der Weerd
Department of Radiology, Leiden University Medical Center, Leiden, the Netherlands
Department of Human Genetics, Leiden University Medical Center, Leiden, the Netherlands

Binbin Nie, Hua Liu and Baoci Shan
Key Laboratory of Nuclear Analysis Techniques, Beijing Engineering Research Center of Radiographic Techniques and Equipment, Institute of High Energy Physics, Chinese Academy of Sciences, Beijing, China

Xiaofeng Jiang
School of Public Health and Family Medicine, Capital Medical University, Beijing, China

Kewei Chen
Banner Alzheimer's Institute, Banner Good Samaritan Positron Emission Tomography Center, Phoenix, Arizona, United States of America
Department of Mathematics and Statistics, Arizona State University, Tempe, Arizona, United States of America

Department of Radiology, University of Arizona, Tucson, Arizona, United States of America
Arizona Alzheimer's Consortium, Phoenix, Arizona, United States of America

Catharina Lange, Winfried Brenner and Ralph Buchert
Department of Nuclear Medicine, Charité – Universitätsmedizin Berlin, Berlin, Germany

Anita Seese, Karen Steinhoff, Osama Sabri and Swen Hesse
Department of Nuclear Medicine, Universitätsklinikum Leipzig, Leipzig, Germany

Sarah Schwarzenböck, Bernd J. Krause and Jens Kurth
Department of Nuclear Medicine, Universitätsmedizin Rostock, Rostock, Germany

Bert Umland-Seidler
GE Healthcare Buchler GmbH & Co. KG, Munich, Germany

Pingxin Lv
Department of Radiology, Beijing Chest Hospital, Capital Medical University, Beijing, China

Zhigang Liang
Department of Radiology, Xuanwu Hospital, Capital Medical University, Beijing, China

Jingjing Wang, Tao Sun, Ni Gao, Yanxia Luo, Qi Gao, Huiping Zhu, Lixin Tao, Xiangtong Liu and Xiuhua Guo
School of Public Health, Capital Medical University, Beijing, China
Beijing Municipal Key Laboratory of Clinical Epidemiology, Beijing, China

Xia Li
School of Public Health, Capital Medical University, Beijing, China
Department of Epidemiology & Public Health, University College Cork, Cork, Ireland

Desmond Dev Menon
School of Medical Sciences, Edith Cowan University, Perth, Australia
School of Exercise and Health Sciences, Edith Cowan University, Perth, Australia

Wei Wang
School of Public Health, Capital Medical University, Beijing, China
Beijing Municipal Key Laboratory of Clinical Epidemiology, Beijing, China
School of Medical Sciences, Edith Cowan University, Perth, Australia

Ping Zhao
The Vanderbilt University Institute of Imaging Science (VUIIS), Vanderbilt University Medical School, Nashville, TN, United States of America

Robert J. Coffey
Department of Medicine, Vanderbilt University Medical School, Nashville, TN, United States of America
Department of Vanderbilt Ingram Cancer Center, Vanderbilt University Medical School, Nashville, TN, United States of America

Eliot T. McKinley
The Vanderbilt University Institute of Imaging Science (VUIIS), Vanderbilt University Medical School, Nashville, TN, United States of America
Department of Biomedical Engineering, Vanderbilt University Medical School, Nashville, TN, United States of America
Department of Medicine, Vanderbilt University Medical School, Nashville, TN, United States of America

M. Kay Washington
Department of Medicine, Vanderbilt University Medical School, Nashville, TN, United States of America
Department of Vanderbilt Ingram Cancer Center, Vanderbilt University Medical School, Nashville, TN, United States of America
Department of Pathology, Vanderbilt University Medical School, Nashville, TN, United States of America

H. Charles Manning
The Vanderbilt University Institute of Imaging Science (VUIIS), Vanderbilt University Medical School, Nashville, TN, United States of America

Department of Biomedical Engineering, Vanderbilt University Medical School, Nashville, TN, United States of America
Department of Vanderbilt Ingram Cancer Center, Vanderbilt University Medical School, Nashville, TN, United States of America
Department of Radiology and Radiological Sciences, Vanderbilt University Medical School, Nashville, TN, United States of America
Department of Neurosurgery, Vanderbilt University Medical School, Nashville, TN, United States of America
Department of Chemical and Physical Biology, Vanderbilt University Medical School, Nashville, TN, United States of America

Jie Huo, Xianfeng Zhu, Xuemin Wang and Gang Wang
Department of Biomedical Engineering, Tianjin University, Tianjin, China

Yang Dong, Zhiyong Yuan and Ping Wang
Department of Radiation Oncology, Tianjin Cancer Hospital, Tianjin, China
Xin-Hua Hu
Department of Physics, East Carolina University, Greenville, North Carolina, United States of America

Yuanming Feng
Department of Biomedical Engineering, Tianjin University, Tianjin, China
Department of Radiation Oncology, Tianjin Cancer Hospital, Tianjin, China
Department of Radiation Oncology, East Carolina University, Greenville, North Carolina, United States of America

Qingjie Ma, Bin Chen, Shi Gao, Tiefeng Ji, Qiang Wen, Yan Song, Zheli Xu and Lin Liu
China-Japan Union Hospital, Jilin University, Changchun, China

Lei Zhu
State Key Laboratory of Molecular Vaccinology and Molecular Diagnostics & Center for Molecular Imaging and Translational Medicine, School of Public Health, Xiamen University, Xiamen, China

Index

9 781632 425560